# Pruritus

Laurent Misery · Sonja Ständer

Editors

# Pruritus

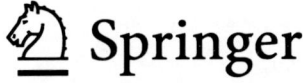 Springer

*Editors*

Laurent Misery
Department of Dermatology
CHU Brest
29200 Brest
France
laurent.misery@chu-brest.fr

Sonja Ständer
Department of Dermatology
Competence Center Pruritus
University Hospital Münster
Von-Esmarch-Str. 58
48149 Münster
Germany
sonja.staender@uni-muenster.de

ISBN 978-1-84882-321-1        e-ISBN 978-1-84882-322-8
DOI 10.1007/978-1-84882-322-8
Springer London Dordrecht Heidelberg New York

Library of Congress Control Number: 2009943295

Printed on acid-free paper

Springer is part of Springer Science+Business Media (www.springer.com)

# Foreword

Toward the end of the last century (1994), I edited the first comprehensive medical textbook on itch. Since that time, clinical interest and research in itch have blossomed. (Afterwards, therefore, because of? A pleasing but grandiose notion.)

There is now an International Forum for the Study of Itch (www.itchforum.net), and it has sponsored four International Workshops for the Study of Itch, where everything from chemical receptors to specific itch neurons to itch inhibitors to treatment in the clinic has been discussed.

Over just the past 15 years there has been progress in every aspect of itch: neuroanatomy, neurophysiology, molecular biology, diagnosis, terminology, classification, and treatment. You will find it all here.

In this book, every imaginable aspect of pruritus,* from bench to bedside, has been covered by experts. Misery and Ständer – both recognized across the globe as leading itch workers – have now produced *the* itch book for the twenty-first century.

Jeffrey D. Bernhard, MD, FRCPedin

---

*"Itch" and "pruritus" are synonymous and may be used interchangeably. According to the great philosopher Willard V.O. Quine, "Faced with two terms for the same thing, one tends to cast about for a distinction."

Most people now agree that giving these two terms different meanings is confusing, not to mention that "itch" is easier to say and to spell.

# Foreword

The American poet Ogden Nash tells us that *"happiness is having a scratch for every Itch"* – and there is much truth in that pithy aphorism. Unfortunately effective and practical solutions for the chronically itchy patient still remain elusive and those of us who work in the clinic are faced all too frequently with the very unhappy patient complaining of excruciating and intractable itching despite our best efforts.

Up to the latter years of my career, itching – though the dominant symptom of skin disease – has attracted little or no attention from physiologists. When it had received attention in the past, it has all too often been relegated to the Cinderella status of a mild form of pain, despite self-evident differences such as the withdrawal reflex response to pain versus the scratch response to itch. Even that acute observer of skin physiology Thomas Lewis in his classic text "The blood vessels of the human skin and their responses", in which he devotes several chapters to the actions of histamine, does not once mention itching.

However, it has been my good fortune, during the new millennium, to witness an upsurge of interest in the mechanisms of itch at a molecular level, resulting in impressive advances in the understanding of the neurophysiology of itching, which offers real prospects of progress in the management of the itchy patient. These advances have been facilitated by the utilisation of advances in neurophysiological technology including microneurography and positron emission tomography of the human brain, and by improved methods of quantifying itch and its deleterious effect on quality of life. The realisation that itch can be generated centrally, by dysregulation of afferent neuronal traffic within the CNS – a concept espoused by the late neurophysiologist Pat Wall – has also had an impact on therapeutic strategies for itch.

Although this book is not the first devoted to bringing together the multiple strands of research on itch, it has the advantage of a more solid foundation of new insights, particularly at a basic molecular level and also realistic prospects for the emergence of treatments. Edited by Laurent Misery and Sonja Ständer, both of whom are in the forefront of current research in this field, the book successfully encapsulates all major advances. Their clinical background accounts for the emphasis placed in the book on translational research and there is much which should be of interest to the practising physician as well as the researcher.

Altogether, this book will prove an invaluable acquisition to the libraries of the laboratory and the clinic alike.

Malcolm W. Greaves
Emeritus Professor of Dermatology, The Cutaneous Allergy Clinic,
St John`s Institute of Dermatology, St Thomas' Hospital,
Lambeth Palace Rd, London SE1 7EH UK

# Foreword

I am delighted to write this foreword for the book – Pruritus – by Laurent Misery MD and Sonja Ständer MD and congratulate both of them on this excellent contribution. For many years they have pioneered clinical and experimental research on cutaneous neurobiology and neuroinflammation which ultimately has resulted in an improved understanding of itch as well as the development of novel therapeutic strategies.

Pruritus or Itch is an important danger signal of the body to external noxious stimuli or a variety of diseases involving many organs, which due to lack of knowledge has been neglected in the past as the "little sister of pain". It may develop to be very distressing, and substantially impairing the quality of life and in some cases may even provoke patients to contemplate suicide. The enormous progress in our understanding of the pathophysiology and molecular basis of pruritus resulted in a new classification of itching. As a consequence, several novel compounds became available and others are currently being investigated to define an individual treatment depending on the underlying cause of itch.

The most current knowledge of the complex epidemiological, clinical, experimental and therapeutic aspects of pruritus is contributed by leading experts in the field. The book has been very thoughtfully divided into three parts, each having a logical sequence of chapters. The first part deals with basic aspects such as neuroanatomy, central and peripheral transmission, neuropeptides and their receptors, neuroimaging, tools for measurement and finally animal models. The chapters of the second part are dedicated to the clinical aspects of the different forms of pruritus as well as diseases associated with itch and psychological aspects. In the third part several chapters address the most up-to-date therapeutic developments with regard to their specific efficacy for the distinct forms of itch.

I am convinced that this excellent book which provides important insights into a rapidly developing field will be a must for any clinician involved in the management of patients suffering from this distressing symptom. For scientists interested in pruritus research this book will provide an excellent update on the most recent developments.

Thomas A. Luger
Professor and Chairman
Department of Dermatology
University of Münster
Münster, Germany

# Preface

Pruritus or itch is an unpleasant sensation that makes a person want to scratch – this definition has remained unchanged for almost 350 years.[1,3] However, pruritus as a protection mechanism will exist as long as animals and human beings have skin or fur. Acute and chronic pruritus is also a common manifestation of dermatologic and non-dermatologic diseases. Recent epidemiological studies have revealed that chronic itch is very frequent (in almost one third of the population ).[2]

All patients suffering from itch know that it is a very disturbing sensation with a high impact on the quality of life. Unfortunately, this major symptom was considered the "little brother" and not severe by comparison to pain until the beginning of the 1990s . The consequences of this paradigm were that research on this field was hindered and development of effective antipruritic drugs delayed. Recently, new concepts and genuine discoveries of itch have completely modified our understanding of itch and suggested new therapeutic modalities. International collaboration is now really effective, with the creation of the first Society dedicated to pruritus research: the International Forum for Studies on Itch (IFSI) – www.itchforum.net.

Our objectives were to provide a book on itch that would be convenient for doctors who are confronted by patients suffering from itch, by giving practical data on the causes and treatments of pruritus and to present all the new data about pathophysiology and therapeutics. This book could not have been completed without experts and friends world-wide; therefore we want to thank all the authors who have contributed to this book.

Laurent Misery
Sonja Ständer

## References

1. Bernhard JD. *Itch. Mechanisms and Management of Pruritus.* Mac Graw-Hill; 1994:454 .
2. Dalgard F, Lien L, Dalen I. Itch in the community: associations with psychosocial factors among adults. *J Eur Acad Dermatol Venereol.* 2007;21:1215–1219.
3. Hafenreffer S. Nosodochium, in quo cutis, eique adhaerentium partium, affectus omnes, singulari methodo, et cognoscendi et curandi fidelissime traduntur. Ulm, Typis & expensis Balthasar. Kühnen, reipubl. ibid. typogr. & biblopolae;1660.

# Contents

## Section 2    Topical

## Section 3    Systemical

## Section 4    Other Approaches

**Section 5    Future Perspectives**

# Contributors

**Heidrun Behrendt**
ZAUM – Center for Allergy and Environment, Division of Environmental Dermatology and Allergy Helmholtz Zentrum/TUM, Technische Universität München, Munich, Germany

**Nora V. Bergasa**
Department of Medicine, Metropolitan Hospital Center, New York, USA

**Ulrich Beuers**
Department of Gastroenterology and Hepatology, Liver Center, Academic Medical Center, University of Amsterdam, Amsterdam, The Netherlands

**Nicholas Boulais**
Laboratory of Skin Neurobiology, Unit of Compared and Integrative Physiology, University Hospital of Brest, Brest, France

**Eric Caumes**
Département des Maladies Infectieuses et Tropicales, Hôpital Pitié-Salpêtrière, Paris, France

**Florence Dalgard**
Institute of General Practice and Community Medicine, University of Oslo and Judge Baker Children's Center, Harvard Medical School, Boston, Massachusetts, USA

**Ulf Darsow**
Department of Dermatology and Allergy Biederstein, Technische Universität München, Munich, Germany

**Deewan Deewan**
Medicine, Woodhull Medical and Mental Health Center, Brooklyn, New York, USA

**Sabine Dutray**
Dermatology, University and Regional Hospital Center, Brest Cedex, France

**Stefan Evers**
Department of Neurology, University of Münster, Münster, Germany

**Alan B. Fleischer, Jr.**
Department of Dermatology, Wake Forest University School of Medicine, Winston-Salem, North Carolina, USA

**Camille Fleuret**
Service de Dermatologie, CHIC Laënnec, Quimper, France

**Caroline Gaudy-Marqueste**
Dermatology Department, STE Marguerite Hospital, Marseille, France

**Tobias Görge**
Department of Dermatology, University Hospital Münster, Münster, Germany

**Matthieu Gréco**
Department of Dermatology, University Hospital, Brest, France

**Wolfgang Hartschuh**
Department of Dermatology, University of Heidelberg, Heidelberg, Germany

**Akihiko Ikoma**
Department of Dermatology, University of California, San Francisco,
San Francisco, USA

**Yozo Ishiuji**
Department of Dermatology, Jikei University School of Medicine, Tokyo, Japan

**Alexander Kapp**
Department of Dermatology and Allergology, Hannover Medical School, Hannover,
Germany

**Malgorzata Krajnik**
Nicolaus Copernicus University, Collegium Medicum, Bydgoszcz, Poland

**Andreas E. Kremer**
Department of Gastroenterology and Hepatology, Liver Center, Academic Medical
Center, University of Amsterdam, Amsterdam, The Netherlands

**Torello Lotti**
Department of Dermatology, Faculty of Medicine, University of Florence, Florence,
Italy

**Thomas A. Luger**
Department of Dermatology, University of Münster, Münster, Germany

**Martin Marziniak**
Department of Neurology, University of Münster, Münster, Germany

**Thomas Mettang**
Nephrology, Deutsche Klinik für Diagnostik, Wiesbaden, Germany

**Laurent Misery**
Department of Dermatology and Laboratory of Skin Neurophysiology, University
of Western Brittany, Brest, France

**Silvia Moretti**
Department of Dermatology, Faculty of Medicine, University of Florence, Florence,
Italy

**Micheline Moyal-Barracco**
Department of Dermatology, Hôpital Ambroise Paré, Boulogne, France

**Ronald P.J. Oude-Elferink**
Department of Gastroenterology and Hepatology, Liver Center, Academic Medical Center, University of Amsterdam, Amsterdam, The Netherlands

**Tejesh Surendra Patel**
Department of Internal Medicine, University of Tennessee Health Science Center, Memphis, Tennessee, USA

**Ulysse Pereira**
Department of Dermatology, University Hospital, Brest, Bretagne, France

**Florian Pfab**
Department of Dermatology and Allergy Biederstein, Technische Universität München, Munich, Germany

**Esther Pogatzki-Zahn**
Department of Anesthesiology, University of Münster, Münster, Germany

**Francesca Prignano**
Department of Dermatology, Faculty of Medicine, University of Florence, Florence, Italy

**Sylvia Proske**
Department of Dermatology, University of Heidelberg, Heidelberg, Germany

**Ulrike Raap**
Department of Dermatology and Allergology, Hannover Medical School, Hannover, Germany

**Adam Reich**
Department of Dermatology, Venereology and Allergology, Wroclaw Medical University, Wroclaw, Poland

**Laurence Richard**
University Hospital of Brest, Brest, France

**Johannes Ring**
Department of Dermatology and Allergy, Technische Universität München, Munich, Germany

**Meinhard Schiller**
University Hospital Münster, Department of Dermatology, Münster, Germany

**Martin Schmelz**
Department Anesthesiology and Intensive Care Medicine, Karl Feuerstein Professorship, Medical Faculty Mannheim, University of Heidelberg, Mannheim, Germany

**Gudrun Schneider**
Department of Psychosomatics and Psychotherapy, University of Münster, Münster, Germany

**Sonja Ständer**
Competence Center Pruritus, Department of Dermatology, University of Münster, Münster, Germany

**Jacek C. Szepietowski**
Department of Dermatology, Venereology and Allergology, Wroclaw Medical
University, Wroclaw, Poland

**Thomas R. Tölle**
Department of Neurology, Technische Universität München, Munich, Germany

**Michael Valet**
Department of Neurology, Technische Universität München, Munich, Germany

**Joanna Wallengren**
Department of Dermatology, University Hospital, Getingev, Lund, Sweden

**Bettina Wedi**
Department of Dermatology and Allergology, Hannover Medical School, Hannover,
Germany

**Elke Weisshaar**
Department of Clinical Social Medicine, Occupational and Environmental
Dermatology, University Hospital of Heidelberg, Heidelberg, Germany

**Gil Yosipovitch**
Departments of Dermatology and Neurobiology and Anatomy, Wake Forest
University School of Medicine, Winston-Salem, North Carolina, USA

**Zbigniew Zylicz**
Dove House Hospice, East Riding of Yorkshire, Hull, UK

# Chapter 1
# Neuroanatomy of Itch

Akihiko Ikoma

## 1.1 Nerves in the Skin

Peripheral tissues that can produce an itching sensation are the skin, the conjunctiva and the mucous membrane. In the skin, sensory nerves innervate the epidermis as well as the dermis and the subcutaneous fat tissue, although the autonomic nerves never innervate the epidermis. However, the sensory nerves causing the itching sensation seem to be located in a restricted part of the skin. Histamine has been known for decades to be a potent pruritogen in human beings and, for example, plays a key role in urticaria-associated pruritus.[1] The sensation induced by experimentally applied histamine is, however, not always itchy. Itch is a sensation mainly induced when histamine is applied to the skin by iontophoresis or by pricking, while it is rather painful when subcutaneously injected.[2] Clinically, release of histamine from mast cells in the upper dermis leads to urticaria that is characterized by wheal, flare and itching sensation. On the other hand, histamine release in the deep dermis or subcutaneous tissue results in angioedema that often associates with pain rather than with itch.[3] The sensation caused by skin-burn also depends on the depth of damage. Itch frequently occurs in such damage in a limited and superficial manner or at the last recovering stage, while almost only pain occurs when there is deeper damage. According to a report published half a century ago, a single spicule taken from cowhage (macuna pruriens) pods induced itch most intensely if inserted to the depth of the basal membrane, while itch was never induced if the epidermis and upper dermis had been removed.[4] Thus, it has been suggested that the peripheral origin of itch is limited to a superficial layer of skin, especially epidermis and upper dermis around the basal membrane.

However, this does not mean that origin of pain is limited to a deeper level. Immunohistochemical ultrastructural investigations have revealed that free nerve endings exist in healthy human epidermis.[5] They elongate into the upper epidermis in many pruritic skin diseases like atopic dermatitis[6] (Fig. 1.1a,b). But the elongation of free ending nerves in the epidermis has also been reported in vulvar vestibulitis[7] that associates with pain sensitization in the genital area. This indicates that elongated nerve endings in the epidermis are involved in intensifying sensation even if it is itch or pain, although one cannot still tell whether elongated nerve endings belong to itch or pain nerves since specific receptors to distinguish itch and pain nerves are not yet identified.

## 1.2 Primary Afferent Nerves for Itch

Sensory nerves that have nerve endings in the skin can be categorized into three groups: $A\beta$, $A\delta$ and C nerves (Table 1.1). $A\delta$ and C nerves are involved in the conduction of thermal and pain/itch sensation, while A-beta nerves conduct touch sensation.[8] Pain sensations originating from the skin surface are of two different types, which are perceived with a time lag. The pain first conducted by the $A\delta$ nerves is often described as "stabbing," while the second one conducted by C nerves, are described as "burning," From the viewpoint of a time course, itch has similar features to the second "burning" pain. Itch was generally believed to occur from weak activation of pain-conveying C-nerves.[9] This hypothesis was called as "intensity theory," However, the hypothesis against this, called "specific theory," that itch and pain are distinct sensations with separate pathways, has been getting more support from

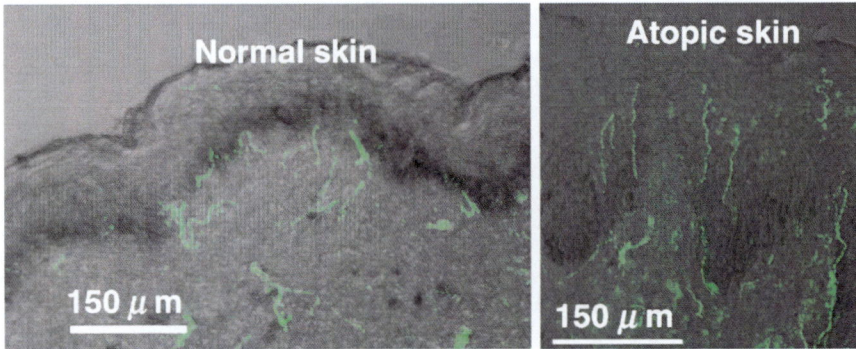

**Fig. 1.1** Elongation of free nerve endings into the epidermis in atopic dermatitis. A larger amount of protein gene product 9.5 (PGP9.5) positive nerves are found in the epidermis of atopic dermatitis (Fig. 1.1b) than in normal skin (Fig. 1.1a) (Courtesy of Prof. Kenji Takamori, Juntendo University, Japan.)

**Table 1.1** Classification of primary sensory nerves

|    | Diameter (μm) | Conduction velocity (m/s) | Sensation |
|----|---------------|---------------------------|-----------|
| Aβ | 6–12          | 33–75                     | Touch, pressure |
| Aδ | 1–5           | 3–30                      | Stabbing pain, thermal sense |
| C  | 0.2–1.5       | 0.5–2                     | Burning pain, itch, thermal sense |

**Table 1.2** Differences between histamine-sensitive and polymodal C nerves

|                                 | Histamine-sensitive C nerves | Polymodal C nerves |
|---------------------------------|------------------------------|--------------------|
| Sensation                       | Itch                         | Pain               |
| Percentage                      | 5                            | 80                 |
| Sensitivity to mechanical stimuli | No                         | Yes                |
| Innervating skin area           | Large                        | Small              |
| Conduction velocity             | 0.5 m/s                      | 0.5–2 m/s          |
| Threshold to electrical stimuli | High                         | Low                |
| Spontaneous activity            | No                           | Yes                |

evidences like opioids reducing pain but inducing itch and electrical stimulation used to elicit itch not transforming into pain at higher frequencies.[10]

Decisive evidence supporting the specific theory has been provided by identification of nerves for histamine-induced itch. Several human microneurography studies in the past had only revealed a weak histamine-induced activation of polymodal C nerves, which failed to explain intense itch. Moreover, the size of their cutaneous receptive field was too small to account for histamine-induced large flare. On the other hand, histamine-sensitive neurons found out among mecha-no-insensitive C nerves (CMi) were activated in parallel to the time course of histamine-induced itch and their receptive field size of CMi nerves was larger than that of polymodal C nerves and therefore consistent with a large flare size.[11] Thus, histamine-induced itch and flare appear to be mediated by these CMi nerves. In addition, histamine-sensitive CMi nerves have different characteristics from polymodal C nerves such as a higher threshold to electrical stimulation, slower conduction velocities and less spontaneous activity, suggesting the presence of an itch-specific neural pathway different from pain pathways (Table 1.2). A later study has shown that they are reactive not only to histamine but, sometimes, also to

capsaicin and other pain mediators, though weakly.[12] On the other hand, histamine activates mechano/heat-sensitive C-nerves (CMH) nerves to some extent. These suggest that substances activating itch-CMi nerves intensely but activating CMH nerves only weakly seem to act a s pruritogens.[13]

Though identification of primary afferents for histamine-induced itch was a breakthrough in itch research, histamine-responsive CMi nerves are not able to explain other types of itch. While histamine-induced itch always accompanies axon-reflex flare, itch without flare is experienced in our daily life. Itch induced by insertion of cowhage spicules to the skin does not accompany any axon-reflex flare. A study, recently reported, supports that cowhage-induced itch appears to be mediated by a subpopulation of capsaicin-sensitive afferent nerves that can be separated from those conducting histamine-induced itch.[14] Another recent report that describes itch evoked by weak transepidermal electrical stimulation of healthy human skin suggests the presence of C-nerves for itch with much lower thresholds to electrical stimulation than histamine-sensitive C-nerves.[15] Thus, there seems to be more than one peripheral neural pathway for itch.

## 1.3  Secondary Afferent Nerves for Itch

The neurons of primary afferent nerves for skin-originating pain are located in the dorsal root ganglions (DRG) and are relatively small among DRG neurons,[16] which is perhaps also true of those for itch. The proximal axon ends of DRG neurons are found in the dorsal horn of the spinal cord. Histamine-sensitive neurons of cats were found in a small subgroup of the lamina I, whose axons run to the contralateral thalamus through the spinothalamic tract (STT).[17] A later study using rats with dry skin also reveals an itch-related c-fos expression in lamina I, but not in lamina II or III, which is different from capsaicin-induced c-fos expression that was observed throughout laminae I, II and III.[18] Similar to histamine-sensitive C-nerves in humans, histamine-sensitive STT tract neurons of cats did not respond to mechanical or thermal stimulation and have slow conduction velocities. Furthermore, they project mainly to the ventral posterior inferior (VPI) nucleus and the ventral periphery of the ventral posterior lateral (vVPL) nucleus of lateral thalamus, while nociceptive STT neurons project mainly to nucleus submedius (SM) of medial thalamus. These findings support the idea that production of histamine-induced itch is due to activation of itch-specific neural elements not only at the primary level but also at the secondary level (Fig. 1.2). A very recent report on gastrin releasing peptide (GRP) and its receptors (GRPR) located in the superficial layer of the dorsal horn shows that GRPR-knockout mice reduce itch-related scratching, but not pain-related behaviors;[19] this also supports the presence of itch-specific transmission mechanism at the spinal level.

In contrast, however, a recent primate study has revealed that histamine-responding wide dynamic range (WDR) neurons antidromically activated from the VPL of thalamus also respond to capsaicin, though they are likely to contribute to pain rather than to itch.[20] Another recent study in monkeys investigating STT neurons reactive to histamine and cowhage has shown

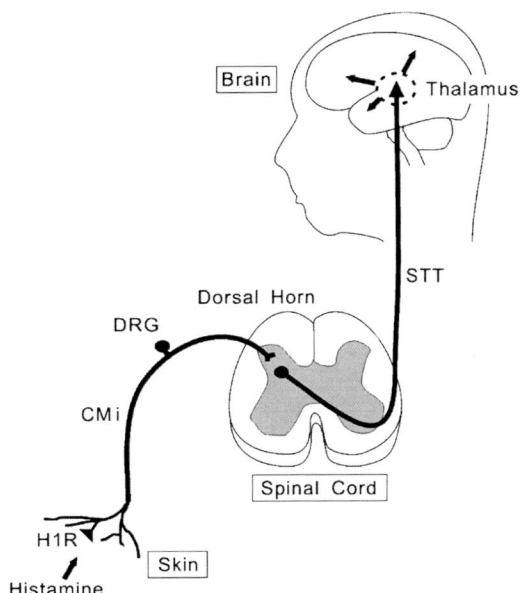

**Fig. 1.2**  Neural pathway for histamine-induced itch. H1R, histamine H1 receptor; CMi, mechano-insensitive C nerve; DRG, dorsal root ganglion; STT, spinothalamic tract

that there are no STT neurons reactive to both histamine and cowhage, suggesting separate STT pathways for histamine- and cowhage-induced itch.[21]

Thus, there are possibly several neuronal pathways for itch in the primary and secondary afferent nerves and so it is still difficult to conclude itch-specificity.

## References

1. Ikoma A, Steinhoff M, Stander S, et al. The neurobiology of itch. *Nat Rev Neurosci.* 2006;7:535–546.
2. Rosenthal SR. Histamine as the chemical mediator for cutaneous pain. *J Invest Dermatol.* 1977;69:98–105.
3. Black AK. Unusual urticarias. *J Dermatol.* 2001;28:632–634.
4. Shelley WB, Arthur RP. Mucunain, the active pruritogenic proteinase of cowhage. *Science.* 1955;122:469–470.
5. Hilliges M, Wang L, Johansson O. Ultrastructural evidence for nerve fibers within all vital layers of the human epidermis. *J Invest Dermatol.* 1995;104:134–137.
6. Urashima R, Mihara M. Cutaneous nerves in atopic dermatitis. A histological, immunohistochemical and electron microscopic study. *Virchows Arch.* 1998;432:363–370.
7. Bohm-Starke N, Hilliges M, Falconer C, et al. Increased intraepithelial innervation in women with vulvar vestibulitis syndrome. *Gynecol Obstet Invest.* 1998;46:256–260.
8. Lawson SN. Phenotype and function of somatic primary afferent nociceptive neurones with C-, Adelta- or Aalpha/beta-fibres. *Exp Physiol.* 2002;87:239–244.

9. von Frey M. Zur Physiologie der Juckempfindung. *Arch Neerland Physiol*. 1922;7:142–145.

10. Tuckett RP. Itch evoked by electrical stimulation of the skin. *J Invest Dermatol*. 1982;79:368–373.

11. Schmelz M, Schmidt R, Bickel A, et al. Specific C-receptors for itch in human skin. *J Neurosci*. 1997;17:8003–8008.

12. Schmelz M, Schmidt R, Weidner C, et al. Chemical response pattern of different classes of C-nociceptors to pruritogens and algogens. *J Neurophysiol*. 2003;89:2441–2448.

13. Schmelz M. Itch – mediators and mechanisms. *J Dermatol Sci*. 2002;28:91–96.

14. Johanek LM, Meyer RA, Hartke T, et al. Psychophysical and physiological evidence for parallel afferent pathways mediating the sensation of itch. *J Neurosci*. 2007;27: 7490–7497.

15. Ikoma A, Handwerker H, Miyachi Y, et al. Electrically evoked itch in humans. *Pain*. 2005;113:148–154.

16. Zimmermann M. Pathobiology of neuropathic pain. *Eur J Pharmacol*. 2001;19:429:23–37.

17. Andrew D, Craig AD. Spinothalamic lamina 1 neurons selectively sensitive to histamine: a central neural pathway for itch. *Nat Neurosci*. 2001;4:72–77.

18. Nojima H, Cuellar JM, Simons CT, et al. Spinal c-fos expression associated with spontaneous biting in a mouse model of dry skin pruritus. *Neurosci Lett*. 2004;361:79–82.

19. Sun YG, Chen ZF. A gastrin-releasing peptide receptor mediates the itch sensation in the spinal cord. *Nature*. 2007;448:700–703.

20. Simone DA, Zhang X, Li J, et al. Comparison of responses of primate spinothalamic tract neurons to pruritic and algogenic stimuli. *J Neurophysiol*. 2004;91:213–222.

21. Davidson S, Zhang X, Yoon CH, et al. The itch-producing agents histamine and cowhage activate separate populations of primate spinothalamic tract neurons. *J Neurosci*. 2007;27:10007–10014.

# Chapter 2
# Neuroreceptors and Neuromediators

Sonja Ständer and Thomas A. Luger

## 2.1 Introduction

The skin has the important sensory function of reacting to external stimuli such as cold, warmth, touch, destruction (pain) and tickling (itch). The modality-specific communication is transmitted to the central nervous system (CNS) by specialized nerve fibers. Dermal myelinated nerve fibers such as Aβ- and Aδ-fibers transmit touch and other mechanical stimuli (e.g., stretching the skin) and fast-conducting pain.[46] Unmyelinated C-fibers in the papillary dermis and epidermis are specialized to stimuli such as cold, warmth, burning or slow conducting pain and itch.[13,14,41,84] In the epidermis, two major classes of sensory nerve fibers can be distinguished (Table 2.1) by their conduction velocity, reaction to trophic stimuli (e.g., nerve growth factor, glial cell-line derived neurotrophic factor), and expression of neuropeptides and neuroreceptors.[3,115,116] This complex system enables the CNS to clearly distinguish between incoming signals from different neurons in quality and localization.[33,77] Moreover, C-fibers have contacts and maintain cross-talk with other skin cells such as keratinocytes, Langerhans cells, mast cells and inflammatory cells.[5,12,31,34,36,37,82,109] This enables sensory nerves, not only to function as an afferent system, which conducts stimuli from the skin to the CNS, but also as an efferent system, which stimulates cutaneous cells by secreting several kinds of neuropeptides.[24,73,105] In addition, sensory sensations can be modified in intensity and quality by this interaction. In this chapter, an overview of the neuroreceptors and mediators of C-fibers involved in the sensory system of the skin and their communication with other skin cells is given.

## 2.2 Histamine Receptors

Histamine and the receptors H1 have been the most thoroughly studied mediator and neuroreceptor for decades (Table 2.2). Lewis reported seventy years ago that intradermal injection of histamine provokes redness, wheal and flare (so called triple response of neurogenic inflammation) accompanied by pruritus.[52] Accordingly, histamine is used for most experimental studies investigating neurogenic inflammation and itching.[78,99] Histamine is stored in mast cells and keratinocytes while H1 to H4 receptors are present in sensory nerve fibers and inflammatory cells.[15,35,100] Thus, histamine-induced itch may be evoked by release from mast cells or keratinocytes. Only recently, it was reported that in addition to H1, H3 and H4 receptors on sensory nerve fibers are also involved in pruritus induction in mice.[6,96] The histamine H4 receptor has a higher affinity for histamine compared with the histamine H1 receptor and appears to be more selectively expressed and is involved in chemotaxis and inflammatory mediator release by eosinophils, mast cells, monocytes, dendritic cells, and T cells. In addition, H4 antagonists have shown promise in experimental models of asthma and pruritus and may represent one new therapeutic option in chronic pruritus.[38] Interestingly, histamine released from mast cells may act on keratinocytes to enhance production and the release of nerve growth factor (NGF).[47] In turn, NGF induces histamine release from mast cells and sensitizes different neuroreceptors including transient receptor potential V1 (TRPV1).[113] Current studies suggest that histamine also regulates SP release via prejunctional histamine H3 receptors that are located on peripheral endings of

L. Misery and S. Ständer (eds.), *Pruritus*,
DOI 10.1007/978-1-84882-322-8_2, © Springer-Verlag London Limited 2010

**Table 2.1** Major classes of epidermal C-fibers

|  | Peptidergic C-fibers | Non-peptidergic C-fibers |
|---|---|---|
| Conducting velocity | 0.5 m/s | 1.0 m/s |
| Diameter | 0.3–1.0 μm | 0.3–1.0 μm |
| Localization in epidermis | Up to stratum spinosum | Up to granular layer |
| Receptors (receptor for growth factors, other receptors) | trkA, p75, e.g., histamine receptor, TRP-group | c-RET, binding of isolectin B4, Mrgprd, TRPV1 |
| Neurotransmitters | Neuropeptides (SP, CGRP) | – |
| Trophic factor (both present in keratinocytes) | Nerve growth factor (NGF) | Glial cell-line derived neurotrophic factor (GDNF) |
| Function | Itch, cold, warmth, burning pain, noxious heat | Mechanical stimuli, warmth, pain |

**Table 2.2** Neuroreceptors on sensory C-fibers and their role in pruritus

| Receptor | Ligand | Function |
|---|---|---|
| Histamine receptors: H1-H4 | Histamine | Pruritus (H1 and H4 receptor), neurogenic inflammation; sensitized by bradykinin, prostaglandins |
| ET receptors: A, B | ET 1, 2, 3 | ETA: Pruritus, mast cell degranulation, inflammation, increase of TNF-alpha, IL-6, VEGF, TGF-beta1<br>ETB: suppression of pruritus |
| TRPV1 | Noxious heat (>42°C), protons, capsaicin, anandamide | Cold, heat, burning pain, burning pruritus, noxious heat sensitized by NGF, galanin, bradykinin |
| TRPM8 | Cold (8°–28°C), menthol, icilin | Cold |
| TRPA1 (AnkTM1) | Noxious cold (<17°C), wasabi, horseradish, mustard | Pain induced by cold, burning |
| PAR-2 | Tryptase, trypsin | Pruritus, neurogenic inflammation |
| Opioid receptors: Mu-, delta-receptor | Endorphins, enkephalins | Suppression of pain, pruritus and neurogenic inflammation |
| Cannabinoid receptors:CB1, CB2 | Cannabinoids<br>CB1: anandamide<br>CB2: PEA | Suppression of itch, pain and neurogenic inflammation, release of opioids |

sensory nerves.[67] This may have an impact on SP-dependent diseases such as atopic dermatitis and ulcerations. Accordingly, a current study demonstrated that mast cell activation and histamine are required for normal cutaneous wound healing.[32,53,106]

## 2.3 Endothelin Receptors

Endothelin (ET) -1, -2 and -3 produced by endothelial cells and mast cells induce neurogenic inflammation associated with burning pruritus.[48,108] ET binds to two different receptors, ET receptor A (ETA) and ETB, which are present on mast cells.[57] When injected into the skin, ET-1 induces mast cell degranulation and mast cell-dependent inflammation.[59] Furthermore, ET-1 induces tumor necrosis factor (TNF)-alpha and interkeukin (IL) -6 production, enhanced vascular endothelial Growth Factor (VEGF) production and transforming growth factor

(TGF)-beta1 expression by mast cells.[57] ET-1 was therefore identified to participate in pathological conditions of various disorders via its multi-functional effects on mast cells under certain conditions. For example, ET-1 contributes to ultraviolet radiation (UVR)-induced skin responses such as tanning or inflammation by involvement of mast cells.[59] Interestingly, it was also identified that ET-1 displays potent pruritic actions in the mouse, mediated to a substantial extent via ETA while ETB exerted an antipruritic role.[101] The effect of ET on human sensory nerve fibers is currently under investigation.

## 2.4 Transient Receptor Potential (TRP) -Family

The TRP family of ion channels is constantly growing and to date comprises more than 30 cation channels, most of which are permeable for $Ca^{2+}$. On the basis of a sequence homology, the TRP family can be divided into seven main subfamilies: the TRPC ("Canonical") family, the TRPV ("Vanilloid") family, the TRPM ("Melastatin") family, the TRPP ("Polycystin") family, the TRPML ("Mucolipin") family, the TRPA ("Ankyrin") family, and the TRPN ("NOMPC") family. Concerning a role in cutaneous nociception, the TRPV and the TRPM groups are both expressed on sensory nerve fibers with different functions.[68]

## 2.5 TRPV1: The Capsaicin Receptor

The TRPV1 receptor (vanilloid receptor, VR1) is expressed on central and peripheral neurons.[19,68] In the skin, the TRPV1 receptor is present on sensory C- and Aδ-fibers.[87] Different types of stimuli activate the receptor such as low pH (<5.9), noxious heat (>42°C), the cannabinoid/endovanilloid anandamide, leukotrien B4 and exogenous capsaicin. TRP receptors act as nonselective cation-channels which open after stimulation and enable ions to move inward into the nerve fiber resulting in depolarization. As a result, e.g., after capsaicin application, TRPV1 is stimulated to either, transmit burning pain or burning pruritus. Due to antidromic activation, C-fibers release neuropeptides which mediate neurogenic inflammation. TRPV1 is a receptor very well known for induction of burning pain. The physiological role of TRPV1 in pruritus induction is still not fully clarified. However, it is speculated that it has several indirect effects. For example, histamine was shown to activate TRPV1 after stimulating the phospholipase A2 and lipoxygenase pathway, leading to the excitation of sensory neurons.[43]

Upon chronic stimulation, such as repeated activation by capsaicin or protons, the $Ca^{2+}$ influx via TRPV1 desensitizes functionally the channel itself, which may represent not only a feedback mechanism protecting the cell from toxic Ca2+ overload, but also likely contributes to the analgesic and antipruritic effect of capsaicin.[111] Moreover, neuropeptides such as SP are depleted from the sensory nerve fiber; the axonal transport of both neuropeptides and NGF in the periphery is slowed down. This mechanism is used therapeutically upon long-term administration of capsaicin for relief of both localized pain and localized pruritus. Clinically, the first days of the

therapy are accompanied by burning, erythema or flare induced by the neurogenic inflammation. After this initial phase, pain and itch sensations are depressed as demonstrated in many studies and case reports.[83] Like the histamine receptor, the TRPV1 receptor may be sensitized by bradykinin and prostaglandins, as well as by NGF,[39,81,113] with lowering of the activation threshold and facilitated induction of pain and itch. For example, instead of noxious heat, moderate warmth may activate a sensitized receptor.

The topical calcineurin inhibitors pimecrolimus and tacrolimus have been introduced during the past years as new topical anti-inflammatory therapies. The only clinically relevant side-effect is initial burning and stinging itch with consequent rapid amelioration of pruritus. This resembles neurogenic inflammation induced by activation of the TRPV1 receptor. Recent animal studies provide evidence that both calcineurin inhibitors bind to the TRPV1.[80,90] It was demonstrated that topical application of pimecrolimus and tacrolimus is followed by an initial release of SP and CGRP from primary afferent nerve fibers in mouse skin.[90] Animal studies proved that the $Ca^{2+}$-dependent desensitization of TRPV1 receptor might be, in part, regulated through channel dephosphorylation by calcineurin.[61,111]

## 2.6 TRPM8, TRPA1: The Cold Receptors

TRPM8 (CMR1) is a cold receptor expressed on unmyelinated C-fibers as well as on myelinated Aδ-fibers that is stimulated by 8°–28°C.[50,98] Menthol and icilin activate the TRPM8 and thereby may act as a therapeutic tool in cold-mediated suppression of itch.[68] Another cold receptor, TRPA1 (ANKTM1), has a lower activation temperature (<17°C) compared to the TRPM8 receptor and is activated by wasabi, horseradish, mustard, bradykinine as well as tetrahydrocannabinol (THC).[45,71,95] Recently, phytocannabinoids and cannabis extracts were shown to exert some of their pharmacological actions by the activation of TRPA1 and TRPM8 channels also, with potential implications for the treatment of pruritus.[18] TRPA1 is found in a subset of nociceptive sensory neurons where it is co-expressed with TRPV1 but not with TRPM8. It was shown that lowering the skin temperature by cooling reduced the intensity of experimentally induced itch.[11] A similar effect was achieved with menthol, although the skin temperature was not decreased.[11] It was concluded that these findings suggest a central inhibitory effect of cold sensitive Aδ-fiber activation on itch. A role in cold hyperalgesia in inflammatory and neuropathic pain is assumed; however, the underlying mechanisms of this enhanced sensitivity to cold are poorly understood.[65] It has been speculated that cold hyperalgesia occurs by NGF mediating an increase in TRPA1 receptors on nerve fibers.

## 2.7 Proteinase-Activated Receptor 2

The proteinase-activated receptor-2 (PAR-2) was demonstrated on sensory nerve fibers and is activated by mast cell mediators such as tryptase.[92,94] Activation leads to induction of pruritus and neurogenic inflammation comparable to effects induced upon histamine release from mast cells.[66,102] In atopic dermatitis (AD), expression of PAR-2 was enhanced on primary afferent nerve fibers in the lesional skin, suggesting that this receptor is involved in the pathophysiology of pruritus in AD.[93] This may also explain the inefficacy of antihistamines in AD as they do not block the tryptase-mast cell axis. Cutaneous mast cells also express PAR-2, suggesting an additional autocrine mechanism.[62] PAR-2 was recently suggested to also be involved in pain mechanisms. Activation of PAR-2 is reported to induce sensitization of primary nociceptors along with hyperalgesia.[21] Together, these results suggest PAR-2 to be involved in cutaneous nociception mainly during inflammation.

## 2.8 Opioid Receptors

Two opioid receptors, the μ- and δ-receptor, have been demonstrated on cutaneous sensory nerve fibers.[85,86] Peripheral opioid receptors differ from central opioid receptors.[8,29,49,76] In the spinal cord, binding of opioids lead to the induction of pruritus leading to the application of opioid antagonists as antipruritic therapy.[60,97] In the skin, opioid peptides such as β-endorphin, enkephalins, and endomorphins act on sensory nerve fibers to inhibit the release of inflammatory neuropeptides such as SP, neurokinin A and CGRP.[51,74] In previous studies, it was shown that peripheral opioid receptors mediate

antinociceptive effects preferentially by the activation of the μ-receptor and less by δ-receptor.[91] Application of peripheral morphine inhibited responses to both mechanical and thermal stimuli in inflamed skin, suggesting that peripheral opioids might modulate inflammatory pain responses.[107] These findings suggest that the peripheral opioid receptors act as inhibitory receptors in the skin. Interestingly, a recent paper described the efficacy of topical application of mu-opioid antagonist in chronic pruritus suggesting a complex role of peripheral opioid receptors in nociception.[5]

## 2.9 Cannabinoid Receptors

Up to now, two cannabinoid receptors, CB1 and CB2, have been defined precisely by their wide expression in the CNS and on immune cells.[20,56,63] CB1 was described as being densely localized in the CNS; recent studies revealed an additional expression of CB1 in peripheral tissue, i.e., primary afferent neurons.[2,16,72] CB2 receptors were mainly found in the periphery, e.g., on T-lymphocytes, mast cells,[26,30] and also on rat spinal cord.[112] Both receptors were recently found to be expressed also on cutaneous sensory nerve fibers, mast cells and keratinocytes.[88]

Anandamide, acting on both, CB1 and TRPV1, was shown to downregulate keratin 1 and 10, transglutaminase 5 and involucrin. Anandamide is also able to decrease differentiating gene expression by increasing DNA methylation in human keratinocytes.[70] Moreover, since cannabinoids inhibit keratinocyte proliferation, a potential role for cannabinoids in the treatment of psoriasis was suggested.[110] Recently it was demonstrated, that the endocannabinoid system including anandamide has a protective role in contact allergy.[42] Moreover, during inflammation, CB1 expression in primary afferent neurons and its transport to peripheral axons is increased and thereby, it contributes to enhanced antihyperalgesic efficacy of locally administered CB1 agonist.[4] Topical application of CB2 agonists leads to antinociceptive effects such as inhibition of pain, pruritus and neurogenic inflammation.[23,58,75,89] In addition, it was demonstrated that injections of the CB2 agonist palmitoylethanolamine (PEA) may inhibit experimental NGF-induced thermal hyperalgesia.[27]

However, the antinociceptive effects of agonists are believed to be mediated in part by opioid and vanilloid mechanisms and not directly by activation of cannabinoid receptors. For example, it was shown that the CB1 agonist anandamide binds to the TRPV1 receptor[114] and that topical cannabinoids directly inhibit TRPV1 functional activities via a calcineurin pathway.[69] Moreover, it was demonstrated that the antinociceptive effects of CB2 agonists can be prevented by the μ-opioid receptor-antagonist naloxone.[28,104] Interestingly, the cannabinoid agonist AM1241 stimulates β-endorphin release from rat skin tissue and from cultured human keratinocytes.[40] In sum, cannabinoid receptors seem to exert a central role in cutaneous nociception mediating direct and indirect effects and therefore represent interesting targets for the development of antinociceptive therapies.

## 2.10  Trophic Factors

### 2.10.1  Nerve Growth Factor (NGF)

In recent years, neurotrophins have been found to play a major role in skin homeostasis and inflammatory diseases. One member of this family, NGF, has several regulatory functions in cutaneous nociception, cutaneous nerve development and reconstruction after injury through action on peptidergic C-fibers.[9,64] In epidermal keratinocytes, NGF production underlies neuropeptide release. After release of neuropeptides by a nociceptive stimulus, an up-regulation of the expression of NGF and NGF secretion from the keratinocytes is induced.[17] Released NGF acts on skin nerves to sensitize neuroreceptors towards noxious thermal, mechanical, and chemical stimuli (see above) and is transported along the axon towards the dorsal root ganglia (DRG) to induce up-regulation of a variety of proteins involved in neuronal growth and sensitivity. These mechanisms lead to altered peripheral nociception, e.g., facilitated induction of pruritus and pain. For example, prolonged treatment of rats with moderate doses of NGF is sufficient to stimulate neuropeptide synthesis in primary afferent neurons without causing long-lasting changes in thermal nociceptive threshold.[79] Moreover, application of NGF also enhances capsaicin-evoked thermal hyperalgesia.[10] In cutaneous inflammatory diseases, NGF was demonstrated to be over-expressed in prurigo nodularis[1] and in AD as well as in allergic diseases, it is speculated to contribute to the neurohyperplasia of the disease.[22,44,64]

## 2.11  Glial Cell Line-Derived Neurotrophic Factor (GDNF)

During embryonic development, nociceptors are dependent on NGF, but a large subpopulation lose this dependence during embryonic and postnatal life and become responsive to the transforming growth factor beta family member, glial cell line-derived growth factor (GDNF). The family comprises members such as artemin and neurturin – which are involved in the induction and maintenance of pain and hyperalgesia.[3] These factors act on non-peptidergic C-fibers[115,116] and expression of GDNF in the skin can change mechanical sensitivity.[3] More importantly, GDNF sensitizes thermal nociceptors towards cold or heat hyperalgesia by the potentiation of TRPV1 signaling or increased expression of TRPA1.[25,54,55] In the DRG, exposure to GDNF, neurturin, or artemin potentate TRPV1 function at doses 10–100 times lower than NGF. Moreover, GDNF family members induced capsaicin responses in a subset of neurons that were previously insensitive to capsaicin.[55] Exposure of nerve fibers to GDNF induces, in addition, expression of the prokineticin receptors (PKR) in the nonpeptidergic population of neurons. These receptors cause heat hyperalgesia by sensitizing TRPV1.[103]

In sum, during the past years, many neuroreceptors, which mediate these sensations and respond to external stimuli were identified on sensory nerve fibers. The chronification of sensations such as pain and itch underlie complex mechanisms such as sensitization of neuroreceptors. Several modern therapies that can interact with these mechanisms and achieve the clinical relief of peripheral pain and pruritus are yet to be identified.

## References

1. Abadia Molina F, Burrows NP, Jones RR, et al. Increased sensory neuropeptides in nodular prurigo: a quantitative immunohistochemical analysis. *Br J Dermatol*. 1992;127: 344–351.
2. Ahluwalia J, Urban L, Capogna M, et al. Cannabinoid 1 receptors are expressed in nociceptive primary sensory neurons. *Neuroscience*. 2000;100:685–688.
3. Albers KM, Woodbury CJ, Ritter AM, et al. Glial cell-line-derived neurotrophic factor expression in skin alters the mechanical sensitivity of cutaneous nociceptors. *J Neurosci*. 2006;26:2981–2990.
4. Amaya F, Shimosato G, Kawasaki Y, et al. Induction of CB1 cannabinoid receptor by inflammation in primary afferent

neurons facilitates antihyperalgesic effect of peripheral CB1 agonist. *Pain.* 2006;124:175–183.

5. Bigliardi PL, Stammer H, Jost G, Rufli T, Büchner S, Bigliardi-Qi M. Treatment of pruritus with topically applied opiate receptor antagonist. *J Am Acad Dermatol.* 2007; 56:979–988.

6. Bell JK, McQueen DS, Rees JL. Involvement of histamine H4 and H1 receptors in scratching induced by histamine receptor agonists in Balb C mice. *Br J Pharmacol.* 2004;142:374–380.

7. Bernstein JE, Swift RM. Relief of intractable pruritus with naloxone. *Arch Dermatol.* 1979;115:1366–1367.

8. Bernstein JE, Grinzi RA. Butorphanol-induced pruritus antagonized by naloxone. *J Am Acad Dermatol.* 1981;5: 227–228.

9. Botchkarev VA, Yaar M, Peters EM, et al. Neurotrophins in skin biology and pathology. *J Invest Dermatol.* 2006;126: 1719–1727.

10. Bowles WR, Sabino M, Harding-Rose C, et al. Chronic nerve growth factor administration increases the peripheral exocytotic activity of capsaicin-sensitive cutaneous neurons. *Neurosci Lett.* 2006;403:305–308.

11. Bromm B, Scharein E, Darsow U, et al. Effects of menthol and cold on histamine-induced itch and skin reactions in man. *Neurosci Lett.* 1995;187:157–160.

12. Chateau Y, Misery L Connections between nerve endings and epidermal cells: are they synapses? *Exp Dermatol.* 2004;13:2–4.

13. Chung MK, Lee H, Caterina MJ. Warm temperatures activate TRPV4 in mouse 308 keratinocytes. *J Biol Chem.* 2003;278:32037–32046.

14. Chung MK, Lee H, Mizuno A, et al. TRPV3 and TRPV4 mediate warmth-evoked currents in primary mouse keratinocytes. *J Biol Chem.* 2004;279:21569–1575.

15. Church MK, el-Lati S, Caulfield JP. Neuropeptide-induced secretion from human skin mast cells. *Int Arch Allergy Appl Immunol.* 1991;94:310–318.

16. Coutts AA, Irving AJ, Mackie K, et al. Localisation of cannabinoid CB(1) receptor immunoreactivity in the guinea pig and rat myenteric plexus. *J Comp Neurol.* 2002;448: 410–422.

17. Dallos A, Kiss M, Polyanka H, et al. Effects of the neuropeptides substance P, calcitonin gene-related peptide, vasoactive intestinal polypeptide and galanin on the production of nerve growth factor and inflammatory cytokines in cultured human keratinocytes. *Neuropeptides.* 2006;40:251–263.

18. De Petrocellis L, Vellani V, Schiano-Moriello A, Marini P, Magherini PC, Orlando P, Di Marzo V. Plant-derived cannabinoids modulate the activity of transient receptor potential channels of ankyrin type-1 and melastatin type-8. *J Pharmacol Exp Ther.* 2008;325:1007–1015.

19. Denda M, Sokabe T, Fukumi-Tominaga T, et al. Effects of skin surface temperature on epidermal permeability barrier homeostasis. *J Invest Dermatol.* 2007;127:654–659.

20. Devane WA, Dysarz FA 3rd, Johnson MR, et al. Determination and characterization of a cannabinoid receptor in rat brain. *Mol Pharmacol.* 1988;34:605–613.

21. Ding-Pfennigdorff D, Averbeck B, Michaelis M. Stimulation of PAR-2 excites and sensitizes rat cutaneous C-nociceptors to heat. *Neuroreport.* 2004;15:2071–2075.

22. Dou YC, Hagstromer L, Emtestam L, et al. Increased nerve growth factor and its receptors in atopic dermatitis: an immunohistochemical study. *Arch Dermatol Res.* 2006;298:31–37.

23. Dvorak M, Watkinson A, McGlone F, et al. Histamine induced responses are attenuated by a cannabinoid receptor agonist in human skin. *Inflamm Res.* 2003;52:238–245.

24. Yaping E, Golden SC, Shalita AR, et al. Neuropeptide (calcitonin gene-related peptide) induction of nitric oxide in human keratinocytes in vitro. *J Invest Dermatol.* 2006;126: 1994–2001.

25. Elitt CM, McIlwrath SL, Lawson JJ, et al. Artemin overexpression in skin enhances expression of TRPV1 and TRPA1 in cutaneous sensory neurons and leads to behavioral sensitivity to heat and cold. *J Neurosci.* 2006;26:8578–8587.

26. Facci L, Dal Toso R, Romanello S, et al. Mast cells express a peripheral cannabinoid receptor with differential sensitivity to anandamide and palmitoylethanolamide. *Proc Natl Acad Sci USA.* 1995;92:3376–3380.

27. Farquhar-Smith WP, Rice AS A novel neuroimmune mechanism in cannabinoid-mediated attenuation of nerve growth factor-induced hyperalgesia. *Anesthesiology.* 2003;99: 1391–1401.

28. Fattore L, Cossu G, Spano MS, et al. Cannabinoids and reward: interactions with the opioid system. *Crit Rev Neurobiol.* 2004;16:147–158.

29. Fjellner B, Hägermark O. Potentiation of histamine-induced itch and flare response in human skin by the enkephalin analogue FK 33–824, beta-endorphin and morphine. *Arch Dermatol Res.* 1982;274:29–37.

30. Galiegue S, Mary S, Marchand J, et al. Expression of central and peripheral cannabinoid receptors in human immune tissues and leukocyte subpopulations. *Eur J Biochem.* 1995;232:54–61.

31. Gaudillere A, Misery L, Souchier C, et al. Intimate associations between PGP9.5-positive nerve fibres and Langerhans cells. *Br J Dermatol.* 1996;135:343–344.

32. Gibran NS, Jang YC, Isik FF, et al. Diminished neuropeptide levels contribute to the impaired cutaneous healing response associated with diabetes mellitus. *J Surg Res.* 2002;108: 122–128.

33. Gray EG. Electron microscopy of presynaptic organelles of the spinal cord. *J Anat.* 1963;97:101–106.

34. Hara M, Toyoda M, Yaar M, et al. Innervation of melanocytes in human skin. *J Exp Med.* 1996;184:1385–1395.

35. Hill SJ. Distribution, properties, and functional characteristics of three classes of histamine receptor. *Pharmacol Rev.* 1990;42:45–83.

36. Hilliges M, Wang L, Johansson O. Ultrastructural evidence for nerve fibers within all vital layers of the human epidermis. *J Invest Dermatol.* 1995;104:134–137.

37. Hosoi J, Murphy GF, Egan CL, et al. Regulation of Langerhans cell function by nerves containing calcitonin gene-related peptide. *Nature.* 1993;363:159–163.

38. Huang JF, Thurmond RL. The new biology of histamine receptors. *Curr Allergy Asthma Rep.* 2008;8:21–27.

39. Hu HJ, Bhave G, Gereau RW 4th. Prostaglandin and protein kinase A-dependent modulation of vanilloid receptor function by metabotropic glutamate receptor 5: potential mechanism for thermal hyperalgesia. *J Neurosci.* 2002;22: 7444–7452.

40. Ibrahim MM, Porreca F, Lai J, et al. CB2 cannabinoid receptor activation produces antinociception by stimulating peripheral release of endogenous opioids. *Proc Natl Acad Sci USA*. 2005;102(8):3093–3098.

41. Ikoma A, Steinhoff M, Ständer S, et al Neurobiology of pruritus. *Nat Rev Neurosci*. 2006;7:535–547.

42. Karsak M, Gaffal E, Date R, Wang-Eckhardt L, Rehnelt J, Petrosino S, Starowicz K, Steuder R, Schlicker E, Cravatt B, Mechoulam R, Buettner R, Werner S, Di Marzo V, Tüting T, Zimmer A. Attenuation of allergic contact dermatitis through the endocannabinoid system. *Science* 2007;316:1494–1497.

43. Kim JC, Kim DB, Seo SI, Park YH, Hwang TK. Nerve growth factor and vanilloid receptor expression, and detrusor instability, after relieving bladder outlet obstruction in rats. *BJU Int*. 2004;94:915–918.

44. Johansson O, Liang Y, Emtestam L Increased nerve growth factor- and tyrosine kinase A-like immunoreactivities in prurigo nodularis skin - an exploration of the cause of neurohyperplasia. *Arch Dermatol Res*. 2002;293:614–619.

45. Jordt SE, Bautista DM, Chuang HH, et al. Mustard oils and cannabinoids excite sensory nerve fibres through the TRP channel ANKTM1. *Nature*. 2004;427:260–265.

46. Julius D, Basbaum AI. Molecular mechanisms of nociception. *Nature*. 2001;413:203–210.

47. Kanda N, Watanabe S Histamine enhances the production of nerve growth factor in human keratinocytes. *J Invest Dermatol*. 2003;121:570–577.

48. Katugampola R, Church MK, Clough GF. The neurogenic vasodilator response to endothelin-1: a study in human skin in vivo. *Exp Physiol*. 2000;85:839–846.

49. Ko MC, Naughton NN. An experimental itch model in monkeys: characterization of intrathecal morphine-induced scratching and antinociception. *Anesthesiology*. 2000;92:795–805.

50. Lee H, Caterina MJ. TRPV channels as thermosensory receptors in epithelial cells. *Pflugers Arch*. 2005;451:160–167.

51. Lembeck F, Donnerer J, Bartho L. Inhibition of neurogenic vasodilation and plasma extravasation by substance P antagonists, somatostatin and [D-Met$^2$, Pro$^5$]-enkephalinamide. *Eur J Pharmacol*. 1982;85:171–176.

52. Lewis T, Grant RT, Marvin HM. Vascular reactions of the skin to injury. *Heart*. 1929;14:139–160.

53. Liang Y, Marcusson JA, Jacobi HH, et al. Histamine-containing mast cells and their relationship to NGFr-immunoreactive nerves in prurigo nodularis: a reappraisal. *J Cutan Pathol*. 1998;25:189–198.

54. Lindfors PH, Voikar V, Rossi J, et al. Deficient nonpeptidergic epidermis innervation and reduced inflammatory pain in glial cell line-derived neurotrophic factor family receptor alpha2 knock-out mice. *J Neurosci*. 2006;26:1953–1960.

55. Malin SA, Molliver DC, Koerber HR, et al. Glial cell line-derived neurotrophic factor family members sensitize nociceptors in vitro and produce thermal hyperalgesia in vivo. *J Neurosci*. 2006;26:8588–8599.

56. Matsuda LA, Lolait SJ, Brownstein MJ, et al. Structure of a cannabinoid receptor and functional expression of the cloned cDNA. *Nature*. 1990;346:561–564.

57. Matsushima H, Yamada N, Matsue H, et al. The effects of endothelin-1 on degranulation, cytokine, and growth factor production by skin-derived mast cells. *Eur J Immunol*. 2004;34:1910–1919.

58. Maekawa T, Nojima H, Kuraishi Y, Aisaka K. The cannabinoid CB2 receptor inverse agonist JTE-907 suppresses spontaneous itch-associated responses of NC mice, a model of atopic dermatitis. *Eur J Pharmacol*. 2006;542:179–183.

59. Metz M, Lammel V, Gibbs BF, et al. Inflammatory murine skin responses to UV-B light are partially dependent on endothelin-1 and mast cells. *Am J Pathol*. 2006;169: 815–822.

60. Metze D, Reimann S, Beissert S, et al. Efficacy and safety of naltrexone, an oral opiate receptor antagonist, in the treatment of pruritus in internal and dermatological diseases. *J Am Acad Dermatol*. 1999;41:533–539.

61. Mohapatra DP, Nau C. Regulation of Ca$^{2+}$-dependent desensitization in the vanilloid receptor TRPV1 by calcineurin and cAMP-dependent protein kinase. *J Biol Chem*. 2005;280: 13424–13432.

62. Moormann C, Artuc M, Pohl E, et al. Functional characterization and expression analysis of the proteinase-activated receptor-2 in human cutaneous mast cells. *J Invest Dermatol*. 2006;126:746–755.

63. Munro S, Thomas KL, Abu-Shaar M. Molecular characterization of a peripheral receptor for cannabinoids. *Nature*. 1993;365:61–65.

64. Nockher WA, Renz H. Neurotrophins in allergic diseases: from neuronal growth factors to intercellular signaling molecules. *J Allergy Clin Immunol*. 2006;117:583–589.

65. Obata K, Katsura H, Mizushima T, et al. TRPA1 induced in sensory neurons contributes to cold hyperalgesia after inflammation and nerve injury. *J Clin Invest*. 2005;115: 2393–2401.

66. Obreja O, Rukwied R, Steinhoff M, et al. Neurogenic components of trypsin- and thrombin-induced inflammation in rat skin, in vivo. *Exp Dermatol*. 2006;15:58–65.

67. Ohkubo T, Shibata M, Inoue M, et al. Regulation of substance P release mediated via prejunctional histamine H3 receptors. *Eur J Pharmacol*. 1995;273:83–88.

68. Patapoutian A. TRP channels and thermosensation. *Chem Senses*. 2005;30(suppl 1):i193–i194.

69. Patwardhan AM, Jeske NA, Price TJ, et al. The cannabinoid WIN 55,212–2 inhibits transient receptor potential vanilloid 1 (TRPV1) and evokes peripheral antihyperalgesia via calcineurin. *Proc Natl Acad Sci USA*. 2006;103: 11393–11398.

70. Paradisi A, Pasquariello N, Barcaroli D, Maccarrone M. Anandamide regulates keratinocyte differentiation by inducing DNA methylation in a CB1 receptor-dependent manner. *J Biol Chem*. 2008;283:6005–6012.

71. Peier AM, Reeve AJ, Andersson DA, et al. A heat-sensitive TRP channel expressed in keratinocytes. *Science*. 2002;296: 2046–2049.

72. Pertwee RG. Evidence for the presence of CB1 cannabinoid receptors on peripheral neurones and for the existence of neuronal non-CB1 cannabinoid receptors. *Life Sci*. 1999; 65:597–605.

73. Quinlan KL, Song IS, Naik SM, et al. VCAM-1 expression on human dermal microvascular endothelial cells is directly and specifically up-regulated by substance P. *J Immunol*. 1999;162:1656–1661.

74. Ray NJ, Jones AJ, Keen P. Morphine, but not sodium cromoglycate, modulates the release of substance P from

capsaicin-sensitive neurones in the rat trachea in vitro. *Br J Pharmacol*. 1991;102:797–800.

75. Rukwied R, Watkinson A, McGlone F, et al. Cannabinoid agonists attenuate capsaicin-induced responses in human skin. *Pain*. 2003;102:283–288.

76. Sakurada T, Sakurada S, Katsuyama S, et al. Evidence that N-terminal fragments of nociceptin modulate nociceptin-induced scratching, biting and licking in mice. *Neurosci Lett*. 2000;279:61–64.

77. Schmelz M, Schmidt R, Bickel A, et al. Innervation territories of single sympathetic C fibers in human skin. *J Neurophysiol*. 1998;79:1653–1660.

78. Schmelz M, Schmidt R, Weidner C, et al. Chemical response pattern of different classes of C-nociceptors to pruritogens and algogens. *J Neurophysiol*. 2003;89: 2441–2448.

79. Schuligoi R, Amann R. Differential effects of treatment with nerve growth factor on thermal nociception and on calcitonin gene-related peptide content of primary afferent neurons in the rat. *Neurosci Lett*. 1998;252:147–149.

80. Senba E, Katanosaka K, Yajima H, et al. The immunosuppressant FK506 activates capsaicin- and bradykinin-sensitive DRG neurons and cutaneous C-fibers. *Neurosci Res*. 2004;50:257–262.

81. Shu X, Medell LM. Nerve growth factor acutely sensitizes the response of adult rat sensory neurons to capsaicin. *J Neurosci*. 1998;18:8947–8959.

82. Singh LK, Pang X, Alexacos N, et al. Acute immobilization stress triggers skin mast cell degranulation via corticotropin releasing hormone, neurotensin, and substance P: A link to neurogenic skin disorders. *Brain Behav Immun*. 1999;13:225–239.

83. Ständer S, Metze D. Treatment of pruritic skin diseases with topical capsaicin. In: Yosipovitch G, Greaves MW, Fleischer AB, McGlone F, eds. *Itch: Basic Mechanisms and Therapy*. New York: Marcel Dekker; 2004:287–304.

84. Ständer S, Schmelz M. Chronic itch and pain – similarities and differences. *Eur J Pain*. 2006;10:473–478.

85. Ständer S, Gunzer M, Metze D, et al. Localization of μ-opioid receptor 1A on sensory nerve fibers in human skin. *Regul Pept*. 2002;110:75–83.

86. Ständer S, Steinhoff M, Schmelz M, et al. Neurophysiology of pruritus. cutaneous elicitation of itch. *Arch Dermatol*. 2003;139:1463–1470.

87. Ständer S, Moormann C, Schumacher M, et al. Expression of vanilloid receptor subtype 1 (VR1) in cutaneous sensory nerve fibers, mast cells and epithelial cells of appendage structures. *Exp Dermatol*. 2004;13:129–139.

88. Ständer S, Schmelz M, Metze D, et al. Distribution of cannabinoid receptor 1 (CB1) and 2 (CB2) on sensory nerve fibers and adnexal structures in human skin. *J Dermatol Sci*. 2005;38:177–188.

89. Ständer S, Reinhardt HW, Luger TA. Topische Cannabinoid-Agonisten: Eine effektive, neue Möglichkeit zur Behandlung von chronischem Pruritus. *Hautarzt*. 2006;57:801–807.

90. Ständer S, Ständer H, Seeliger S, et al. Topical pimecrolimus (SDZ ASM 981) and tacrolimus (FK 506) transiently induces neuropeptide release and mast cell degranulation in murine skin. *Br J Dermatol*. 2007;156:1020–1026.

91. Stein C, Millan MJ, Shippenberg TS, et al. Peripheral opioid receptors mediating antinociception in inflammation.

Evidence for involvement of mu, delta and kappa receptors. *J Pharmacol Exp Ther*. 1989;248:1269–1275.

92. Steinhoff M, Vergnolle N, Young SH, et al. Agonists of proteinase-activated receptor 2 induce inflammation by a neurogenic mechanism. *Nat Med*. 2000;6:151–158.

93. Steinhoff M, Neisius U, Ikoma A, et al. Proteinase-activated receptor-2 mediates itch: a novel pathway for pruritus in human skin. *J Neurosci*. 2003;23:6176–6180.

94. Steinhoff M, Stander S, Seeliger S, et al. Modern aspects of cutaneous neurogenic inflammation. *Arch Dermatol*. 2003;139: 1479–1488.

95. Story GM, Peier AM, Reeve AJ, et al. ANKTM1, a TRP-like channel expressed in nociceptive neurons, is activated by cold temperatures. *Cell*. 2003;112:819–829.

96. Sugimoto Y, Iba Y, Nakamura Y, et al. Pruritus-associated response mediated by cutaneous histamine H3 receptors. *Clin Exp Allergy*. 2004;34:456–459.

97. Summerfield JA. Pain, itch and endorphins. *Br J Dermatol*. 1981;105:725–726.

98. Takashima Y, Daniels RL, Knowlton W, Teng J, Liman ER, McKemy DD. Diversity in the neural circuitry of cold sensing revealed by genetic axonal labeling of transient receptor potential melastatin 8 neurons. *J Neurosci*. 2007;27: 14147–14157.

99. Thomsen JS, Sonne M, Benfeldt E, et al. Experimental itch in sodium lauryl sulphate-inflamed and normal skin in humans: a randomized, double-blind, placebo-controlled study of histamine and other inducers of itch. *Br J Dermatol*. 2002;146:792–800.

100. Togias A. H1-receptors: localization and role in airway physiology and in immune functions. *J Allergy Clin Immunol*. 2003;112(suppl):S60–S68.

101. Trentin PG, Fernandes MB, D'Orleans-Juste P, et al. Endothelin-1 causes pruritus in mice. *Exp Biol Med (Maywood)*. 2006;231:1146–1151.

102. Ui H, Andoh T, Lee JB, et al. Potent pruritogenic action of tryptase mediated by PAR-2 receptor and its involvement in anti-pruritic effect of nafamostat mesilate in mice. *Eur J Pharmacol*. 2006;530:172–178.

103. Vellani V, Colucci M, Lattanzi R, et al. Sensitization of transient receptor potential vanilloid 1 by the prokineticin receptor agonist Bv8. *J Neurosci*. 2006;26:5109–5116.

104. Vigano D, Rubino T, Parolaro D. Molecular and cellular basis of cannabinoid and opioid interactions. *Pharmacol Biochem Behav*. 2005;81:360–368.

105. Weidner C, Klede M, Rukwied R, et al. Acute effects of substance P and calcitonin gene-related peptide in human skin - a microdialysis study. *J Invest Dermatol*. 2000;115: 1015–1020.

106. Weller K, Foitzik K, Paus R, et al. Mast cells are required for normal healing of skin wounds in mice. *FASEB J*. 2006;publ. online Sept. 11th 2006.

107. Wenk HN, Brederson JD, Honda CN. Morphine directly inhibits nociceptors in inflamed skin. *J Neurophysiol*. 2006;95:2083–2097.

108. Wenzel RR, Zbinden S, Noll G, et al. Endothelin-1 induces vasodilation in human skin by nociceptor fibres and release of nitric oxide. *Br J Clin Pharmacol*. 1998;45:441–446.

109. Wiesner-Menzel L, Schulz B, Vakilzadeh F, et al. Electron microscopal evidence for a direct contact between nerve fibres and mast cells. *Acta Derm Venereol*. 1981;61:465–469.

110. Wilkinson JD, Williamson EM. Cannabinoids inhibit human keratinocyte proliferation through a non-CB1/CB2 mechanism and have a potential therapeutic value in the treatment of psoriasis. *J Dermatol Sci*. 2007;45:87–92.

111. Wu ZZ, Chen SR, Pan HL. Transient receptor potential vanilloid type 1 activation down-regulates voltage-gated calcium channels through calcium-dependent calcineurin in sensory neurons. *J Biol Chem*. 2005;280:18142–51.

112. Zhang J, Hoffert C, Vu HK, et al. Induction of CB2 receptor expression in the rat spinal cord of neuropathic but not inflammatory chronic pain models. *Eur J Neurosci*. 2003;17:2750–2754.

113. Zhang X, Huang J, McNaughton PA. NGF rapidly increases membrane expression of TRPV1 heat-gated ion channels. *EMBO J*. 2005;24:4211–4223.

114. Zygmunt PM, Petersson J, Andersson DA, et al. Vanilloid receptors on sensory nerves mediate the vasodilator action of anandamide. *Nature*. 1999;400:452–457.

115. Zylka MJ. Nonpeptidergic circuits feel your pain. *Neuron*. 47:771–772 (Comment on: *Neuron*. 2005;47: 787–793.

116. Zylka MJ, Rice FL, Anderson DJ. Topographically distinct epidermal nociceptive circuits revealed by axonal tracers targeted to Mrgprd. *Neuron*. 2005;45:17–25.

# Chapter 3
# The Brain in the Skin: Neuro-Epidermal Synapses

Nicholas Boulais and Laurent Misery

For the past few years, an impressive amount of data has come into view conveying new insights into the sensory capability of the whole epidermis.[1,2] Because the epidermis appeared as a sensory tissue, investigations about the tight connections that blend epidermis and sensory neurones were fostered. In some cases, these contacts were so closed that synaptic-like communications were supposed. Structural evidences fulfil this idea.[3] Furthermore, epidermal cells produce numerous receptors like those expressed by sensory neurons. Most of these receptors are coupled with calcium channels, whose activation leads to increases in intracellular calcium concentration, which is associated with signal transduction, cell-excitability, and neurotransmitter release. On sensory neurons, these receptors are involved in the recognition of environmental stimulations such as mechanical stress, osmotic pressure, temperature, and chemical stimuli thereafter transduced into electric signal. The presence of such receptors at the surface of epidermal cells may allow them to sense the same type of stimulations. Hence, as epidermal cells express the molecular components of the stimuli perception and, moreover, of the information transduction, it suggests that epidermis could be the first step of the signal integration within the skin. According to this hypothesis, cutaneous stimulations as well as chemical mediators would be first sensed by epidermal cells and, thereafter, may or may not be transmitted to the nerve terminals, which would give rise to action potentials. Action potentials would be further conveyed to the central nervous system where we become aware of the stimulation.

With neurogenic, neuropathic or psychogenic pruritus, the itch sensation, even when appearing anatomically localized, results in brain-generated signals directly by the central nervous system.[4] This phenomenon may occur through the decrease in activity of the itch-inhibitory nociceptive pathway in the spinothalamic tract,[5] which connects the lamina I of the medulla to the thalamus.[6] In contrast, the cutaneous-derived itch, called pruritogenic pruritus, is more likely to occur throughout the peripheral stimulations, localized within the skin. Actually, convincing arguments establish that pruritus-specific neurons are anatomically and functionally distinct from those of the pain pathway.[6] Pruriceptive primary afferent nerve fibers are mainly unmyelinated, mechanically insensitive, histaminergic C-fibers. However, we have to keep in mind that they could be activated by various biochemical agents referred to as pruritogens, whose histamine is the best known member.[5,7] As such fibers often reach the basal and suprabasal layers of the epidermis. It is interesting to consider that pruritus may involve neuro-epidermal synaptic-like connections to activate or to sensitize pruriceptive neurons. The molecular mechanisms leading epidermal cells to activate sensory neurons are poorly known so far. Recently published data describe ATP as a possible candidate.[8] ATP is able to spread from keratinocytes to induce a calcium wave into neighbouring cells as well as neurites of sensory neurones. The intracellular increase in calcium concentration would be able to sensitize nociceptive as well as pruriceptive neuron. This could explain the broad overlap of both the systems. Furthermore, since pruritus is based on the activity of pruriceptors and the decrease in activity of the pain-mediating nociceptors,[9] the itch induced by molecules of the pain-pathway, like neurokinins or capsaicin,[4,9–11] elicits the close involvement of the epidermis in the pruritogenesis. Indeed, pruritogens can lead to the release of neuropeptides involved in pain transmission, such as substance P (SP) and calcitonin gene-related peptide (CGRP).[12] Once released by pruriceptive neurons, they bind their reciprocal receptors on neuronal and non-neuronal cutaneous cells which, in turn, release pruritogens, thus generating a positive regulatory loop.[10,13] Moreover, in patients with atopic dermatitis (AD), application of noxious stimuli like warmth, scratching or pain-mediating neuropeptides do not inhibit pruritus in opposition to what usually happened.[14] Conversely, endogenous algogens like bradykinin, serotonin or even SP turn into potent pruritogens in the lesional skin of AD.[12] These works steadily support the concept that epidermis itself can act as an itch modulator, especially because they express a wide range of neuropeptide mediators and receptors which appear to be involved in pruritus.[1,2,15]

Histamine is well-known to lead to pruritus following intracutaneous injection at significant dose. The histamine-induced pruritus involves specific histamine receptors, which appear to be different between humans and mice.[16] In humans, the histamine H1 and H2 receptors seem to be more important in the pathogenesis of itch,[7,10] whereas the itch behaviour in mice rather implies histamine H1 and H4 receptors.[17] These receptors, and particularly the histamine H1 receptor, are expressed at the surface of pruriceptive neurons.[18] Strikingly, they are also expressed by human keratinocytes.[19,20] Thus, histamine released by mast cells, basophils and platelets after stimulation may activate keratinocytes in addition to sensory neurons. In fact, the histamine thereby released plays pleiotropic effects like oedema and erythema in addition to itch, thus supporting the idea that pruriceptors are not only directly activated. Indeed, in AD patients, antihistamines (H1-receptor blockers) do not always stop pruritus,[12,21] suggesting that mediators other than histamine are involved in itch. The participation of keratinocytes in the initiation of itch may explain why severe pruritic diseases respond poorly to the histamine H1 receptor antagonist.[22] Moreover, it may explain why patients with AD or lesional skin feel an intensive pruritus after repetitive noxious stimuli or scratching, whereas these stimuli usually decrease the itch intensity in healthy skin.[14]

Neuropeptides takes a great part in cutaneous physiology, in the regulation of skin functions and the transmission of pain.[16,23] They also take part in the regulation of pruritus. SP is released from pruriceptors in response to histamine stimulation. On the other hand, SP stimulates mast cells leading them to release histamine.[24] Thus, there is an amplifying loop, between mast cells and pruriceptors, which leads to an increase in the number of cells recruited. In fact, keratinocytes also produce and release histamine,[25] SP[26] and their corresponding

receptors.[19,27,28] Given their location, keratinocytes are the first cells impacted by these exchanges and they probably take part in this communication. Likewise, it was demonstrated that SP-stimulated keratinocytes produce SP, and this autocrine capability would be required to further convey and amplify the stimulation until the mast cells.[26] In addition, SP triggers the cutaneous release of pruritogens like nitric oxide which enhances the SP-induced itch-associated response.[29] Interestingly, neurokinin receptors, which are involved in the regulating loop of pruritus as described above, are over-expressed in the skin in case of AD, which are associated with tough pruritus.[30] This observation endorses the place of SP in pruritus.

CGRP was shown to inhibit pruritus rather than amplify it because it increases the SP-induce itch latency.[31] However, this mediator is overexpressed in skin with pruritic diseases suggesting a participation in the itch modulation. On the other hand, bradykinin is a mediator of pain when it binds bradykinin B2 receptors expressed on sensory neurons. Nevertheless, it can induce itch throughout the induction of histamine release from mast cells. Bradykinin also binds keratinocytes what enhances SP, CGRP and prostaglandin E2 release,[32] thereby provoking the sensitisation of cutaneous nerve endings, including pruriceptors.

Vasoactive intestinal peptide (VIP) is strongly expressed by Merkel cells while its expression is absent from other epidermal cell types.[33] This neuropeptide is involved in blood flow regulation, sweat production and exhibits anti-inflammatory properties.[34] However, some data challenge this idea: in several pathologic conditions, an enhanced release of VIP led to local inflammatory processes partly mediated via the release of histamine from cutaneous mast cells.[33] The participation of VIP in pruritus was also highlighted in a case of aquadynia, a water-related cutaneous pain associated to aquagenic pruritus. In this disease of low prevalence, immunohistochemical investigations had not revealed neuropeptide disorders excepted for VIP which was overexpressed by epidermal cells. This impressive finding is a convincing argument for the relationship between the skin and the brain and the involvement of epidermal cells in pruritus.

Inflammatory mediators such as TNFα, prostaglandins, leukotrienes and interleukins are still known to decrease the activation threshold of pruriceptors but the pathways implied are not clearly defined. In many cases, epidermal cells have to be considered. For example, injection of IL-2 induces pruritus by activation of histaminergic neurons but it also actives bradykinin-responsive neurons, thus implying the bradykinin pathway.[35] Keratinocytes only weakly express IL-2 receptors.[36] However it was demonstrated that IL-2 release was enhanced by SP stimulation at least in T cells.[37] Hence, since keratinocytes strongly express SP, factors affecting keratinocytes would be able to modulate pruritus induced by IL-2. Otherwise, IL-4 overexpressing mice spontaneously developed a pruritic inflammatory skin disease while an enhanced mRNA expression of IL-4 was found in AD lesional skin.[38] Furthermore, tacrolimus, a calcineurin inhibitor efficiently inhibits pruritus and decreases IL-4 mRNA level in the skin.[38,39] IL-6 was found in nerve fibers of patients with prurigo nodularis and is also overexpressed in keratinocytes of pruritic psoriasis.[40] IL-31, which is increased in patients with AD, induces a severe pruritus and dermatitis in mice models.[41] Arachidonic acid derivatives like prostaglandins E2,[42] leukotriene B4[43] and tromboxane A2[44] were shown to induce itch, mainly by lowering the activation threshold of pruriceptors. Indeed a major participation of these molecules is supported since their antagonists can inhibit SP-induced itch. This was partially explained by the increase in leukotrien B4 and prostaglandine E2 concentrations in keratinocytes after SP injections.[43]

Neurotrophins also take part in the multidirectional connection that generates cutaneous pruritus, in addition to playing a crucial role in cutaneous nerve development, survival and regeneration.[45] Nerve growth factor (NGF) is expressed by mast cells, keratinocytes, Merkel cells,[46] fibroblasts and nerves endings. In injured skin, NGF is over-expressed and acts as an inflammatory mediator thus initiating an acute sensitization of afferent C-fibers. Onto pruriceptive neurons, NGF is able to upregulate the expression of pruritogens such as SP and CGRP and the transient receptor potential vanilloid 1 (TRPV1), it induces mast cells degranulation and it was found to induce pruritus itself once administrated therapeutically.[10] Thereby NGF-releasing keratinocytes are able to stimulate pruriceptors. And this capability seems important since histamine enhances the production of NGF in human keratinocytes, through activation of the histamine H1 receptor.[47] Furthermore, the level of NGF was found to be increased in patient with AD,[48] prurigo nodularis[49] and in pruritic lesions of patients with psoriasis.[50]

Proteinase-activated receptors (PAR) are metabotropic G protein-coupled receptors expressed by afferent nerve fibers and also by keratinocytes. In patients with AD, the intracutaneous injection of PAR-2 agonist like tryptase or kallikreins led to a strong pruritus without increase in the concentration of histamine. This fact is interesting because it argues for a key role of these receptors in the pathophysiology of the pruritus through their own pathway. Indeed, it was demonstrated that keratinocytes upregulate PAR-2 during AD.[51] Thus it is more likely that protease activate keratinocytes, which then stimulate pruriceptors.

TRP channels are now considered as putative itch receptors because they transduce sensation, they are sensitive to temperature, and they are widely expressed by sensory neurons and epidermal cells; while pruritus is a thermosensitive sensation implying bidirectional brain-skin connections.[10,52] TRPV1 is the best known receptor of the TRP family. It is a non-specific cation channel which, once activated, leads to neurons depolarization and action potential firing along with neuropeptides and pruritogenic cytokines release.[53] Its interest in pruritus was investigated since it was observed to be dramatically overexpressed in the keratinocytes of prurigo nodularis patients.[54] Thereafter, histamine-responsive sensory neurons were also found to express TRPV1, which emphasise its capabilities to participate in itch, in addition to pain.[11] In these pruriceptors, the inhibition of TRPV1 by specific antagonists inhibits histamine-stimulation induced calcium influx.[55] Hence, TRPV1 act in the pruritus downstream of histamine receptors. TRPV1 can be activated by capsaicin extracted from chilli peppers, but numerous endogenous substances referred to as endovanilloids are able to activate or, at least, sensitize TRPV1. Thus exposition to endovanilloids may be able to provoke itch. Among these molecules, amandamide is an endocannabinoids with analgesic and antipruritic properties after the binding of the cannabinoid receptors (CB-R). This particularity is interesting because inhibition of pruritus after the CB-R stimulation goes with neuropeptides depletion as found after a strong activation of TRPV1.[56] Keratinocytes may take part in this phenomenon because they also expressed CB-R; and they react to their activation by the release of the analgesic β-endorphin and antipruritic neuropeptides such as proopiomelanocortin.[57] Thus keratinocytes are in close relationships with pain and pruritus and factor modulating one of these pathways can have an impact on the other one. All these new insights support the idea of a strong connexion between the pain-processing TRPV1 channel and pruritus, and also between TRPV1-expressing epidermal cells and pruriceptors.

Thus keratinocytes appear to take an essential participation in activation, or at less sensitization of pruriceptors. Even if histamine-producing cells like mast cells and T cells are important in the initiation of this process, epidermal cells clearly belong to the signalling pathway, which leads to pruritus, particularly, keratinocytes relaying pruriceptive signals until the pruriceptive fibers are capable of modulating the information. In some conditions, they might be able to transduce itch without histamine stimulation.

# References

1. Boulais N, Pereira U, Lebonvallet N, Misery L. The whole epidermis as the forefront of the sensory system. *Exp Dermatol*. 2007;16(8):634–635.
2. Denda M, Nakatani M, Ikeyama K, Tsutsumi M, Denda S. Epidermal keratinocytes as the forefront of the sensory system. *Exp Dermatol*. 2007;16(3):157–161.
3. Chateau Y, Misery L. Connections between nerve endings and epidermal cells: are they synapses? *Exp Dermatol*. 2004;13(1):2–4.
4. Paus R, Schmelz M, Biro T, Steinhoff M. Frontiers in pruritus research: scratching the brain for more effective itch therapy. *J Clin Invest*. 2006;116(5):1174–1186.
5. Schmelz M. A neural pathway for itch. *Nat Neurosci*. 2001;4(1):9–10.
6. Andrew D, Craig AD. Spinothalamic lamina I neurons selectively sensitive to histamine: a central neural pathway for itch. *Nat Neurosci*. 2001;4(1):72–77.
7. Schmelz M, Schmidt R, Bickel A, Handwerker HO, Torebjork HE. Specific C-receptors for itch in human skin. *J Neurosci*. 1997;17(20):8003–8008.
8. Koizumi S, Fujishita K, Inoue K, Shigemoto-Mogami Y, Tsuda M, Inoue K. Ca$^{2+}$ waves in keratinocytes are transmitted to sensory neurons: the involvement of extracellular ATP and P2Y2 receptor activation. *Biochem J*. 2004;380(Pt 2):329–338.
9. Steinhoff M, Bienenstock J, Schmelz M, Maurer M, Wei E, Biro T. Neurophysiological, neuroimmunological, and neuroendocrine basis of pruritus. *J Invest Dermatol*. 2006;126(8):1705–1718.
10. Biro T, Toth BI, Marincsak R, Dobrosi N, Geczy T, Paus R. TRP channels as novel players in the pathogenesis and therapy of itch. *Biochim Biophys Acta*. 2007;1772(8):1004–1021.
11. Ikoma A, Steinhoff M, Stander S, Yosipovitch G, Schmelz M. The neurobiology of itch. *Nat Rev Neurosci*. 2006;7(7):535–547.
12. Hosogi M, Schmelz M, Miyachi Y, Ikoma A. Bradykinin is a potent pruritogen in atopic dermatitis: a switch from pain to itch. *Pain*. 2006;126(1–3):16–23.
13. Paus R, Theoharides TC, Arck PC. Neuroimmunoendocrine circuitry of the 'brain-skin connection'. *Trends Immunol*. 2006;27(1):32–39.
14. Ishiuji Y, Coghill RC, Patel TS, et al. Repetitive scratching and noxious heat do not inhibit histamine-induced itch in atopic dermatitis. *Br J Dermatol*. 2008;158(1):78–83.
15. Inoue K, Koizumi S, Fuziwara S, Denda S, Inoue K, Denda M. Functional vanilloid receptors in cultured normal human epidermal keratinocytes. *Biochem Biophys Res Commun*. 2002;291(1):124–129.
16. Roosterman D, Goerge T, Schneider SW, Bunnett NW, Steinhoff M. Neuronal control of skin function: the skin as a neuroimmunoendocrine organ. *Physiol Rev*. 2006;86(4):1309–1379.
17. Bell JK, McQueen DS, Rees JL. Involvement of histamine H4 and H1 receptors in scratching induced by histamine receptor agonists in Balb C mice. *Br J Pharmacol*. 2004;142(2):374–380.
18. Kashiba H, Fukui H, Senba E. Histamine H1 receptor mRNA is expressed in capsaicin-insensitive sensory neurons with neuropeptide Y-immunoreactivity in guinea pigs. *Brain Res*. 2001;901(1–2):85–93.
19. Giustizieri ML, Albanesi C, Fluhr J, Gisondi P, Norgauer J, Girolomoni G. H1 histamine receptor mediates inflammatory responses in human keratinocytes. *J Allergy Clin Immunol*. 2004;114(5):1176–1182.
20. Ashida Y, Denda M, Hirao T. Histamine H1 and H2 receptor antagonists accelerate skin barrier repair and prevent epidermal hyperplasia induced by barrier disruption in a dry environment. *J Invest Dermatol*. 2001;116(2):261–265.
21. Rukwied R, Lischetzki G, McGlone F, Heyer G, Schmelz M. Mast cell mediators other than histamine induce pruritus in atopic dermatitis patients: a dermal microdialysis study. *Br J Dermatol*. 2000;142(6):1114–1120.
22. Andoh T. Importance of epidermal keratinocytes in itching. *Yakugaku Zasshi*. 2006;126(6):403–408.
23. Slominski A, Wortsman J. Neuroendocrinology of the skin. *Endocr Rev*. 2000;21(5):457–487.
24. Ebertz JM, Hirshman CA, Kettelkamp NS, Uno H, Hanifin JM. Substance P-induced histamine release in human cutaneous mast cells. *J Invest Dermatol*. 1987;88(6):682–685.
25. Fitzsimons C, Engel N, Duran H, et al. Histamine production in mouse epidermal keratinocytes is regulated during cellular differentiation. *Inflamm Res*. 2001;50(suppl 2):S100–S101.
26. Bae S, Matsunaga Y, Tanaka Y, Katayama I. Autocrine induction of substance P mRNA and peptide in cultured normal human keratinocytes. *Biochem Biophys Res Commun*. 1999;263(2):327–333.
27. Liu JY, Hu JH, Zhu QG, Li FQ, Sun HJ. Substance P receptor expression in human skin keratinocytes and fibroblasts. *Br J Dermatol*. 2006;155(4):657–662.
28. Staniek V, Doutremepuich J, Schmitt D, Claudy A, Misery L. Expression of substance P receptors in normal and psoriatic skin. *Pathobiology*. 1999;67(1):51–54.
29. Andoh T, Kuraishi Y. Nitric oxide enhances substance P-induced itch-associated responses in mice. *Br J Pharmacol*. 2003;138(1):202–208.
30. Staniek V, Liebich C, Vocks E, et al. Modulation of cutaneous SP receptors in atopic dermatitis after UVA irradiation. *Acta Derm Venereol*. 1998;78(2):92–94.
31. Ekblom A, Lundeberg T, Wahlgren CF. Influence of calcitonin gene-related peptide on histamine- and substance

P-induced itch, flare and weal in humans. *Skin Pharmacol.* 1993;6(3):215–222.

32. Averbeck B, Reeh PW. Interactions of inflammatory mediators stimulating release of calcitonin gene-related peptide, substance P and prostaglandin E2 from isolated rat skin. *Neuropharmacology.* 2001;40(3):416–423.

33. Hartschuh W, Reinecke M, Weihe E, Yanaihara N. VIP-immunoreactivity in the skin of various mammals: immuno-histochemical, radioimmunological and experimental evidence for a dual localization in cutaneous nerves and merkel cells. *Peptides.* 1984;5(2):239–245.

34. Gomariz RP, Juarranz Y, Abad C, Arranz A, Leceta J, Martinez C. VIP-PACAP system in immunity: new insights for multitarget therapy. *Ann N Y Acad Sci.* 2006;1070:51–74.

35. Martin HA. Bradykinin potentiates the chemoresponsiveness of rat cutaneous C-fibre polymodal nociceptors to interleukin-2. *Arch Physiol Biochem.* 1996;104(2):229–238.

36. Grone A. Keratinocytes and cytokines. *Vet Immunol Immunopathol.* 2002;88(1–2):1–12.

37. Calvo CF, Chavanel G, Senik A. Substance P enhances IL-2 expression in activated human T cells. *J Immunol.* 1992;148(11):3498–3504.

38. Inagaki N, Shiraishi N, Igeta K, et al. Inhibition of scratching behavior associated with allergic dermatitis in mice by tacrolimus, but not by dexamethasone. *Eur J Pharmacol.* 2006;546(1–3):189–196.

39. Stander S, Weisshaar E, Luger TA. Neurophysiological and neurochemical basis of modern pruritus treatment. *Exp Dermatol.* 2007.

40. Polat M, Lenk N, Yalcin B, et al. Efficacy of erythromycin for psoriasis vulgaris. *Clin Exp Dermatol.* 2007;32(3):295–297.

41. Takaoka A, Arai I, Sugimoto M, et al. Involvement of IL-31 on scratching behavior in NC/Nga mice with atopic-like dermatitis. *Exp Dermatol.* 2006;15(3):161–167.

42. Futaki N, Arai I, Sugimoto M, et al. Role of prostaglandins on mechanical scratching-induced cutaneous barrier disruption in mice. *Exp Dermatol.* 2007;16(6):507–512.

43. Andoh T, Katsube N, Maruyama M, Kuraishi Y. Involvement of leukotriene B(4) in substance P-induced itch-associated response in mice. *J Invest Dermatol.* 2001;117(6):1621–1626.

44. Andoh T, Nishikawa Y, Yamaguchi-Miyamoto T, Nojima H, Narumiya S, Kuraishi Y. Thromboxane A2 induces itch-associated responses through TP receptors in the skin in mice. *J Invest Dermatol.* 2007;127(8):2042–2047.

45. Botchkarev VA, Yaar M, Peters EM, et al. Neurotrophins in skin biology and pathology. *J Invest Dermatol.* 2006;126(8):1719–1727.

46. Vos P, Stark F, Pittman RN. Merkel cells in vitro: production of nerve growth factor and selective interactions with sensory neurons. *Dev Biol.* 1991;144(2):281–300.

47. Kanda N, Watanabe S. Histamine enhances the production of nerve growth factor in human keratinocytes. *J Invest Dermatol.* 2003;121(3):570–577.

48. Toyoda M, Nakamura M, Makino T, Hino T, Kagoura M, Morohashi M. Nerve growth factor and substance P are useful plasma markers of disease activity in atopic dermatitis. *Br J Dermatol.* 2002;147(1):71–79.

49. Johansson O, Liang Y, Emtestam L. Increased nerve growth factor- and tyrosine kinase A-like immunoreactivities in prurigo nodularis skin – an exploration of the cause of neurohyperplasia. *Arch Dermatol Res.* 2002;293(12):614–619.

50. Chang SE, Han SS, Jung HJ, Choi JH. Neuropeptides and their receptors in psoriatic skin in relation to pruritus. *Br J Dermatol.* 2007;156(6):1272–1277.

51. Buddenkotte J, Stroh C, Engels IH, et al. Agonists of proteinase-activated receptor-2 stimulate upregulation of intercellular cell adhesion molecule-1 in primary human keratinocytes via activation of NF-kappa B. *J Invest Dermatol.* 2005;124(1):38–45.

52. Boulais N, Misery L. The epidermis: a sensory tissue. *Eur J Dermatol.* 2008;18(2):119–127.

53. Southall MD, Li T, Gharibova LS, Pei Y, Nicol GD, Travers JB. Activation of epidermal vanilloid receptor-1 induces release of proinflammatory mediators in human keratinocytes. *J Pharmacol Exp Ther.* 2003;304(1):217–222.

54. Stander S, Moormann C, Schumacher M, et al. Expression of vanilloid receptor subtype 1 in cutaneous sensory nerve fibers, mast cells, and epithelial cells of appendage structures. *Exp Dermatol.* 2004;13(3):129–139.

55. Kim BM, Lee SH, Shim WS, Oh U. Histamine-induced Ca(2+) influx via the PLA(2)/lipoxygenase/TRPV1 pathway in rat sensory neurons. *Neurosci Lett.* 2004;361(1–3):159–162.

56. Dvorak M, Watkinson A, McGlone F, Rukwied R. Histamine induced responses are attenuated by a cannabinoid receptor agonist in human skin. *Inflamm Res.* 2003;52(6):238–245.

57. Ibrahim MM, Porreca F, Lai J, et al. CB2 cannabinoid receptor activation produces antinociception by stimulating peripheral release of endogenous opioids. *Proc Natl Acad Sci USA.* 2005;102(8):3093–3098.

# Chapter 4
# Central Transmission: From Skin to Brain

Tejesh Surendra Patel and Gil Yosipovitch

**Processing" and would read** – "The central processing of pruritus has been shown to activate brain areas implicated in sensory and motor function as well as emotion".

## 4.1 Introduction

Since 1660, itch has been defined as "an unpleasant sensation associated with the desire to scratch."[1] This definition encompasses both sensory and cognitive aspects of the itch experience. However, the manner in which this sensory stimulus transmits from the skin to the brain for processing has only recently been elucidated. This chapter will describe the flow of neural information that pertains to pruritus from the peripheral to the central nervous system.

## 4.2 Neural Theories of Itch

Several theories have been proposed for the neural encoding of itch:

### 4.2.1 Intensity Theory

According to this theory, weak noxious stimuli causes minor activation of nerve fibers which is felt as itch, whereas stronger noxious stimuli excite nerve fibers to a greater degree, evoking pain.[2] Against this theory, the application of low concentrations of algogens do not generally result in itch, just less intense pain.[3] Microneurography has also helped to challenge the validity of this theory by demonstrating that the stimulation of afferent nerve fibers induces either pain or itch. Importantly, decreasing the stimulation frequency reduces the intensity of pain or itch, but does not result in transition from one sensory modality to the other.[4,5] The above evidence means that the "intensity theory" of itch has largely been abandoned.

### 4.2.2 Gate-Control Theory

This theory is an extension of the "gate control theory" of pain. It postulates that the stimulation of large diameter nerve fibers by pain impairs pruritic C nerve fiber transmission by activating the inhibitory neurons of the spinal cord.[6] Numerous painful stimuli such as heat, cold, electrical and mechanical stimuli have been shown to inhibit itch.[7] Scratching, which in itself is painful and the behavioral response to itch also reduces itch. Against this theory lies the abundance of treatment modalities that inhibit pain but induce itch and vice versa. This is exemplified by the effects of μ-opiods that inhibit pain but aggravate itch.

### 4.2.3 Specificity Theory

This hypothesis suggests the existence of primary sensory neurons that respond to pruritic stimuli only. In support of an itch specific sensory pathway are the findings of pruriceptive primary afferent and spinothalamic projection neurons that are both histamine sensitive.[8,9] In addition, recent evidence suggests the existence of other specific primary afferents that mediate nonhistaminergic itch and may be more clinically relevant to pathological itch.[10]

L. Misery and S. Ständer (eds.), *Pruritus*,
DOI 10.1007/978-1-84882-322-8_4, © Springer-Verlag London Limited 2010

### 4.2.4 *Selectivity Theory*

It is argued that the histamine sensitive itch fibers are not "itch specific" but "itch selective" because they are also excited by pure allogens such as capsaicin.[11] This is supported by studies using noxious stimuli, including thermal, mechanical, and chemical (bradykinin) that induce itch rather than pain in patients with chronic pruritus.[12,13]

Current understanding favors the "specificity" or "selectivity" theories of itch.

## 4.3  Pruriceptive Innervation of the Skin

The skin is the most richly innervated organ of the human body and is served by a variety of sensory and motor nerve endings throughout all of its layers. Sensory innervation of the skin allows humans to sense thermal, touch, vibration, painful and pruritic stimuli. The majority of skin cell types express receptors for neuromediators and the skin itself is an important source of these molecules. Besides neurotrophic activity, neuromediators in the skin are involved in cutaneous homeostasis, trophism and stress responses.[14]

A distinctive feature of itch is that it is restricted to the skin, mucous membranes and cornea – no other tissue experiences pruritus.[15] Current evidence suggests the itch sensation emanates from activity in nerve fibers located in the epidermis. Although a specific receptor for itch has not yet been identified within this layer, the following evidence supports this notion:

- Removal of the epidermis abolishes perception of pruritus.[16]
- Inflammation in the reticular dermis and subcutaneous fat (such as that seen in panniculitis and cellulites) typically cause pain but not pruritus – it is assumed nerve fibers located in deeper layers of the reticular dermis and subcutaneous fat do not transmit pruritus.[17]
- Over expression in pruritic dermatoses of intraepidermal nerve fibers with "free" non-specialized nerve endings extending into the stratum granulosum. Many of these fibers stain positively for neuropeptides implicated in the mediation of itch (e.g., substance P, somatostatin, vasoactive intestinal polypeptide and neuropeptide Y) suggesting that pruritus is transmitted in the epidermis by these nerve fibers.[17]

## 4.4  Specific Histamine Sensitive Pruriceptive C Nerve Fibers

Histamine-sensitive afferent nerve fibers that convey histamine-induced itch have been identified.[9] These histamine-sensitive C nerve fibers are characterized by low conduction velocities, large innervation territories, mechanical unresponsiveness, high transcutaneous electrical thresholds and generation of an axon reflex erythema. Importantly, the response pattern of these fibers to histamine matched the time course of itch sensation reported by human subjects.[9] Furthermore, these nerve fibers have shown spontaneous activity in a recent microneurographic study of a patient with chronic pruritus.[18] Histamine-sensitive nerve fibers represent no more than 5% of all nociceptors in the skin.[3] Of note: the vast majority of C fibres are sensitive to mechanical and heat stimuli and are entirely insensitive to histamine.[19]

## 4.5  Histamine Independent Pruriceptive C Nerve Fibers

Histamine-sensitive nerve fibers cannot account for all aspects of the peripheral transmission of itch. There is growing evidence for the existence of histamine-independent pruriceptive C nerve fibers. Anti-histamines do not relieve chronic itch in many pruritic dermatoses suggesting histamine is not the main mediator.[20,21] Furthermore, itch can be produced by mechanical, punctuate heat and electrical stimuli as well as spicules of cowhage, all of which are unlikely to activate the histamine-sensitive C nerve fiber.[2,10,16,22] In addition, electrical stimuli and spicules of cowhage can induce itch in the absence of a flare reaction (axon-reflex erythema) implying that the underlying nerve fibers may be particularly relevant to chronic itch conditions (that are typically without flare reactions).[10,22] Importantly, a recent study has shown cowhage itch is signaled through a population of capsaicin-sensitive afferent nerve fibers that is distinct from the histamine-sensitive C fibers mediating histamine-induced itch.[10]

## 4.6 Pruriceptive Spinothalamic Neuron Projections

In the spinal cord, primary afferent C neurons synapse with the second order neurons in the gray matter of the dorsal horn. These neurons then cross over and ascend in the lateral spinothalamic tract to the thalamus. A subclass of lamina I spinothalamic tract neurons specifically and selectively excited by iontophoretically administered histamine have been identified in the cat using microneurography.[8] These neurons are similar to the histamine-sensitive C nerve fibers in that they are mechanically insensitive and respond to histamine with a typical prolonged activation. Interestingly, a recent study has shown that the gastrin-releasing peptide receptor (GRPR) plays an important part in mediating itch (but not pain) sensation in the dorsal spinal cord.[23] All the above evidence extends the concept of a dedicated neural pathway existing for itch not only in the peripheral but also in the central nervous system.

## 4.7 Higher Central Nervous System Structures Involved with Itch Processing

The pruritus selective spinothalamic neurons project from lamina I of the spinal cord to the ventrocaudal part of the nucleus medialis dorsalis of the thalamus, which in turn projects to higher CNS structures.[7] This higher central processing of itch has been demonstrated using the neuroimaging techniques of positron emission tomography (PET) and functional magnetic resonance imaging (fMRI) in healthy humans. In these studies, histamine-induced itch coactivates the anterior cingulate and insular cortex, premotor and supplementary motor areas, cerebellum, primary somatosensory cortex and thalamus.[24–28] The central processing of pruritus has been shown to activate brain areas implicated in sensory and motor function as well as emotion. Thus, the multiple brain areas involved with the central processing of pruritus are believed to be reflective of the multidimensional aspects of this distressing symptom. Brain areas activated by pruritus are also involved with the central processing of pain, implying that the neural networks activated by these two sensory stimuli are not distinct but reflect a different activation pattern.[29]

## 4.8 Conclusion

Our understanding of how the sensation of itch transmits from the skin to the brain has increased tremendously over the past decade. Future studies that further delineate the neural pathway of itch will ultimately facilitate the development of novel therapies for this most distressing symptom.

## References

1. Haffenreffer S., De pruritu, Nosodochium in Quo Cutis, Eique Adhaerentium Partium, Affectus Omnes, Singulari Methodo, Et Cognoscendi Et Curandi Fidelissime Traduntur, Kuhnen Balthasar, Ulm (1660) p. 98–102.
2. von Frey M. Zur Physiologie der Juckempfindung. *Arch Neerland Physiol.* 1922;7:142–145.
3. Schmelz M, Handwerker H. Neurophysiologic basis of itch. In: Yosipovitch G, Greaves MW, Fleischer AB Jr, McGlone F, eds. *Itch. Basic Mechanisms and Therapy.* New York: Marcel Dekker, Inc; 2004:5–12.
4. Torebjork HOJ. Pain and itch from C fiber stimulation. *Neurosci Abstr.* 1981;7:28.
5. Tuckett RP. Itch evoked by electrical stimulation of the skin. *J Invest Dermatol.* 1982;79(6):368–373.
6. Biro T, Ko MC, Bromm B, et al. How best to fight that nasty itch – from new insights into the neuroimmunological, neuroendocrine, and neurophysiological bases of pruritus to novel therapeutic approaches. *Exp Dermatol.* 2005;14(3):225–240.
7. Biro T, Toth BI, Marincsak R, Dobrosi N, Geczy T, Paus R. TRP channels as novel players in the pathogenesis and therapy of itch. *Biochim Biophys Acta.* 2007 Aug;1772(8):1004–1021.
8. Andrew D, Craig AD. Spinothalamic lamina I neurons selectively sensitive to histamine: a central neural pathway for itch. *Nat Neurosci.* 2001;4(1):72–77.
9. Schmelz M, Schmidt R, Bickel A, Handwerker HO, Torebjork HE. Specific C-receptors for itch in human skin. *J Neurosci.* 1997;17(20):8003–8008.
10. Johanek LM, Meyer RA, Hartke T, et al. Psychophysical and physiological evidence for parallel afferent pathways mediating the sensation of itch. *J Neurosci.* 2007;27(28):7490–7497.
11. Ikoma A, Steinhoff M, Stander S, Yosipovitch G, Schmelz M. The neurobiology of itch. *Nat Rev Neurosci.* 2006;7(7):535–547.
12. Hosogi M, Schmelz M, Miyachi Y, Ikoma A. Bradykinin is a potent pruritogen in atopic dermatitis: a switch from pain to itch. *Pain.* 2006;126(1–3):16–23.
13. Ikoma A, Fartasch M, Heyer G, Miyachi Y, Handwerker H, Schmelz M. Painful stimuli evoke itch in patients with chronic pruritus: central sensitization for itch. *Neurology.* 2004;62(2):212–217.
14. Pincelli C, Bonte F. The "beauty" of skin neurobiology. *J Cosmet Dermatol.* 2003;2(3–4):195–198.

15. Charlesworth EN, Beltrani VS. Pruritic dermatoses: overview of etiology and therapy. *Am J Med*. 2002; 113(suppl 9A):25S–33S.

16. Shelley WB, Arthur RP. The neurohistology and neurophysiology of the itch sensation in man. *AMA Arch Derm*. 1957;76(3):296–323.

17. Yosipovitch G. The pruritus receptor unit: a target for novel therapies. *J Invest Dermatol*. 2007;127(8):1857–1859.

18. Schmelz M, Hilliges M, Schmidt R, et al. Active "itch fibers" in chronic pruritus. *Neurology*. 2003;61(4):564–566.

19. Schmelz M, Schmidt R, Weidner C, Hilliges M, Torebjork HE, Handwerker HO. Chemical response pattern of different classes of C-nociceptors to pruritogens and algogens. *J Neurophysiol*. 2003;89(5):2441–2448.

20. Dawn A, Yosipovitch G. Treating itch in psoriasis. *Dermatol Nurs*. 2006;18(3):227–233.

21. Klein PA, Clark RA. An evidence-based review of the efficacy of antihistamines in relieving pruritus in atopic dermatitis. *Arch Dermatol*. 1999;135(12):1522–1525.

22. Ikoma A, Handwerker H, Miyachi Y, Schmelz M. Electrically evoked itch in humans. *Pain*. 2005;113(1–2):148–154.

23. Sun YG, Chen ZF. A gastrin-releasing peptide receptor mediates the itch sensation in the spinal cord. *Nature*. 2007; 448(7154):700–703.

24. Darsow U, Drzezga A, Frisch M, et al. Processing of histamine-induced itch in the human cerebral cortex: a correlation analysis with dermal reactions. *J Invest Dermatol*. 2000; 115(6):1029–1033.

25. Drzezga A, Darsow U, Treede RD, et al. Central activation by histamine-induced itch: analogies to pain processing: a correlational analysis of O-15 $H_2O$ positron emission tomography studies. *Pain*. 2001;92(1–2):295–305.

26. Hsieh JC, Hagermark O, Stahle-Backdahl M, et al. Urge to scratch represented in the human cerebral cortex during itch. *J Neurophysiol*. 1994;72(6):3004–3008.

27. Leknes SG, Bantick S, Willis CM, Wilkinson JD, Wise RG, Tracey I. Itch and motivation to scratch: an investigation of the central and peripheral correlates of allergen- and histamine-induced itch in humans. *J Neurophysiol*. 2007; 97(1):415–422.

28. Mochizuki H, Tashiro M, Kano M, Sakurada Y, Itoh M, Yanai K. Imaging of central itch modulation in the human brain using positron emission tomography. *Pain*. 2003; 105(1–2):339–346.

29. Paus R, Schmelz M, Biro T, Steinhoff M. Frontiers in pruritus research: scratching the brain for more effective itch therapy. *J Clin Invest*. 2006;116(5):1174–1186.

# Chapter 5
# Modulation of Pruritus: Peripheral and Central Sensitisation

Martin Schmelz

## 5.1 Introduction

Sensitization of nociceptors has been identified as the crucial mechanism in chronic pain conditions. The sensitization processes can be mediated in peripheral tissues not only by inflammatory mediators but also by directly amplifying the processing of noxious information in the central nervous system. In pruritus, research was mainly focused on peripheral mediators of itch that would activate pruriceptive neurons and would represent the ideal target for therapeutic intervention. However, modulation of pain and itch processing by sensitization in the periphery and the central nervous system shared many unexpected similarities and therefore the broad knowledge of sensitization mechanisms in pain might be used also in itch research and possibly in antipruritic therapeutic approaches.

## 5.2 Peripheral Sensitization

Numerous endogenous inflammatory mediators that can activate and sensitize nociceptive nerve endings have been identified.[1] It is interesting to note that it has been demonstrated that many of the classic inflammatory mediators like bradykinin, serotonin, histamine and prostaglandins, which are released in a wide range during inflammation, not only acutely sensitize nociceptors,[2] but also activate pruriceptors.

The complex effects of inflammatory mediators are even more complicated by their interactions: supra-additive effects are known for various combinations such as between prostaglandin E2 and histamine.[3] Moreover, sensitization of the Capsaicin receptor TRPV1 by various mediators – among them proteinase-activated receptor 2 (PAR-2)[4] – provide evidence for possible underlying mechanisms of cross-sensitization.

However, even though acute effects of combinations of mediators can explain sensitization of primary afferent nerve fibers, it remains problematic to correlate these acute effects to the long-lasting hypersensitivity observed in the patients, as adaptation and tachyphylaxis processes are operational in the primary afferent nerve endings and desensitize them.[5]

Thus, in addition to acute sensitization, long lasting structural changes are required to mediate clinical states of hypersensitivity. Neurotrophins not only induce acute sensitization,[6] but also cause lasting structural changes (sprouting) of nociceptors. The expression of nerve growth factor (NGF) is high in injured and inflamed tissues and activation of the NGF receptor, tyrosine kinase trkA, on nociceptive neurons triggers and potentiates pain-signaling by multiple mechanisms.[7]

Sprouting of epidermal nerve fibers initiated by increased NGF is not only found in combination of localized pain and hyperalgesia like vulvar dysesthesia,[8] but also in atopic dermatitis.[9] In addition, remarkably increased serum levels of NGF and substance P have been found to correlate with the severity of the disease in atopic dermatitis.[10] The sources of NGF were mainly keratinocytes and mast cells.[11] Increased fiber density and higher local NGF concentrations were also found in patients with pruritic contact dermatitis,[12] while increased NGF and trkA immunoreactivity was found in prurigo nodularis[13] and also in patients with pruritic lesions of psoriasis.[14] These similarities between localized painful and pruritic lesions might suggest that similar mechanisms of neuronal sprouting and sensitization exist both for pain and pruritus on a peripheral level. Anti-NGF strategies have already been used in animal pain models,[15] and also in patients with pain.[16]

L. Misery and S. Ständer (eds.), *Pruritus*,
DOI 10.1007/978-1-84882-322-8_5, © Springer-Verlag London Limited 2010

Therapeutic anti-NGF approaches against pruritus have been performed in animal models of atopic dermatitis only.[17] In this model (NC/Nga mice) increased epidermal NGF expression has been shown.[18,19]

NGF is known to up regulate neuropeptides, especially substance P (SP) and calcitonin gene related peptide (CGRP).[20] For SP an important role in the induction of pain and hyperalgesia has been found in rodents,[21] although there has not been much evidence for the clinical analgesic efficacy of NK1 antagonists.[22] There is no confirmation for SP as an acute pruritogen in humans,[23] but it might contribute to itch by neuronal sensitization and by its long-term interaction with mast cells.[24] A sensitizing effect on nociceptors has also been found for CGRP in rodents,[25,26] but its role in pruritus is unclear.[27] Interestingly, increased SP levels coexist with reduced CGRP levels in the NC/Nga mice, an atopic dermatitis mouse model.[28] Given that heat and pain sensitivity correlates to CGRP levels,[26] and pain sensitivity negatively correlates to sensitivity in itch models,[29] one might speculate about a preferred role of CGRP for nociception and SP for itch.

As of today most data on the role of neurotrophins in itch relate to NGF. However, brain derived neurotrophic factor (BDNF), Neurotrophin 3 and 4, and glia cell derived neurotrophic factor are also important modulators of intraepidermal nerve fibers and may be involved in chronic itch conditions.[30,31]

## 5.3 Central Sensitization

Noxious neuronal input to the spinal cord is known to sensitize pain processing in the spinal cord and is termed as "central sensitization."[32] This consists of hypersensitivity to touch ("allodynia") and punctates mechanical stimuli ("punctate hyperalgesia"). Two types of mechanical hyperalgesia can be differentiated. Non-noxious touch stimuli in the uninjured surroundings of a trauma can be felt as painful "touch or brush-evoked hyperalgesia," or allodynia. Though this sensation is mediated by myelinated mechanoreceptor units, it requires ongoing activity of the primary afferent C-nociceptors.[33] The second type of mechanical hyperalgesia results in slightly painful pinprick stimulation being perceived as being more painful in the secondary zone around a focus of inflammation. This type has been termed "punctate hyperalgesia." The latter does not require ongoing activity

of primary nociceptors for its maintenance. It can persist for hours following a trauma, usually much longer than touch or brush-evoked hyperalgesia.[34]

A strikingly similar pattern of central sensitization is observed in the itch pathway: touch or brush-evoked pruritus around an itching site and has been termed "itchy skin."[35,36] Like allodynia, it requires ongoing activity in primary afferents and is most probably elicited by low threshold mechanoreceptors (A-β fibers).[36,37] Also more intense prick-induced itch sensation in the surroundings, "hyperknesis," has been reported following histamine iontophoresis in healthy volunteers.[38]

The existence of central sensitization for itch can greatly improve our understanding of clinical itch. Under the conditions of central sensitization, normally painful stimuli are perceived as itching. This phenomenon has already been described in patients suffering from atopic dermatitis, who perceive normally painful electrical stimuli as itching when applied inside their lesional skin.[39] Furthermore, acetylcholine and bradykinin provoke itch instead of pain in patients with atopic dermatitis[40,41] indicating that pain-induced inhibition of itch might be compromised in these patients.

The exact mechanisms and roles of the central sensitization for itch in specific clinical conditions still need to be explored, whereas a major role of central sensitization in patients with chronic pain is generally accepted. It should be noted that, in addition to the parallels between experimentally induced secondary sensitization phenomena, there is also emerging evidence for corresponding phenomena in patients with chronic pain and chronic itch. It has recently been reported that in patients with neuropathic pain histamine-iontophoresis resulted in burning pain instead of pure itch, which would be induced by this procedure in healthy volunteers.[42,43] This phenomenon is of special interest as it demonstrates spinal hypersensitivity to C-fiber input in chronic pain. Conversely, normally painful electrical, chemical, mechanical and thermal stimulation is perceived as itching when applied in or close to lesional skin of atopic dermatitis patients[41,44] suggesting that there is also spinal hypersensitivity to C-fiber input in chronic itch. Histamine prick tests in non-lesional skin of atopic dermatitis patients provoked less intense itching as compared to healthy controls. However, when applied inside their lesions, itch ratings were enhanced and lasted very long, whereas the axon reflex erythema was even smaller when compared to the controls.[37] Thus, in addition to

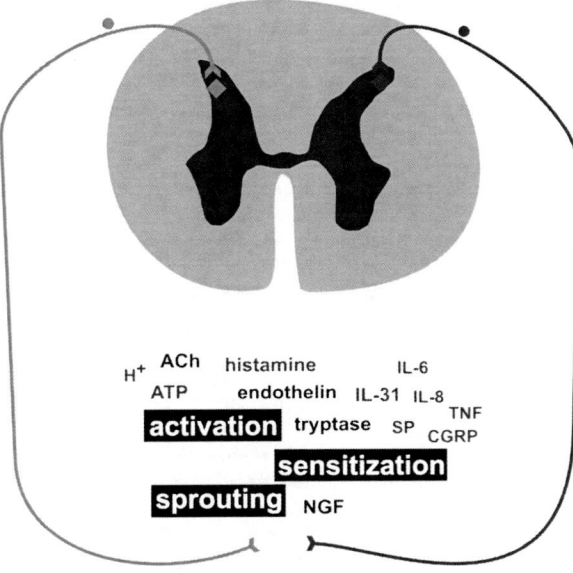

touch evoked allodynia   touch evoked alloknesis
punctate hyperalgesia   punctate hyperknesis
"itch allodynia"   "pain allokknesis"

H⁺ ACh   histamine       IL-6
ATP       endothelin   IL-31   IL-8
                                         TNF
**activation**   tryptase   SP   CGRP
           **sensitization**
**sprouting**   NGF

**Fig. 5.1** Peripheral and central mechanisms of sensitization of pain and itch processing are shown. In the periphery, inflammatory mediators can activate and sensitization nociceptive and pruriceptive nerve endings. In addition to acute sensitization, trophic factors, such as nerve growth factor (NGF) induce long term sensitivity changes along with structural alterations (sprouting). In the spinal cord itch and pain processing can be sensitized such that touch stimuli evoke itch (alloknesis) or pain (touch allodynia), that punctate mechanical stimuli evoke more intense pricking pain (punctate hyperalgesia) or itch (punctate hyperknesis). Moreover, normally painful stimuli can be misinterpreted as itch in chronic itch patients ("pain allokknesis") or normally itching stimuli can be misinterpreted as pain in chronic pain patients ("itch allodynia")

peripheral sensitization, there is evidence for a central sensitization of itch in chronic pruritus (Fig. 5.1).

## 5.4 Neuropathic Itch vs. Neuropathic Pain

The similar patterns of central sensitization in itch and pain have led to antiprurite therapeutic approaches using drugs usually applied in neuropathic pain. Thus far, there have been no controlled studies; however, anecdotal reports show success with carbamazepine, gabapentin and the recently developed pregabalin.[45] Gabapentin and pregabalin inhibit the alpha[2] delta sub-unit of voltage-dependent $Ca(^{2+})$ channels.[46] Gabapentin has also been proven to be effective for the treatment of neuropathic pruritus, particularly in the case of brachioradial pruritus and multiple sclerosis-related itch.[47,48] Gabapentin seems to alter the sensation of itch as well as the pruritus related to nerve damage in cutaneous and systemic diseases.[49]

The combination of neuropathic itch and neuropathic pain is present in some neuropathies, but only rarely has been investigated with a focus on the relationship between the two: the intimate link between neuropathic pain and neuropathic itch has been shown in postherpetic itch,[50] but data on the therapeutic implications are still rare. It will be of major interest to more closely study neuropathic diseases such as postherpetic neuralgia, meralgia paresthetica, and brachioradial pruritus in respect to the occurrence of central and peripheral sensitization in the pain and in the itch pathway, combining efforts of dermatologists, neurologists and anesthesiologists.

## References

1. Reeh PW, Kress M. Effects of classical algogens. *Semin Neurosci.* 1995;7:221–226.
2. Kidd BL, Urban LA. Mechanisms of inflammatory pain. *Br J Anaesth.* 2001;87(1):3–11.
3. Nicolson TA, Foster AF, Bevan S, Richards CD. Prostaglandin E(2) sensitizes primary sensory neurons to histamine. *Neuroscience.* 2007;150(1):22–30.
4. Amadesi S, Cottrell GS, Divino L, et al. Protease-activated receptor 2 sensitizes TRPV1 by protein kinase Cepsilon-and A-dependent mechanisms in rats and mice. *J Physiol.* 2006;575(pt 2):555–571.
5. Liang YF, Haake B, Reeh PW. Sustained sensitization and recruitment of rat cutaneous nociceptors by bradykinin and a novel theory of its excitatory action. *J Physiol.* 2001;532 (pt 1):229–239.
6. Zhang X, Huang J, McNaughton PA. NGF rapidly increases membrane expression of TRPV1 heat-gated ion channels. *EMBO J.* 2005;24(24):4211–4223.
7. Hefti FF, Rosenthal A, Walicke PA, et al. Novel class of pain drugs based on antagonism of NGF. *Trends Pharmacol Sci.* 2006;27(pt 2):85–91.
8. Bohm-Starke N, Hilliges M, Falconer C, Rylander E. Increased intraepithelial innervation in women with vulvar vestibulitis syndrome. *Gynecol Obstet Invest.* 1998;46(4): 256–260.
9. Urashima R, Mihara M. Cutaneous nerves in atopic dermatitis – a histological, immunohistochemical and electron microscopic study. *Virchows Arch Int J Pathol.* 1998;432(4): 363–370.

10. Toyoda M, Nakamura M, Makino T, Hino T, Kagoura M, Morohashi M. Nerve growth factor and substance P are useful plasma markers of disease activity in atopic dermatitis. *Br J Dermatol*. 2002;147(1):71–79.

11. Groneberg DA, Serowka F, Peckenschneider N, et al. Gene expression and regulation of nerve growth factor in atopic dermatitis mast cells and the human mast cell line-1. *J Neuroimmunol*. 2005;161(1–2):87–92.

12. Kinkelin I, Motzing S, Koltenzenburg M, Brocker EB. Increase in NGF content and nerve fiber sprouting in human allergic contact eczema. *Cell Tissue Res*. 2000;302(1): 31–37.

13. Johansson O, Liang Y, Emtestam L. Increased nerve growth factor- and tyrosine kinase A-like immunoreactivities in prurigo nodularis skin – an exploration of the cause of neurohyperplasia. *Arch Dermatol Res*. 2002;293(12):614–619.

14. Choi JC, Yang JH, Chang SE, Choi JH. Pruritus and nerve growth factor in psoriasis. *Korean J Dermatol*. 2005;43(6): 769–773.

15. Halvorson KG, Kubota K, Sevcik MA, et al. A blocking antibody to nerve growth factor attenuates skeletal pain induced by prostate tumor cells growing in bone. *Cancer Res*. 2005;65(20):9426–9435.

16. Lane N, Webster L, Lu SP, Gray M, Hefti F, Walicke P. Proceedings American College of Rheumatology, San Diego (Abstract).

17. Takano N, Sakurai T, Kurachi M. Effects of anti-nerve growth factor antibody on symptoms in the NC/Nga mouse, an atopic dermatitis model. *J Pharmacol Sci*. 2005;99(3): 277–286.

18. Tanaka A, Matsuda H. Expression of nerve growth factor in itchy skins of atopic NC/NgaTnd mice. *J Vet Med Sci*. 2005;67(9):915–919.

19. Tominaga M, Ozawa S, Ogawa H, Takamori K. A hypothetical mechanism of intraepidermal neurite formation in NC/Nga mice with atopic dermatitis. *J Dermatol Sci*. 2007;46(3):199–210.

20. Verge VM, Richardson PM, Wiesenfeld-Hallin Z, Hokfelt T. Differential influence of nerve growth factor on neuropeptide expression in vivo: a novel role in peptide suppression in adult sensory neurons. *J Neurosci*. 1995;15(3 pt 1):2081–2096.

21. Laird JM, Roza C, De Felipe C, Hunt SP, Cervero F. Role of central and peripheral tachykinin NK1 receptors in capsaicin-induced pain and hyperalgesia in mice. *Pain*. 2001; 90(1–2):97–103.

22. Hill R. NK1 (substance P) receptor antagonists - why are they not analgesic in humans? *Trends Pharmacol Sci*. 2000;21(7):244–246.

23. Weidner C, Klede M, Rukwied R, et al. Acute effects of substance P and calcitonin gene-related peptide in human skin – a microdialysis study. *J Invest Dermatol*. 2000;115(6): 1015–1020.

24. Yosipovitch G, Greaves M, Schmelz M. Itch. *Lancet*. 2003;361:690–694.

25. Sun RQ, Tu YJ, Lawand NB, Yan JY, Lin Q, Willis WD. Calcitonin gene-related peptide receptor activation produces PKA- and PKC-dependent mechanical hyperalgesia and central sensitization. *J Neurophysiol*. 2004;92(5):2859–2866.

26. Mogil JS, Miermeister F, Seifert F, et al. Variable sensitivity to noxious heat is mediated by differential expression of the CGRP gene. *Proc Natl Acad Sci USA*. 2005;102(36): 12938–12943.

27. Ekblom A, Lundeberg T, Wahlgren CF. Influence of calcitonin gene-related peptide on histamine- and substance P-induced itch, flare and weal in humans. *Skin Pharmacol*. 1993;6(3):215–222.

28. Katsuno M, Aihara M, Kojima M, et al. Neuropeptides concentrations in the skin of a murine (NC/Nga mice) model of atopic dermatitis. *J Dermatol Sci*. 2003;33(1):55–65.

29. Green AD, Young KK, Lehto SG, Smith SB, Mogil JS. Influence of genotype, dose and sex on pruritogen-induced scratching behaviour in the mouse. *Pain*. 2006;124:50–58.

30. Grewe M, Vogelsang K, Ruzicka T, Stege H, Krutmann J. Neurotrophin-4 production by human epidermal keratinocytes: increased expression in atopic dermatitis. *J Invest Dermatol*. 2000;114(6):1108–1112.

31. Hon KL, Lam MC, Wong KY, Leung TF, Ng PC. Pathophysiology of nocturnal scratching in childhood atopic dermatitis: the role of brain-derived neurotrophic factor and substance P. *Br J Dermatol*. 2007;157(5):922–925.

32. Koltzenburg M. Neural mechanisms of cutaneous nociceptive pain. *Clin J Pain*. 2000;16(3 suppl):S131–S138.

33. Torebjörk HE, Schmelz M, Handwerker HO. Functional properties of human cutaneous nociceptors and their role in "Neurobiology of Nociceptors" Cervero F, Belmonte C, Oxford University Press, Oxford 1996:349–369.

34. LaMotte RH, Shain CN, Simone DA, Tsai EFP. Neurogenic hyperalgesia psychophysical studies of underlying mechanisms. *J Neurophysiol*. 1991;66:190–211.

35. Bickford RGL. Experiments relating to itch sensation, its peripheral mechanism and central pathways. *Clin Sci*. 1938;3:377–386.

36. Simone DA, Alreja M, LaMotte RH. Psychophysical studies of the itch sensation and itchy skin ("alloknesis") produced by intracutaneous injection of histamine. *Somatosens Mot Res*. 1991;8(3):271–279.

37. Heyer G, Ulmer FJ, Schmitz J, Handwerker HO. Histamine-induced itch and alloknesis (itchy skin) in atopic eczema patients and controls. *Acta Derm Venereol (Stockh )*. 1995;75(5):348–352.

38. Atanassoff PG, Brull SJ, Zhang J, Greenquist K, Silverman DG, LaMotte RH. Enhancement of experimental pruritus and mechanically evoked dysesthesiae with local anesthesia. *Somatosens Mot Res*. 1999;16(4):291–298.

39. Nilsson HJ, Schouenborg J. Differential inhibitory effect on human nociceptive skin senses induced by local stimulation of thin cutaneous fibers. *Pain*. 1999;80(1–2):103–112.

40. Vogelsang M, Heyer G, Hornstein OP. Acetylcholine induces different cutaneous sensations in atopic and non-atopic subjects. *Acta Derm Venereol*. 1995;75(6):434–436.

41. Hosogi M, Schmelz M, Miyachi Y, Ikoma A. Bradykinin is a potent pruritogen in atopic dermatitis: a switch from pain to itch. *Pain*. 2006;126(1–3):16–23.

42. Birklein F, Claus D, Riedl B, Neundorfer B, Handwerker HO. Effects of cutaneous histamine application in patients with sympathetic reflex dystrophy. *Muscle Nerve*. 1997;20(11): 1389–1395.

43. Baron R, Schwarz K, Kleinert A, Schattschneider J, Wasner G. Histamine-induced itch converts into pain in neuropathic hyperalgesia. *Neuroreport*. 2001;12(16):3475–3478.

44. Ikoma A, Fartasch M, Heyer G, Miyachi Y, Handwerker H, Schmelz M. Painful stimuli evoke itch in patients with chronic pruritus: central sensitization for itch. *Neurology*. 2004;62(2):212–217.

45. Summey BT, Jr., Yosipovitch G. Pharmacologic advances in the systemic treatment of itch. *Dermatol Ther*. 2005;18(4): 328–332.

46. Rogawski MA, Loscher W. The neurobiology of antiepileptic drugs for the treatment of nonepileptic conditions. *Nat Med*. 2004;10(7):685–692.

47. Bueller HA, Bernhard JD, Dubroff LM. Gabapentin treatment for brachioradial pruritus. *J Eur Acad Dermatol Venereol*. 1999;13(3):227–228.

48. Winhoven SM, Coulson IH, Bottomley WW. Brachioradial pruritus: response to treatment with gabapentin. *Br J Dermatol*. 2004;150(4):786–787.

49. Yesudian PD, Wilson NJ. Efficacy of gabapentin in the management of pruritus of unknown origin. *Arch Dermatol*. 2005;141(12):1507–1509.

50. Oaklander AL, Bowsher D, Galer B, Haanpää M, Jensen MP. Herpes zoster itch: Preliminary epidemiologic data. *J Pain*. 2003;4(6):338–343.

# Chapter 6
# Interaction of Pruritus and Pain

Martin Schmelz

## 6.1 Introduction

Pruritus and pain are clearly distinct sensations linked to a characteristic reflex pattern: a withdrawal of pain and scratching for itch. Physiologically, a well known antagonism between pain and itch is used commonly to reduce itch by scratching. Interestingly, the mirror image of this interaction is also of clinical importance: reduction of pain can provoke itch as can be induced by spinal opioids.

Acute behavioural responses to pain and pruritus are fairly well conceived and protect the integrity of the body; however, in the pathophysiological state, chronic pain and itch lead to suffering of the patients without any obvious benefit, and the mechanisms underlying chronic itch and pain are poorly understood.

## 6.2 Itch Modulation by Painful and Non-Painful Stimuli

It is common experience that the itch sensation can be reduced by the painful sensations caused by scratching. The inhibition of itch by painful stimuli has been experimentally demonstrated by the use of various painful thermal, mechanical, and chemical stimuli.[1] Painful electrical stimulation reduced histamine-induced itch for hours in an area exceeding the stimulated site by 10 cm, suggesting a central mode of action.[2] Recent results suggest that noxious heat stimuli and scratching produce a stronger itch inhibition than noxious cold stimuli.[3] Consistent with these results, itch is suppressed inside the secondary zone of capsaicin-induced mechanical hyperalgesia.[4] This central effect of nociceptor excitation by capsaicin should be

clearly distinguished from the neurotoxic effect of higher concentrations of capsaicin which destroy most C-fiber terminals, including fibers that mediate itch.[5] The latter mechanism, therefore, also abolishes pruritus locally, until the nerve terminals have regenerated.

Itch can be reduced by painful stimuli, but vice versa analgesia may reduce this inhibition and thus enhance itch.[6] This phenomenon is particularly relevant to spinally administered μ-opioid receptor agonists, which induce segmental analgesia often combined with segmental pruritus.[7] Given that μ-opioids can induce itch, it is not surprising that μ-opioid antagonists have antipruritic effects in experimental itch[8] and also in patients with cholestatic itch. It is remarkable, that in some of the cholestatic patients the reduction of itch by naloxone is accompanied by the induction of pain[9] and withdrawal-like reactions,[10] suggesting an upregulation of endogenous opioids in these patients. Conversely, in animal experiments *kappa*-opioid antagonists enhanced itch.[11] In line with these results, κ- opioid agonists have been shown to reduce experimental cholestatic itch,[12] and also μ-opioid induced pruritus in man[13] and primates.[14] This new therapeutic concept has already been tested successfully in chronic itch patients.[15]

## 6.3 Opioid Receptors in the Epidermis

While effects of opioids in the spinal cord and central nervous system have been investigated for decades, local production of opioids in the skin is a recent finding.

After detection of *peripheral* opioid receptors in the skin, research tended to focus on peripheral analgesic effects[16] whereas investigations on opioid effects other than analgesia remained sparse.[17] However, finally discovery of endogenous opioid production in the skin,

L. Misery and S. Ständer (eds.), *Pruritus*,
DOI 10.1007/978-1-84882-322-8_6, © Springer-Verlag London Limited 2010

such as β-endorphin, promoted studies on different functions, e.g. control of hair growth and pigmentation[18], including wound healing and differentiation.[19] We are just beginning to understand which stimuli such as cannabinoid receptor (CB2) activation induce epidermal opioid release [20] and how they may contribute to control growth and differentiation, and also inflammation and modulation of neuronal excitability.

## 6.4  Primary Afferent Nerve Fibers for Itch and Pain

In the past, a low level activation of nociceptors was thought to induce pruritus and a higher discharge frequency to induce pain.[21] Consistent with this theory was the observation that the intradermal application of high concentrations of pruritogens, e.g. histamine, may cause pain. Firing frequency in nociceptors cannot therefore account for the differentiation between pain and itch. It must be assumed that pruritogens preferentially excite a distinct subgroup of C-fibres, which give rise to itch. Such C-fibres have been discovered among mechano-insensitive C-nociceptors which respond to histamine iontophoresis parallel to the itch ratings of the subjects.[22] In contrast, the most common type of C-fibres, mechano-heat nociceptors (CMH or polymodal nociceptors) are either insensitive to histamine or only weakly activated by it.[23] They cannot account for the prolonged itch induced by the intradermal application of histamine.

Only a few mediators can induce histamine-independent pruritus, such as prostaglandins,[24] serotonin[25] or acetylcholine.[26] In normal skin the relative potency of the best known pruritogens is histamine >> prostaglandin $E_2$ > acetylcholine = serotonin. Prostaglandin $E_2$ responses were restricted to a subpopulation of the mechano-insensitive fibers, namely those which were also responsive to histamine when tested in another part of their receptive field. In contrast, mechano-insensitive units which were negative to histamine also did not respond to prostaglandin $E_2$. All mechano-responsive units were also negative to prostaglandin $E_2$ application. Thus, histamine and prostaglandin $E_2$ induced itch can be attributed to the activation of the same subpopulation of mechano-insensitive afferents.[27]

In the light of the pruritogenic effects of PgE$_2$, activation of histamine-responsive chemoreceptors by this mediator provides a strong argument for a fairly specific neuronal system for itch, different from the pain pathway. However, the histamine-responsive fibres are also excited by at least one specific algogen, namely capsaicin. The observation that capsaicin induces not only pain but also activates itch fibres, may be explained by an inhibition of itch by pain in the central nervous system. On the other hand topical capsaicin also is known to provoke itch in humans[28] and thus cannot be regarded as a pure pain provoking substance. In this unclear situation, itch processing neurons have been termed "itch selective."[29] Most importantly, activation of itch neurons by algogens like capsaicin does not contradict a "labeled line" for itch suggested by the discovery of histamine-sensitive central neurons.[30] Recent data from the tests conducted on the monkeys, however, question the existence of specific histamine-sensitive spinal projection neurons, but nevertheless propose two separate itch processing pathways, one being activated by histamine, the other being activated by cowhage.[31, 32]

Confirming the existence of different itch processing pathway, in an early study using papain, itch was induced in the absence of an axon reflex flare.[33] Furthermore, itch can be elicited by weak electrical stimulation without evoking an axon reflex flare,[34, 35] providing further evidence that the sensation of itch can be dissociated from cutaneous vasodilation. Because of the long delay between electrical stimulation and sensation (>1s) Ikoma et al. suggested that C-fibers might be the nerve fiber class involved.[35] Therefore, C fiber afferents with electrical thresholds lower than those of CMi[36] are likely to convey itch sensation, but are not able to produce an axon reflex flare.

Cowhage spicules inserted into human skin produce itch comparable to that following histamine application. Mechano-responsive "polymodal" C-fiber afferents, usually assumed to be pure nociceptors, can be activated by cowhage in the cat[37] and according to a recent study also in non-human primates.[38] Polymodal C-fibers are the most frequent type of afferent C-fibers in human skin nerves[39] and they are not involved in sustained axon reflex flare reactions.[40] This is consistent with the observation that cowhage induced itch is not accompanied by a widespread axon reflex flare.[41-43]

Given that cowhage spicules can activate a large proportion of polymodal nociceptors, we are facing a major problem in explaining why activation of these fibers by heat or by scratching is actually inhibiting itch, whereas activation by cowhage is producing it.

Further research is required to clarify as to how the spatial activation patterns of very focal epidermal stimuli are processed locally and in the spinal cord: focal activation of a small population of afferents may lead to a reduced surround inhibition which already has been proposed as an explanation for pruritus following very localized stimulation.[44] This would fit the observation that punctate mechanical, heat and electrical stimuli can cause the sensation of itch.[35,45]

While for histamine-induced itch a specific neuronal pathway can be described, cowhage induced itch is mediated most probably by mechanisms involving classical nociceptors. The discussion on specificity might appear as purely academic and interesting mainly for neuroscientists, however, it is crucial to identify those neurons in the skin that are mediating the itch sensation especially in chronic itch patients. Therefore, studies investigating structures and staining patterns of different primary afferent nerve fiber classes in the epidermis[46] are required for humans to understand how pain and pruritic stimuli are processed in the epidermis.

# References

1. Ward L, Wright E, McMahon SB. A Comparison of the effects of noxious and innocuous counterstimuli on experimentally induced itch and pain. *Pain*. 1996;64:129–138.
2. Nilsson HJ, Levinsson A, Schouenborg J. Cutaneous field stimulation (CFS): a new powerful method to combat itch. *Pain*. 1997;71(1):49–55.
3. Yosipovitch G, Fast K, Bernhard JD. Noxious heat and scratching decrease histamine-induced itch and skin blood flow. *J Invest Dermatol*. 2005;125(6):1268–1272.
4. Brull SJ, Atanassoff PG, Silverman DG, Zhang J, LaMotte RH. Attenuation of experimental pruritus and mechanically evoked dysesthesiae in an area of cutaneous allodynia. *Somatosens Mot Res*. 1999;16(4):299–303.
5. Simone DA, Nolano M, Johnson T, Wendelschafer-Crabb G, Kennedy WR. Intradermal injection of capsaicin in humans produces degeneration and subsequent reinnervation of epidermal nerve fibers: correlation with sensory function. *J Neurosci*. 1998;18(21):8947–8954.
6. Atanassoff PG, Brull SJ, Zhang J, Greenquist K, Silverman DG, LaMotte RH. Enhancement of experimental pruritus and mechanically evoked dysesthesiae with local anesthesia. *Somatosens Mot Res*. 1999;16(4):291–298.
7. Andrew D, Schmelz M, Ballantyne JC. Itch – mechanisms and mediators. In: Dostrovsky JO, Carr DB, Koltzenburg M, eds. *Progress in Pain Research and Management*. Seattle: IASP Press; 2003:213–226.
8. Heyer G, Dotzer M, Diepgen TL, Handwerker HO. Opiate and H1 antagonist effects on histamine induced pruritus and alloknesis. *Pain*. 1997;73(2):239–243.
9. McRae CA, Prince MI, Hudson M, Day CP, James OF, Jones DE. Pain as a complication of use of opiate antagonists for symptom control in cholestasis. *Gastroenterology*. 2003;125(2):591–596.
10. Jones EA, Neuberger J, Bergasa NV. Opiate antagonist therapy for the pruritus of cholestasis: the avoidance of opioid withdrawal-like reactions. *QJM*. 2002;95(8):547–552.
11. Kamei J, Nagase H. Norbinaltorphimine, a selective kappa-opioid receptor antagonist, induces an itch-associated response in mice. *Eur J Pharmacol*. 2001;418(1–2):141–145.
12. Inan S, Cowan A. Nalfurafine, a kappa opioid receptor agonist, inhibits scratching behavior secondary to cholestasis induced by chronic ethynylestradiol injections in rats. *Pharmacol Biochem Behav*. 2006;85(1):39–43.
13. Kjellberg F, Tramer MR. Pharmacological control of opioid-induced pruritus: a quantitative systematic review of randomized trials. *Eur J Anaesthesiol*. 2001;18(6):346–357.
14. Lee H, Naughton NN, Woods JH, Ko MC. Effects of butorphanol on morphine-induced itch and analgesia in primates. *Anesthesiology*. 2007;107(3):478–485.
15. Delmez JA. Efficacy and safety of a new kappa-opioid receptor agonist for the treatment of uremic pruritus. *Nat Clin Pract Nephrol*. 2006;2(7):358–359.
16. Stein C, Schafer M, Machelska H. Attacking pain at its source: new perspectives on opioids. *Nat Med*. 2003;9(8):1003–1008.
17. Braz J, Beaufour C, Coutaux A, et al. Therapeutic efficacy in experimental polyarthritis of viral-driven enkephalin overproduction in sensory neurons. *J Neurosci*. 2001;21(20):7881–7888.
18. Schmelz M, Paus R. Opioids and the skin: "itchy" perspectives beyond analgesia and abuse. *J Invest Dermatol*. 2007;127(6):1287–1289.
19. Bigliardi-Qi M, Gaveriaux-Ruff C, Pfaltz K, et al. Deletion of mu- and kappa-opioid receptors in mice changes epidermal hypertrophy, density of peripheral nerve endings, and itch behavior. *J Invest Dermatol*. 2007;127(6):1479–1488.
20. Ibrahim MM, Porreca F, Lai J, et al. CB2 cannabinoid receptor activation produces antinociception by stimulating peripheral release of endogenous opioids. *Proc Natl Acad Sci USA*. 2005;102(8):3093–3098.
21. v.Frey M. Zur Physiologie der Juckempfindung. *Arch Neerl Physiol*. 1922;7:142–145.
22. Schmelz M, Schmidt R, Bickel A, Handwerker HO, Torebjörk HE. Specific C-receptors for itch in human skin. *J Neurosci*. 1997;17(20):8003–8008.
23. Handwerker HO, Forster C, Kirchhoff C. Discharge patterns of human C-fibers induced by itching and burning stimuli. *J Neurophysiol*. 1991;66(1):307–315.
24. Woodward DF, Nieves AL, Hawley SB, Joseph R, Merlino GF, Spada CS. The pruritogenic and inflammatory effects of prostanoids in the conjunctiva. *J Ocul Pharmacol Ther*. 1995;11(3):339–347.
25. Hägermark O. Peripheral and central mediators of itch. *Skin Pharmacol*. 1992;5(1):1–8.
26. Vogelsang M, Heyer G, Hornstein OP. Acetylcholine induces different cutaneous sensations in atopic and non-atopic subjects. *Acta Derm Venereol*. 1995;75(6):434–436.
27. Schmelz M, Schmidt R, Weidner C, Hilliges M, Torebjork HE, Handwerker HO. Chemical response pattern of different classes of C-nociceptors to pruritogens and algogens. *J Neurophysiol*. 2003;89(5):2441–2448.

28. Green BG, Shaffer GS. The sensory response to capsaicin during repeated topical exposures: differential effects on sensations of itching and pungency. *Pain*. 1993;53(3):323–334.

29. McMahon SB, Koltzenburg M. Itching for an explanation. *Trends Neurosci*. 1992;15(12):497–501.

30. Craig AD, Andrew D. Responses of spinothalamic lamina I neurons to repeated brief contact heat stimulation in the cat. *J Neurophysiol*. 2002;87(4):1902–1914.

31. Davidson S, Zhang X, Yoon CH, Khasabov SG, Simone DA, Giesler GJ, Jr. The itch-producing agents histamine and cowhage activate separate populations of primate spinothalamic tract neurons. *J Neurosci*. 2007;27(37):10007–10014.

32. Simone DA, Zhang X, Li J, et al. Comparison of responses of primate spinothalamic tract neurons to pruritic and algogenic stimuli. *J Neurophysiol*. 2004;91(1):213–222.

33. Hagermark O. Influence of antihistamines, sedatives, and aspirin on experimental itch. *Acta Derm Venereol*. 1973; 53(5):363–368.

34. Shelley WB, Arthur RP. The neurohistology and neurophysiology of the itch sensation in man. *AMA Arch Derm*. 1957;76(3):296–323.

35. Ikoma A, Handwerker H, Miyachi Y, Schmelz M. Electrically evoked itch in humans. *Pain*. 2005;113(1–2):148–154.

36. Weidner C, Schmelz M, Schmidt R, Hansson B, Handwerker HO, Torebjork HE. Functional attributes discriminating mechano-insensitive and mechano-responsive C nociceptors in human skin. *J Neurosci*. 1999;19(22):10184–10190.

37. Tuckett RP, Wei JY. Response to an itch-producing substance in cat. II. Cutaneous receptor population with unmyelinated axons. *Brain Res*. 1987;413:95–103.

38. Johanek LM, Meyer RA, Hartke T, et al. Psychophysical and physiological evidence for parallel afferent pathways mediating the sensation of itch. *J Neurosci*. 2007;27(28):7490–7497.

39. Schmidt R, Schmelz M, Forster C, Ringkamp M, Torebjork E, Handwerker H. Novel classes of responsive and unresponsive C nociceptors in human skin. *J Neurosci*. 1995; 15(1 pt 1):333–341.

40. Schmelz M, Michael K, Weidner C, Schmidt R, Torebjork HE, Handwerker HO. Which nerve fibers mediate the axon reflex flare in human skin? *Neuroreport*. 2000;11(3): 645–648.

41. Shelley WB, Arthur RP. Studies on cowhage (*Mucuna pruriens*) and its pruritogenic proteinase, mucunain. *AMA Arch Derm*. 1955;72(5):399–406.

42. Shelley WB, Arthur RP. The neurohistology and neurophysiology of the itch sensation in man. *AMA Arch Derm*. 1957;76(3):296–323.

43. Johanek LM, Meyer RA, Hartke T, et al. Psychophysical and physiological evidence for parallel afferent pathways mediating the sensation of itch. *J Neurosci*. 2007; 27(28): 7490–7497.

44. Greaves MW, Wall PD. Pathophysiology of itching. *Lancet*. 1996;348(9032):938–940.

45. Wahlgren CF, Hagermark O, Bergstrom R. Patients' perception of itch induced by histamine, compound 48/80 and wool fibres in atopic dermatitis. *Acta Derm Venereol*. 1991;71(6): 488–494.

46. Zylka MJ, Rice FL, Anderson DJ. Topographically distinct epidermal nociceptive circuits revealed by axonal tracers targeted to Mrgprd. *Neuron*. 2005;45(1):17–25.

# Chapter 7
# Neuroimaging

Florian Pfab, Michael Valet, Thomas Tölle, Heidrun Behrendt, Johannes Ring, and Ulf Darsow

## 7.1 Introduction

Itch is a complex and unpleasant sensory experience that induces the urge to scratch.[1] It is the most prevalent symptom of inflammatory skin diseases[2,3] and difficult to be measured objectively. With its well-known psychophysiological aspects it has substantial impact on the quality of life of the patients.[4] Its pathophysiology remains poorly understood in spite of numerous studies.[2]

Quantity and quality of perceived itch show specific characteristics in different pruritic skin diseases. Clinical observations point to differences in the processing of pruritus by the central nervoussystem. The multidimensional "Eppendorf Itch Questionnaire" (EIQ)[5] was used in hospitalized patients suffering from atopic eczema (AE, n = 62) and chronic urticaria (CU, n = 58). Total scores (127 items), emotional and sensory ratings, reactive behavior and visual analogue scale (VAS) ratings for itch intensity were evaluated. The mean VAS ratings of itch intensity showed no significant difference between the two diseases. In contrast, the total EIQ score was significantly higher in the AE group with 231.6 ± 11.5 vs. 175.2 ± 9.4. In 34 of 127 items, a significantly different rating was obtained, mostly with a higher load for the affective and some sensory items in AE. Significant differences were also seen in the description of the scratch response. Thus, itch perception in AE and CU differs on a qualitative level, influencing items relevant for quality of life. Similar findings were perceived in a study investigating the preventive effect of acupuncture on experimental itch - showing a preventive point-specific effect on emotional items of the EIQ.[6] These findings accentuate the emotional component of the itch sensation; with possibly differences in Central Nervous System (CNS) processing.

Itch can easily be elicited experimentally – most effectively via a histamine stimulus.[7] With its mainly subjective characteristics itch has some psychophysiological similarity to pain. Although some degree of overlap is present, recent neurophysiological studies have confirmed that itch pathways are clearly distinct from pain pathways.[8–10] In recent years, progress in the central nervous system imaging technologies have had substantial impact on itch research. New models to measure itch may also be useful for the development of new therapeutic strategies against pruritus.

## 7.2 Neuroimaging of Itch by Positron Emission Tomography (PET)

Objective covariates of itch and differences to pain processing were shown using imaging techniques for the CNS: a complex pattern of cerebral activation after experimental itch induction with histamine dihydrochloride (0.03–8%) at the right lower arm in healthy volunteers was observed in a $H^{2(15)}O$ PET correlation study (n = 6).[8] Subtraction analysis of histamine versus control condition revealed significant activation of the primary sensory cortex and motor-associated areas, predominantly left-sided activations of the frontal, orbitofrontal and superior temporal cortex and anterior cingulate cortex. Compared to activation patterns induced by pain stimuli[11] itch did not lead to thalamus activation, but significant activation was there in the insula region and differences in sensory, motor and cingulate areas.

Mochizuki et al.[12] investigating the central modulation of histamine-itch by application of a contralateral cold pain stimulus, showed significant increases in regional cerebral blood flow in the anterior cingulate cortex, the thalamus, the parietal cortex, the dorsolateral prefrontal cortex and the premotor cortex.

These results give evidence for central nervous processing of itch, and clearly demonstrate the differences to pain processing. Planning of a scratch response is mirrored by extensive activation of the motor areas in the cortex, and other areas may be involved in the emotional evaluation of pruriception.

## 7.3 New Methodology Enabling Itch Measurement by fMRI

Until recently functional magnetic resonance imaging (fMRI) studies on itch had been hampered by the lack of a phasic stimulus. In contrast to pain, no method had been described to elicit and stop the sensation of itch within seconds. In a recent study the itch sensation was investigated using a methodology with short term temperature changes for the modulation of histamine-induced itch.[13]

In nine healthy right-handed male volunteers, 1% histamine dihydrochloride was used as evaluated itch stimulus[5] on the right forearm with subsequent modulation of the temperature of the target skin area by a

Medoc TSA thermode. The latter is capable of heating or cooling the skin and was placed exactly above the stimulus area. Using a boxcar design 14 equal cycles were applied: Each cycle started with a warm block producing a constant skin temperature of 32°C for 20 s then changing within 1.5 s (ramp 5°C/s) to a cold block of 25°C also lasting for 20 s.

Subjective scales were recorded using a computerized VAS ranging from 0 to 100 at 4 s intervals. At one-third of the VAS (33/100) the intervention point "scratch threshold" was installed. Above this threshold each individual felt the clear-cut desire to scratch; this, however, was not permitted nor done. Itch intensity was quantitatively expressed as a percent of the maximum VAS value.

All subjects reported itch without pain within 40 s after histamine application. None of the volunteers ever felt a sensation of pain during the whole experiment.

In each individual subject as well as in the total group, significant differences between VAS rating intervals concerning itch intensity were noted. In each cycle, itch intensity was generally perceived as higher during 25°C-blocks than during 32°C-blocks. Mean itch intensity was 50.6% ± 3.5% during the 25°C-block (intervals 6–10) and 33.8% ± 3.9% during the 32°C-block (intervals 1–5) with a highly significant difference (p < 0.0001) between the two temperature blocks (Fig. 7.1).

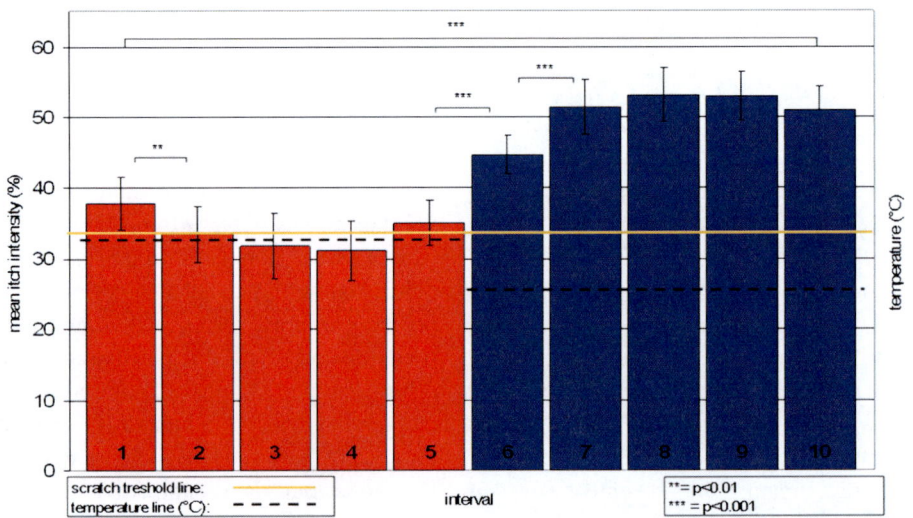

**Fig. 7.1** Stimulus model, showing one cycle: Mean itch intensity (VAS) of both sessions at the various temperature intervals (n = 9). As indicated by the dotted line the red columns numbered 1–5 indicate 32°C-temperature intervals, whereas the blue columns numbered 6–10 mark 25°C-temperature intervals, each lasting 4 s. The yellow line represents the scratch threshold (33% itch-intensity). Asterisks indicate significant differences between intervals **p < 0.01, ***p < 0.001 (adapted from Pfab et al.[13])

Alternating changes in mean itch perception comparing warm and cold blocks were remarkably reproducible.

In spite of the common knowledge that intensive cold inhibits itch sensation, a reproducible, significant enhancement of histamine-induced itch by short term moderate cooling was shown. This effect might be explained by peripheral and central adaptation processes triggered by abnormal afferent activity patterns.

This method allows controlled and rapid modulation of itch. Short term cooling enhances histamine-induced itch, providing the possibility of further and more detailed investigations of itch by functional imaging methods such as fMRI.

## 7.4 Cerebral Processing of Histamine-Induced Itch Using Short-Term Alternating Temperature Modulation – An fMRI Study

Using the previously established biphasic temperature stimulus model, we investigated the cerebral activation pattern of itch processing in 12 healthy volunteers with functional Magnetic Resonance Imaging (MRI).[14]

Itch was provoked on the right forearm with 1% histamine-dihydrochloride. Local temperature modulation allowed reproducible itch provocation above scratch threshold (defined as 33/100 on a VAS) during 25°C whereas itch declined below scratch threshold during the 32°C stimulation period. No itch sensation was reported using 0.9% saline with temperature modulation.

The calculation of itch-specific activation maps for the first 4, 8, 12, 16 and 20 s of the 25°C stimulation period confirmed that the changes during the first 8 s are reflected by the higher brain activations during this time period than during the other time periods. Focusing on the first 8 s of 25°C stimulation, the thalamus, pre-Supplementary Motor Area (SMA), lateral prefrontal cortex, anterior insular cortex and inferior parietal cortex were more active than during the saline condition (p < 0.001; Fig. 7.2). The medial frontal cortex, the orbito-frontal cortex, the dorsal part of the anterior cingulate cortex (dACC) and the primary motor cortex (M1) were less active during histamine induced itch than during the saline condition (p < 0.001; Fig. 7.2).

So far this is the only imaging study on itch using a phasic supra-threshold itch model comparing itch and non-itch phases.

## 7.5 Further Neuroimaging Studies

Neuroimaging studies on itch have been done using analysis in PET[8,12,15–17] and more recently fMRI.[18,19] Table 7.1 summarizes the findings of current neuroimaging studies.

Taking the results of these studies together key centers of histamine-itch perception in healthy volunteers seem to be ipsilaterally the pre-motor and supplementary motor area and contralaterally the cingulate cortex, the insular cortex, the thalamus and the frontal inferior gyrus (inferior parietal and dorsolateral prefrontal cortex).

So far one study[19] has investigated the effect of allergen-induced itch in patients with mucosal atopy showing similarities to histamine-itch (Table 7.1). Mochizuki et al.[18] directly compared itch and pain stimuli with fMRI in healthy volunteers: Neural activity in the posterior cingulated cortex and the posterior insula associated with itch was significantly higher than that associated with pain; pain in contrast to itch induced an activation of the thalamus.

## 7.6 Key Anatomic Brain Regions of Itch and Their Function

### 7.6.1 Insular Cortex

The anterior insula is assumed to subserve subjective feelings[20] and to integrate sensory and emotional experiences.[21] It has been suggested that the insular cortex is part of an interoceptive system providing the basis for a cortical image of homeostatic activity that reflects all aspects of the physiological condition.[22] In this context, the activation of the insular cortex might indicate an interference by the sensation of itch, on the homeostatic balance, leading to the desire to scratch.[13,19]

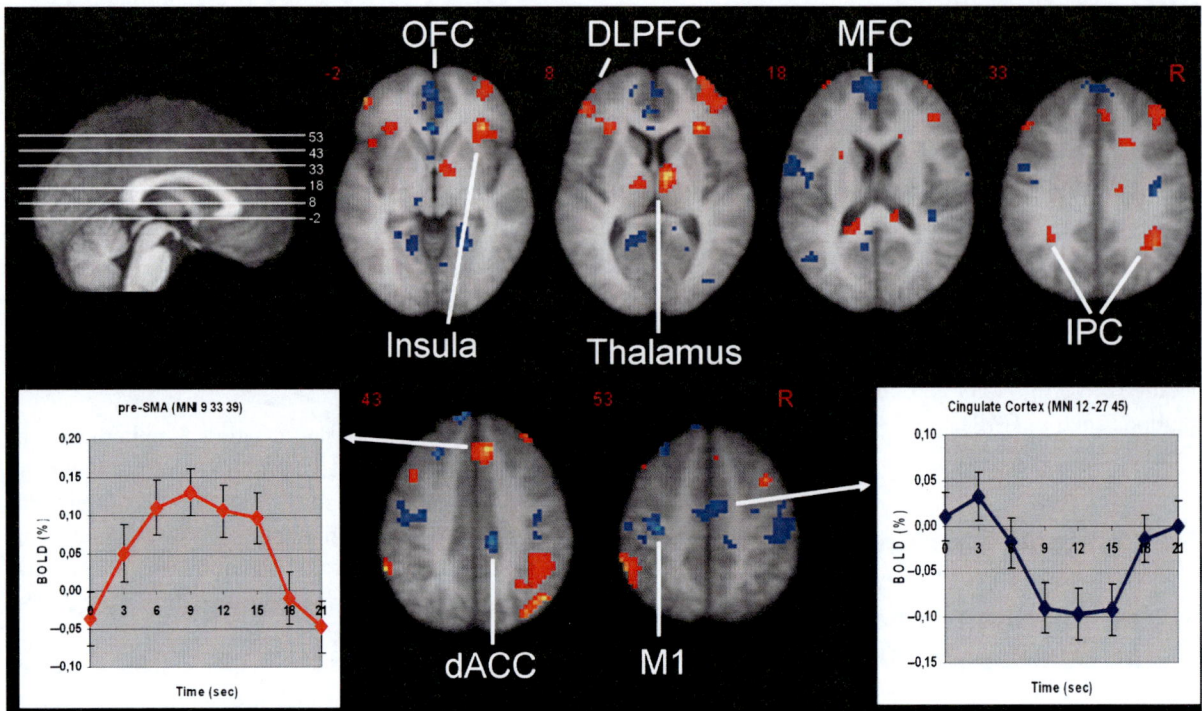

**Fig. 7.2** The increase of histamine induced itch during the first 8 s of the 25°C stimulation periods (as compared to saline) is associated with an increase (*red*) and decrease (*blue*) of activation in various brain structures subserving sensory, emotional, cognitive and motivational aspects of itch processing. As an example, the averaged relative fMRI BOLD signal of all subjects during 20 s of the 25°C period is presented – for the pre-SMA region with increased and the cingulate cortex with decreased activation in comparison to saline. OFC, orbitofrontal cortex; DLPFC, dorsolateral prefrontal cortex; MFC, medial frontal cortex; IPC, inferior parietal cortex; dACC, dorsal anterior cingulate cortex; M1, primary motor cortex; R, right side of the brain (adapted from Valet et al.[14])

### 7.6.2 Pre-Supplementary Motor Area and Primary Motor Cortex, Motor Part of the Cingulate Cortex

The pre-SMA is thought to encode motor actions prior to self-initiated voluntary movements and during imagination of motor action.[23] M1 is typically involved in motor planning and execution highlighting the definition of itch which includes the intention to scratch.[1] As the subjects were not allowed to scratch the deactivation might indicate a suppression of motor activity. The dorsal anterior cingulated cortex (dACC) is also thought to be engaged in premotor planning[24,25] as well as in stimulus intensity encoding.[26,27] Translating this information from pain to itch processing, we hypothesize that the dual function of the dACC and the anatomical neighboring to M1 is advantageous for the generation of an adequate motor response to the itching stimulus (planning of a scratch response) in relation to the processed sensory information.

### 7.6.3 Thalamus and Primary Somatosensory Cortex

The activation of the thalamus and S1 cortex can be attributed to sensory aspects of itch processing. The ability to locate itch (S1) plays an important role in the initiation of withdrawal behavior. These brain structures are fulfilling important functions regarding detection, localization, discrimination and intensity encoding of sensory stimuli.[28]

### 7.6.4 Inferior Parietal Cortex and Dorsolateral Prefrontal Cortex

The inferior parietal cortex is known to be involved in the spatial representation of the intra- and extrapersonal space (body scheme) and regarded as polymodal association area integrating multisensory information

**Table 7.1** Summarizing findings of current neuroimaging studies. Activation in the corresponding region is marked by I (ipsilateral) or C (contralateral); the minus (−) indicates reduced activation in comparison to a saline control stimulus

| Brain region | Histamine-itch | | | | | | | Allergen-itch |
| --- | --- | --- | --- | --- | --- | --- | --- | --- |
| | Hsieh et al.[16] PET | Drzezga et al.[15] PET | Mochizuki et al.[12] PET | Walter et al.[17] fMRI | Leknes et al.[19] fMRI | Valet et al.[14] fMRI | Mochizuki et al.[18] fMRI | Leknes et al.[19] fMRI |
| Primary somatosens. cortex (BA 1–3) | I,C | I,C | | | | C- | | C |
| Primary motor cortex (BA 4) | | C | | | | | | C |
| Somatosens. assoc./par. cortex (BA 5,7) | I,C | I,C | I | | | | | |
| Pre-motor and suppl. motor cortex (BA 6) | I,C | I,C | I | | | I | I | C |
| Prefrontal cortex (BA 9) | | C | | | | | | |
| Frontopolar and orbitofrontal area (BA 10–12) | | C | | I,C | | I,C- | I | I,C |
| Insular cortex (BA 13,14) | | C | | | I,C | C | C | |
| Temporal gyrus (BA 20–22) | | | | C | | | | |
| Cingulate cortex (BA 23,24,25,32) | C | I,C | C | C | I,C | I- | C | I,C |
| Temporal lobe/Wernickes area (BA 38–40) | | | I | | | I,C | | C |
| Inf. par. & dorsolat. prefrontal cortex (BA 45,46) | | C | I,C | | | I,C | | |
| Cerebellum | I,C | | | C | | | | |
| Thalamus | | | C | | I,C | I,C | | I,C |
| Basal ganglia | | | | | I | | | I,C |

I, ipsilateral; C, contralateral; somatosens, somatosensory; assoc., association; par, parietal; suppl, supplementary; inf, inferior; dorsolat, dorsolateral.

from the thalamus, insula, anterior cingulate cortex and prefrontal cortex.[29] It is known that lesions of this region in the non-dominant hemisphere are highly associated with neglect and inattention syndromes. Activation of this region may therefore reflect a spatially directed attention to the itching stimulus.

The dorsolateral prefrontal cortex is associated with cognitive evaluative, attention-dependent, working memory and executive functions.[30] Besides the input from the thalamus and cingulate cortex, it receives and processes multisensory information mainly from the inferior parietal cortex.[30] The sensory convergence and integration is required in the preparation of motor action.

## 7.7 Conclusion

The itch sensation is processed by a network of brain regions contributing to the encoding of sensory, emotional, attention-dependent, cognitive-evaluative and motivational patterns. It now seems possible to further analyze the specific effects of various therapies on these significant activation patterns.

## References

1. Hafenreffer S. In: Kuhnen, ed. Nosodochium, in quo cutis, eique adaerentium partium, affectus omnes, singulari methodo, et cognoscendi e curandi fidelissime traduntur. Ulm; 1660:98–102.
2. Charlesworth EN, Beltrani VS. Pruritic dermatoses: overview of etiology and therapy. *Am J Med.* 2002;113(suppl 9A): 25S–33S.
3. Behrendt H, Krämer U, Schäfer T, Kasche A, Eberlein-König B, Darsow U. Allergotoxicology – a research concept to study the role of environmental pollutants in allergy. *ACI Int.* 2001;13:122–128.
4. Staender S, Weisshaar E, Mettang T, et al. Clinical classification of itch: a position paper of the international forum for the study of itch. *Acta Derm Venereol.* 2007;87(4):291–294.
5. Darsow U, Scharein E, Simon D, Walter G, Bromm B, Ring J. New aspects of itch pathophysiology: component analysis of atopic itch using the "Eppendorf Itch Questionaire". *Int Arch Allergy Immunol.* 2001;124:326–331.
6. Pfab F, Hammes M, Backer M, et al. Preventive effect of acupuncture on histamine-induced itch: a blinded, randomized, placebo-controlled, crossover trial. *J Allergy Clin Immunol.* 2005;116(6):1386–1388.
7. Darsow U, Ring J, Scharein E, Bromm B. Correlations between histamine-induced wheal, flare and itch. *Arch Dermatol Res.* 1996;288(8):436–441.
8. Darsow U, Drzezga A, Frisch M, et al. Processing of histamine-induced itch in the human cerebral cortex: a correlation analysis with dermal reactions. *J Invest Dermatol.* 2000;115 (6):1029–1033.
9. Schmelz M, Schmidt R, Bickel A, Handwerker HO, Torebjoerk HE. Specific C-receptors for itch in human skin. *J Neurosci.* 1997;17(20):8003–8008.
10. Ikoma A, Steinhoff M, Stander S, Yosipovitch G, Schmelz M. The neurobiology of itch. *Nat Rev.* 2006;7(7):535–547.
11. Sprenger T, Ruether K, Boecker H, et al. Altered metabolism in frontal brain circuits in cluster headache. *Cephalgia* 2007;27:1033–1042.
12. Mochizuki H, Tashiro M, Kano M, Sakurada Y, Itoh M, Yanai K. Imaging of central itch modulation in the human brain using positron emission tomography. *Pain.* 2003;105 (1–2):339–346.
13. Pfab F, Valet M, Sprenger T, et al. Short-term alternating temperature enhances histamine-induced itch: a biphasic stimulus model. *J Invest Dermatol.* 2006;126(12): 2673–2678.
14. Valet M, Pfab F, Sprenger T, et al. Cerebral processing of histamine-induced itch using short-term alternating temperature modulation – an fMRI study. *J Invest Dermatol.* 2008; 128:426–433.
15. Drzezga A, Darsow U, Treede RD, et al. Central activation by histamine-induced itch: analogies to pain processing: a correlational analysis of O-15 H$_2$O positron emission tomography studies. *Pain.* 2001;92(1–2):295–305.
16. Hsieh JC, Hagermark O, Stahle-Backdahl M, et al. Urge to scratch represented in the human cerebral cortex during itch. *J Neurophysiol.* 1994;72(6):3004–3008.
17. Walter B, Sadlo MN, Kupfer J, et al. Brain activation by histamine prick test-induced itch. *J Invest Dermatol.* 2005;125 (2):380–382.
18. Mochizuki H, Sadato N, Saito DN, et al. Neural correlates of perceptual difference between itching and pain: a human fMRI study. *NeuroImage.* 2007;36(3):706–717.
19. Leknes SG, Bantick S, Willis CM, Wilkinson JD, Wise RG, Tracey I. Itch and motivation to scratch: an investigation of the central and peripheral correlates of allergen-and histamine-induced itch in humans. *J Neurophysiol.* 2007;97(1): 415–422.
20. Singer T, Seymour B, O'Doherty J, Kaube H, Dolan RJ, Frith CD. Empathy for pain involves the affective but not sensory components of pain. *Science.* 2004;303(5661):1157–1162.
21. Gracely RH, Geisser ME, Giesecke T, et al. Pain catastrophizing and neural responses to pain among persons with fibromyalgia. *Brain.* 2004;127(pt 4):835–843.
22. Craig AD. Interoception: the sense of the physiological condition of the body. *Curr Opin Neurobiol.* 2003;13(4): 500–505.
23. Cunnington R, Windischberger C, Moser E. Premovement activity of the pre-supplementary motor area and the readiness for action: studies of time-resolved event-related functional MRI. *Hum Mov Sci.* 2005;24(5–6):644–656.
24. Vogt BA. Pain and emotion interactions in subregions of the cingulate gyrus. *Nat Rev.* 2005;6(7):533–544.
25. Kwan CL, Crawley AP, Mikulis DJ, Davis KD. An fMRI study of the anterior cingulate cortex and surrounding medial wall activations evoked by noxious cutaneous heat and cold stimuli. *Pain.* 2000;85(3):359–374.

26. Tölle TR, Kaufmann T, Siessmeier T, et al. Region-specific encoding of sensory and affective components of pain in the human brain: a positron emission tomography correlation analysis. *Ann Neurol.* 1999;45(1):40–47.

27. Buchel C, Bornhovd K, Quante M, Glauche V, Bromm B, Weiller C. Dissociable neural responses related to pain intensity, stimulus intensity, and stimulus awareness within the anterior cingulate cortex: a parametric single-trial laser functional magnetic resonance imaging study. *J Neurosci.* 2002;22(3):970–976.

28. Apkarian AV, Bushnell MC, Treede RD, Zubieta JK. Human brain mechanisms of pain perception and regulation in health and disease. *Eur J Pain (London, England).* 2005;9(4): 463–484.

29. Freund HJ. The parietal lobe as a sensorimotor interface: a perspective from clinical and neuroimaging data. *NeuroImage.* 2001;14(1 pt 2):S142–S146.

30. Fuster JM. *The Prefrontal Cortex. Anatomy, Physiology and Neuropsychology of the Frontal Lobe.* Philadelphia: Lippincott-Raven; 1997.

# Chapter 8
# Measurement of Itch

Joanna Wallengren

Itch is a major symptom of skin disease. Yet, until the last thirty years the investigation of itch has been ignored by researchers. One important reason has been the lack of reliable and sensitive measurement. We can only indirectly measure different aspects of itch perception which is performed on several levels of the nervous system. Physiological itch participates in the defence of the organism from harmful agents and involves multiple steps including the peripheral receptor, the afferent nerve transmitting the impulse to the spinal cord, the signal processing in the dorsal horn and finally transmission to higher cerebral centres in the thalamus and the cortex.[1] The perceived itch induces scratching with the purpose of removing harmful agents from the skin. Scratching has for a long time been recognised as the most objective and reliable measurement of itch.[2] This chapter provides a historical and critical review of the objective and subjective methods of itch measurement both in experimental and in clinical setting.

## 8.1 Quantification of Scratching in Patients

Pioneering clinical studies of itch were designed to objectively evaluate itch in order to measure the effects of antipruritic agents. As interference with sleep has been regarded as a rough guide to the severity of pruritus, nocturnal scratching was registered in patients in a sleep laboratory of Savin and co-workers.[3] Here, the recordings were made of all-night electroencephalogram, electro-oculogram and electromyogram. Muscle potentials from both hands were recorded using two electrodes taped to the ulnar side of the ventral part of the forearm in order to register scratching movements. This technique could reveal the frequency and duration of bouts of scratching during each stage of sleep and the proportion of sleep spent scratching. The limitation of this method is that it requires a sleep laboratory and that the wires attached to the electromyography may disturb the subject's sleep. Felix and Shuster introduced vibration transducers attached to the bed in order to measure movements of the body during sleep.[4] In addition, they measured the movements of both legs and hands using a "self-winding watch."[4] Later trails revealed that all scratch movements were not recorded by this technique.[5] An electromagnetic limb movement meter was therefore constructed to record the cumulative time spent moving, along with the registration of all scratch movements of the patients with itch and of controls.[5] Another approach to register nocturnal scratching was by the use of a paper gauge attached to the dorsum of each hand and an amplifier.[6] The limitation of these techniques is that with a self-winding watch or paper gauge attached to the patient's wrist, some patients may get disturbed in sleep. In addition, all these early scratch recordings were performed on subjects at the hospital. Therefore, another technique using a sensor, "a radar," positioned at a distance from the sleepers hands was designed.[7] The intention was to register the rapid movements typical of scratching and filter out larger movements of the limbs and body. Unfortunately only one study employing this technique has been published.[7]

Further studies on scratch activity were performed in the patients' own homes. The gold standard here was infrared videotaping of the patients movements at night.[8] A new instrument called accelerometer (Actiwatch Plus, Cambridge Neurotechnology,

Cambridge, United Kingdom) placed on the dominant wrist, to be worn at night, was developed to record the intensity, amount, and duration of scratching stimuli.[9] Accelerometer was validated against videotaping of children with atopic dermatitis.[9] Analysis of the videos showed that not only scratch movements but also writhing, rubbing at slow speeds, as well as movements under the covers were registered by the accelerometer, but all these movements were regarded as a symptom of the disease.[9] In a later study on adult patients, the authors found a negative correlation between objective movement activity and self-reported quality of sleep.[10] Another monitor of nocturnal movements on the market is DigiTrac (IM Systems, Baltimore, MD, USA) to be worn on the dominant wrist during sleeping.[11]

In many skin diseases, such as atopic eczema, nocturnal scratching is crucial and therefore recordings of scratching at night are very useful. During other circumstances, such as evaluation of anti-pruritic therapy in clinical trails, scratching activity at both day and night or mean hourly scratching may be important. Therefore a new instrument called Pruritometer 2 was constructed to register and store scratching during a 24 h period.[12] The instrument processes the signals of a piezoelectric vibration sensor, fixed on the midfinger of the patient's dominant hand, to a counter worn by the patient like a wristwatch.[12] A statistically good correlation between measured (Pruritometer) and visually counted scratches was demonstrated.[12] To obtain satisfactory 24 h recordings, the patient must continue to wear the device during the night which requires compliance and acceptance by the patient.

## 8.2 Quantification of Scratching in Animal Models

Small animal models, common in studies of inflammatory mediators, have also been employed in the investigation of itch. Scratching behaviour in response to intradermal injection of pruritogens has been studied in different ways. In a Japanese study, experimental mice were equipped with magnets inserted into both hind paws. Scratching behaviour

was thereafter induced and the animals were put into a small round chamber surrounded by a coil (MicroAct, Neuroscience, Inc, Tokyo, Japan).[13] A chamber was constructed to detect and amplify electric current induced by the movements of the mouse legs through the magnets.[6] The difficult part of this study was to differentiate the scratching from other movements of the legs and the authors found that scratching induced characteristic waves.[13] In other studies iontophoresis was used to minimize the pain of intradermal administration of mediators studied and the behaviour of animals (mice and guinea pigs) was followed by a video camera.[14] Here administration of capsaicin induced not only scratching but also changes in resting, feeding, drinking and grooming behaviour.[14] Therefore, the same group developed a programmed micro-controller to discriminate between non-specific movement, grooming behaviour, and scratching movements made by animals's hind limbs.[15] However, scratching may actually also occur as a response to pain in both mice and rats.[16,17] Thus, in animal studies, counting of scratch bouts alone cannot be used to evaluate the sensations induced by different itch mediators or to evaluate the effects of potential antipruritic drugs.

## 8.3 Measurement of the Threshold, Duration and Intensity of Itch

In early experimental studies of mediators of pruritus, substances were administered topically on scarified skin,[18] by intradermal injections[19] and later by intradermal microdialysis in order to reduce the pain of an injection.[20] The threshold for itch induction[18] or the duration of itch[19] was measured.

In the clinical setting, especially in clinical trails, the intensity and quality of itch, and how it responds to different therapies are major issues. Medical records contain descriptions of both the quality of itch such as burning, stinging, pricking or sensations of insects crawling over the skin and of the severity of itch such as mildly, moderately or severely disturbing sleep. Therefore rating scales have been introduced for a quantitative grading of itch and questionnaires have been designed to measure the qualitative aspects of the itch sensation.

## 8.4  Rating Scales

Here follows a review of rating scales commonly used in dermatology. In addition, a few other scales, common in pain research, are described and adapted to the investigation of itch.

### 8.4.1  Verbal Rating Scales

Verbal rating scales (VRS) comprise a list of adjectives to denote increasing itch intensities. In the four-point scale (VRS-4) the most common words are none, mild, moderate and severe. For ease of recordings these adjectives are assigned numbers, so the least intense descriptor is usually given a score of 0, the next a score of 1 and so on. These rank numbers may suggest that the differences between the scale steps are equal, which is not necessarily the case.[21] It means that VRS is an ordinal scale and the data collected using VRS can only be analysed with non-parametric statistical methods with loss of power. On the other hand, VRS is probably the easiest to use in retrospective studies.

Another 6-point behavioural rating scale (BRS-6) is widely used in pain research.[21] It consists of a list of statements which describe the intensity of pain in terms of interference with daily life activities. With respect to itch, the points on the rating scale could be as follows: (0) no itch, (1) itch present, but can easily be ignored, (2) itch present, cannot be ignored, but does not interfere with every day activities (3) itch present, cannot be ignored, interferes with concentration, (4) itch present, cannot be ignored, interferes with all tasks except taking care of basic needs such as toileting and eating, (5) itch present, cannot be ignored, incapacitating (the person does not know what to do with himself or herself).

A comparison of these three methods revealed that the BRS-4 gave the highest number of correct responses followed by the BRS-5, while the BRS-6 gave the lowest number.[21]

Little is known about children's ability to assess itch, although self report may be obtained from children of three years.[22] A seven-point scale named "face's pain scale" (FPS) is the most preferred by children and healthcare professionals over other pain assessment measures because they are easy to use and reproduce.[22,23] This scale consisting of schematic faces with different expression has been demonstrated to be valid and reliable in measuring pain in children although they have not been employed in the rating of itch.

### 8.4.2  Numerical Rating Scales

Numerical rating scales are based on the assumption that there is a true zero-point and may be presented graphically as lines (Visual Analogue Scale, VAS) or boxes (Box scale) with their boundaries clearly defined as the extremes of the feeling from "none" to "worst possible." The main advantage of the numerical rating scales is that they allow parametric statistics.

The simplest to administer and score is the numerical rating scale (NRS-101).[21] The patient is asked to rate his or her perceived level of itch intensity on an imaginary numerical scale from 0–100 with 0 "no itch" and 100 indicating "itch as bad as it could be," and to choose only one number. This number can be written by the patient or communicated verbally to the investigator. When VAS; Box and NRS were compared with each other, NRS-101 was suggested as the most sensitive in comparisons of treatment outcome.[21]

Box scales are more common in pain research than in itch research. The Box Scale 11 (BS-11) consists of 11 numbers (0 through 10) surrounded by boxes.[21] The boxes are being placed close to each other on a horizontal line. The patient is told that that 0 represents one extreme of pain and 10 the other and is asked to place an "X" through the number representing his or her pain level. According to some studies 11-point scales are the most popular for the patients when they are asked to quantify their pain.[24]

Visual analogue scale (VAS) is the oldest graphical rating scale and has been used in the measurement of feelings since 1960.[25] In the rating of itch it is by far the most used scale. It is presented as a 100 mm line anchored by verbal descriptors, which usually are "no itch" and "worst imaginable itch." The patient is asked to put an "X" on the line to indicate itch intensity.[21] Evaluation may differ between individuals; there are also cultural differences in expressing feelings. However within an individual it is convenient to compare VAS at different time points, such as in the evaluation of therapy.

VAS may be difficult to use without supervision and explanation especially among older patients and children.[21] However, when supervised, children, aged 6–12 years, were able to discriminate between different itch stimuli in a dose dependent manner.[26]

The line is usually placed horizontally which is the most natural position in Western countries. Interestingly, in Chinese patients the vertical scale demonstrated less error.[24] This suggests that the graphic orientation of the VAS should be decided according to the normal reading tradition of the population on which it is being used.[24]

In children a vertical VAS, the so called colour analogue scale (CAS) which looks like a thermometer has been used to evaluate pediatric patients at emergency department.[23] The bottom, where the thermometer is small and white means no pain and the top where it is wider and red means the most imaginable pain. The children were supervised and asked to put a marker to the spot on the thermometer that shows the pain they were having at the moment.[23]

Ratings of pain or itch as of "right now," such as at the emergency department, are probably more reliable than retrospective ratings after an interval of time. Therefore a microcomputer based system, Pain-Track (Autenta AB, Uppsala, Sweden), was constructed to be worn by the patient all day for hourly assessment of pain.[27] This instrument, called "Symtrack," was further developed for assessment of itch.[28] It is a microcomputer data logger to be carried by the patient all day with a switch indicating conditions of being awake or asleep. Every hour during the day there is a signal to remind the patient to rate their itch by moving a lever along a 100 mm VAS.

## 8.5 Measurement of the Quality of Itch

The milestone in the rating of the quality of pain has been the McGill Pain Questionnaire, which according to PubMed has been used in about 32,000 publications since 1975 when it was described by Ronald Melzack at the McGills University of Montreal.[29] The questionnaire was constructed to collect quantitative information that can be treated statistically, and is sufficiently sensitive to detect differences among different methods to relieve pain.[29] It consists primarily of three major classes of word descriptors: sensory, affective and evaluative. In the primary version of McGill questionnaire the questions were read loud to the patients by a research assistant. In the sensory and affective part of the questionnaire the patients should describe what the pain feels like by choosing words that best describe it; out of 78 words within 20 categories. Categories that were not suitable should be omitted and only one word within a category should be used. In the next part, the patients should describe how their pain changes with time and what kind of things relieve their pain and what increases it. In the last part, the patients were asked to rate their pain using a five point verbal rating scale (VRS-5). This scale includes the following five points: mild, discomforting, distressing, horrible and excruciating, respectively, at different time points: right now, when it is at its worst, and when it is at its least.

In analogy to the McGill pain questionnaire, Darsow and co-workers developed a questionnaire for analysing atopic itch, that is, the Eppendorf itch questionnaire.[30] Here, several descriptors of pain were replaced by descriptors of itch. Altogether 40 adjectives describing sensory aspects of itch and 40 adjectives describing affective aspects of itch were included and rated on a five point verbal rating scale (VRS-5) ranging from 0 = "not true" to 4 = "describes exactly my itch sensation." In the next part the patients should describe how their itch changes with time, what kind of things relieve their itch and what increases it. In the last part the patients were asked to rate their pain using VAS. Although this questionnaire was designed for atopic patients it is also suitable for other patients with itch.

In 1987, Melzack published a short form of the McGill questionnaire consisting of 11 sensory descriptors and 4 affective ones which were rated on a 4- point verbal rating scale as 0 = none, 1 = mild, 2 = moderate or 3 = severe.[31] The intensity of the present pain was then rated on the five point verbal rating scale (VRS-5) as in the long form McGill questionnaire and in addition on the VAS to assess the overall intensity scores.

In analogy with the short-form McGill questionnaire, Yosipovitch and co-workers constructed an itch questionnaire to evaluate uremic pruritus.[32] It consists of six sensory descriptors and four affective ones which were rated on a 4-point verbal rating scale (see above). The overall intensity was assessed by the VAS. In addition, descriptors on the effect on sleep as well as on daily activities and habits were included. The last part included behavioural aspects of coping with pruritus and quality of life measures.

## 8.6 Measurement of the Impact of Itch on the Quality of Daily Life

The health-related quality of life parameter is presently recognized as a primary outcome in clinical trials and in population studies. Dermatologists have long recognized the impact of skin disease on a patient's quality of life which can now be measured using a dermatology quality of life index.[33] This questionnaire consists of 10 questions assessing the magnitude of skin problems over the previous week. The questions concern itching, embarrassment, interference with: domestic activities, clothes, social activities, sporting, working, relations with the partner, and close friends, sexual difficulties and the impact of the treatment on daily life. The answers are rated on a 4-point scale.

In a recent study, Verhoeven at al found that approximately 50% of their 492 dermatology patients experience itch and fatigue and 25% suffer from severe symptoms.[34] Occurrence of these symptoms was significantly associated with lower disease-related quality of life and a more severe skin disease. These results indicate the importance of both qualitative and quantitative assessment of itch.

## References

1. Wallengren J. Neuroanatomy and neurophysiology of itch. *Dermatol Ther*. 2005;18:292–303.
2. Rees JL, Laidlaw A. Pruritus: more scratch than itch. *Clin Exp Dermatol*. 1999;24(6):490–493.
3. Savin JA, Paterson WD, Oswald I. Scratching during sleep. *Lancet*. 1973;2(7824):296–297.
4. Felix R, Shuster S. A new method for the measurement of itch and the response to treatment. *Br J Dermatol*. 1975;93(3): 303–312.
5. Summerfield JA, Welch ME. The measurement of itch with sensitive limb movement meters. *Br J Dermatol*. 1980; 103(3):275–281
6. Aoki T, Kushimoto H, Hisikawa Y, et al. Nocturnal scratching and its relationship to the disturbed sleep of itchy subjects. *Clin Exp Dermatol*. 1991;16(4):268–272
7. Mustakallio KK, Räsanen T. Scratch radar. *Skin Pharmacol* 1989;2:233.
8. Ebata T, Aizawa H, Kamide R. An infrared video camera system to observe nocturnal scratching in atopic dermatitis patients. *J Dermatol*. 1996;23(3):153–155
9. Benjamin K, Waterston K, Russell M, Schofield O, Diffey B, The development of an objective method for measuring scratch in children with atopic dermatitis suitable for clinical use. *J Am Acad Dermatol*. 2004;50(1):33–40
10. Bringhurst C, Waterston K, Schofield O, et al. Measurement of itch using actigraphy in pediatric and adult populations. *J Am Acad Dermatol*. 2004;51(6):893–898
11. Hon KLE, Lam MC, Leung WY, et al. Nocturnal wrist movements are correlated with objective clinical scores and plasma chemokine levels in children with atopic dermatitis. *Br J Dermatol*. 2006;154(4):629–635
12. Bijak M, Mayr W, Rafolt D, et al. Pruritometer 2: portable recording system for the quantification of scratching as objective criterion for the pruritus. *Biomed Tech (Berl)*. 2001;46(5):137–141.
13. Inagaki N, Igeta K, Shiraishi N, et al. Evaluation and characterization of mouse scratching behavior by a new apparatus, *MicroAct. Skin Pharmacol Appl Skin Physiol*. 2003;16(3): 165–175.
14. Rees JL, Flecknell P, Laidlaw A. Production of acute and chronic itch with histamine and contact sensitizers in the mouse and guinea pig. *Exp Dermatol*. 2002;11(4): 285–291.
15. Brash HM, McQueen DS, Christie D, et al. A repetitive movement detector used for automatic monitoring and quantification of scratching in mice. *J Neurosci Methods*. 2005; 142(1):107–114.
16. Seo YJ, Kwon MS, Shim EJ, et al. Changes in pain behavior induced by formalin, substance P, glutamate and pro-inflammatory cytokines in immobilization-induced stress mouse model. *Brain Res Bull*. 2006;71(1–3):279–286.
17. Osborne MG, Coderre TJ. Nociceptive effects of intrathecal administration of sulphur-containing amino acids. *Behav Brain Res*. 2003;144(1–2):105–110.
18. Greaves MW, McDonald-Gibson W. Itch. Role of prostaglandins. *Br Med J*. 1973;3(5881):608–609.
19. Fjellner B, Hägermark O. Studies on pruritogenic and histamine-releasing effects of some putative peptide neurotransmitters. *Acta Derm Venereol*. 1981;61(3): 245–250.
20. Rukwied R, Lischetzki G, McGlone F, et al. Mast cell mediators other than histamine induce pruritus in atopic dermatitis patients: a dermal microdialysis study. *Br J Dermatol*. 2000;142(6):1114–1120.
21. Jensen MP, Karoly P, Braver S. The measurement of clinical pain intensity: a comparison of six methods. *Pain*. 1986;27: 117–126.
22. Belville RG, Seupaul RA. Pain measurement in pediatric emergency care: a review of the faces pain scale-revised. *Pediatr Emerg Care*. 2005;21(2):90–93.
23. Bulloch B, Tenenbein M. Validation of the Ottawa Knee Rule in children: a multicenter study. *Ann Emerg Med*. 2003;42(1):48–55.
24. Williamson A, Hoggart B. Pain: a review of three commonly used pain rating scales. *J Clin Nurs*. 2005;14(7):798–804.
25. Aitken RCB. A growing edge of measurement of feelings. *Proc R Soc Med*. 1969;62:989–993.
26. Wahlgren CF. Children's rating of itch: an experimental study. *Pediatr Dermatol*. 2005;22(2):97–101.

27. Wahlgren CF, Ekblom A, Hägermark O. Some aspects of the experimental induction and measurement of itch. *Acta Derm Venereol.* 1989;69(3):185–189.

28. Hagermark O, Wahlgren CF. Some methods for evaluating clinical itch and their application for studying pathophysiological mechanisms. *J Dermatol Sci.* 1992;4(2):55–62.

29. Melzack R. The McGill Pain Questionnaire: major properties and scoring methods. *Pain.* 1975;1(3):277–299.

30. Darsow U, Scharein E, Simon D, Walter G, Bromm B, Ring J. New aspects of itch pathophysiology: component analysis of atopic itch using the 'Eppendorf Itch Questionnaire'. *Int Arch Allergy Immunol.* 2001;124(1–3):326–331.

31. Melzack R. The short-form McGill Pain Questionnaire. *Pain.* 1987;30(2):191–197.

32. Yosipovitch G, Zucker I, Boner G, Gafter U, Shapira Y, David M. A questionnaire for the assessment of pruritus: validation in uremic patients. *Acta Derm Venereol.* 2001;81(2):108–111

33. Finlay AY, Khan GK. Dermatology Life Quality Index (DLQI) - a simple practical measure for routine clinical use. *Clin Exp Dermatol.* 1994;19(3):210–216.

34. Verhoeven EW, Kraaimaat FW, van de Kerkhof PC, et al. Prevalence of physical symptoms of itch, pain and fatigue in patients with skin diseases in general practice. *Br J Dermatol.* 2007;156(6):1346–1349.

# Chapter 9
# Experimental Models of Itch

Ulysse Pereira and Laurent Misery

## 9.1 Introduction

Pruritus can be defined as an unpleasant cutaneous sensation that leads to the need to scratch. This "umbrella definition" was proposed more than 360 years ago by the German physician Samuel Hafenreffer and does not describe the complexity of this phenomenon. Activation and control of pruritus may occur at different levels of the skin–brain connection[1] like pruritoceptive itch, neurogenic itch, neuropathic itch and psychogenic itch. Because they are different types of pruritus, it is impossible to develop a "universal model of pruritus" and so, different categories of models, according to the purpose of the study, are available. It is obvious that no model is perfect. Each model exhibits advantages for a particular kind of study, and is also restricted by limitations that impede its use in other studies.

## 9.2 Human Studies

This approach is the only one to study the psychogenic itch[2] and serves as a reference to confirm the relevance of other models. Human studies can be performed:

1. On healthy volunteers
   Clinical trials can be used to understand the physiological process of itch with a number of invasive technical approaches like skin prick test or ionotophoresis associated (or not) with different medical imaging techniques[3-5] or the use of transcutaneous electrical stimulations[6-8] or microdialysis studies.[9]

2. On patients with pruritus
   The interest of these studies is to better understand different causes of the itching[10-16] and to evaluate treatments[17-19] (see Chapter 8 of this part)

Studies on humans have many limitations. Firstly, medical studies are strongly regulated for legal and ethical reasons. Secondly, the cost of the logistics are very high. Thirdly, such research presents scientific limitations like the size of the group studied (difficulty in finding a cohort). Difficulties to perform studies on humans make the use of experimental models necessary.

## 9.3 Animal Models

The legislation of studies on laboratory animals is based on the principle that, under certain conditions, it is morally acceptable to use animals for scientific or experimental purposes. That is why, most of our knowledge of biochemistry, physiology and pharmacology comes from studies on animals. However, are animals good models for human biology and disease? Is it possible to substitute it by another model? "There is simply no way that we are even within decades of being able to replace the complexity of living organism with a tissue culture dish or a silicon chip."[20] In this context, the choice of species can be critical, must be well thought-out and may be fundamental to the validity of extrapolations from animals to humans. For example, "Is this model simply reproducing the clinical signs of a disease, or reflecting the actual cause of the disease, such as the reflecting agent or the genetic defect? Animal species with similar

L. Misery and S. Ständer (eds.), *Pruritus*,
DOI 10.1007/978-1-84882-322-8_9, © Springer-Verlag London Limited 2010

genetic predispositions, or metabolic pathways, or those that show similar diseases as human may be better models. For pruritus, researchers have developed different animal models (normal or pathological) of itch (or the pathological source of pruritus) that they would study. Animal models present lots of interest but before starting any work, it is important to appraise if the specific approach of a given study is appropriate for the scientific objectives. There are three points to establish before beginning any animal study:

1. Can I use another alternative method to obtain my result or has the model been validated, if so how, and is it scientifically acceptable?
2. The choice of the animal is the critical step. Which species must I choose?
3. The last question is about whether adequate facilities are available locally to create the model.

### 9.3.1 Rodents

The rodents are commonly used for their multiple facilities. These species are easily available, fast in reproduction, small in size, cost less and easy to handle. For example, guinea pig is used in animal testing to discover treatments against allergic conjunctivitis, a source of pruritus. This model is based on a conjunctivitis induced by repeated sensitizations of the *Hartley guinea* pigs eyes by ovalbumine and by the observation of the ocular itch-scratch response.[21–23] Rat is also used for allergic conjunctivitis[24,25] or studies on cholestasis,[26] Dolichos pruriens,[27] dermatis[28] and spinal cord cavernous hemangioma.[29] These models differ by the methods employed to induce the symptoms and they are based on the observation of hind limb scratch. This measure is based on a scratching behavior that typically manifests as multiple bouts of variable duration, with each bout consisting of rapid back-and-forth movements of the toenails of the hind paw across the region of treated skin, usually of the nape of neck.[30] Rats, were also used to expand our knowledge of physiological itching like pruritoceptive itch[31–33] or neurogenic itch[34–36] and neuropathic itch.[37] However, in the rodent family the mice are the most used rodents to explore the physiological pathway of itch in the skin[38–43] or in the central nervous system.[44,45] Mice with induced (or constitutional) diseases could

be used to elucidate mechanisms and to develop new, appropriate drugs for therapy, for example: atopic dermatis,[46–48] auto-immune disease,[49] diisocyanate-induced asthma,[50] cholestatsis.[51] Actually, four different groups of mouse models can be distinguished:

1. Mouse models with spontaneous development of the disease.[52]
2. Genetically engineered mice (transgenic, knockout).[53,54]
3. Disease induced by protein sensitization.[55,56]
4. Humanized mouse models.[57]

One of the major interests of mouse models is the genetic tools which allow characterizing the implication of a gene in pathology.[58–60] An example of this application is the study of Carstens team on the application of the SP in the central neurotransmission of itch. For that, they use knockout mice (KO) with the deletion of the pre-protachykinin A gene and they compare the pruritus activity of serotonine to that of the wild mice.[61]

Despite these advantages, small animals differ from humans in a number of anatomical and physiological ways. For example, these animals have a dense layer of body hair, thin epidermis and dermis. Furthermore, rodents present significant differences in pruritoceptive and neurogenic itch in comparison with humans. For example, neuropeptide like substances P, which can evoke scratching in humans are not able to do so in rodent or are needed in different intensity. These species difference in the in vivo pharmacology of itch significantly contribute to different results and interpretations. The most representative example is unmistakably histamine the most famous human pruritogenious. This active substance does not evoke itching in rodents.[32,62–64] On the other hand, some substance induce itching in rodents and not in humans.[65] In the same manner at the CNS level, the spinal administration of morphine evokes intense long lasting itching sensation in humans but not in rodents.[66,67] Furthermore, some scratching responses in rodents can be induce by pain and attenuated by morphine and do not reflect an itching sensation.

### 9.3.2 Pig

Large animals are less used in animal research in consideration of their cost and also of their size, housing, and reproduction. These limitations have limited their use but pig is being increasingly exploited for modeling human disease. Because, porcine organs are physiologically very similar to those of humans and a variety of human diseases also occur in pigs. Pigs present a very intriguing large animal model to study cutaneous disease[68] because the structure and the morphology of pig skin is very similar to that of the human skin.[69] Both pig and humans have a thick epidermis. Human epidermis ranges from 50 to 120 μm and the pig's from 30 to 140 μm and the measure of dermal–epidermal thickness ratio ranges from 10:1 to 13:1 in the two species.[70] Furthermore, they show well-developed rete-rigdes and dermal papillary bodies, and abundant subdermal adipose tissue.[71,72] However, although the pig stratum corneum is most similar to the human corneum in terms of lipid composition, they differ in terms of thickness.[73] Nevertheless, the thickness of newborn pig stratum corneum is considerably thinner than that of adult pig and closest to that of human skin. Another element reinforcing the use of swine model is the similarity of the neurogenic inflammation.[74] In fact, contrary to rodents, pigs react for the same molecule and in the same intensity like humans. The best example of that is the impact of histamine, which induced an INC associated with neuropeptides release.[75] This measure agrees with the study of the porcine TRPV1 which demonstrates the very close response between human and swine.[76] Furthermore pigs are used for the study of human neuropathology.[77] All these elements contribute to develop porcine models in neuro-cutaneous studies. Actually, pigs are currently used in the permeation studies[78–80] or for decontamination models[81] and inflammation models[82–85] and also for atopic dermatis models.[86]

### 9.3.3 Non-Human Primates

In the animal kingdom, non-human primates are the closest to humans for their sensory system. Humans and monkeys have similar thresholds for detecting stimuli and for neural treatment of stimuli.[87] For the example of pruritus, monkeys have scratching responses when they receive histamine or spinal administration of morphine in the same intensity as human, This homology of spinal behavior allows the study of the impacts of intrathecal injection of morphinergic and itching.[88,89] However, ethical and financial reasons strongly reduce the use of primates for research.

To avoid wasteful animal experiment, most scientific communities and governments are agreeing with a growing ethical practice. In this option, the Three Rs were proposed by Russell and Burch (1959). These texts are the guiding principles for the use of animals in research in many countries.

*R*efinement: Those methods which avoid, alleviate, or minimize the potential pain, distress, or other adverse effects suffered by the animals involved, or which enhance animal wellbeing.

*R*educe: Refers to methods that enable researchers to obtain comparable levels of information from fewer animals, or to obtain more information from the same number of animals.

*R*eplacement: Refers to the preferred use of non-animal methods over animal methods whenever it is possible to achieve the same scientific aim. This last point introduces the interest of in vitro studies.

## 9.4 In Vitro Models

In the light of the directive 67/548/EEC of the European commission and at the same time pursuing the goal of reducing the number of laboratory animals used, the scientists try to develop reliable in vitro tests. However, the modeling of itching is very complex because it is impossible to assemble in the same dish all actors of the pruritus. In fact, the purpose of in vitro models is not to recreate the whole pathophysiogeny of itch but more simple degrees of complexity (multi cellular, cell, and receptor). In vitro studies on itch are not dissociable from studies on inflammation. This more restricted environment allows for a strict control of conditions with the possibility to repeat experimentations.

The first described difference between pruritoceptors and nociceptors was by the strong responses of pruritoceptors to histamine.[90] Histamine is undoubtedly the best-known pruritogen and has been regarded as the main target for antipruritic therapies. However, the histamine-sensitive fiber subclass cannot account for all aspects of itch, especially when pruritus is induced mechanically or without the characteristic flare reaction. Thus, other subgroups of primary afferents must be involved in the generation of pruritus.[8] Studies of sensory neurons involved in itching are obvious and there is no currently known difficulty. But there is no specific tag of prurito-neurons. Nevertheless, these in vitro studies give lots of information through electrophysiology,[91] calcium measure,[92] Elisa test of neuropeptides,[93] or immunofluocytology.[94]

Neurons are not the only cells involved in pruritus. The skin is a major sensory organ. The whole epidermis is the forefront of the sensory system[95,96] (see Chapter 3 of this part). A new approach, of pruritus is to study receptors on skin cells like TRPV1, or PAR 2[97,98] or mediators (NGF, neuropeptides, cytokines, etc.) are implicated. These studies can give clues for the understanding of the cellular communication between nerves and cells like keratinocytes,[99] Merkel cells, melanocytes, mast cells,[100] or endothelial cells.[101]

Mast cells are of particular interest because they are the main producer of histamine and are able to release a wide variety of other inflammatory mediators implied in itching like proteases, TNF-alpha, and interleukins. The first approach of an in vitro model of pruritus was to test the impact of different molecules on mast cell degranulation induced by compound 48/80. This degranulation can be studied by different methods: Measurement of histamine release by the *o*-phtaldialdehyde spectrofluorometric procedure,[102,103] or interleukins, TNF-alpha or protease release by enzyme-linked immunosorbent assay (ELISA).[104,105] The second approach on mast cells was the study of the impact of molecules on these mediators of inflammation by RT-PCR[106] or on the presence on the transcription factor (NF)-kB in the nuclear compartment by Western blot.[107] Activation of mast cell leads to phosphorylation of tyrosine kinase and mobilization of internal $Ca^{2+}$ followed by activation of protein kinase C, mitogen-activated protein kinases (MAPKs), and nuclear factors such as NF-kB. MAPK and NF-kB are thought to play an important role in the regulation of pro-inflammatory molecule synthesis on cellular responses, especially TNF-alpha, IL-1 beta and IL-6.

Nevertheless, pruritus is based on a cellular communication. The next step for a better model is to assemble different cells types in the same environment in co-culture systems. Mast cells were included in the first co-cultures systems. Interactions of mast cells and neurites were established in 1999.[108–111]

Because pruritoceptors appear located in the epidermis, a more reliable model of pruritus must mimic these contacts between epidermis and fiber nerves. The major problem of such cultures is the difficulty to establish a shared environment. Keratinocytes need a low-calcium level to proliferate in vitro contrary to neurons, which need a higher calcium level for their axonal growth.[112] Nonetheless, in vitro studies of the interactions between keratinocytes and sensory neurons in co-cultures are possible. Primary new born spinal cord cells were grown in special 35 mm dishes with primary rat astrocytes conditioned medium. Reproducing in vivo conditions in the dishes by using three different compartments, for Keratinocytes (the skin), sensory neurons (the dorsal root ganglia) and spinal cord cells (the spinal cord)., connected by microchannels was tried. Sensory neurons spontaneously emit neurites toward epidermal and spinal compartments. This approach permitted the first studies of the communication between the keratinocytes and sensory neurons.[113] This interesting model showed some limitations for studies on itch. The conditioned medium used presented a high variability among each of the experimentations. The format of the dishes was incompatible with multiple series of tests. The number of contacts between keratinocytes and neurites was not reproducible A co-culture of human and rat cells might induce artifacts.

For studies on itch, a single-species model was chosen. The easiest could be to develop a model with rodent cells but the bibliographical study of the in vivo observations demonstrated that the rodent was a very bad choice to study the pruritus.[32,62–64] Pork cells appear more pertinent because this choice was based on its similarity with the human and neurogenic inflammation and this (similarity) is extended to itching.[76] This new model was performed for screening conditions. Keratinocytes and the sensory neurons were pooled in 96-wheel plaques. After 1 week of co-culture, an enzyme immunoassay (EIA) of SP, one marker of neurogenic inflammation was performed. Basal concentration of SP released in the medium after incubation was compared with compounds which are known to induce the neurogenic inflammation like capsaicin or proteases. Furthermore, this induced SP-release as in in vivo conditions can be amplified by pre-treatment with prostaglandin E2 (an itch inducer) or decreased by the pre-treatment with ruthenium red (antagonist of calcium channels). Hence, we are able to test the capacity of molecules to modulate SP release and the artificial CNI induced by addition of capsaicin. This model could be a reliable tool for screening new molecules with anti-inflammatory or apaisant or anti-pruritic effects.

Another in vitro model of itch is based on a compartmented model with integrated electrodes (Fig. 9.1).

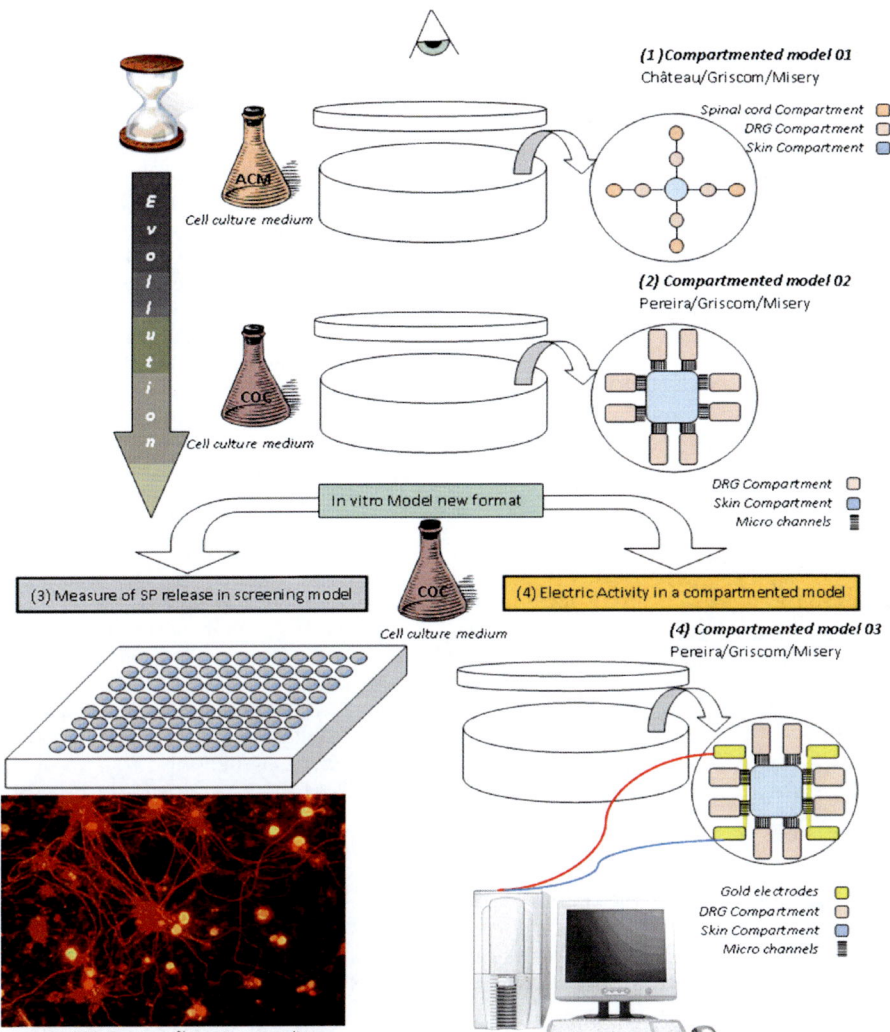

**Fig. 9.1** Evolution of an in vitro model of skin and nerve interactions, like pruritus The primary format (1) of *in vitro* model of the interactions between keratinocytes and sensory neurons in co-cultures tried to reproduce *in vivo* conditions by three different compartments, connected by micro-channels. Human keratinocytes (the skin), rat sensory neurons (the dorsal root ganglia) and rat spinal cord cells (the spinal cord). Cells were grown in special dishes with primary rat astrocytes conditioned medium (ACM). The first evolution of this model (2) was to cancel the spinal cord compartment and to develop a porcine model in reproducible co-culture medium (COC). This new format was incompatible with multiple series of tests. To get around this problem a new format of non compartmented model was performed to screening conditions (3). This in vitro model associated with substance P ELISA could be a reliable tool for screening new molecules with anti-inflammatory or apaisant or anti-pruritic effects. Another alternative model of itch (4) is based on a compartmented format with integrated electrodes where the nerves impulse resulting of stimulation in keratinocyte compartment could be measured through gold electrodes

In this alternative model, the nerve impulse resulting in stimulations in the keratinocyte compartment could be measured through gold electrodes.

In vivo and in vitro experimental approaches are complementing. To understand the pathways in the interacting networks (like in pruritus), integration of the numerous information from genomics, transcriptomics, proteomics, metabolomics, clinical, and epidemiological data by using *in silico* models might be necessary.

## 9.5 In Silico and in Virtuo Models

Biological systems are complex systems consisting of numerous dynamic networks of biochemical reactions and signaling interactions between cellular components. This complexity makes it virtually unanalyzable by traditional methods. *In silico* models allows merging of different information. In the near future, these models will be used to reproduce experimental data or to estimate hidden system parameters that might be not experimentally accessible.

Now, no *in silico* model is available for the study of itching. Such models require comprehensive databases for merging information from different kinds of studies. For example, we can cite these:

1. The study of the mast cells specific genes.[114] This project rests on applied microarray technologies involved in allergic diseases. The objective is to create a database, which would allow constructing human mast cell models *in silico* by analyzing integrative information regarding the genome, transcriptome and proteome of mast cells.
2. *In virtuo* model for research on allergic reaction. This project uses mathematical modeling to reproduce the different steps of allergy in the skin after histamine injection.[115] This model is based on the the reification of interactions into the autonomous active objects.

Actually, alternative methods cannot wholly substitute animal research about itch because they cannot mimic the complex interactions that occur within a living organism. The in vitro and *in silico* models are convenient research tools for screening.

## References

1. Pereira U, Misery L. Understanding pruritus. *Keratin.* 2006;11:12–18.
2. Misery L, Alexandre S, Detray S et al. Functional itch disorder or psychogenic pruritus: suggested diagnosis criteria from the French psychodermatology group. *Acta Derm Venereol.* 2007;87(4):341–344.
3. Walter B, et al. Brain activation by histamine prick test-induced itch. *J Invest Dermatol.* 2005;125(2):380–382.
4. Valet M, et al. Cerebral processing of histamine-induced itch using short-term alternating temperature modulation – an fMRI study. *J Invest Dermatol.* 2008; 128(2):426–433.
5. Mochizuki H, et al. Neural correlates of perceptual difference between itching and pain: a human fMRI study. *Neuroimage.* 2007;36(3):706–717.
6. Dundas JE, Thickbroom GW, Mastaglia FL. Perception of comfort during transcranial DC stimulation: effect of NaCl solution concentration applied to sponge electrodes. *Clin Neurophysiol.* 2007;118(5):1166–1170.
7. Ozawa M, et al. Neuroselective transcutaneous electric stimulation reveals body area-specific differences in itch perception. *J Am Acad Dermatol.* 2006;55(6):996–1002.
8. Ikoma A, et al. Electrically evoked itch in humans. *Pain.* 2005;113(1–2):148–154.
9. Blunk, JA, et al. Opioid-induced mast cell activation and vascular responses is not mediated by mu-opioid receptors: an in vivo microdialysis study in human skin. *Anesth Analg.* 2004;98(2):364–370, table of contents.
10. Yosipovitch G, et al. Skin barrier structure and function and their relationship to pruritus in end-stage renal disease. *Nephrol Dial Transplant.* 2007;22(11):3268–3272.
11. Hosogi M, et al. Bradykinin is a potent pruritogen in atopic dermatitis: a switch from pain to itch. *Pain.* 2006;126(1–3):16–23.
12. Namura K, et al. Relationship of serum brain-derived neurotrophic factor level with other markers of disease severity in patients with atopic dermatitis. *Clin Immunol.* 2007;122(2):181–186.
13. Raychaudhuri SP, Raychaudhuri SK. Role of NGF and neurogenic inflammation in the pathogenesis of psoriasis. *Prog Brain Res.* 2004;146:433–437.
14. Toyoda M, et al. Localization and content of nerve growth factor in peripheral blood eosinophils of atopic dermatitis patients. *Clin Exp Allergy.* 2003;33(7):950–955.
15. Toyoda M, et al. Nerve growth factor and substance P are useful plasma markers of disease activity in atopic dermatitis. *Br J Dermatol.* 2002;147(1):71–79.
16. Patel T, Ishiuji Y, Yosipovitch G. Nocturnal itch: why do we itch at night? *Acta Derm Venereol.* 2007;87(4):295–298.
17. Legroux-Crespel E, Cledes J, Misery L. A comparative study on the effects of naltrexone and loratadine on uremic pruritus. *Dermatology.* 2004;208(4):326–330.
18. Misery L, Cambazard F. Pruritis (with treatment). Diagnostic approach. *Rev Prat.* 2002;52(10):1139–1144.
19. Shohrati M, et al. Cetirizine, doxepine, and hydroxyzine in the treatment of pruritus due to sulfur mustard: a randomized clinical trial. *Cutan Ocul Toxicol.* 2007;26(3):249–255.
20. Kim L. Of mice and men. Momentum 2002;4(3):1–10.
21. Kato M, et al. Apafant, a potent platelet-activating factor antagonist, blocks eosinophil activation and is effective in the chronic phase of experimental allergic conjunctivitis in guinea pigs. *J Pharmacol Sci.* 2004;95(4):435–442.
22. Woodward DF, Nieves AL, Friedlaender MH. Characterization of receptor subtypes involved in prostanoid-induced conjunctival pruritus and their role in mediating allergic conjunctival itching. *J Pharmacol Exp Ther.* 1996;279(1):137–142.
23. Woodward DF, et al. Characterization of a behavioral model for peripherally evoked itch suggests platelet-activating factor as a potent pruritogen. *J Pharmacol Exp Ther.* 1995;272(2):758–765.

24. Minami K, Kamei C. A chronic model for evaluating the itching associated with allergic conjunctivitis in rats. *Int Immunopharmacol*. 2004;4(1):101–108.

25. Minami K, Fujii Y, Kamei C. Participation of chemical mediators in the development of experimental allergic conjunctivitis in rats. *Int Immunopharmacol*. 2004;4(12): 1531–1535.

26. Inan S, Cowan A. Nalfurafine, a kappa opioid receptor agonist, inhibits scratching behavior secondary to cholestasis induced by chronic ethynylestradiol injections in rats. *Pharmacol Biochem Behav*. 2006;85(1):39–43.

27. de Paula Coelho C, et al. Therapeutic and pathogenetic animal models for Dolichos pruriens. *Homeopathy*. 2006;95(3): 136–143.

28. Hayashi K, et al. Effects of olopatadine hydrochloride on the cutaneous vascular hyperpermeability and the scratching behavior induced by poly-L-arginine in rats. *Jpn J Pharmacol*. 2001;87(2):167–170.

29. Dey DD, Landrum O, Oaklander AL. Central neuropathic itch from spinal-cord cavernous hemangioma: a human case, a possible animal model, and hypotheses about pathogenesis. *Pain*. 2005;113(1–2):233–237.

30. Nojima H, Carstens E. Quantitative assessment of directed hind limb scratching behavior as a rodent itch model. *J Neurosci Methods*. 2003;126(2):137–143.

31. Thomsen JS, et al. The effect of topically applied salicylic compounds on serotonin-induced scratching behaviour in hairless rats. *Exp Dermatol*. 2002;11(4):370–375.

32. Thomsen JS, et al. Scratch induction in the rat by intradermal serotonin: a model for pruritus. *Acta Derm Venereol*. 2001; 81(4):250–254.

33. Nojima H, Carstens MI, Carstens E. c-fos expression in superficial dorsal horn of cervical spinal cord associated with spontaneous scratching in rats with dry skin. *Neurosci Lett*. 2003;347(1):62–64.

34. Jinks SL, Carstens E. Superficial dorsal horn neurons identified by intracutaneous histamine: chemonociceptive responses and modulation by morphine. *J Neurophysiol*. 2000;84(2):616–627.

35. Carstens E. Responses of rat spinal dorsal horn neurons to intracutaneous microinjection of histamine, capsaicin, and other irritants. *J Neurophysiol*. 1997;77(5):2499–2514.

36. Nojima H, et al. Opioid modulation of scratching and spinal c-fos expression evoked by intradermal serotonin. *J Neurosci*. 2003;23(34):10784–10790.

37. Gingold AR, Bergasa NV. The cannabinoid agonist WIN 55, 212–2 increases nociception threshold in cholestatic rats: implications for the treatment of the pruritus of cholestasis. *Life Sci*. 2003;73(21):2741–2747.

38. Andoh T. Importance of epidermal keratinocytes in itching. *Yakugaku Zasshi*. 2006;126(6):403–408.

39. Yamaoka J, et al Erratum to "changes in cutaneous sensory nerve fibers induced by skin-scratching in mice". *J Dermatol Sci*. 2007;47(2):172–182.

40. Yamaoka J, et al. Changes in cutaneous sensory nerve fibers induced by skin-scratching in mice. *J Dermatol Sci*. 2007;46(1):41–51.

41. Yamashita H, et al. Pharmacological characterization of a chronic pruritus model induced by multiple application of 2,4,6-trinitrochlorobenzene in NC mice. *Eur J Pharmacol*. 2007;563(1–3):233–239.

42. Costa SK, et al. How important are NK1 receptors for influencing microvascular inflammation and itch in the skin? Studies using Phoneutria nigriventer venom. *Vascul Pharmacol*. 2006;45(4):209–214.

43. Shimada SG, Shimada KA, Collins JG. Scratching behavior in mice induced by the proteinase-activated receptor-2 agonist, SLIGRL-NH2. *Eur J Pharmacol*. 2006;530(3): 281–283.

44. Sun YG, Chen ZF. A gastrin-releasing peptide receptor mediates the itch sensation in the spinal cord. *Nature*. 2007;448(7154):700–703.

45. Umeuchi H, et al. Involvement of central mu-opioid system in the scratching behavior in mice, and the suppression of it by the activation of kappa-opioid system. *Eur J Pharmacol*. 2003;477(1):29–35.

46. Yatsuzuka R, et al. Development of new atopic dermatitis models characterized by not only itching but also inflammatory skin in mice. *Eur J Pharmacol*. 2007;565(1–3): 225–231.

47. Akamatsu H, et al. The effect of fexofenadine on pruritus in a mouse model (HR-ADf) of atopic dermatitis. *J Int Med Res*. 2006;34(5):495–504.

48. Sasakawa T, et al. Topical application of FK506 (tacrolimus) ointment inhibits mite antigen-induced dermatitis by local action in NC/Nga mice. *Int Arch Allergy Immunol*. 2004; 133(1):55–63.

49. Umeuchi H, et al. Spontaneous scratching behavior in MRL/lpr mice, a possible model for pruritus in autoimmune diseases, and antipruritic activity of a novel kappa-opioid receptor agonist nalfurafine hydrochloride. *Eur J Pharmacol*. 2005;518(2–3):133–139.

50. Herrick CA, et al. A novel mouse model of diisocyanate-induced asthma showing allergic-type inflammation in the lung after inhaled antigen challenge. *J Allergy Clin Immunol*. 2002;109(5):873–878.

51. Nelson L, et al. Endogenous opioid-mediated antinociception in cholestatic mice is peripherally, not centrally, mediated. *J Hepatol*. 2006;44(6):1141–1149.

52. Onishi N, et al. A new immunomodulatory function of low-viscous konjac glucomannan with a small particle size: its oral intake suppresses spontaneously occurring dermatitis in NC/Nga mice. *Int Arch Allergy Immunol*. 2005;136(3): 258–265.

53. Baiou D, et al. Neurochemical characterization of insulin receptor-expressing primary sensory neurons in wild-type and vanilloid type 1 transient receptor potential receptor knockout mice. *J Comp Neurol*. 2007;503(2): 334–347.

54. Tzavara ET, et al. Endocannabinoids activate transient receptor potential vanilloid 1 receptors to reduce hyperdopaminergia-related hyperactivity: therapeutic implications. *Biol Psychiatry*. 2006;59(6):508–515.

55. Spergel JM, et al. Epicutaneous sensitization with protein antigen induces localized allergic dermatitis and hyperresponsiveness to methacholine after single exposure to aerosolized antigen in mice. *J Clin Invest*. 1998;101(8):1614–1622.

56. Nojima H, et al. Spinal c-fos expression associated with spontaneous biting in a mouse model of dry skin pruritus. *Neurosci Lett*. 2004;361(1–3):79–82.

57. Gunther C, et al. CCL18 is expressed in atopic dermatitis and mediates skin homing of human memory T cells. *J Immunol*. 2005;174(3):1723–1728.

58. Bigliardi-Qi M, et al. Deletion of mu- and kappa-opioid receptors in mice changes epidermal hypertrophy, density of peripheral nerve endings, and itch behavior. *J Invest Dermatol.* 2007;127(6):1479–1488.

59. Matesic LE, et al. Itch genetically interacts with Notch1 in a mouse autoimmune disease model. *Hum Mol Genet.* 2006;15(24):3485–3497.

60. Deumens R, et al. Mice lacking L1 have reduced CGRP fibre in-growth into spinal transection lesions. *Neurosci Lett.* 2007;420(3):277–281.

61. Cuellar JM, et al. Deletion of the preprotachykinin A gene in mice does not reduce scratching behavior elicited by intradermal serotonin. *Neurosci Lett.* 2003;339(1):72–76.

62. Thomsen JS, et al. Experimental itch in sodium lauryl sulphate-inflamed and normal skin in humans: a randomized, double-blind, placebo-controlled study of histamine and other inducers of itch. *Br J Dermatol.* 2002;146(5):792–800.

63. Simone DA, et al. The magnitude and duration of itch produced by intracutaneous injections of histamine. *Somatosens Res.* 1987;5(2):81–92.

64. Jinks SL, Carstens E. Responses of superficial dorsal horn neurons to intradermal serotonin and other irritants: comparison with scratching behavior. *J Neurophysiol.* 2002;87(3):1280–1289.

65. Kamei A, Hayashi S. Properties of partially purified beta-N-acetylglucosaminidase from bovine crystalline lens. *Biol Pharm Bull.* 1999;22(8):866–869.

66. Palmer CM, et al. Dose-response relationship of intrathecal morphine for postcesarean analgesia. *Anesthesiology.* 1999;90(2):437–444.

67. Lee H, et al. Characterization of scratching responses in rats following centrally administered morphine or bombesin. *Behav Pharmacol.* 2003;14(7):501–508.

68. Dunstan RW, Rosser EJ Jr. Does a condition like human pityriasis rosea occur in pigs? *Am J Dermatopathol.* 1986;8(1):86–89.

69. Meyer W, Schwarz R, Neurand K. The skin of domestic mammals as a model for the human skin, with special reference to the domestic pig. *Curr Probl Dermatol.* 1978;7:39–52.

70. Vardaxis NJ, et al. Confocal laser scanning microscopy of porcine skin: implications for human wound healing studies. *J Anat.* 1997;190(Pt 4):601–611.

71. Morris GM, Hopewell JW. Epidermal cell kinetics of the pig: a review. *Cell Tissue Kinet.* 1990;23(4):271–282.

72. Montagna W, Yun JS. The skin of the domestic pig. *J Invest Dermatol.* 1964;42:11–21.

73. Hammond SA, et al. Transcutaneous immunization of domestic animals: opportunities and challenges. *Adv Drug Deliv Rev.* 2000;43(1):45–55.

74. Rukwied R, et al. Nociceptor sensitization to mechanical and thermal stimuli in pig skin in vivo. *Eur J Pain.* 2008;12(2):242–250.

75. Sann H, Pierau FK. Efferent functions of C-fiber nociceptors. *Z Rheumatol.* 1998;57(suppl 2):8–13.

76. Ohta T, et al. Molecular cloning, functional characterization of the porcine transient receptor potential V1 (pTRPV1) and pharmacological comparison with endogenous pTRPV1. *Biochem Pharmacol.* 2005;71(1–2):173–187.

77. Gillespie JI, Markerink-van Ittersum M, de Vente J. *Sensory collaterals, intramural ganglia and motor nerves in the guinea-pig bladder: evidence for intramural neural circuits.Cell Tissue Res.* 2006;325(1):33–45.

78. Cilurzo F, Minghetti P, Sinico C. Newborn pig skin as model membrane in in vitro drug permeation studies: a technical note. *AAPS Pharm Sci Tech.* 2007;8(4):E94.

79. Sekkat N, Kalia YN, Guy RH. Development of an in vitro model for premature neonatal skin: biophysical characterization using transepidermal water loss. *J Pharm Sci.* 2004;93(12):2936–2940.

80. Sekkat N, Kalia YN, Guy RH. Porcine ear skin as a model for the assessment of transdermal drug delivery to premature neonates. *Pharm Res.* 2004;21(8):1390–1397.

81. Taysse L, et al. Skin decontamination of mustards and organophosphates: comparative efficiency of RSDL and Fuller's earth in domestic swine. *Hum Exp Toxicol.* 2007;26(2):135–141.

82. Monteiro-Riviere NA, Inman AO, Riviere JE. Skin toxicity of jet fuels: ultrastructural studies and the effects of substance P. *Toxicol Appl Pharmacol.* 2004;195(3):339–347.

83. Sabourin CL, et al. Cytokine, chemokine, and matrix metalloproteinase response after sulfur mustard injury to weanling pig skin. *J Biochem Mol Toxicol.* 2002;16(6):263–272.

84. Jancso G, Pierau FK, Sann H. Mustard oil-induced cutaneous inflammation in the pig. *Agents Actions.* 1993;39(1–2):31–34.

85. Nair X, et al. Swine as a model of skin inflammation. Phospholipase A2-induced inflammation. *Inflammation.* 1993;17(2):205–215.

86. Simonsen L, Fullerton A. Development of an in vitro skin permeation model simulating atopic dermatitis skin for the evaluation of dermatological products. *Skin Pharmacol Physiol.* 2007;20(5):230–236.

87. LaMotte RH, Campbell JN. Comparison of responses of warm and nociceptive C-fiber afferents in monkey with human judgments of thermal pain. *J Neurophysiol.* 1978;41(2):509–528.

88. Ko MC, et al. Activation of kappa-opioid receptors inhibits pruritus evoked by subcutaneous or intrathecal administration of morphine in monkeys. *J Pharmacol Exp Ther.* 2003;305(1):173–179.

89. Ko MC, et al. The role of central mu opioid receptors in opioid-induced itch in primates. *J Pharmacol Exp Ther.* 2004;310(1):169–176.

90. Schmelz M, et al. Chemical response pattern of different classes of C-nociceptors to pruritogens and algogens. *J Neurophysiol.* 2003;89(5):2441–2448.

91. Zhu W, et al. Activin acutely sensitizes dorsal root ganglion neurons and induces hyperalgesia via PKC-mediated potentiation of transient receptor potential vanilloid I. *J Neurosci.* 2007;27(50):13770–13780.

92. Shim WS, et al. TRPV1 mediates histamine-induced itching via the activation of phospholipase A2 and 12-lipoxygenase. *J Neurosci.* 2007;27(9):2331–2337.

93. Tang HB, Nakata Y. The activation of transient receptor potential vanilloid receptor subtype 1 by capsaicin without extracellular $Ca^{2+}$ is involved in the mechanism of distinct substance P release in cultured rat dorsal root ganglion neurons. *Naunyn Schmiedebergs Arch Pharmacol.* 2008;377(46):325–332.

94. Liu M, et al. Differential pH and capsaicin responses of Griffonia simplicifolia IB4 (IB4)-positive and IB4-negative small sensory neurons. *Neuroscience.* 2004;127(3):659–672.

95. Denda M, et al. Epidermal keratinocytes as the forefront of the sensory system. *Exp Dermatol.* 2007;16(3):157–161.

96. Boulais N, et al. The whole epidermis as the forefront of the sensory system. *Exp Dermatol.* 2007;16(8):634–635.

97. Stander S, et al. Expression of vanilloid receptor subtype 1 in cutaneous sensory nerve fibers, mast cells, and epithelial cells of appendage structures. *Exp Dermatol.* 2004;13(3):129–139.

98. Biro T, et al. TRP channels as novel players in the pathogenesis and therapy of itch. *Biochim Biophys Acta.* 2007; 1772(8):1004–1021.

99. Southall, MD, et al. Activation of epidermal vanilloid receptor-1 induces release of proinflammatory mediators in human keratinocytes. *J Pharmacol Exp Ther.* 2003;304(1): 217–222.

100. Moormann C, et al. Functional characterization and expression analysis of the proteinase-activated receptor-2 in human cutaneous mast cells. *J Invest Dermatol.* 2006;126(4): 746–755.

101. McQueen DS, Noble MA, Bond SM. Endothelin-1 activates ETA receptors to cause reflex scratching in BALB/c mice. *Br J Pharmacol.* 2007;151(2):278–284.

102. Kim, SH, Shin TY. Amomum xanthiodes inhibits mast cell-mediated allergic reactions through the inhibition of histamine release and inflammatory cytokine production. *Exp Biol Med (Maywood).* 2005;230(9):681–687.

103. Shore PA, Burkhalter A, Cohn, Jr VH. A method for the fluorometric assay of histamine in tissues. *J Pharmacol Exp Ther.* 1959;127:182–186.

104. Kim EK, et al. Lithospermi radix extract inhibits histamine release and production of inflammatory cytokine in mast cells. *Biosci Biotechnol Biochem.* 2007;71(12): 2886–2892.

105. Albrecht M, et al. Ionizing radiation induces degranulation of human mast cells and release of tryptase. *Int J Radiat Biol.* 2007;83(8):535–541.

106. Park HH, et al. Anti-inflammatory activity of fisetin in human mast cells (HMC-1). *Pharmacol Res.* 2007;55(1):31–37.

107. Shin TY, et al. Anti-allergic effects of Lycopus lucidus on mast cell-mediated allergy model. *Toxicol Appl Pharmacol.* 2005;209(3):255–262.

108. De Jonge F, et al. In vitro activation of murine DRG neurons by CGRP-mediated mucosal mast cell degranulation. *Am J Physiol Gastrointest Liver Physiol.* 2004;287(1):G178–G191.

109. Suzuki R, et al. Direct neurite-mast cell communication in vitro occurs via the neuropeptide substance P. *J Immunol.* 1999;163(5):2410–2415.

110. Suzuki R, et al. Bi-directional relationship of in vitro mast cell-nerve communication observed by confocal laser scanning microscopy. *Biol Pharm Bull.* 2001;24(3):291–294.

111. Mori N, et al. Nerve-mast cell (RBL) interaction: RBL membrane ruffling occurs at the contact site with an activated neurite. *Am J Physiol Cell Physiol.* 2002;283(6):C1738–C1744.

112. Ulmann L, et al. Trophic effects of keratinocytes on the axonal development of sensory neurons in a coculture model. *Eur J Neurosci.* 2007;26(1):113–125.

113. Chateau Y, et al. In vitro reconstruction of neuro-epidermal connections. *J Invest Dermatol.* 2007;127(4):979–981.

114. Saito H. Mast cell-specific genes – new drug targets/pathogenesis. *Chem Immunol Allergy.* 2005;87:198–212.

115. Desmeulles G, et al. In virtuo model for research on allergic reaction. *Ann Dermatol Venereol.* 2005;132(8–9 pt 1):697–701.

# Part II
# Clinics

# Chapter 10
# Pruritus, Pain and Other Abnormal Skin Sensations

Laurent Misery

In the past, itch was frequently considered as a minor pain but it is clearly a wrong idea. Pain and itch have some similarities and can be associated, but they have many differences.[1]

## 10.1 Definitions

*Pruritus* can be defined as an unpleasant cutaneous sensation that leads to the need to scratch. *Pain* is defined by the International Association for the Study of Pain (IASP) as "an unpleasant sensory and emotional experience associated with actual or potential tissue damage, or described in terms of such damage."

Experiences that resemble pain or itch but are not unpleasant, e.g., pricking or tickling, should not be called pain or itch. *Tickle* is a sensation with two components: a light pre-noxious sensation (*knismesis*) and laughter-associated sensation (*gargalesis*).[2]

Unpleasant abnormal experiences (dysesthesias) may also be pain but are not necessarily so because, subjectively, they may not have the usual sensory qualities of pain. *Dysesthesias* are abnormal sensations, whether spontaneous or evoked, such as burning, wetness, sensations of pins and needles, etc. *Paresthesias* are sensations of tingling, pricking or numbness of a person's skin with no apparent long-term physical effect.

Many people report pain in the absence of tissue damage or any likely pathophysiological cause; usually this happens for psychological reasons. There is usually no way to distinguish their experience from that due to tissue damage if we take the subjective report. If they regard their experience as pain, and if they report it in the same ways as pain caused by tissue damage, it should be accepted as pain. This definition avoids linking pain to the stimulus. Activity induced in the nociceptor and nociceptive pathways by a noxious stimulus is not pain, which is always a psychological state, even though we may well appreciate that pain most often has a proximate physical cause. *Nociception* (synonyms: nociperception, physiological pain) is the afferent activity produced in the peripheral and central nervous system by stimuli that have the potential to damage tissue.

Itch, pain, nausea, cough, dyspnea or other unpleasant sensations are causes of *suffering*,[3] which can be defined by an individual's basic affective experience of unpleasantness and aversion associated with harm or threat of harm.

From the patient's point of view, it is frequently difficult to distinguish itch from pain or other abnormal sensations. It depends on his/her personal feeling and the sociocultural context. In some languages, there are no different words for itch and pain.

## 10.2 Similarities

Itch and pain share similarities in their transmission from the skin to the brain: C-fibers, sensory nerves, dorsal horn, thalamus and then cerebral cortex. At each level, itch or pain can be initiated, and itch or pain can be neuropathic, neurogenic or psychogenic. From the macroscopic anatomical point of view, they have common areas in the spinal cord (dorsal horn and the brain thalamus, anterior cingulate and insular cortex, somatosensory cortex and even motor areas). Many mediators are able to induce both itch and pain: endothelins, substance P, vasoactive intestinal peptide (VIP), neuropeptide Y, neurotensin, prostaglandins and opioid peptides. The activation of transient receptor potential vanilloid 1 (TRPV1) by protons or capsaicin

L. Misery and S. Ständer (eds.), *Pruritus*,
DOI 10.1007/978-1-84882-322-8_10, © Springer-Verlag London Limited 2010

may induce burning, pain and/or pruritus, and then can inhibit them.[1,4]

Sensitization appears as a common phenomenon for itch and pain.[4] Inflammatory mediators are known to sensitize nociceptors chemically, and a similar mechanism is probably observed with pruriceptors. As a result, inflammation facilitates both pain and itch. Chronic sensitization is more related to neurotrophins. Trophic factors also initiate nerve sprouting and change neuron morphology, facilitating itch or pain. For example, chronic scratching induces the release of nerve growth factor (NGF), which is responsible for neuronal growth and sensitization of nociceptors and pruriceptors.[5,6]

Clinically, peripheral and central sensitization leads to the abnormal perception of normal stimuli, which can be perceived as pain (allodynia) or pruritus (alloknesis). Patients with chronic itch consistently report more itch, while patients with chronic pain report more pain, in response to analogous somatosensory stimuli than healthy controls.[7]

As chronic sensations, itch and pain tend to generalize over the whole skin, to develop sensitization and have a strong impact of quality of life, with the final induction of depression. Some treatments may act on both pain and itch: capsaicin, cannabinoids, gabapentin, pregabalin and other novel anticonvulsivant drugs[8] or antidepressants.

## 10.3 Differences

### 10.3.1 Clinical Aspects

Clinical differences between itch and pain are usually obvious. Nonetheless, it can be useful to know some clinical differences that could be very useful in some cases:

- Itch induces scratching whereas pain induces withdrawal.
- Itch is soothed by cold and aggravated by warmth whereas pain is aggravated by cold and soothed by warmth.
- Itch may be soothed by anti-pruritic treatments, such as antihistamines, but never by analgesics whereas pain is never soothed by anti-pruritics but is eased by antalgics.
- Itch is restricted to the skin and some mucosa whereas pain is ubiquitous.
- Itch is usually triggered by stimuli which are weaker than those which induce pain.

#### 10.3.1.1 Pathogenesis

Itch and pain serve different purposes.[9] The neuronal apparatus might develop itch as a nocifensive system for removal of irritating objects and agents assaulting the skin (parasites, insects, allergens) and thereby preserve the body's integrity. While withdrawal is useful for avoiding pain, scratching appears more appropriate for suppressing external factors.

There are specific pruriceptors in the skin such as mechano-insensitive and pain-insensitive, and theses can be activated by histamine.[10] Histamine-independent pruriceptors defined by their activation by cowhage have been recently described.[11] A specialized class of dorsal horn neurons projecting to the thalamus has been evidenced.[12] Another population of neurons is dedicated to the transmission of cowhage-induced itch in the spinal cord.[13]

Thus the combination of dedicated central and peripheral neurons with a unique response pattern to pruritic mediators and anatomically distinct projections to the thalamus provides the basis of specialized neuronal pathway of itch.[1] These neurons have a very high affinity for histamine, tryptase and prostaglandin E2, whereas pain receptors have a high affinity for bradykinin, ATP, adenosine or acetylcholine. In the brain, itch and pain share common centers, although itch processing is characterized by weaker activation of primary and secondary somatosensory cortexes but relatively stronger activation of ipsilateral motor areas.[14] At the molecular levels, peptides such as opioids are able to induce pruritus through mu receptors and to inhibit it through kappa receptors, with opposite effects on pain.

## 10.4 Interactions

Itch is very well known to be inhibited by painful sensations. Noxious heat stimuli and scratching produce stronger itch reduction than noxious cold stimuli.[15] On the other hand, opioid analgesics can induce itch.

Itch and pain are very frequently associated, especially in women, as demonstrated in a Norwegian study.[16]

# References

1. Ständer S, Schmelz M. Chronic itch and pain – similarities and differences. *Eur J Pain*. 2006;10:473–478.
2. Seledn ST. Tickle. *J Am Acad Dermatol*. 2004; 50:93–97.
3. Misery L. Are pruritus and scratching the cough of the skin? *Dermatology*. 2008;216:3–5.
4. Ikoma A, Steinhoff M, Stander S, Yosipovitch G, Schmelz M. The neurobiology of itch. *Nat Rev*. 2006;7:535–547.
5. Bohm-Starke N, Hilliges M, Brodda-Jansen G, Rylander E, Toerbjörk E. Psychophysical evidence of nociceptor sensitization in vulvar vestibulitis syndrome. *Pain*. 2001;94:177–183.
6. Zhang X, Huang J, Mac Naughton PA. NGF rapidly increases membrane expression of TRPV1 heat-gated ion channels. *EMBO J*. 2005;24:4211–4223.
7. Van Laarhoven AIM, Kraaimaat FW, Wilder-Smith OH, et al. Generalzed and symptom-specific sensitization of chronic itch and pain. *J Eur Acad Dermatol Venereol*. 2007;21:1187–1192.
8. Stefan H, Feuerstein TJ. Novel anticonvulsivant drugs. *Pharmacol Ther*. 2007;113:165–183.
9. Paus R, Schmelz M, Biro T, Steinhoff M. Frontiers in pruritus research: scartching the brain for more effective therapy. *J Clin Invest*. 2006;116:1174–1185.
10. Schmelz M, Schmidt R, Bickel A, Handwerker HO, Torebjörk HE. Specific C-receptors for itch in human skin. *J Neurosci*. 1997;17:2003–2008.
11. Johanek LM, Meyer RA, Hartke T, et al. Psychopysical and physiological evidence for parallel afferent pathways mediating the sensation of itch. *J Neurosci*. 2007;27:7490–7497.
12. Andrew D, Craig AD. Spiothalamaic lamina 1 neurons selectively sensitive to histamine: a central neural pathway for itch. *Nat Neurosci*. 2001;4:72–77.
13. Davidson S, Zhang X, Yoon CH, Khasabov SG, Simone DA, Giesler GJ. The itch-producing agents histamine activate separate populations of primate spinothalaamic tract neurons. *J Neurosci*. 2007;27:10007–10014.
14. Drzezga A, Darsow U, Treede RD, et al. Central activation by histamine-induced itch: analogies to pain processing: a correlational analysis of $O^{15}$ $H_2O$ poistron emission tomography studies. *Pain*. 2001;92:295–305.
15. Yosipovitch G, Fast K, Berhard JD. Noxious heat and scratching decrease histamine-induced itch and skin blood flow. *J Invest Dermatol*. 2005;125:1268–1272.
16. Dalgard F, Dawn AG, Yosipovitch G. Are itch and chronic pain associated in adults? Results of a large population survey in Norway. *Dermatology*. 2007;214:305–309.

# Chapter 11
# The Epidemiology of Pruritus

Florence Dalgard and Elke Weisshaar

## 11.1  Itch in the Community

Epidemiology is the discipline concerned with disease frequency and the associations between risk factors and outcome in the population. Assessment of disease in the community is an important measure not only for the purpose of health planning but also for the understanding of associations between diseases and factors in the environment, as well as meeting the demands and investigating factors of importance to prevent disease in the population.[1, 2]

Individuals presenting themselves to doctors tend to have more severe disease, and so the patient population represents only the tip of the iceberg of the ill health at the community level.[1, 3] Clinical populations are highly selective and depend, for instance, on perceived severity of symptoms and access to health services. The study of a symptom such as itch at the community level can give precious information on associations with demographical factors, psychosocial factors and eventually other diseases in the community. This perspective is different from the clinical one and has the advantage of adding information on the risk factors for itch that cannot be explored so easily in patient populations. The purpose of this chapter is to describe what we know about the distribution of itch in the general population. For information on the distribution in patient populations, refer to the specific chapters in this book.

### 11.1.1  The Prevalence of Itch

Recently, a larger population survey in a Western urban population was conducted which enabled for the first time collection of data on the prevalence of itch. The study was cross-sectional and took place in Oslo in 2000–2001, and a total of 40,888 adult men and women were invited to participate.[4] The questionnaires provided information on sociodemographic factors, self-reported health, various aspects of health behavior, and psychosocial factors. Acute itch was part of a questionnaire on skin complaints.[5]

The question asked was as follows: "In the last week, have you had itchy skin?" The possible answers were: no; yes, a little; yes, quite a lot; yes, very much (Table 11.1). The answers were dichotomized in the descriptive analysis of the prevalence of itch.

The prevalence of acute itch in the general population was found to be 8.4%.[4] It is the most prevalent symptom of all reported skin complaints. This result was derived from a dichotomized answer in which "quite a lot of itching" and "very much itching" were taken into consideration. When looking at the prevalence of the severity of itch, 18.7% of adults reported a little itching, 5.9% quite a lot of itching and 2.5% very much itching. In another community study from 1976 among 2,180 adults (the Lambeth study),[6] prurigo and allied conditions showed a prevalence of 8.2%. A German pilot study of chronic itch in a sample of the general population (n=200) showed a point prevalence of 13.9%. In this study, 16.5% had experienced chronic itch within the last 12 months, and the lifetime prevalence of chronic itch was 22.6%. This indicates a possible higher prevalence of chronic itch in the general population than reported previously.[7] In such studies, any method of assessment will show limitations because, per definition, a subjective experience can only be partly transcribed by an objective measurement.[7, 8]

L. Misery and S. Ständer (eds.), *Pruritus*,
DOI 10.1007/978-1-84882-322-8_11, © Springer-Verlag London Limited 2010

**Table 11.1** Prevalence of reported itch in the general population ($N = 18,747$)

| Total prevalence (itch yes/no) | Itch (%) |
|---|---|
| Severity | 8.4 |
| Yes, a little | 18.7 |
| Yes, quite a lot | 5.9 |
| Yes, very much | 2.5 |

**Table 11.2** The associations of itch and sociodemographic factors in the general population ($N = 18,747$)

| Sociodemographic factors | Itch (%) |
|---|---|
| *Gender* | |
| Males | 7 |
| Females | 9 |
| *Age (years)* | |
| 30 | 11 |
| 40–45 | 8 |
| 59–60 | 7 |
| 75–76 | 6 |
| *Ethnicity* | |
| Norway | 8 |
| Other Western countries | 9 |
| Eastern Europe | 10 |
| Middle East | 14 |
| Indian subcontinent | 13 |
| East Asia | 14 |
| Sub-Saharan Africa | 7 |
| Central and South America | 10 |
| *Socioeconomic status (income)* | |
| Low | 10 |
| Medium | 8 |
| High | 7 |

## 11.2 Itch and Sociodemographic Factors

### 11.2.1 Itch and Demographical Factors

Although gender differences have been little explored in the field of dermatology, the overreport of itch among women confirms other studies.[6, 10, 11] In the Norwegian study, individuals reporting itch were also younger and had a lower household income (Table 11.2).[4]

There is a worldwide variation of itch while considering the age group. Pruritus in children is mainly caused by atopic dermatitis (AD). The prevalence rates of AD vary from 17 to 22% in highly affected countries like Japan, United States, Denmark and Singapore to 7% in Tanzania and 4.3% in Turkey. This most likely explains the differing prevalence of pruritus in children throughout the world. There are no studies investigating the prevalence of pruritus in children alone.

Epidemiological studies focusing on the prevalence of pruritus during pregnancy unrelated to skin diseases are limited. Interestingly, pruritus is described as the main dermatological symptom during pregnancy and is observed in approximately 18% of pregnancies. A French prospective study of 3,192 pregnant women revealed that 1.6% had pruritus. Seventeen cases (0.5%) had pruritus gravidarum; all other cases were pregnancy-specific dermatoses.[12] The prevalence of pruritus in pregnancy was 4.6% in an Indian study of 500 pregnant women, but except 4 cases of pruritus gravidarum all suffered from specific dermatosis of pregnany.[13] The prevalence of pruritus gravidarum was 0.8%.[13] Intrahepatic cholestasis was found to be higher in Chile depending on ethnic predisposition and dietary factors. A prevalence rate of 13.2% was found for pruritus gravidarum and 2.4% for cholestatic jaundice of pregnancy.[14]

Only a small number of studies have investigated pruritus in elderly persons. They are characterized by differing case numbers and differing aims (pruritic skin disease instead of pruritus). A Turkish study detected that pruritus ranked first within the distribution of skin diseases when investigating 4,099 elderly patients. In this study, 11.5% complained about pruritus. Women were more affected (12.0%) than men (11.2%).[15] According to the age group, patients older than 85 years showed the highest prevalence rate (19.5%). When looking at seasonal variations, pruritus was among the five most frequent diagnoses in all seasons, being the most frequent in winter (12.8%) and autumn (12.7%).[15] Pruritic diseases were the most common in a study from Thailand (41%), identifying xerosis (which for the authors was identical with senescent pruritus) as the most frequent (38.9%) form in a total of 149 elderly patients.[16]

### 11.2.2 Itch and Ethnicity

Research in the field of "health and ethnicity" has been difficult because of a lack of standards in defining ethnicity,[17–19] but studies have demonstrated increased mortality rates and cardiovascular morbidity among immigrants. Low socioeconomic position among the immigrants is an important explanatory factor.[17, 20, 21]

Human migration is an increasing phenomenon, and people move into cities in the West, both from rural areas and also from other parts of the globe, forming a multiethnic society.[17–22]

The report of itch seems to be associated with ethnic background in Western communities. The distribution of the report of itch among ethnic groups was slightly different: people from the Middle East and North Africa, as well as those from the Indian subcontinent, report more itch. The ethnic differences with respect to itch are difficult to interpret. Other studies have shown ethnic differences in morbidity, and this is also true for the reporting of itch.[17, 23]

### 11.2.3 Itch and Socioeconomic Status

Itch is more prevalent among people of lower socioeconomic status. Many health outcomes have strong social determinants. The poor and under-resourced carry a higher burden of many diseases.[24–26] The relationship between health and socioeconomic inequality has been shown for mortality, cardiovascular disease, mental health and rheumatoid arthritis.[20, 28, 29] How could social circumstances influence health outcomes? Several explanations have been suggested. The first explanation is social selection: the weakest individuals are over-represented in the lowest socioeconomic classes.[27] A second explanation is cultural factors:life style explains unhealthy health behaviors, for instance concerning diet, smoking, alcohol consumption or physical activity. A third explanation is material use: poor materials used for housing might affect health. Lastly, psychosocial factors related to socioeconomic status have been suggested as an explanation to health inequalities, with stress as a mediating factor.[2]

### 11.3 Itch and Psychosocial Factors

At a community level there is significantly more reporting of itch among persons with mental distress and those who have experienced more than two negative life events. There are more individuals with poor social support among those who reported itch.

It has previously been shown that itch is associated with stress (Table 11.3).[30, 31] The association of itch and

**Table 11.3** The association of itch with psychosocial factors in the general population ($N = 18,747$)

| Psychosocial factors | Itch (%) |
|---|---|
| *Mental distress (Hopkin symptom check list)* | |
| Yes | 16 |
| No | 7 |
| *Negative life events* | |
| None | 6 |
| One event | 9 |
| Two or more | 12 |
| *Social support* | |
| One or none good friend | 10 |
| Two or three | 10 |
| More than four | 8 |

the number of life events is lower for individuals with a good social network than for those with a poor one suggesting a buffer effect of social support. The results of the logistic regression in the same study showed that independently of distress there was an association with negative life events; this association was more significant when the person had experienced several negative events. This indicates that life events might explain the itch itself without giving stress symptoms. The influence of psychosocial environmental factors on health has been widely explored.[25, 32, 33] The effect of negative life events on mortality and cardiovascular disease has been shown,[34] as well as the impact of social support as a protective effect.[35–38] These environmental influences are also true for itch and will need to be explored in the future.

### 11.4 Itch and the Quality of Life

There is a worldwide variation of quality of life (QoL) in patients with pruritus. Health-related quality of life (HRQoL) measures are important for patients with pruritus but may not be appropriate for all ethnic groups. Many studies have shown that HRQoL impact increases with disease severity. This relationship is not necessarily a linear one but is dependent upon various factors, e.g., body site and a person's coping abilities. One study detected that generalized pruritus had a greater impact on life than other dermatological diseases such as acne, basal carcinoma and viral warts.[39] Our own studies in Germany showed that the QoL in patients with pruritus in systemic disease was less impaired. This may be explained by the fact that all these patients had a severe underlying disease that might have provoked better coping strategies. This is in accordance with the findings of others that in 52% of uremic patients pruritus did not have any effect on mood, and only 8% reported depression related to pruritus.[40] There is no doubt that renal failure lowers the patients' QoL, but the importance of pruritus might be lower within the disease course. Another aspect to consider could be the patients' age. In patients suffering from skin diseases after renal transplantation, the younger ones were more likely to experience a poorer QoL.[41] Quite interestingly, a very recent study on QoL in older patients with skin diseases showed that people older than 65 years suffering from rashes had significantly poorer QoL than patients with lesions, even those with skin cancer.[42] It was striking that patients with pruritus due to dermatoses were significantly younger and were significantly more depressed than patients with systemic pruritus.[43] Impairment of QoL in patients with various types of pruritic diseases has been described; e.g., those with psoriasis and chronic idiopathic urticaria were found to be more agitated, depressed and had difficulties in concentration.[44, 45] Previous studies showed that patients with AD described themselves as being more anxious, more aroused, more depressed and less energetic.[46] Interestingly, this group was characterized by less intense itching and scratching.[46] According to our own studies, patients with AD in Germany tended to be more aggressive and depressed, but this was in a smaller number of patients. Pruritus in patients with AD in China was also reported to cause depression, agitation and difficulties in concentrating.[47]

Patients with eczema in Uganda were less impaired compared to German patients in our own study.[43] It could be shown that QoL was more impaired in patients who were HIV positive compared to those who were HIV negative. QoL impairment associated with certain diagnoses such as eczema seems to be different in different ethnic groups. Another study showed that QoL in Turkish patients with skin diseases had higher scores for psoriasis, urticaria and acne compared to eczema in the emotional life domain.[48] Pruritus of unknown origin appears to especially impair the QoL in German patients with pruritus.[43]

Table 11.4 shows that at a community level also itch has a significant impact on the well-being and QoL.[49] QoL research in dermatology has high-

**Table 11.4** Affected quality of life among individuals reporting itch and those who do not, in a Western community (N = 18,747)

| Measures of quality of life | Itch (%) | No itch (%) |
| --- | --- | --- |
| Poor well-being | 34 | 21 |
| Affected work abilities | 8 | 1 |
| Affected leisure activities | 10 | 1 |
| Affected social life | 8 | 1 |

lighted the impact of skin disease on life and demonstrated the burden of skin disease. Active research in this field in the last decade, with the development and use of questionnaires among dermatological patients, has pointed out the effect of skin symptoms on feelings, daily activities, work and personal relationships.[39, 50–56]

## 11.5 Epidemiology of Pruritic Diseases

### 11.5.1 Pruritus in Systemic Diseases and Pruritus of Unknown Origin

There is a worldwide variation in the epidemiology of itch in systemic diseases. Studies such as the one in a German population resemble those in patients attending a dermatologic clinic and may therefore be different in comparison to, e.g., an internal medicine department. Nevertheless, this reflects the real situation quite well because pruritus is not only the most frequently described symptom in dermatology but most primarily attributed to a skin disease.

In 10–50% of patients with pruritus, a systemic disease can be found resembling the underlying etiology.[43, 57–59] In about 8% of the patients, the cause of pruritus remains unclear in spite of intensive diagnostic investigations.[43] According to a French study investigating patients with generalized pruritus, 40% had an underlying systemic etiology.[57] Interestingly, toxocariasis was the most frequently found disease. American studies showed that 22–30% of patients with generalized pruritus had a systemic disease.[58, 59] In a German population, 36% had an underlying systemic disease, and in Uganda none of the patients with pruritus had a systemic disease.[43] Also in HIV, pruritus was caused by dermatoses. It is known that patients with HIV/AIDS are prone to develop a number of pruritic dermatoses. It is likely that the Ugandan patients with severe diseases, e.g., renal failure, did not have a chance of survival allowing the development of pruritus. Access to certain therapies such as hemodialysis may be more limited, but no reports have been found on this issue. The lack of systemic pruritus in Uganda can be explained in terms of some facts about the Ugandan healthcare system.

Uganda ranks among the 10 poorest countries in Africa, and this is reflected also in its healthcare system. In 2001, every citizen could spend only US$12 for health care. Among the 2,000 physicians registered in 1998, only 3 were dermatologists, but due to better training facilities the situation is slowly improving.[60] Overall, about one-fifth of the Ugandan study population was HIV positive (against none in the German study population).[43] According to a study, 28% of all Ugandan patients suffered from prurigo, 71.4% of which were HIV positive.[60] This is in accordance with earlier observations showing a high association between prurigo and HIV. In 2002, 88% of the HIV-tested prurigo patients were found positive.[60] It is striking that in both populations (German and Ugandan) eczema and prurigo were the most frequently observed dermatoses. According to the Ugandan ministry of health, 7% of the adult population in Uganda is HIV-infected, but others feel that this number is much higher in reality.[60] No information has been given about the burden of skin disease in patients with AIDS. There are also no epidemiological data existing on pruritus in Uganda, but according to the high frequency of skin diseases among HIV patients the prevalence rate is supposedly high. The management of HIV and AIDS is still poor, with inadequate resources and capacity as well as weak institutional and logistical framework.[60]

## 11.5.2 Pruritus in Specific Diseases

According to a survey by questionnaire among 17,000 members of the American Psoriasis Foundation, pruritus was the second most frequent symptom experienced by 79% of the interviewed patients with psoriasis.[61] In a study in Singapore on 101 patients with psoriasis, 84% reported generalized pruritus, 77% reporting daily occurrence.[44] Renal pruritus in patients undergoing dialysis is a considerable problem and affected up to 85% of these patients in the 1970s

and 1980s. Due to improved dialysis techniques, it decreased to 22% in Germany.[62] According to recent studies, regional differences need to be taken into account; however, the prevalence of pruritus was assessed 66% in Israel and 51.9% in Turkey.[63, 64] In another study on patients with pruritus, the number of renal pruritus was quite high.[43] This may be attributed to the fact that this type of pruritus is long lasting, most bothersome and quite therapy-refractory, so that these patients are frequently referred to a dermatologist within a German university department. Pruritus accompanying diabetes mellitus affected 2.7% of a diabetic population in the United States.[65] Generalized pruritus as a presenting symptom of diabetes may occur, but is not significantly more frequent than in nondiabetic patients. Localized pruritus, especially in the genital and perianal areas, was significantly more common in women diabetic patients and significantly associated with poor diabetes control.[65] Pruritus vulvae were significantly more common in diabetic women (18.4%) than in controls (5.6%). In Israel, 2% of diabetic patients are affected by pruritus.[66] A study from Kuwait described pruritus to be the second most common presenting symptom in 49% of diabetic patients.[67] Medications can lead to considerable pruritus, which is frequently accompanied by specific skin efflorescences (e.g., urticarial drug eruption), but may also present on unaffected skin. In an American prospective study with hospitalized patients, pruritus without skin lesions occurred in 5% of drug-induced cutaneous side effects.[68] Drug-induced pruritus without skin lesions should be considered especially when investigating pruritus of undetermined origin. Hydroxyethyl-starch (HES) induced pruritus, which may occur in up to 50% of the patients treated with HES, needs to be considered.[69] In tropical regions, chloroquine-induced pruritus in malaria therapy during pregnancy is frequent, with a prevalence rate of 64.5%. It is reported to be severe in more than 60%, and occurring within 24 h after consumption in 75% of those affected.[70]

The population-based approach is complementary to the biological approach. The exploration of the interactions between the individual and the social context adds arguments to the connection between itch and the environment, highlighting the link between the symptom itch and sociodemographic as well as psychosocial factors.[71]

# References

1. Rose G. *The Strategy of Preventive Medicine.* Oxford: Oxford University Press, 1992.
2. Marmot MG. *Social Determinants of Health.* Oxford: Oxford University Press, 2001.
3. Last JM. The iceberg "completing the clinical picture" in general practice. The *Lancet,* 1963;282(7297):28–31.
4. Dalgard F, Svensson Å, Holm JØ, et al. Self-reported skin morbidity in Oslo: associations with socio-demographic factors among adults in a cross sectional study. *Br J Dermatol.* 2004;151:452–457.
5. Dalgard F, Svensson A, Holm JO, et al. Self-reported skin complaints: validation of a questionnaire for population surveys. *Br J Dermatol.* 2003;149:794–800.
6. Rea JN, Newhouse ML, Halil T. Skin disease in Lambeth. A community study of prevalence and use of medical care. *Br J Prevent Soc Med.* 1976;30:107–114.
7. Matterne U, Strassner T, Apfelbacher C, Diepgen TL, Weisshaar E: Measuring the prevalence of itch in the general population: a pilot study. *Acta Derm Venereol* 2009; 89: 250–256.
8. Yosipovitch G. Assessment of itch: more to be learned and improvements to be made. *J Invest Dermatol.* 2003;121(6): xiv–xv.
9. Wahlgren CF. Measurement of itch. *Semin Dermatol.* 1995;14(4):277–284.
10. Meding B, Liden C, Berglind N. Self-diagnosed dermatitis in adults. Results from a population survey in Stockholm. *Contact Dermatitis.* 2001;45(6):341–345.
11. Lomholt G. Prevalence of skin diseases in a population. *Danish Med Bull.* 1964;11:1–7.
12. Roger D, Vaillant L, Fignon A, et al. Specific pruritic dermatoses of pregnancy. A prospective study of 3192 pregnant women. *Arch Dermatol.* 1994;130:734–739.
13. Shanmugam S, Thappa DM, Habeebullah S: Pruritus gravidarum: a clinical and laboratory study. *J Dermatol.* 1998;25:582–586.
14. Reyes H, Gonzales MC, Ribalta J, et al. Prevalence or intrahepatic cholestasis of pregnancy in Chile. *Ann Int Med.* 1978;88:487–493.
15. Yalcm B, Tamer E, Toy GG, et al. The prevalence of skin diseases in the elderly: analysis of 4099 geriatric patients. *Int J Dermatol.* 2006;45:672–676.
16. Thaipisuttikul Y: Pruritic skin diseases in the elderly. *J Dermatol.* 1998;25:153–157.
17. Macbeth HP, S. *Health and Ethnicity,* Vol. Chapter 4. London and New York: Taylor and Francis; 2001.
18. Oppenheimer GM. Paradigm lost: race, ethnicity, and the search for a new population taxonomy. *Am J Publ Health.* 2001;91:1049–1055.
19. Rook A. *Textbook of Dermatology.,* Vol. 1, Chapter 6. Malden, MA: Blackwell Science; 1998.
20. Nazroo JY. South Asian people and heart disease: an assessment of the importance of socioeconomic position. *Ethnicity Dis.* 2001;11(3):401–411.
21. Marmot MG, Adelstein AM, Bulusu L. Lessons from the study of immigrant mortality. *Lancet.* 1984;1(8392):1455–1457.
22. Vlahov D, Galea S. Urban health: a new discipline. *Lancet.* 2003;362:1091–1092.
23. Bhopal R, Hayes L, White M, et al. Ethnic and socio-economic inequalities in coronary heart disease, diabetes and risk factors in Europeans and South Asians. *J Publ Health Med.* 2002;24:95–105.
24. Murray CJ, Lopez AD. Global mortality, disability, and the contribution of risk factors: global burden of disease study. *Lancet.* 1997;349:1436–1442.
25. Marmot MG, Smith GD, Stansfeld S, et al. Health inequalities among British civil servants: the Whitehall II study. *Lancet.* 1991;337:1387–1393.
26. Siegrist J, Marmot M. Health inequalities and the psychosocial environment-two scientific challenges. *Soc Sci Med.* 2004;58(8):1463–1473.
27. Townsend P, Davidson N. *The Black Report.* London: Penguin; 1992.
28. Brekke M, Hjortdahl P, Kvien TK. Severity of musculoskeletal pain: relations to socioeconomic inequality. *Soc Sci Med.* 2002;54(2):221–228.
29. Brekke M, Hjortdahl P, Thelle DS, et al. Disease activity and severity in patients with rheumatoid arthritis: relations to socioeconomic inequality. *Soc Sci Med.* 1999;48(12):1743–1750.
30. Lonne-Rahm S, Berg M, Marin P, et al. Atopic dermatitis, stinging, and effects of chronic stress: a pathocausal study. *J Am Acad Dermatol.* 2004;51(6):899–905.
31. Dalgard F, Svensson Å, Sundby J, et al. Skin morbidity and mental health. A population survey among adults in a Norwegian city. *Br J Dermatol.* 2005;153: 145–149.
32. Stansfeld SA, Head J, Fuhrer R, et al. Social inequalities in depressive symptoms and physical functioning in the Whitehall II study: exploring a common cause explanation. *J Epidemiol Commun Health.* 2003;57(5):361–367.
33. Berkman Lisa KI. *Social Epidemiology.* Oxford: University Press; 2000.
34. Rosengren A, Hawken S, Ounpuu S, et al. Association of psychosocial risk factors with risk of acute myocardial infarction in 11 119 cases and 13648 controls from 52 countries (the INTERHEART study): case-control study. [see comment]. *Lancet.* 2004;364(9438):953–962.
35. Kawachi I, Colditz GA, Ascherio A, et al. A prospective study of social networks in relation to total mortality and cardiovascular disease in men in the USA. *J Epidemiol Commun Health.* 1996;50:245–251.
36. Rosengren A, Orth-Gomer K, Wedel H, et al. Stressful life events, social support, and mortality in men born in 1933. *Br Med J.* 1993;307(6912):1102–1105.
37. Penninx BW, van Tilburg T, Kriegsman DM, et al. Effects of social support and personal coping resources on mortality in older age: the longitudinal aging study Amsterdam. *Am J Epidemiol* 1997;146:510–519.
38. Olsen O. Impact of social network on cardiovascular mortality in middle aged Danish men. *J Epidemiol Commun Health.* 1993;47:176–180.
39. Finlay AY, Khan GK. Dermatology life quality index (DLQI) – a simple practical measure for routine clinical use. *Clin Exp Dermatol.* 1994;19:210–216.
40. Yosipovitch G, Zucker I, Boner G, et al. A questionnaire for the assessment of pruritus: validation in uremic patients. *Acta Derm Venereol.* 2001;81:108–111.
41. Moloney FJ, Keane S, O'Kelly P, et al. The impact of skin disease following renal transplantation on quality of life. *Br J Dermatol.* 2005;153:574–578.

42. Shah M, Coates M. An assessment of the quality of life in older patients with skin disease. *Br J Dermatol.* 2006;154:150–153.

43. Weisshaar E, Apfelbacher CJ, Jäger G, et al. Pruritus as a leading symptom – clinical characteristics and quality of life in German and Ugandan patients. *Br J Dermatol.* 2006;155:957–964.

44. Yosipovitch G, Goon A, Wee J, et al. The prevalence and clinical characteristics of pruritus among patients with extensive psoriasis. *Br J Dermatol.* 2000;143:969–973.

45. Yosipovitch G, Ansari N, Goon A, et al. Clinical characteristics of pruritus in chronic idiopathic urticaria. *Br J Dermatol.* 2002;147:32–36.

46. Gieler U, Ehlers A, Höhler T, et al. The psychosocial status of patients with endogenous eczema. A study using cluster analysis for the correlation of psychological factors with somatic findings. *Hautarzt.* 1990;41:416–423.

47. Yosipovitch G, Goon ATJ, Wee J, et al. Itch characteristics in Chinese patients with atopic dermatitis using a new questionnaire for the assessment of pruritus. *Int J Dermatol.* 2002;41:212–216.

48. Gurel SM, Yanik M, Simsek Z, et al.: Quality of life instrument for Turkish people with skin diseases. *Int J Dermatol.* 2005;44:933–938.

49. Dalgard F, Svensson A, Holm JO, et al. Self reported skin morbidity among adults. Associations with quality of life and general health in a Norwegian study. *J Invest Dermatol.* 2004;9:120–125.

50. Richards HL, Fortune DG, Main CJ, et al. Stigmatization and psoriasis. *Br J Dermatol.* 2003;149(1):209–211.

51. Zachariae R, Zachariae C, Ibsen HH, et al. Psychological symptoms and quality of life of dermatology outpatients and hospitalized dermatology patients. *Acta Dermato-Venereologica.* 2004;84(3):205–212.

52. Wahl A, Loge JH, Wiklund I, et al. The burden of psoriasis: a study concerning health-related quality of life among Norwegian adult patients with psoriasis compared with general population norms. *J Am Acad Dermatol.* 2000;43:803–808.

53. Lasek RJ, Chren MM. Acne vulgaris and the quality of life of adult dermatology patients. *Arch Dermatol.* 1998;134(4):454–458.

54. Jemec GB, Wulf HC. Patient-physician consensus on quality of life in dermatology. *Clin Exper Dermatol.* 1996;21:177–179.

55. Finlay AY. Quality of life measurement in dermatology: a practical guide. *Br J Dermatol.* 1997;136:305–314.

56. Chren MM, Lasek RJ, Quinn LM, et al. Skindex, a quality-of-life measure for patients with skin disease: reliability, validity, and responsiveness. *J Invest Dermatol.* 1996;107:707–713.

57. Afifi Y, Azubin F, Puzenat E, et al. Pruritus sine materia: a prospective study of 95 patients. *La Revue de Medicine Interne.* 2004;25:490–493.

58. Kantor GR, Lookingbill DP. Generalised pruritus and systemic disease. *J Am Acad Dermatol.* 1983;9:375–382.

59. Zirwas MJ, Seraly MP: Pruritus of unknown origin: A retrospective study. *J Am Acad Dermatol.* 2001; 45:892–896.

60. Schmidt E, Rose C, Mulyowa GK, et al. Dermatology at the University Hospital of Mbarara, Uganda. *J Dtsch Dermatol Ges.* 2004;2:920–927.

61. Krueger G, Koo J, Lebwohl M, et al.. The impact of psoriasis on quality of life. Results of a 1998 National Psoriasis Foundation patient membership survey. *Arch Dermatol.* 2001;137:280–284.

62. Mettang T, Pauli-Magnus C, Alscher DM. Uraemic pruritus-new perspectives and insights from recent trials. *Nephrol Dial Transplant.* 2002;17:1558–1563.

63. Zucker I, Yosipovitch G, David M, et al. Prevalence and characterization of uremic pruritus in patients undergoing hemodialysis: uremic pruritus is still a major problem for patients with end-stage renal disease. *J Am Acad Dermatol.* 2003;49:842–846.

64. Mistik S, Utas S, Ferahbas A, et al. An epidemiology study of patients with uremic pruritus. *JEADV.* 2006; 20: 672–678.

65. Neilly JB, Martin A, Simpson N, et al. Pruritus in diabetes mellitus: investigation of prevalence and correlation with diabetes control. *Diabetes Care.* 1986;9:273–275.

66. Yosipovitch G, Hodak E, Vardi P, et al. The prevalence of cutaneous manifestations in IDDM patients and their association with diabetes risk factors and microvasculature complications. *Diabetes Care.* 1998;21:506–509.

67. Al-Mutari N, Zaki A, Sharma AK, et al. Cutaneous manifestations of diabetes mellitus. *Med Princ Pract.* 2006;15:427–430.

68. Bigby M, Jack S, Jick H, et al. Drug-induced cutaneous reactions. A report from the Boston Collaborative Drug Surveillance Program on 15438 consecutive inpatients, 1975–1982. *JAMA.* 1986;256:3358–3363.

69. Bork K. Pruritus precipitated by hydroxyethyl starch: a review. *Br J Dermatol.* 2005;152:3–12.

70. Olayemi O, Fehintola FA, Osungbade A, et al. Pattern of chloroquin-induced pruritus in antenatal patients of the University College Hospital Ibadan. *J Obstet Gynacol.* 2003;23:490–495.

71. Adler HM. Might a psychosocial approach improve our understanding of itching and scratching? *Int J Dermatol.* 2003;42(2):160–163.

# Chapter 12
# Classification

Sonja Ständer

The research focusing on the neurobiology and clinics of pruritus is young but growing. As a consequence, most of the old terms and definitions currently used for different types of pruritus need to be redefined and approved by an international expert team. This is one aim of the Special Interest Group (SIG) of the International Forum for the Study of Itch (IFSI). Here we present the terms, definitions and classification that have been defined between 2005 and 2008.[1-3]

## 12.1 Terms and Definitions

- Pruritus is currently distinguished between **acute** (up to 6 weeks) and **chronic itch** (lasting for 6 weeks and longer).
- It is generally accepted that **pruritus and itch** can be used synonymously.
- The term **pruritus sine materia** produced much confusion since it was used to describe different conditions (e.g., pruritus in systemic disease, pruritus on non-diseased skin). The term should be avoided.
- In patients with unknown origin of pruritus the term **pruritus of unknown origin or pruritus of undetermined origin (PUO)** should be used instead. This term can be used interchangeably with "**itch of undetermined origin (IUO)**" to describe (a) patients in whom no diagnosis is reached and history does not suggest the origin of pruritus; and (b) patients with pruritus whose origin is unknown even after the diagnosis.
- The term **somatoform pruritus** describes pruritus of psychosomatic/psychiatric origin.
- **Pruritus of advanced aging** or **pruritus in the elderly** replaces the term **senile pruritus.**
- Several synonyms are currently accepted and discussed for the term **uremic pruritus: pruritus of CKD (chronic kidney disease), renal pruritus, nephrogenic itch.**

## 12.2 Neurophysiological Classification of Pruritus

A neurophysiologically based classification was proposed in 2003.[4] Twycross et al. classified itch according to its origin as follows:

- **Pruritoceptive:** Pruritogenic nerves are activated by pruritogens at their sensory endings.
- **Neuropathic:** Diseased or lesioned pruritogenic neurons generate itch.
- **Neurogenic:** Itch is induced by mediators acting centrally in the absence of neural damage.
- **Psychogenic**

This classification is beneficial for neurobiological itch research to describe the neuroanatomical mechanism underlying pruritus. The classification cannot be applied clinically since several diseases such as atopic dermatitis and cholestatic pruritus fall under more than one category.

## 12.3 Clinical Classification of Pruritus

An internationally accepted clinical classification was defined by the IFSI in 2007.[1-3] This classification is focused on the clinical presentation of the patient and distinguishes between disorders with or without primary or secondary skin lesions. In the first part of the classification, three groups of conditions were defined according to the history and skin investigation of patients with pruritus.

L. Misery and S. Ständer (eds.), *Pruritus*,
DOI 10.1007/978-1-84882-322-8_12, © Springer-Verlag London Limited 2010

**Table 12.1** Categories of underlying diseases (from ref.[3])

| Category | Diseases |
|---|---|
| I. Dermatologic | Arising from "diseases of the skin" such as psoriasis, atopic dermatitis, dry skin, scabies and urticaria |
| II. Systemic | Arising from "diseases of organs" other than the skin, such as liver (e.g., primary biliary cirrhosis), kidney (e.g., chronic renal failure), blood (e.g., Hodgkin's disease) and certain multifactorial states (e.g., metabolic) or drugs |
| III. Neurologic | Arising from "diseases or disorders of the central or peripheral nervous system," e.g., nerve damage, nerve compression, nerve irritation |
| IV. Psychogenic/ Psychosomatic | Somatoform pruritus with comorbidity of "psychiatric and psychosomatic diseases" |
| V. Mixed | Overlapping and coexistence of several diseases |
| VI. Other | Undetermined origin |

**Fig. 12.1**

1. step – history and clinical investigation

the patient can be readily assigned to one group

2. step – histological, laboratory and radiological investigation

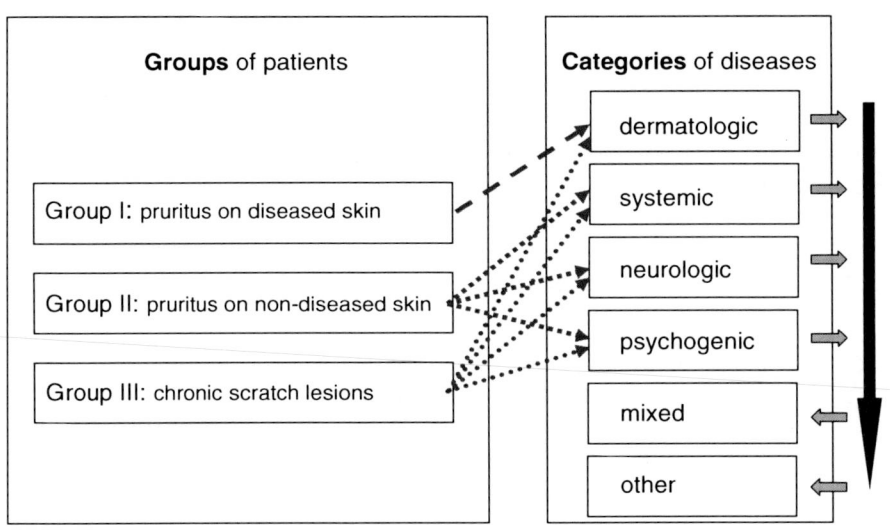

First group: **Pruritus on primary diseased skin** represents pruritic dermatoses and comprises inflammatory, infectious, or autoimmune cutaneous diseases, genodermatoses, drug reactions, dermatoses of pregnancy and skin lymphomas, all leading to specific skin changes.

**Second group: Pruritus on primary non-diseased (normal) skin** arises from systemic diseases and includes endocrine and metabolic disorders, infections, hematological and lymphoproliferative diseases, solid neoplasms, neurologic diseases, psychiatric diseases and drug-induced pruritus.

**Third group: Severe chronic secondary scratch lesions** such as prurigo nodularis or lichen simplex.

The next step is categorizing the patients according to the underlying disease. For this, several categories have been defined (Table 12.1).

This two-step classification can be used in the medical care of patients aiming to avoid unnecessary laboratory and radiological investigations of the patients (Fig. 12.1). For example, in patients with a typical history of an itch-inducing dermatosis, laboratory investigation is mostly not necessary.

## References

1. Bernhard JD. Itch and pruritus: what are they, and how should itches be classified? *Dermatol Ther.* 2005;18:288–291.
2. Ständer S, Weisshaar E, Mettang T, et al. Klinische Klassifikation von chronischem Pruritus: Interdisziplinärer Konsensusvorschlag für einen diagnostischen Algorithmus. *Hautarzt.* 2006;57:390–394.
3. Ständer S, Weisshaar E, Mettang T, et al. Clinical classification of itch: a position paper of the International Forum for the Study of Itch. *Acta Dermatol Venerol.* 2007;87:291–294.
4. Twycross R, Greaves MW, Handwerker H, et al. Itch: scratching more than the surface. *QJM.* 2003;96:7–26.

# Chapter 13
# Examination of Patients*

Elke Weisshaar

## 13.1 Taking the History in Patients Suffering from Pruritus

Precise history, clinical examination and laboratory as well as radiological diagnostics are of high importance in diagnosing pruritus. The intensity of pruritus, onset, time course, quality (burning, painful, stinging, prickling), localization and trigger factors (e.g., physical activity, contact with water, own observation) should be assessed. The patient's own theory should be enquired into because this enables determination of important differential diagnoses. Special attention should also be paid to the time relationship of events or preceding events (e.g., prodromal pruritus especially on the neck minutes before an asthma attack; pruritus following bathing). It is important to ask the patient for his/her own initiative to combat or relieve pruritus such as showering, or use of brushes and other objects. This may explain clinically striking findings such as the absence of secondary skin lesions in the mid-back area known as the "butterfly sign." This shows that the patient cannot reach and scratch this region by hand.

Precise history-taking includes preexisting diseases and operations, known allergies, medications, over-the-counter drugs, present and past therapies for pruritus and atopic disposition. History of medications includes ones taken presently and those taken in the recent past (at least one year), as well as infusions such as hydroxyethyl starch, opioids and blood transfusions. A study showed that drug-induced pruritus without a rash accounted for approximately 5% of adverse cutaneous reactions in prospectively followed-up hospitalized patients. Adverse cutaneous reactions occurred in 3% of patients.[1] During pregnancy,

on average 3–8 different medications may be taken which are partly self-medicated and partly prescribed by a physician.[2] Strong pruritus can lead to considerable psychological impairment. The physician should not underestimate the psychological implications of pruritus and should also address the patient's psychological impairment. Chronic pruritus frequently goes along with reduced quality of life, behavioral/adjustment dysfunction and a withdrawal from social and work life.[3] In these cases, psychosomatic counseling is required. In contrast to these cases, chronic pruritus or chronic scratch lesions including self-mutilation can be caused by psychiatric diseases such as delusional state of parasitosis, needing psychiatric examination and, if necessary, treatment. A solely psychosomatic/psychiatric cause of pruritus should not be diagnosed without psychiatric examination.

By precise history-taking, the clinical evaluation and examination can be made easier.

- When multiple family members are affected, scabies or other parasites should be considered.
- The relationship between pruritus and special activities is important: pruritus during physical activity can resemble cholinergic pruritus. Pruritus provoked by the skin cooling after emerging from a warm shower/bath can be a sign of aquagenic pruritus or polycythemia vera.
- Nocturnal generalized pruritus in association with chills, fatigue, tiredness and B symptoms (weight loss, fever and nocturnal sweating) can be a sign of a malignant disease such as Hodgkin's disease.
- While psychogenic/somatoform pruritus rarely interferes with sleep, most pruritic diseases cause nocturnal wakening.
- Seasonal pruritus frequently occurs as so-called "winter pruritus," mostly representing pruritus caused by exsiccation eczema in the elderly.

* No funding sources supported for these book chapters. The author has no conflict of Interest.

## 13.2 Clinical Examination of Patients Suffering from Pruritus

The examination of the patient includes a thorough inspection of the entire skin including mucous membranes, scalp, hair, nails and anogenital region (Table 13.1). Primary and secondary efflorescences have to be distinguished. Primary skin lesions in patients with pruritus may vary from erythema and urticae to papules, nodules, blisters, vesicules and pustules. Secondary skin lesions are excoriations, erosions, necrosis, ulcerations, scaling, atrophy, scars, hyper- and hypopigmentations of the skin. They are almost exclusively caused by scratching. The morphology of skin lesions, their distribution pattern, skin color, lichenification and xerosis of the skin should be carefully ruled out. Any skin signs of systemic diseases have to be assessed. According to clinical experience, scratch artifacts are especially pronounced in children. A general physical examination should include palpation of the liver, kidneys, spleen, lymph nodes, as well as pelvic and rectal areas. One cannot conclude that

generalized pruritus is significantly associated with malignancy.[4] Generalized pruritus may present years before the onset of the symptoms of malignancy.[4] It should be remembered that if the initial evaluation does not reveal an origin, it is advisable to reevaluate the patient periodically.

It would be very helpful for clinicians if there were characteristics that helped to predict the likelihood of a systemic etiology in patients with pruritus. As previously shown, there are no clinical characteristics that would allow the clinician to classify a patient as a high-risk patient.[3] The distribution and type of secondary scratch lesions give no clue to the underlying etiology.[5] According to one study, patients with systemic diseases were older, had evening and nocturnal intermittent pruritus and had more associated complaints such as sleeplessness, weakness and dizziness when compared to patients suffering from pruritus due to a dermatological disease.[3] Pruritus over the whole body was more frequent in pruritus caused by dermatoses when compared to pruritus caused by systemic diseases.[3] Pruritus during pregnancy

**Table 13.1** Laboratory and additional diagnostics in patients with chronic pruritus of unknown etiology (from ref.[21])

| | |
|---|---|
| Initial laboratory tests | • Erythrocyte sedimentation rate (ESR) |
| | • Complete blood cell count with differential leukocyte count |
| | • Calcium, phosphate |
| | • Creatinine (urea only in elderly patients) |
| | • Liver transaminases, alkaline phosphatase, bilirubin, hepatitis serology |
| | • Protein, glucose (or HbA1c, if patient has not fastened) |
| | • Thyroid-stimulating hormone (TSH) |
| | • Prostate-specific antigen (PSA) |
| | • Iron, transferrin, ferritin, vitamin B12, folic acid, zinc |
| | • Urine status |
| | • Stool for occult blood test |
| | • Stool for ova and parasites, worms (only in case of anal pruritus) |
| | • Skin biopsy (histology, immunofluorescence, electron microscopy) |
| Initial apparatus diagnostics | Chest X-ray, sonography of abdomen and lymph nodes |
| Further tests depending on history, symptoms and prior findings | • Protein electrophoresis (paraproteins if required) |
| | • IgM, antinuclear antibodies (ANA), antimitochondrial antibodies (AMA), indirect immunofluorescence, anti-gliadin, anti-transglutaminase antibodies |
| | • Sodium, potassium, parathormone, porphyrins |
| | • HIV status |
| | • Tryptase, urinary excretion of 5-hydroxyindolacetic acid, mast cell metabolites |
| | • Creatinine clearance |
| | • Bacteriological and mycological stainings |
| | • Test for scabies mites |
| | • Allergological diagnostics: total IgE, prick tests for atopy, patch testing, specific allergological diagnostics (e.g. drugs, additives) |
| Further apparatus diagnostics | In case of suspicious findings: |
| | CT, MR, bone marrow biopsy, endoscopic examinations |
| | In case of neuropathic findings: neurology and MR, chest X-ray (cervical rib) |
| | In case of aquageneous pruritus: lactose intolerance test |
| Co-treatment of patients (symptoms- and findings-associated) | Internal medicine, neurology, urology, gynecology, paediatrics, psychosomatics, psychiatry |

unrelated to skin diseases including pregnancy-specific dermatoses and presenting without any skin lesions can occur as pruritus gravidarum without and with intrahepatic cholestasis (Table 13.2).[2] This may be associated with clinical jaundice. There is no clear terminology. Some authors name them *pruritus gravidarum* and *intrahepatic cholestasis* of pregnancy. Both may lead to scratching resulting in, for example, papules, nodules, excoriations and crusts. Some suggest that pruritus gravidarum in women with atopic predisposition can result in prurigo of pregnancy.

## 13.3 Documentation and Measuring of Pruritus

There is no standardized and generally accepted method of documenting pruritus. The sensation of pruritus is subjective, varying inter- and intraindividually due to, for example, tiredness, anxiety, stress or depression. The intensity of pruritus can be assessed by using questionnaires or various scales. These methods have not yet been included into clinical routine and are at present predominantly used in experimental studies.

Several modalities have been proposed to aid the clinician.

*Categorical scales:* These are the most commonly employed research scales and consist of discrete divisions of the frequency of the measured dimension. They can also be employed to assess the impact of pruritus upon the life of the affected patient. Examples: pruritus – never, rarely, occasionally, frequently, always.

*Interval scales:* These describe pruritus by choosing a number on a fixed or limited scale, such as 0–10, having the advantage of equidistant points between response categories. Examples: pain track - a computerized system with a 7-step-graded, fixed-point, nonverbal scale.

*Continuous scales:* The visual analog scale (VAS) is the most common scale in experimental and clinical pruritus research. The patient is requested to document the individual itch intensity by marking a line. It is a line of defined length (in most studies 100 mm) with descriptive anchors at the extremes, e.g., "no pruritus" and "pruritus as bad as it could be." The subjects can precisely describe the itch sensation without limitation to a few discrete categories, thereby providing continuous data for analysis. It may represent the most sensitive approach to measuring pruritus intensity. Disadvantages need to be considered. The definition of "10" is variable. In some studies "10" has been defined as "strongest pruritus ever experienced." The VAS scale does not consider the frequent occurrence of itch attacks during the course of a day or night. For patients with severe and unclear courses of pruritus, the use of a daily diary can be helpful for the physician to attribute and interpret pruritus.

*Scratch-behavior measurement:* This reflects the symptom in a limited way, as some pruritic diseases such as urticaria and mastocytosis rarely cause scratching (rather rubbing or pressing). Clinicians usually evaluate scratch behavior by registration of secondary scratch lesions. There are several measurement characteristics.

- *Self-report of scratching behavior:* patients can be provided with hand-activated counters to record their scratching,[6] but recording of nocturnal scratching is not possible.
- *Direct observation:* these are expensive and time-consuming, and the potential for scratching behavior underneath covers goes unnoticed.
- *Nocturnal bed movements:* body movement at night is measured by a vibration transducer on a bed leg.

**Table 13.2** Pruritus in pregnancy not related to dermatoses

| Pregnancy dermatoses | Occurrence | Etiology and laboratory findings | Fetal risk | Localization of pruritus |
|---|---|---|---|---|
| Pruritus gravidarum (without cholestasis) | 1. Trimenon | Not clear, increased bile acids and decreased itch threshold due to prostaglandins, normal liver function | No | Generalized |
| Pruritus gravidarum (with cholestasis) | 2 and 3. Trimenon | Not clear, genetic predisposition and alterated bile duct and hepatocytes, increased bile acids, transaminases, alkaline phosphatase, cholesterol, lipids | Yes | Generalized, especially hands and feet, deterioration during night |
| Prurigo gestationis | Early and late form possible | Not clear (atopy?) | No | Extensor sides of extremities |

Limb activity is measured with movement-sensitive meters.[7,8] Nocturnal scratching can also be measured by using an infrared video camera, providing very interesting and impressive data, but this method is not suitable for routine monitoring in clinical use.[9]

- *Limb activity meters*: patients responding to nocturnal pruritus tend to move their arms more than their legs, and a careful analysis of this ratio provides insight into the scratching behavior. Investigations, especially in children suffering from AD, with sensors fixed to their extremities demonstrated that objectively assessed data (limb movements, disease-specific skin lesions) do not correlate with subjective symptoms such as insomnia and parents' report.[10]
- *Forearm activity meters*: rhythmic muscle potentials can be recorded at the same time as an electroencephalogram records sleep activity.

*Questionnaires*: During the past years, questionnaires to assess and document pruritus have been designed and applied. They should also include the assessment of life quality, as this can be significantly impaired, especially in patients with pruritus of unknown origin.[3] There is no single questionnaire that fulfills all clinical and experimental needs, especially concerning the evaluation of therapy effects.

The Eppendorf Itch Questionnaire (Eppendorfer Juckreizfragebogen) was developed in cooperation between dermatology and neurophysiology.[11] This is a multidimensional questionnaire modified according to the McGill Pain Questionnaire. It is very informative in pruritus description but does not include characteristics such as the effect of, for example, daily life habits, physical activities on pruritus or antipruritics. The Eppendorf Itch Questionnaire was validated in patients with pruritus suffering from atopic dermatitis (AD).[12]

A questionnaire for uremic patients is based on the short form of the McGill Pain Questionnaire.[13] In 145 patients suffering from uremic pruritus, dialysis was not found to influence uremic pruritus, which tends to be prolonged, frequently intense, and a major source of distress to the patient. A modified form of this questionnaire has been used for evaluating patients with psoriasis, chronic idiopathic urticaria and AD, and found to be reliable and reproducible.[13–16]

Another pruritus questionnaire is available in English and German assessing various clinical symptoms and quality of life. It has been successfully applied in German and Ugandan patients.[3] A German pruritus cognition questionnaire assesses the cognitions that are favorable for coping with pruritus sensations (scale coping strategies) and the ones adverse for coping (scale catastrophic thinking/helplessness).[17] Further questionnaires have been developed for children and adolescents, investigating their disease coping and their pruritus cognition (JUCKKI, JUCKJU).[18] According to our own experiences, questionnaires are useful for providing a more meaningful and structured approach to the care of patients with pruritus. Besides, it is perceived as a positive indication of the physician's interest by the patient.

## 13.4 Laboratory Diagnostics

In patients with chronic, unclear pruritus, systemic causes should carefully be ruled out by laboratory testing (Table 4.1). Blood tests, bacteriological and mycological stains as well as a skin biopsy should be carried out depending on the patient's history, physical examination and differential diagnoses. In cases of unclear or suspicious dermatosis or a dermatosis modified by scratch artifacts, a skin biopsy should be performed, if necessary with direct immunofluorescence. In spite of intensive efforts, the cause of pruritus may not be identified in 5–14% of affected patients.[3,19,20]

## 13.5 Further Diagnostics

Further diagnostic procedures may be required for the clarification of systemic pruritus and depend on the individual symptom constellation (Table 4.1). Radiological examinations such as chest X-ray, computer tomography (CT) of chest and abdominal organs or magnetic resonance tomography, sonographic examinations (e.g., sonography of abdomen/lymph nodes), endoscopic examinations and bone marrow biopsy may be required for further evaluation of specific symptoms (e.g., cerebral CT to exclude a cerebral tumor in case of facial pruritus).

As chronic pruritus may go along with behavioral/ adjustment dysfunction, psychosomatic counseling may be required. In these cases, chronic pruritus or chronic scratch lesions including self-mutilation can be caused by a psychiatric disease such as delusional state of parasitosis. These patients will need psychiatric examination and, if necessary, treatment. A solely psychological cause of pruritus should not be diagnosed without psychiatric examination.

# References

1. Bigby M, Jack S, Jick H, et al. Drug-induced cutaneous reactions. A report from the Boston Collaborative Drug Surveillance Program on 15438 consecutive inpatients, 1975–1982. *JAMA.* 1982;56:3358–3363.

2. Weisshaar E, Diepgen TL, Luger TA, et al. Pruritus in pregnancy and childhood – do we really consider all relevant differential diagnoses? *Eur J Dermatol.* 2005;15(5):320–331.

3. Weisshaar E, Apfelbacher CJ, Jäger G, et al. Pruritus as a leading symptom – clinical characteristics and quality of life in German and Ugandan patients. *Br J Dermatol.* 2006; 55:957–964.

4. Lober CW. Should the patient with generalized pruritus be evaluated for malignancy? *J Am Acad Dermatol.* 1988;19: 350–352.

5. Sommer F, Hensen P, Böckenholt B, et al. Underlying diseases and co-factors in patients with severe chronic pruritus: a 3-year retrospective study. *Acta Derm Venereol.* 2007;87(6):510–516.

6. Melin L, Frederikson T, Noren P, et al. Behavioural treatment of scratching in patients with atopic dermatitis. *Br J Dermatol.* 1986;115:467–474.

7. Felix R, Shuster S. A new method for the measurement of itch and the response to treatment. *Br J Dermatol.* 1975;93: 303–312.

8. Bringhurst C, Waterston K, Schofield O, et al. Measurement of itch using actigraphy in pediatric and adult populations. *J Am Acad Dermatol.* 2004;51:893–898.

9. Ebata T, Iwasaki S, Kamide R, et al. Use of a wrist activity monitor for the measurement of nocturnal scratching in patients with atopic dermatitis. *Br J Dermatol.* 2001;144:305–309.

10. Hon KLE, Leung TF, Wong Y, et al. Lessons from performing SCORADs in children with atopic dermatitis: subjective symptoms do not correlate well with disease extent or intensity. *Int J Dermatol.* 2006;45:728–730.

11. Darsow U, Mautner VF, Bromm B, et al. Der Eppendorfer Juckreizfragebogen. *Hautarzt.* 1997;48:730–733.

12. Darsow U, Scharein E, Simon D, et al. New aspects of itch pathophysiology: component analysis of atopic itch using the "Eppendorf Itch Questionnaire". *Int Arch Allergy Immunol.* 2001;124:326–331.

13. Yosipovitch G, Zucker I, Boner G, et al. A questionnaire for the assessment of pruritus: validation in uremic patients. *Acta Derm Venereol.* 2001;81:108–111.

14. Yosipovitch G, Goon A, Wee J, et al. The prevalence and clinical characteristics of pruritus among patients with extensive psoriasis. *Br J Dermatol.* 2000;143:969–973.

15. Yosipovitch G, Ansari N, Goon A, et al. Clinical characteristics of pruritus in chronic idiopathic urticaria. *Br J Dermatol.* 2002;147:32–36.

16. Yosipovitch G, Goon AT, Wee J, et al. Itch characteristics in Chinese patients with atopic dermatitis using a new questionnaire for the assessment of pruritus. *Int J Dermatol.* 2002;41:212–216.

17. Ehlers A, Stangier U, Dohn D, et al. Kognitive Faktoren beim Juckreiz: Entwicklung und Validierung eines Fragebogens. *Verhaltenstherapie.* 1993;3:112–119.

18. Kupfer J, Keins P, Brosig B, et al. Development of questionnaires on coping with disease and itching cognitions for children and adolescents with atopic eczema. *Dermatol Psychosom.* 2003;4:79–85.

19. Kantor GR, Lookingbill DP. Generalised pruritus and systemic disease. *J Am Acad Dermatol.* 1983;9:375–382.

20. Zirwas MJ, Seraly MP: Pruritus of unknown origin: A retrospective study. *J Am Acad Dermatol.* 2001;45:892–896.

21. Ständer S, Streit M, Darsow U, et al. Diagnostic and therapeutic procedures in chronic pruritis. *J Dtsch Dermatol Ges.* 2006;4:350–370.

**Section 2**
**Dermatology**

# Chapter 14
# Inflammatory Diseases

Jacek C. Szepietowski and Adam Reich

## 14.1 Introduction

Local inflammatory mechanisms may induce pruritus in many dermatoses. Mild to severe pruritus accompanies numerous inflammatory skin disorders including, but not limited to, atopic dermatitis (AD), eczema, psoriasis and lichen planus. The frequency of pruritus in skin diseases may vary depending on the entity and studied population. In AD pruritus occurs as a main diagnostic symptom. In other dermatoses such as allergic and irritant contact dermatitis, nummular or dyshydrotic eczema, itching is a frequent but not obligatory symptom.[1] Among inflammatory diseases itch has been studied in detail in AD and psoriasis.

## 14.2 Atopic Dermatitis

### 14.2.1 Frequency and Clinical Manifestation of Pruritus

Itching is a cardinal symptom of AD, and is included in four major diagnostic criteria of AD proposed by Hanifin and Rajka[2] as well as in AD diagnostic criteria used in the UK.[3] Assessment of itching intensity also plays an important role in the evaluation of AD severity.[4] It is generally believed that every patient with AD suffers from pruritus.[5] According to Yosipovitch et al.,[6] 87% of patients with AD experienced itching on a daily basis, 8% several times a week and only 5% reported itching less frequently, but at least every second week. Mean itch duration was 10.7 months. The majority of patients with AD had only short time periods without pruritus: in 38% of subjects the periods without pruritus were shorter than 1 week and in a further

23% it was longer than 1 week but shorter than 1 month. Ten percent of patients had pruritus-free periods of 1–6 months' duration and only 1% of investigated patients declared that the periods without itching lasted longer than half a year. In contrast, 28% declared that they never experience pruritus-free periods.[7,8] The average body surface area involved by itching was 29%. Pruritus was located mainly on lower extremities (78% of patients) and in flexural areas (72%), but less commonly it was observed on upper extremities (67%), neck (61%) and back (59%). The scalp and genitals were the least frequently involved (13% each).[6] In 43% of subjects pruritus was described as symmetrical. The mean intensity of pruritus according to the visual analog scale (VAS) ranged between 7.9 and 9 points.[6–8] The most intense itching was reported mainly at night (65%) and much less commonly in the morning (20%). In another study, the most intensive itching was experienced in the evening (53%) and at night (38%), and only 11% of patients reported the most severe itching in the morning.[7,8] High severity of pruritus at night resulted in significant sleeping problems. Eighty-four percent of patients declared difficulties in falling asleep, 79% awakening in the night and 38% the necessity of taking sleeping medications.[6] Problems in falling asleep were noted by 81% of subjects and the use of sleeping medication was observed in 31% of participants.[7,8] In a study conducted among children with AD, 62 scratching episodes were observed on average during every night, lasting in total 48 min, which constitutes about 8% of the whole sleeping time.[9] In addition, both shorter (8.5 vs. 2 awakenings) and longer awakening episodes (5.5 vs. 1 awakenings) were more frequently observed in children with AD compared to healthy controls; thus the sleep efficacy was significantly decreased in children with AD.[9] Based on the VAS results, it seems that itching in AD should be con-

L. Misery and S. Ständer (eds.), *Pruritus*,
DOI 10.1007/978-1-84882-322-8_14, © Springer-Verlag London Limited 2010

sidered as one of the most severe, compared to other entities, e.g., psoriasis (VAS = 5) or uraemic pruritus (VAS = 7.2).[10,11]

The most commonly mentioned factors aggravating pruritus in AD were sweating (88–96%), skin dryness (71–90%), physical effort (66–73%), stress (71%), specific fabrics (e.g., wool) (64%), hot water (48–55%) and diet (57%).[6–8] On the other hand, the most commonly used treatment modalities reported by Polish patients with AD to reduce or alleviate itching were as follows: emollients (80.9%), antihistaminics (77.5%), topical corticosteroids (68.5%), cold air (37.1%), cool bath (23.6%) and relaxation (20.2%).[7,8] However, emollients provide a long-term antipruritic effect only in 26% of patients, and 62% of subjects noted only short-term reduction of pruritus; in a further 4%, emollients did not influence itching at all (8% did not have any opinion regarding emollients usage).[7,8] Similarly, long-term antipruritic effect after antihistaminics usage was observed only in 14% of patients, short-term effect in 65% and no effect in a further 14% of study participants.[7,8]

### 14.2.2 Pathogenesis of Pruritus in Atopic Dermatitis

Pathogenesis of pruritus in AD remains unclear. It seems that pruritus is generated in the skin by activation of pruriceptors, but the injury of peripheral nerves and central mechanisms may also play a significant role.[5] According to the most widely accepted hypothesis, patients with AD show decreased threshold for pruritogenic stimuli, as many substances may provoke itching in them at much lower concentrations than in control subjects.[12] Moreover, AD skin shows increased number of nerve fibers, increased number of neurofilaments as well as altered levels of β-endorphin, substance P (SP), neuropeptide Y (NPY) and calcitonin gene-related peptide (CGRP).[12–14] SP and brain-derived neurotrophic factor serum levels correlated with childhood AD severity and with the nocturnal wrist movements.[15] Due to increased excretion of nerve growth factor (NGF) by the basal layer of epidermis, an increased number of hyperplastic nerve fibers with enlarged axons was observed in AD skin.[12] On the other hand, Bigliardi-Qi et al.[16] observed that in AD the epidermal nerve endings are thin and run straight through the epidermis, while in normal skin the epidermal nerve endings are rather thick.[16] The important role of altered innervations in the pathogenesis of AD pruritus may be supported by the observation of itching reduction after capsaicin treatment.[17]

It could be also speculated that neuropeptides in atopic skin may induce expression and/or activity of dermal proteases, which, acting via proteinase activated receptors (PARs), might be responsible for pruritus.[18,19] Recent findings suggested that proteases not only are degrading enzymes but rather represent a group of mediators communicating with nerves, thereby modulating inflammation, pain and pruritus.[19,20] A massive itch behavior was noted in mice overexpressing epidermal kallikrein-7.[19] Tryptase and microbial proteases induced itch by the PAR-2-mediated neurogenic mechanism.[19,21] Activation of PAR-2 induced itching both in mice and in humans.[19–22] Because PAR-2 is irreversibly activated by proteinases, it might also be a good candidate for the explanation of chronic itch. In addition, a significant correlation was found between the pruritus intensity and the number of tryptase-positive mast cells in lesional atopic skin, and the imbalance of tryptase and chymase activity in mast cells was suggested to play an important role in the pathogenesis of AD.[23]

Histamine may also play a role in the pathogenesis of itching in AD; however, its role seems to be less important as was suggested in the past. Although increased levels of histamine in the skin and blood were noted in patients with AD,[24,25] protein extravasation induced by histamine in these patients was significantly reduced compared to healthy controls.[26] Moreover, blockade of H1 receptors by cetirizine did not diminish experimentally induced pruritus in AD subjects.[26] Histamine receptors in AD skin also showed lower affinity to histamine than in healthy skin.[5] Regarding the results of clinical trials on the efficacy of antihistaminics in the reduction of pruritus, some authors have shown that they may bring some relief of itching,[25,27] while other showed no benefit over placebo[26,28] (see also below).

There is also a long list of other possible mediators that might contribute to itching. Several cytokines, mainly interleukin (IL)-2 and IL-6, were suspected to induce pruritus in AD.[29] Intradermal injection of IL-2 induced itching in humans, and the appearance of pruritus was faster in patients with AD than in controls.[29] The severity of itching after IL-2 injection was increased by bradykinin but reduced by cyclosporin A.[29] Recently, a novel cytokine, IL-31, was suggested to play important role in pruritus of AD, as IL-31 caused the itch-associated scratching behavior in conventional NC/Nga mice, which is an experimental animal model for AD.[30]

Pruritus in AD subjects may be elucidated by the opioid system as well, as significantly altered μ- and κ-opioid receptor expression was observed in the epidermis of AD skin, showing mainly downregulation of κ-opioid system, which is believed to have itch-suppressive properties.[16,31] Psoralen and ultraviolet A radiation (PUVA) treatment, a frequently applied and effective therapy of AD, was shown to reconstitute the altered opioid receptor distribution in AD epidermis.[31] Opioids may also induce pruritus acting in the central nervous system. It was shown that intrathecal administration of morphine may elicit pruritus, and both naloxone and naltrexone, the potent opioid receptor antagonists, reduced histamine-induced pruritus in AD subjects to a greater extent than antihistaminic drugs.[32,33] Although it was suggested that opioid receptor antagonists act in AD mainly via the central nervous system,[34] recently it was clearly demonstrated that topically applied opioid receptor antagonist may also be useful for the treatment of AD itching.[35]

Another candidate for pruritus mediator in AD is acetylcholine. This substance injected intradermally was demonstrated to elicit pure pruritus in AD patients with acute eczema, and a "mixture" of pain and itch in the atopics just free from eczema, instead of pain, which is usually observed in healthy controls.[36] Moreover, an increased concentration of acetylcholine was found in AD skin.[12] Pruritus in AD may also be related to the decreased ability of producing prostaglandin D$_2$ (PGD$_2$) by atopic skin. PGD$_2$ was shown to possess antipruritic activity.[37,38] In the mouse model of AD, the impaired scratch-induced cutaneous PGD$_2$ production resulted in no suppression of scratching and aggravated the dermatitis.[37,38]

## 14.2.3  Therapy of Pruritus in Atopic Dermatitis

The efficacious control of pruritus in AD subjects remains a major challenge during therapy of AD. As mentioned above, data regarding the usage of antihistaminics in

patients with AD are not conclusive. "It must also be underlined that well designed, randomised, placebo-controlled studies assessing efficacy of antihistaminics in AD are still lacking."[39] The majority of trials are flawed in terms of the sample size or study design.[39] However, it seems that antihistaminics could be of some help at least in a subgroup of patients with AD. Drake et al.[40–42] reported that topically applied doxepin reduced pruritus in AD to a greater extent than the vehicle alone, and this treatment was generally well tolerated. Sometimes, local irritation may be noted.[43] Doxepin is used as a 5% cream and should be applied three to four times a day to a maximum of 10% of body surface (the total daily dose of doxepin should not exceed 3 g per day). The therapeutic effect is noticeable about 15 min after application. Regarding the oral administration, it seems that the first generation of antihistaminics might bring better relief of pruritus due to their additional sedative properties. However, the necessary doses are usually high and therefore they may produce significant sedation of patients.[44,45] Among the newer antihistaminics, cetirizine seems to be the best choice; however, the efficacy is strictly related to administered dose of the drug.[44,46–48] The significant reduction of pruritus was observed for the dose of at least 20 mg per day of cetirizine.[45] A dose of 10 mg cetirizine twice daily was shown to be more effective in reducing pruritus than 60 mg terfenadine twice daily.[49] Other antihistaminics, including loratidine, epinastine, fexofenadine, ketotifen or oxatomide, may also be of help in improving pruritus in AD subjects.[25,27,50–52] It is probable that the reduction of pruritus in case of some antihistaminics is related not only to histamine blockade, but may also be connected with counteracting eosinophil migration or inhibition of the platelet-activating factor.[53–56]

Improvement of pruritus in patients with AD was also noted after the use of calcineurin inhibitors (tacrolimus, pimecrolimus).[5] The probable antipruritic mechanism is related to IL-2 blockade and inhibition of histamine release from mast cells.[5] Pimecrolimus may also directly act on nerve endings, although this pathway has not been studied well so far.[57] After topical application of calcineurin inhibitors, transient irritation with burning or itching sensation is frequently observed.[5,57] This effect is probably connected with the binding of pimecrolimus and tacrolimus to ion channels, such as transient receptor potential vanilloid 1 or receptors involved in nociception, and a subsequent release of neuropeptides from dermal nerve endings. After prolonged use of topical calcineurin inhibitors, the density of these receptors decreases and their affinity to pimecrolimus or tacrolimus becomes lower, and finally the initially observed irritation disappears.[58] Calcineurin inhibitors may also reduce pruritus by the direct inhibition of IgE-mediated degranulation of mast cells.[5] The efficacy of topical calcineurin inhibitors in the therapy of AD pruritus was confirmed in clinical trials and was dependent on the concentration as well as the frequency of application.[59–62] Despite the initial irritation, the antipruritic effect of calcineurin inhibitors was evident as quickly as 2–3 days after beginning of the treatment.[59,63] Calcineurin inhibitors significantly diminished the intensity of pruritus both in adults and children with AD, the efficacy increased with the duration of the treatment and maximal efficacy is observed about 40–45 days after beginning of the therapy.[59,64,65]

Significant reduction of pruritus was also achieved when emollients were used in combination with topical corticosteroids.[66–68] Moreover, the regular use of emollients during the periods of remission decreases the risk of AD relapse and enables prevention of pruritus flare when topical corticosteroids are discontinued.[68] It is important to remember that not all emollients may be suitable for patients with AD, and some formulations may even deteriorate the skin condition as, for instance, emulsifiers may weaken the skin barrier.[69] However, many formulations have been shown to be well tolerated by patients with AD or similar skin conditions.[68] It is also worth mentioning that topical preparation containing N-palmitoylethanolamine, an endocannabinoid, was recently shown to significantly improve itching in AD patients.[70] A good option for patients with severe AD is cyclosporin A.[28,71–73] In severe, intractable pruritus, psychotropic drugs may also be tried.[74]

## 14.3 Psoriasis

### 14.3.1 Frequency and Clinical Manifestation of Pruritus

Psoriasis is one of the most common chronic inflammatory skin diseases with a complex, multifactor and still not fully understood etiopathogenesis. About 70–90%

of patients with psoriasis suffer from itching,[10,75–80] and many of them (at least 30%) have generalized pruritus.[10,77] The mean intensity of this symptom assessed according to the 10-point VAS ranged between 3.7 and 6.4 points,[77,78,81–83] which is markedly less than the intensity observed in AD or uremic pruritus.[8,11] The mean surface area involved in itch was 24%.[77] It seems that patients with pruritus suffer from more severe psoriasis,[10,76,79] although some authors did not find any relationship between the pruritus intensity and psoriasis severity.[77,83] The presence and intensity of itching was independent of age, gender, marital status, family history of psoriasis or atopy, type of psoriasis, alcohol or smoking habits and duration of the disease, as well as duration of the last outbreak of psoriasis.[10,76,79]

Pruritus tended to appear more at night and in the evening than in the morning or at noon.[77] Pruritus in psoriatic subjects was also very frequent; it appeared on a daily basis in 77%, on a weekly basis in 18% and less frequently in 5% of patients.[77] The most commonly affected body areas were trunk as well as lower and upper extremities.[10,77] The scalp was observed to be pruritic in less than 40% of individuals and face was only sporadically reported to be itchy.[10,77] The itch location was not related to handedness.[77] In about 70–80% of patients itching was limited to psoriatic lesions and in the remaining ones it also involved the non-lesional skin.[10,79] According to patients' own evaluation, the most intensive itching was observed during the appearance of skin lesions or the extension of psoriatic lesions.[10] The majority of pruritic individuals stated that relief of itching was associated with total disappearance of psoriatic lesions and, less commonly, when psoriatic scales were removed or just after introduction of topical antipsoriatic treatment.[10]

Pruritus was very often mentioned as the most bothersome symptom of psoriasis.[76] Moreover, in many patients pruritus was associated with difficulty in falling asleep and awakenings.[77] On analyzing psychosocial parameters it was noted that pruritus intensity significantly correlated with degree of quality of life impairment, level of stigmatization and the presence and severity of depressive symptoms.[83] As a result of pruritus, 35% of the patients became more agitated, 24% became depressed, 30% had difficulty in concentrating, 23% changed their eating habits and 35% reported their sexual function to be decreased or nonexistent.[77] It was also demonstrated that the degree of depressive psychopathology discriminated between the mild, moderate, and severe pruritus groups at admission.[76] Prospectively, the change in depression scores correlated with the change in pruritus.[76] The presence and intensity of itching was also related to the severity of stress experienced before the exacerbation of the disease.[78,83] It could be concluded that pruritus has a big negative influence on the psychosocial well-being of patients with psoriasis.

## 14.3.2  The Pathogenesis of Pruritus

The pathogenesis of itching in psoriasis remains unclear. Histamine, which is one of the major mediators of pruritus, does not seem to be involved in its development in psoriasis, as there was no correlation between pruritus intensity and plasma histamine level in psoriasis, and there was no difference in plasma histamine levels between pruritic and non-pruritic patients with psoriasis.[81] The most often discussed theory mentioned the importance of altered innervations and neuropeptide imbalance in psoriatic skin. Several studies demonstrated changed expression and distribution within various layers of skin of several neuropeptides and their receptors including SP, CGRP, vasoactive intestinal peptide (VIP), somatostatin or pituitary adenylate cyclase activating polypeptide (PACAP) in psoriasis.[18,84–91] Neuropeptides may degranulate mastocytes, activate dendritic cells, lymphocytes, macrophages and neutrophils, and may produce vascular changes in the skin by inducing angiogenesis, dilatation of vessels and stimulation of synthesis of nitric oxide.[18] They also stimulate synthesis and release of many proinflammatory cytokines from mast cells, lymphocytes, dendritic cells, fibroblasts and keratinocytes, induce expression of vascular adhesion molecules on endothelium and may exert hyperproliferative effect on keratinocytes.[18] Regarding pruritus in psoriasis, Nakamura et al.[92] observed an increased number of mast cells in the papillary dermis in pruritic psoriatic skin among the various cellular components examined, including resident cells and infiltrating cells in the skin lesions. Ultrastructural examination showed that these mast cells possessed degranulating specific granules, indicating that mast cells in pruritic psoriatic skin were activated. The particularly characteristic finding of mast cells in lesional skin from patients with pruritus was the presence of free mast cell granules in close

apposition to the perineurium surrounding unmyelinated nerve fibers. These findings were never observed in skin from patients without pruritus.[92] In addition, pruritic psoriatic skin demonstrated significantly increased numbers of NGF-immunoreactive keratinocytes, NGF contents in lesional skin, expression of high-affinity receptor for NGF (Trk-A) in the epidermis and dermal nerve fibres, protein gene product (PGP) 9.5-immunoreactive nerve fibers in the epidermis and in the upper dermal areas and SP-containing nerves in the perivascular areas as well as decreased expression of neutral endopeptidase in the epidermal basal layer and in the endothelia of blood vessels.[92] The pruritus intensity correlated with the number of PGP 9.5-immunoreactive intraepidermal nerve fibers, NGF-immunoreactive keratinocytes and expression of TrkA in the epidermis.[92] Nakamura et al.[92] did not find any differences between pruritic and non-pruritic psoriatics regarding the skin expression of brain-derived neurotrophic factor, neurotrophin-3, VIP, NPY, somatostatin, low-affinity receptor for NGF and angiotensin-converting enzyme. In another study,[79] a hyperproliferation of small cutaneous nerves was found in the lesional skin of pruritic psoriatic subjects. Keratinocytes in the psoriatic plaques of patients with pruritus also showed consistently increased expression of SP receptor, TrkA and CGRP receptor, but the immunoreactivity for SP, CGRP, VIP and PACAP was independent of the occurrence of pruritus. Similarly, the expression of NGF, neurotrophin-4, low-affinity receptor for NGF, receptor for PACAP as well as neutral endopeptidase did not differ between pruritus and nonpruritus groups.[79] Interestingly, Remröd et al.[82] did not find any relationship between SP-positive fibers or cells and the degree of pruritus. In addition, the plasma NPY level was significantly decreased in patients with pruritus compared to patients without pruritus.[80] Plasma levels of SP, CGRP and VIP did not differ significantly between patients with and without pruritus; however, a tendency to lower SP and VIP plasma levels in patients with itching was noted.[80] Moreover, a significant negative correlation between pruritus severity and SP as well as VIP plasma levels was found. In another study, it was noted that CGRP plasma level was significantly elevated in pruritic psoriatic patients and that the CGRP plasma level correlated with itching intensity in some subgroups of psoriatics.[81] The important role of altered innervation and neuropeptide imbalance in pruritus accompanying psoriasis may also be supported by the observations that topically applied capsaicin, which is a potent SP depletory, effectively treated pruritus in psoriatics.[93,94] Increased innervation in the skin of psoriatic patients with pruritus may lead to a lower threshold for pruritic stimuli compared to patients without pruritus, but this hypothesis still requires further studies and confirmation.

Regarding other possible mediators of pruritus in psoriasis, Nakamura et al.[92] found an increased number of IL-2 immunoreactive cells in pruritic versus non-pruritic lesions of psoriasis. There were no significant differences in the expression of other cytokines (INF-$\gamma$, TNF-$\alpha$, IL-1$\alpha$, IL-1$\beta$, IL-4, IL-5, IL-6, IL-8, IL-10, IL-12).[92] These authors also observed a marked increase in the density of endothelial leukocyte adhesion molecule (ELAM)-1-positive venules in patients with pruritus.[92] There was no statistical difference in the number of vessels immunoreactive for intercellular cell adhesion molecule (ICAM)-1, vascular cell adhesion molecule (VCAM)-1 or platelet endothelial cell adhesion molecule (PECAM)-1 in the upper dermis or in the expression of ICAM-1 in the epidermis.[92] Moreover, a significant correlation was demonstrated between the itching intensity and the density of E-selectin immunoreactive vessels.[92] Madej et al.[95] found an increased serum concentration of soluble vascular adhesion protein (VAP)-1 in psoriatic subjects with pruritus compared to patient free of this symptom. These observations suggest that vascular alterations found in psoriatic lesions may also contribute to the development of itching.

### 14.3.3 Treatment of Pruritus in Psoriasis

As the pathogenesis of pruritus in psoriasis remains undetermined, no specific and effective antipruritic treatment has been developed to date for this group of patients. In the questionnaire study conducted among Polish psoriatics, over 80% of participants declared that they used various treatment modalities to control itching.[10] The most commonly applied therapy were various emollients and moisturizers or systemic antihistaminic agents.[10] However, only less than 20% of studied subjects stated that these kinds of the therapies were highly effective. For the vast majority of patients these treatment modalities appeared to be ineffective or caused only temporary relief.[10] It seems that only

sedating antihistaminics should be administered in pruritic psoriatics, as the histamine blockade alone does not prevent pruritus. In a recent review by Dawn and Yosipovitch,[96] several types of remedies were mentioned to be of help to control pruritus in psoriasis: tar products, topical corticosteroids, topical salicylates, agents that alter skin sensation, phototherapy, vitamin D analogs, topical immunomodulators, methotrexate, oral mirtazapine and biologics. Most of them were oriented towards the improvement of psoriatic lesions and concomitant decrease of itching intensity, as it has already been shown that the vast majority of patients noted reduction of pruritus with the disappearance of skin lesions.[10,96] However, it is important to mention that well-designed studies confirming the advantages of these treatment modalities over placebo in controlling pruritus in psoriasis are still lacking. Narrow-band ultraviolet B (UVB) was shown to be effective in treating psoriatic itch;[97] however, treatment with UVB may actually aggravate itch during the first 2–3 weeks of therapy.[96] It is important to use moisturizers or emollients throughout phototherapy treatment.[96] In case of severe pruritus, oral antidepressants, mainly mirtazapine (15 mg at night), should be tried. Mirtazapine relieves itch even in cases of severe pruritus associated with erythrodermic psoriasis.[96,98] Mirtazapine has a sedative effect due to its H$_1$-antihistamine properties, but it also acts as an antagonist on noradrenergic $\alpha$2-receptors and 5HT$_2$ and 5HT$_3$ serotonin receptors.[96] Summarizing, the therapy of psoriatic itch remains an important goal and, for sure, no single therapy will be effective for all psoriasis patients with itch. For many patients a good option will be even combining two or more strategies. Most treatments that relieve psoriatic itch also treat psoriasis in general; however, the primary goal is to alleviate itch before clearance of visible lesions is achieved with topical and systemic therapies.[96]

## 14.4 Conclusions

Summarizing, it could be stated that pruritus is an important symptom of inflammatory skin diseases. To date, the best data are available for AD, but many aspects of itching in AD have not been clarified. Recently, several studies have been undertaken to elucidate the clinical manifestation and pathogenesis of pruritus accompanying psoriasis. However, this is just a beginning, and similarly to AD we still need further data to better understand and treat this symptom in patients with psoriasis. Data regarding itching in other inflammatory skin conditions are very limited and any conclusion is hard to be established, although this symptom has been well recognized for decades in such disorders as lichen planus. Therefore, clinical and molecular studies on itching in inflammatory skin conditions are highly warranted, as many items need to be clarified.

# References

1. Ständer S, Streit M, Darsow U, et al. Diagnostisches und therapeutisches Vorgehen bei chronischem Pruritus. *J Dtsch Dermatol Ges*. 2006;4:350–370.
2. Hanifin JM, Rajka G. Diagnostic features of atopic dermatitis. *Acta Dermatol Venereol (Stockh)*. 1980;92(suppl):44–7.
3. Williams HC, Burney PG, Pembroke AC et al. The U.K. working party's diagnostic criteria for atopic dermatitis. III. Independent hospital validation. *Br J Dermatol*. 1994;131:406–16.
4. European Task Force on Atopic Dermatitis. Severity scoring of atopic dermatitis: the SCORAD index. *Dermatology*. 1993;186:23–31.
5. Szepietowski J, Reich A, Białynicki-Birula R. Itching in atopic dermatitis: clinical manifestation, pathogenesis and the role of pimekrolimus in itch reduction. *Dermatol Klin*. 2004;6:173–6.
6. Yosipovitch G, Goon ATJ, Wee J, et al. Itch characteristics in Chinese patients with atopic dermatitis using a new questionnaire for the assessment of pruritus. *Int J Dermatol*. 2002;41:212–6.
7. Chrostowska-Plak D, Salomon J, Reich A, Szepietowski JC. Clinical aspects of itch in adult atopic dermatitis patients. *Acta Derm Venereol*. 2009;89:379–383.
8. Chrostowska-Plak. *Analysis of Itching in Patient Suffering from Atopic Dermatitis*. [PhD thesis]. Wroclaw: Akademia Medyczna; 2006.
9. Stores G, Burrows A, Crawford C. Physiological sleep disturbance in children with atopic dermatitis: a case control study. *Pediatr Dermatol*. 1998;15:264–268.
10. Szepietowski JC, Reich A, Wiśnicka B. Itching in patients suffering from psoriasis. *Acta Dermatovenerol Croat*. 2002;10:221–226.
11. Szepietowski JC, Sikora M, Kusztal M et al. Uremic pruritus: a clinical study of maintenance hemodialysis patients. *J Dermatol*. 2002;29:621–627.
12. Ständer S, Steinhoff M. Pathophysiology of pruritus in atopic dermatitis: an overview. *Exp Dermatol*. 2002;11:12–24.
13. Glinski W, Brodecka H, Glinska-Ferenz M et al. Increased concentration of beta-endorphin in the sera of patients with severe atopic dermatitis. *Acta Derm Venereol*. 1995;75:9–11.
14. Salomon J, Baran E. The role of selected neuropeptides in pathogenesis of atopic dermatitis. *J Eur Acad Dermatol Venereol*. 2008;22:223–228.
15. Hon K-L, Lam M-CA, Wong K-Y et al. Pathophysiology of nocturnal scratching in childhood atopic dermatitis: the role of brain-derived neurotrophic factor and substance P. *Br J Dermatol*. 2007;157:922–925.
16. Bigliardi-Qi M, Lipp B, Sumanovski LT et al. Changes of epidermal mu-opiate receptor expression and nerve endings in chronic atopic dermatitis. *Dermatology*. 2005;210:91–99.
17. Reitamo S, Ansel JC, Luger TA. Itch in atopic dermatitis. *J Am Acad Dermatol*. 2001;45:S55–S56.
18. Reich A, Orda A, Wiśnicka B et al. Plasma concentration of selected neuropeptides in patients suffering from psoriasis. *Exp Dermatol*. 2007;16:421–428.
19. Steinhoff M, Bienenstock J, Schmelz M et al. Neurophysiological, neuroimmunological, and neuroendocrine basis of pruritus. *J Invest Dermatol*. 2006;126:1705–1718.
20. Steinhoff M, Neisius U, Ikoma A et al. Proteinase-activated receptor-2 mediates itch: a novel pathway for pruritus in human skin. *J Neurosci*. 2003;23:6176–6180.
21. Ui H, Andoh T, Lee J-B et al. Potent pruritogenic action of tryptase mediated by PAR-2 receptor and its involvement in anti-pruritic effect of nafamostat mesilate in mice. *Eur J Pharmacol*. 2006;530:172–178.
22. Shimada SG, Shimada KA, Collins JG. Scratching behavior in mice induced by the proteinase-activated receptor-2 agonist, SLIGRL-NH$_2$. *Eur J Pharmacol*. 2006;530:281–283.
23. Kapelko K, Cislo M. Tryptase and chymase-positive mast cells in atopic dermatitis. *J Eur Acad Dermatol Venereol*. 1999;13(suppl 2):159.
24. Hanifin JM. Pharmacophysiology of atopic dermatitis. *Clin Rev Allergy*. 1986;4:43–65.
25. Imaizumi A, Kawakami T, Murakami F et al. Effective treatment of pruritus in atopic dermatitis using H1 antihistamines (second-generation antihistamines): changes in blood histamine and tryptase levels. *J Dermatol Sci*. 2003;33:23–29.
26. Rukwied R, Lischetzki G, McGlone F et al. Mast cell mediators other than histamine induce pruritus in atopic dermatitis patients: a dermal microdialysis study. *Br J Dermatol*. 2000;142:1114–1120.
27. Kawashima M, Tango T, Noguchi T et al. Addition of fexofenadine to a topical corticosteroid reduces the pruritus associated with atopic dermatitis in a 1-week randomized, multicentre, double-blind, placebo-controlled, parallel-group study. *Br J Dermatol*. 2003;148:1212–1221.
28. Wahlgren CF. Itch and atopic dermatitis: clinical and experimental studies. *Acta Derm Venereol Suppl (Stockh)*. 1991;165:1–53.
29. Lippert U, Hoer A, Moller A et al. Role of antigen-induced cytokine release in atopic pruritus. *Int Arch Allergy Immunol*. 1998;116:36–39.
30. Takaoka A, Arai I, Sugimoto M et al. Involvement of IL-31 on scratching behavior in NC/Nga mice with atopic-like dermatitis. *Exp Dermatol*. 2006;15:161–167.
31. Tominaga M, Ogawa H, Takamori K. Possible role of epidermal opioid systems in pruritus of atopic dermatitis. *J Invest Dermatol*. 2007;127:2228–2235.
32. Heyer G, Dotzer M, Diepgen TL et al. Opiate and H1 antagonist effects on histamine induced pruritus and alloknesis. *Pain*. 1997;73:239–243.
33. Heyer G, Groene D, Martus P. Efficacy of naltrexone on acetylcholine-induced alloknesis in atopic eczema. *Exp Dermatol*. 2002;11:448–455.

34. Maekawa T, Yamaguchi-Miyamoto T, Nojima H et al. Effects of naltrexone on spontaneous itch-associated responses in NC mice with chronic dermatitis. *Jpn J Pharmacol.* 2002;90:193–196.

35. Bigliardi PL, Stammer H, Jost G et al. Treatment of pruritus with topically applied opiate receptor antagonist. *J Am Acad Dermatol.* 2007;56:979–988.

36. Heyer GR, Hornstein OP. Recent studies of cutaneous nociception in atopic and non-atopic subjects. *J Dermatol.* 1999;26:77–86.

37. Sugimoto M, Arai I, Futaki N et al. Increased scratching counts depend on a decrease in ability of cutaneous prostaglandin D$_2$ biosynthesis in NC/Nga mice with atopic dermatitis. *Exp Dermatol.* 2005;14:898–905.

38. Takaoka A, Arai I, Sugimoto M et al. Role of scratch-induced cutaneous prostaglandin D$_2$ production on atopic-like scratching behaviour in mice. *Exp Dermatol.* 2007;16:331–339.

39. Klein PA, Clark RAF. An evidence-based review of the efficacy of antihistamines in relieving pruritus in atopic dermatitis. *Arch Dermatol.* 1999;135:1522–1525

40. Drake LA, Fallon JD, Sober A. Relief of pruritus in patients with atopic dermatitis after treatment with topical doxepin cream. The Doxepin Study Group. *J Am Acad Dermatol.* 1994;31:613–616.

41. Drake LA, Millikan LE. The antipruritic effect of 5% dexepin cream in patients with eczematous dermatitis. The Doxepin Study Group. *Arch Dermatol.* 1995;131:1403–1408.

42. Drake LA, Cohen L, Gillies R et al. Pharmacokinetics of doxepin in subjects with pruritic atopic dermatitis. *J Am Acad Dermatol.* 1999;41:209–214.

43. Taylor JS, Praditsuwan P, Handel D, Kuffner G. Allergic contact dermatitis from doxepin cream. One-year patch test clinic experience. *Arch Dermatol.* 1996;132:515–518.

44. Zuberbier T, Henz BM. Use of cetirizine in dermatologic disorders. *Ann Allergy Asthma Immunol.* 1999;83:476–480.

45. Wahlgreen C-F, Hägermark Ö, Bergström R. The antipruritic effect of sedative and a non-sedative antihistamine in atopic dermatitis. *Br J Dermatol.* 1990;122:545–551.

46. Diepgen TL. Long-term treatment with cetirizine of infants with atopic dermatitis: a multi-country, double blind, randomized, placebo controlled trial (the ETAC? trial) over 18 months. *Pediatr Allergy Immunol.* 2002;13:278–286.

47. Hannuksela M, Kalimo K, Lammintausta K et al. Dose running study: cetirizine in the treatment of atopic dermatitis in adults. *Ann Allergy.* 1993;70:127–133.

48. La Rosa M, Ranno C, Musarra I et al. Double-blind study of cetirizine in atopic eczema in children. *Ann Allergy.* 1994;73:117–122.

49. Behrendt H, Ring J. Histamine, antihistamines and atopic eczema. *Clin Exp Allergy.* 1990;20(suppl 4):25–30.

50. Langeland T, Fagertun HE, Larsen S. Therapeutic effect of loratadine on pruritus in patients with atopic dermatitis. A multi-crossover-designed study. *Allergy.* 1994;49:22–26.

51. Falk ES. Ketotifen in the treatment of atopic dermatitis. Results of a double blind study. *Riv Eur Sci Med Farmacol.* 1993;15:63–66.

52. Yoshida H, Niimura M, Ueda H et al. Clinical evaluation of ketotifen syrup on atopic dermatitis: a comparative multicenter double-blind study of ketotifen and clemastine. *Ann Allergy.* 1989;62:507–512.

53. Slater JW, Zechnich D, Haxby DG. Second-generation antihistamines. A comparative review. *Drugs.* 1999;57:31–47.

54. Amon U, Gibbs BF, Buss G et al. In vitro investigations with the histamine H1 receptor antagonist, epinastine (WAL 801 CL), on isolated human allergic effector cells. *Inflamm Res.* 2000;49:112–116.

55. Marone G, Granata F, Spadaro G et al. Antiinflammatory effects of oxatomide. *J Investig Allergol Clin Immunol.* 1999;9:207–214.

56. Abdelaziz MM, Devalia JL, Khair OA et al. Effect of fexofenadine on eosinophil-induced changes in epithelial permeability and t, Wozel G et al. Pimecrolimus cream in the long-term management of atopic dermatitis in adults: a six month study. *Dermatology.* 2000;205:271–277.

61. Luger T, van Leent EJM, Graeber M et al. SDZ ASM 981: an emerging safe and effective treatment for atopic dermatitis. *Br J Dermatol.* 2001;144:788–794.

62. Ashcroft DM, Dimmock P, Garside R et al. Efficacy and tolerability of topical pimecrolimus and tacrolimus in the treatment of atopic dermatitis: meta-analysis of randomised controlled trials. *Br Med J.* 2005;330:516.

63. Kaufmann R, Bieber T, Helgesen AL et al. Onset of pruritus relief with pimecrolimus cream 1% in adult patients with atopic dermatitis: a randomized trial. *Allergy.* 2006;61:375–381.

64. Eichenfield LF, Lucky AW, Boguniewicz M et al. Safety and efficacy of pimekrolimus (ASM 981) cream 1% in the treatment of mild and moderate atopic dermatitis in children and adolescents. *J Am Acad Dermatol.* 2002;46:495–504.

65. Boguniewicz M, Fiedler VC, Raimer S et al. A randomized, vehicle-controlled trial of tacrolimus ointment for treatment of atopic dermatitis in children. *J Allergy Clin Immunol.* 1998;102:637–644

66. Hanifin JM, Hebert AA, Mays SR et al. Effects of a low-potency corticosteroid lotion plus a moisturizing regimen in the treatment of atopic dermatitis. *Curr Ther Res.* 1998;59:227–233.

67. Grimalt R, Mengeaud V, Cambazard F. Study Investigators' Group. The steroid-sparing effect of an emollient therapy in infants with atopic dermatitis: a randomized controlled study. *Dermatology.* 2007;214:61–67.

68. Reich A, Szczepanowska J, Szepietowski J. The role of emollients in the treatment of atopic dermatitis. *Dermatol Klin.* 2007;9:153–156.

69. Loden M. Role of topical emollients and moisturizers in the treatment of dry skin barrier disorders. *Am J Clin Dermatol.* 2003;4:771–788.

70. Eberlein B, Eicke C, Reinhardt H-W et al. Adjuvant treatment of atopic eczema: assessment of an emollient containing N-palmitoylethanolamine (ATOPA study). *J Eur Acad Dermatol Venereol.* 2008;22:73–82.

71. Wahlgren CF, Scheynius A, Hägermark O. Antipruritic effect of oral cyclosporin A in atopic dermatitis. *Acta Derm Venereol.* 1990;70:323–329.

72. Berth-Jones J, Graham-Brown RA, M.arks R et al. Long-term efficacy and safety of cyclosporin in severe adult atopic dermatitis. *Br J Dermatol.* 1997;136:76–81.

73. Harper JI, Ahmed I, Barclay G et al. Cyclosporin for severe childhood atopic dermatitis: short course versus continuous therapy. *Br J Dermatol.* 2000;142:52–58.

74. Mahtani R, Parekh N, Mangat I et al. Alleviating the itch-scratch cycle in atopic dermatitis. *Psychosomatics.* 2005;46:373–374.

75. Newbold PCH. Pruritus in psoriasis. In: Farber EM, Cox AJ, eds. *Psoriasis: Proceedings of the Second International Symposium.* New York: Yorke Medical Books; 1997:334–336.

76. Gupta MA, Gupta AK, Kirby S et al. Pruritus in psoriasis. A prospective study of some psychiatric and dermatologic correlates. *Arch Dermatol.* 1988;124:1052–1057.

77. Yosipovitch G, Goon A, Wee J et al. The prevalence and clinical characteristics of pruritus among patients with extensive psoriasis. *Br J Dermatol.* 2000;143:969–973.

78. Reich A, Szepietowski JC, Wiśnicka B et al. Does stress influence itching in psoriatic patients? *Dermatol Psychosom.* 2003;4:151–155.

79. Chang S-E, Han S-S, Jung H-J et al. Neuropeptides and their receptors in psoriatic skin in relation to pruritus. *Br J Dermatol.* 2007;156:1272–1277.

80. Reich A, Orda A, Wiśnicka, et al. Plasma neuropeptides and perception of pruritus in psoriasis. *Acta Derm Venereol (Stockh).* 2007;87:299–304.

81. Wiśnicka B, Szepietowski JC, Reich A et al. Histamine, substance P and calcitonin gene-related peptide plasma concentration and pruritus in patients suffering from psoriasis. *Dermatol Psychosom.* 2004;5:73–78.

82. Remröd C, Lonne-Rahm S, Nordlind K. Study of substance P and its receptor neurokinin-1 in psoriasis and their relation to chronic stress and pruritus. *Arch Dermatol Res.* 2007;299:85–91.

83. Reich A, Hrechorow E, Szepietowski JC. Negative influence of itching on psoriatic patients' well-being. *Acta Derm Venereol (Stockh).* 2007;87:478–479.

84. Eedy DJ, Johnston CF, Shaw, et al. Neuropeptides in psoriasis: an immunocytochemical and radioimmunoasay study. *J Invest Dermatol.* 1991;96:434–438.

85. Naukkarinen A, Harvima I, Paukkonen K et al. Immunohistochemical analysis of sensory nerves and neuropeptides, and their contacts with mast cells in developing and mature psoriatic lesions. *Arch Dermatol Res.* 1993; 285:341–346.

86. Chan J, Smoller BR, Raychauduri SP et al. Intraepidermal nerve fiber expression of calcitonin gene-related peptide, vasoactive intestinal peptide and substance P in psoriasis. *Arch Dermatol Res.* 1997;287:611–616.

87. Jiang W-Y, Raydchaudhuri SP, Farber EM. Double-labeled immunofluorescence study of cutaneous nerves in psoriasis. *Int J Dermatol.* 1998;37:572–574.

88. Raychaudhuri SP, Jiang W-Y, Farber EM. Psoriatic keratinocytes express high levels of nerve growth factor. *Acta Derm Venereol (Stockh).* 1998;78:84–86.

89. Staniek V, Doutremepuich J-D, Schmitt D et al. Expression of substance P receptors in normal and psoriatic skin. *Photobiology.* 1999;67:51–54.

90. Steinhoff M, McGregor GP, Radleff-Schlimme A et al. Identification of pituitary adenylate cyclase activating polypeptide (PACAP) and PACAP type 1 receptor in human skin: expression of PACAP-38 is increased in patients with psoriasis. *Regul Pept.* 1999;80:49–55.

91. He Y, Ding G, Wang X et al. Calcitonin gene-related peptide in Langerhans cells in psoriatic plaque lesions. *Chin Med J.* 2000;113:747–751.

92. Nakamura M, Toyoda M, Morohashi M. Pruritogenic mediators in psoriasis vulgaris: comparative evaluation of itch-associated cutaneous factors. *Br J Dermatol.* 2003;149: 718–730.

93. Bernstein JE, Parish LC, Rapaport M et al. Effects of topically applied capsaicin on moderate and severe psoriasis vulgaris. *J Am Acad Dermatol.* 1986;15:504–507.

94. Ellis CN, Berberian B, Sulica VI et al. A double-blind evaluation of topical capsaicin in pruritic psoriasis. *J Am Acad Dermatol.* 1993;29:438–442.

95. Madej A, Reich A, Orda A et al. Vascular adhesion protein-1 (VAP-1) is overexpressed in psoriatic patients. *J Eur Acad Dermatol Venereol.* 2007;21:72–78.

96. Dawn A, Yosipovitch G. Treating itch in psoriasis. *Dermatol Nurs.* 2006;18:227–233.

97. Gupta G, Long J, Tillman DM. The efficacy of narrowband ultraviolet B phototherapy in psoriasis using objective and subjective outcome measures. *Br J Dermatol.* 1999;140: 887–890.

98. Hundley JL, Yosipovitch G. Mirtazapine for reducing nocturnal itch in patients with chronic pruritus: a pilot study. *J Am Acad Dermatol.* 2004;50:889–891.

# Chapter 15
# Pruritus in Autoimmune Diseases

Yozo Ishiuji and Alan B. Fleischer, Jr.

## 15.1 Introduction

Autoimmune diseases are a collection of more than 80 individual diseases that are estimated to affect more than 3% of the U.S. population.[1] Underlying this diverse group of diseases is one common pathology: the malfunction of the immune system, resulting in the destruction of self-tissue. The etiology of autoimmune diseases is thought to have both genetic and environmental contributions.

Several types of autoimmune diseases have cutaneous symptoms. Pruritus is a common, distressing and difficult-to-manage complication of such autoimmune diseases. The pathogenesis of this symptom is unknown, and there are limited treatment options available; e.g., antihistamines are not effective.[2]

## 15.2 Connective Tissue Diseases

### 15.2.1 Dermatomyositis

Dermatomyositis (DM) is a rare inflammatory myopathy with characteristic skin manifestations and muscular weakness. The disease can be categorized as adult idiopathic, juvenile or amyopathic DM as well as that associated with a connective tissue disease or a malignancy.

Classic signs and symptoms include proximal muscle weakness and cutaneous symptoms. Other systemic manifestations include pulmonary disease (usually diffuse interstitial fibrosis),[3] cardiac involvement,[4] nonerosive arthritis (more common with juvenile onset DM)[5] and increased risk of internal malignancy.[6]

Cutaneous symptoms include a heliotrope cutaneous eruption, periungual telangectasias, cuticular dystrophy, nail fold infarcts, poikiloderma, photosensitivity and Gottron's papules.[7] Patients may present with pruritus and photosensitivity. Pruritus is a prominent feature in DM noted by clinicians. A case review of 20 patients with juvenile DM showed that 38% had a report of pruritus.[8] It has been suggested that pruritus is a feature that can help distinguish patients with DM from those with systemic lupus erythematosis, in which pruritus is uncommon.[9]

The primary skin change of DM is highly characteristic: often pruritic, symmetric, confluent, macular violaceous erythema variably affecting the skin overlying the extensor aspect of fingers, hands, forearms, arms, deltoid areas, posterior shoulders and neck, the "V" area of the anterior neck and upper chest, the central aspect of the face, periorbital areas, the forehead and the scalp.[10] Subjects had a mean score of 44.6 on the 100-mm visual analog scale (VAS) in response to effect of itching on daily life.[11] Pruritus has also a significant correlation with declining quality of life (QoL). The effect of pruritus was significant in both the models for the Dermatology Life Quality Index (DLQI) and Skindex-16. Because of its significant impact on QoL, pruritus management is an important component of DM management.[12] Clinicians need to be aware of the significant pruritus associated with this inflammatory disease and use appropriate topical and systemic antiinflammatory treatement to bring the muscle and skin disease under control as well as to improve QoL. One possible explanation of the significant pruritus may be related to the inflammatory component of DM. The immunopathology of cutaneous DM includes a variable degree of immunoglobulin and the complement deposition at the dermal–epidermal junction.[13]

L. Misery and S. Ständer (eds.), *Pruritus*,
DOI 10.1007/978-1-84882-322-8_15, © Springer-Verlag London Limited 2010

## 15.2.2 Lupus Erythematosus

Lupus erythematosus (LE) ranges from life-threatening manifestations of acute systemic lupus erythematosus (SLE) to the limited and exclusive skin involvement in chronic cutaneous lupus erythematosus (CCLE). More than 85% of patients with LE have skin lesions, which can be classified into LE specific and LE nonspecific. The prevalence of SLE is estimated to be 17–48 per 100,000 population worldwide. This serious multisystem autoimmune disease is based on polyclonal B cell immunity, which involves connective tissue and blood vessels. The common clinical manifestations of SLE include skin lesions, fever and arthritis, as well as central nervous system (CNS), renal, cardiac and pulmonary disease.[14]

Pruritus and skin burning are felt only occasionally by LE patients.[11] It has been reported that 45% of the patients with SLE had a report of pruritus,[14,15] but the true prevalence may be substantially lower. Discoid lesions, more commonly found in CCLE, are often quite pruritic, whereas the inflammatory photosensitive eruption of SLE more commonly presents as burning.

Some patients with systemic LE have selective loss of small-diameter nerve fibers, while larger nerve fibers are unaffected.[14,16] The sensory neuropathy from this loss, as well as neuropathy secondary to vasculitis, can occasionally contribute to pruritus sensations.

## 15.2.3 Systemic Sclerosis

Scleroderma is a multisystem disorder characterized by inflammatory, vascular and sclerotic changes of the skin and various internal organs including the lungs, the heart and the gastrointestinal (GI) tract. Systemic sclerosis (SSc) can be divided into two subsets: limited systemic scleroderma and diffuse systemic scleroderma. The autoantibodies classically associated with SSc include anti-centromere antibodies (ACA) and anti-Scl-70 (otherwise known as antitopoisomerase I or anti-topo I).[17] Anti-Scl-70 antibodies are associated with diffuse cutaneous involvement, increased frequency of pulmonary fibrosis and higher mortality.[18] Anti-Scl-70 antibodies are very useful in the diagnosis and clinical management of SSc patients and also to establish prognosis in these patients, particularly those with diffuse skin involvement.[19]

Pruritus has been reported to be sometimes present in early stages of the disease.[20] There is a tendency for a higher density of neuropeptide Y-positive nerve fibers in the forearm skin.[20] It should be noted that as the disease progresses, occasional patients may be seen with severe, unremitting, diffuse pruritus. This severe pruritus seems to be akin to itching observed in scarring phenomena, likely due to the compression of cutaneous nerves. The prognosis of SSc depends chiefly on the extent of the skin lesions, which correlates with the severity of the cardiovascular, pulmonary, and renal manifestations.[21]

## 15.2.4 Sjögren's Syndrome

Sjögren's syndrome (SS) is an autoimmune disease that is characterized by exocrine gland involvement and dryness of the mucous membrane of the eyes, nose, mouth and vagina. Salivary, lacrimal and sweat glands are infiltrated by T lymphocytes leading to xerostomia, keratoconjunctivitis sicca and xerosis. SS may occur alone (primary SS) or in association with other connective tissue diseases and rhumatoid arthritis (secondary SS).

Cutaneous manifestations of SS consist of pruritus, xerosis, angular cheilitis, eyelid dermatitis, cutaneous vasculitis (frequently manifesting as palpable purpura) and erythema annulare. It is reported that the skin is affected in nearly one-half of SS patients. Most of them are nonspecific and less severe than the oral, ocular, or musculoskeletal symptoms.[22] SS patients also complain of dryness of their hair and note a decrease in luster, and severe dryness of the skin is frequently accompanied by pruritus.[23] A recent study has demonstrated that there are significant difference in the presence of xerosis ($p = 0.009$) (56% versus 26%) between primary SS patients and those with secondary SS. A significant association of xerosis with anti-SSA + SSB ($p = 0.03$) antibodies was also demonstrated. Xerosis is the most frequent and characteristic cutaneous manifestation of primary SS. It is not linked to decreased sebaceous or sweat gland secretion, but more probably to a specific alteration of the protective function of the stratum corneum.[24]

## 15.3 Autoimmune Bullous Diseases

Autoimmune bullous diseases are associated with autoimmunity against structural components maintaining cell-cell and cell-matrix adhesion in the skin and mucous membranes. There is increasing evidence for a critical role of autoreactive T cells in the regulation of the production of pathogenic autoantibodies of autoimmune bullous disorders.[25]

## 15.3.1 Pemphigus

### 15.3.1.1 Pemphigus Vulgaris

Pemphigus vulgaris is a rare autoimmune blistering disease of the skin and the mucous membranes. In pemphigus, IgG autoantibodies against desmoglein 3 (Dsg3) and Dsg1 lead to loss of desmosomal adhesion of epidermal keratinocytes and intraepidermal blister formation.[25] Typically, the disease begins as oral mucosal sloughing and can spread quickly until all areas of the body are affected. Slight pressure or rubbing can cause skin separation. Immunofluorescent staining of biopsy specimens also can confirm the presence of intracellular autoantibodies. Pemphigus diseases are characterized by autoantibodies against the intercellular junctions and intraepithelial blisters.[26] A hallmark of these disorders is the presence of IgG and occasionally IgA autoantibodies that target distinct adhesion structures of the epidermis, dermoepidermal basement membrane and anchoring fibrils of the dermis.[25]

Pain and sore throat were the most common presenting symptoms. Thus, the skin lesions in pemphigus vulgaris are rarely pruritic but are often painful.[27]

## 15.3.2 Bullous Pemphigoid

Bullous pemphigoid (BP) is an autoimmune disorder presenting as a chronic bullous eruption, mostly in patients over 60 years of age. In the pemphigoid disease, IgG autoantibodies against components of the dermoepidermal basement membrane such as BP antigen 180 (BP180; also referred to as BP antigen 2 and type XVII collagen), BP antigen 230 (BP230; also referred to as BP antigen 1) and laminin 5 interfere with the adhesion of basal epidermal keratinocytes to the dermoepidermal basement membrane zone.[25]

Pruritus is a common feature of BP; it may be mild or quite severe. It is also a common initial manifestation of BP, which is an autoimmune blistering disease of the skin and mucosae occurring predominantly in elderly individuals. Erythematous, papular or urticarial lesions may precede bullae formation by days to months. Bullae that are large, tense, firm-topped, oval or round may arise in normal or erythematous skin and contain serous or hemorrhagic fluid. The eruption may be localized or generalized, usually scattered but also grouped in arciform and serpiginous patterns. Bullae rupture less easily than in pemphigus, but sometimes large, bright red, oozing and bleeding erosions become a major problem. Usually, however, the originally tense bullae collapse and transform into crusts.

Occasionally, patients may develop generalized pruritus without blisters as a prodrome of BP. This presentation could be described as "pruritic pemphigoid," because it joins the remarkable clinical finding of generalized pruritus with the underlying diagnosis of BP. Elderly patients with severe or persistent unexplained generalized pruritus may merit immunofluorescence biopsy testing to exclude BP as the cause of the generalized pruritus. Similarly, the urticarial phase of BP may present with significant pruritus, and unlike true urticaria lesions last longer than 24 h. A rare variant, pemphigoid nodularis, can mimic prurigo nodularis, and may merit further histologic evaluation. Establishing an early diagnosis permits the prompt institution of effective therapy with anti-inflammatory agents with an excellent prognosis for complete control of the disease.

## 15.3.3 Dermatitis Herpetiformis Duhring

Dermatitis herpetiformis (DH) is characterized by an intensely itchy, chronic, papulovesicular eruption that is usually distributed symmetrically on the scalp, buttocks, shoulders, front of the knees and backs of the elbows (pressure points).[28] Although this condition is an autoimmune blistering disease, the intense itch of the eruption with resultant scratching behavior makes finding intact vesicles uncommon. It is most common in early to middle adulthood. DH is a rare cause of itch, but certainly needs to be kept in mind when a patient presents with a very itch rash in characteristic distribution.[29]

Though the cause of the etiopathogenesis has not been completely elucidated, DH is frequently associated with gluten (a protein found in cereals) sensitivity in the small bowel. Gluten plays a critical role in the pathogenesis of DH and a related condition, celiac sprue. Subclinical cases of both conditions may be more common than is recognized.

### 15.3.4 Pemphigoid Gestationes

Pemphigoid gestationis (PG; also known as herpes gestationis) is a rare autoimmune subepidermal blistering disorder associated with pregnancy. Pruritus is the leading dermatological symptom during pregnancy. It is a rare vesiculobullous eruption that develops during the last trimester or even postpartum and creates severe pruritus. Other than its onset in pregnancy, the clinical, histopathologic and immunopathologic features of PG are similar to those of the pemphigoid group of disorders, and these diseases may be related.[30,31]

Because of potential effects on the fetus, the treatment of pruritus in pregnancy requires prudent consideration. The use of topical and systemic treatments depends on the underlying etiology of pruritus and the stage and status of the skin. In general, emollients and bland topical antipruritic agents appear to be the safest options for mild forms of the condition. Topical tacrolimus – now allowed during pregnancy – and topical corticosteroid agents may be appropriate as the disease increases in severity, whereas systemic corticosteroids and a restricted number of antihistamines may be administered in severe cases.

### 15.3.5 Linear IgA Dermatitis

Linear IgA dermatitis is a rare immune-mediated blistering skin disease that is defined by the presence of homogeneous linear deposits of IgA at the cutaneous basement membrane.

Clinical manifestations are very similar to those of DH, but there is more blistering. Patients present with combinations of annular or grouped papules, vesicles and bullae that are distributed symmetrically. The lesions are very pruritic, resulting in numerous crusted papules. However, the degree of pruritus is variable, and, in general, less severe than those of DH. Linear IgA dermatosis is not associated with gluten-sensitive enteropathy as is DH.[32]

### 15.3.6 Epidermolysis Bullosa Acquisita

Epidermolysis bullosa acquisita (EBA) is a chronic subepidermal bullous disease associated with autoimmunity to the type VII collagen within the anchoring fibrils in the basement membrane zone.[33] In the classical mechanobullous presentation, it is a noninflammatory blistering eruption with acral distribution that heals with scarring and milia formation.

Large areas of inflamed skin may be seen without any blisters, and only erythema or urticarial plaques are seen. These patients often complain of pruritus and do not demonstrate prominent skin fragility, scarring or milia formation. This clinical constellation is more reminiscent of BP than mechanobullous disorder.[34]

## 15.4 Summary

Pruritus is a cardinal symptom not only in many dermatological disorders but also in the autoimmune diseases. The therapeutic options are those related to the disease condition itself and are not directed to the sensation of pruritus. In some autoimmune diseases, such as DH, the pruritus sensations rapidly come under complete control. By contrast, the pruritus of SSc may be severe and unremitting, and may not respond to any therapy. Clinicians should carefully evaluate their patients with pruritic conditions and consider autoimmune diseases as one of the possible etiologies.

## References

1. Jacobson DL, Gange SJ, Rose NR, Graham NM. Epidemiology and estimated population burden of selected autoimmune diseases in the United States. *Clin Immunol Immunopathol.* 1997;84(3):223–243.
2. Levy C, Lindor KD. Management of primary biliary cirrhosis. *Curr Treat Options Gastroenterol.* 2003;6(6):493–498.
3. Sigurgeirsson B, Lindelof B, Edhag O, Allander E. Risk of cancer in patients with dermatomyositis or polymyositis. A population-based study. *N Engl J Med.* 1992;326(6):363–367.
4. Chow WH, Gridley G, Mellemkjaer L, McLaughlin JK, Olsen JH, Fraumeni JF, Jr. Cancer risk following polymyositis and dermatomyositis: a nationwide cohort study in Denmark. *Cancer Causes Control.* 1995;6(1):9–13.
5. Ytterberg SR. Infectious agents associated with myopathies. *Curr Opin Rheumatol.* 1996;8(6):507–513.
6. Caro I. Dermatomyositis. *Semin Cutan Med Surg.* 2001;20(1):38–45.
7. Kurzrock R, Cohen PR. Cutaneous paraneoplastic syndromes in solid tumors. *Am J Med.* 1995;99(6):662–671.
8. Peloro TM, Miller OF, III, Hahn TF, Newman ED. Juvenile dermatomyositis: a retrospective review of a 30-year experience. *J Am Acad Dermatol.* 2001;45(1):28–34.

9. Sontheimer RD. Dermatomyositis: an overview of recent progress with emphasis on dermatologic aspects. *Dermatol Clin*. 2002;20(3):387–408.

10. Sontheimer RD. Dermatomyositis: an overview of recent progress with emphasis on dermatologic aspects. *Dermatol Clin*. 2002;20(3):387–408.

11. Shirani Z, Kucenic MJ, Carroll CL, et al. Pruritus in adult dermatomyositis. *Clin Exp Dermatol*. 2004;29(3):273–276.

12. Hundley JL, Carroll CL, Lang W, et al. Cutaneous symptoms of dermatomyositis significantly impact patients' quality of life. *J Am Acad Dermatol*. 2006;54(2):217–220.

13. Crowson AN, Magro CM. The role of microvascular injury in the pathogenesis of cutaneous lesions of dermatomyositis. *Hum Pathol*. 1996;27(1):15–19.

14. Patel P, Werth V. Cutaneous lupus erythematosus: a review. *Dermatol Clin*. 2002;20(3):373–85, v.

15. Kapadia N, Haroon TS. Cutaneous manifestations of systemic lupus erythematosus: study from Lahore. *Pakistan Int J Dermatol*. 1996;35(6):408–409.

16. Goransson LG, Brun JG, Harboe E, Mellgren SI, Omdal R. Intraepidermal nerve fiber densities in chronic inflammatory autoimmune diseases. *Arch Neurol*. 2006;63(10):1410–1413.

17. Ho KT, Reveille JD. The clinical relevance of autoantibodies in scleroderma. *Arthritis Res Ther*. 2003;5(2):80–93.

18. Cepeda EJ, Reveille JD. Autoantibodies in systemic sclerosis and fibrosing syndromes: clinical indications and relevance. *Curr Opin Rheumatol*. 2004;16(6):723–732.

19. Basu D, Reveille JD. Anti-scl-70. *Autoimmunity*. 2005;38(1):65–72.

20. Wallengren J, Akesson A, Scheja A, Sundler F. Occurrence and distribution of peptidergic nerve fibers in skin biopsies from patients with systemic sclerosis. *Acta Derm Venereol*. 1996;76(2):126–128.

21. Meyer O. Prognostic markers for systemic sclerosis. *Joint Bone Spine*. 2006;73(5):490–494.

22. Soy M, Piskin S. Cutaneous findings in patients with primary Sjogren's syndrome. *Clin Rheumatol*. 2007;26(8):1350–1352.

23. Provost TT, Watson R. Cutaneous manifestations of Sjogren's syndrome. *Rheum Dis Clin North Am*. 1992;18(3):609–616.

24. Bernacchi E, Amato L, Parodi A, et al. Sjogren's syndrome: a retrospective review of the cutaneous features of 93 patients by the Italian Group of Immunodermatology. *Clin Exp Rheumatol*. 2004;22(1):55–62.

25. Hertl M, Eming R, Veldman C. T cell control in autoimmune bullous skin disorders. *J Clin Invest*. 2006;116(5):1159–1166.

26. Mihai S, Sitaru C. Immunopathology and molecular diagnosis of autoimmune bullous diseases. *J Cell Mol Med*. 2007;11(3):462–481.

27. Woldegiorgis S, Swerlick RA. Pemphigus in the southeastern United States. *South Med J*. 2001;94(7):694–698.

28. Caproni M, Feliciani C, Fuligni A, et al. Th2-like cytokine activity in dermatitis herpetiformis. *Br J Dermatol*. 1998;138(2):242–247.

29. Amerio P, Verdolini R, Giangiacomi M, et al. Expression of eotaxin, interleukin 13 and tumour necrosis factor-alpha in dermatitis herpetiformis. *Br J Dermatol*. 2000;143(5):974–978.

30. Engineer L, Bhol K, Ahmed AR. Pemphigoid gestationis: a review. *Am J Obstet Gynecol*. 2000;183(2):483–491.

31. Castro LA, Lundell RB, Krause PK, Gibson LE. Clinical experience in pemphigoid gestationis: report of 10 cases. *J Am Acad Dermatol*. 2006;55(5):823–828.

32. Chan LS, Traczyk T, Taylor TB, Eramo LR, Woodley DT, Zone JJ. Linear IgA bullous dermatosis. Characterization of a subset of patients with concurrent IgA and IgG anti-basement membrane autoantibodies. *Arch Dermatol*. 1995;131(12):1432–1437.

33. Sitaru C. Experimental models of epidermolysis bullosa acquisita. *Exp Dermatol*. 2007;16(6):520–531.

34. Pai S, Marinkovich MP. Epidermolysis bullosa: new and emerging trends. *Am J Clin Dermatol*. 2002;3(6):371–380.

# Chapter 16
# Urticaria

Ulrike Raap, Alexander Kapp, and Bettina Wedi

## 16.1 Introduction

Several chronic or acute inflammatory skin diseases such as urticaria, atopic dermatitis and psoriasis are associated with pruritus. Interestingly, the clinical presentation of pruritus in these skin diseases is completely different. While patients with atopic dermatitis develop excessive scratching resulting in excoriation and bleeding of the skin, patients with urticaria rather rub their lesions, explaining why excoriation is not a consequence of urticaria.

The clinical characteristics of itch in patients with urticaria have been described with stinging, tickling and burning, which is usually worse in the evening or at night. Patients with urticaria describe their itch as bothersome, annoying, unbearable and worrisome. Itch intensity can be assessed by the visual analog score (VAS) and the verbal intensity score. Of note, sensory and affective scores positively correlate with the worst intensity of itch.[1] Itch intensity in chronic urticaria (CU) is related to stress. However, this relation is significantly less strong than in other pruritic dermatoses including psoriasis.[2] The most frequently involved areas with itch in patients with chronic idiopathic urticaria were the arms ($n = 86$), the back ($n = 78$) and the legs ($n = 75$) as shown in a study of 100 patients.[1]

Urticaria is one of the most common skin diseases and affects 15–25% of the population once in their lifetime.[3] The causes of urticaria are multiple. In more than 80%, urticaria is triggered by an inflammatory focus, a subclinical infection or autoimmune reactions.[4, 5] In addition, nonspecific pharmacological or toxin-mediated release of inflammatory mediators from basophils or mast cells can trigger urticaria. In daily practice, stress has been regarded as an important trigger factor for urticaria. Urticaria symptoms affect everyday life, limiting and impairing physical and emotional functioning, leading to an indirect burden on life satisfaction underlining the major impact on health-related quality of life.[6] Interestingly, urticaria had already been described by Hippocrates as an annoying itchy skin disease.

## 16.2 Urticaria Definition

The main characteristic clinical feature of urticaria is the rapid appearance of itchy, short-lived (duration up to 24 h) wheals defined by pale centers surrounded by a red flare (Fig. 16.1). The wheal is a result of the transudation of fluid due to increased vascular permeability. Degranulation products of mast cells releasing histamine, prostaglandins, leukotrienes, proteases and cytokines are the main mediators leading to itchy swellings of superficial layers of the dermis, clinically seen as wheals. The size of the wheals can rise from a few millimeters to several centimeters in diameter anywhere on the skin. In contrast, swellings of the deep dermis, subcutaneous or submucosal tissues which can persist up to 72 h are often painful rather than itchy and are defined as angioedema. Angioedema coexists in approximately 50% of urticaria cases but can also occur alone.[7]

## 16.3 Urticaria Histopathology

The initiation of the inflammatory process in urticaria is certainly triggered by the degranulation of skin mast cells. Skin affected by urticaria is characterized by a

L. Misery and S. Ständer (eds.), *Pruritus*,
DOI 10.1007/978-1-84882-322-8_16, © Springer-Verlag London Limited 2010

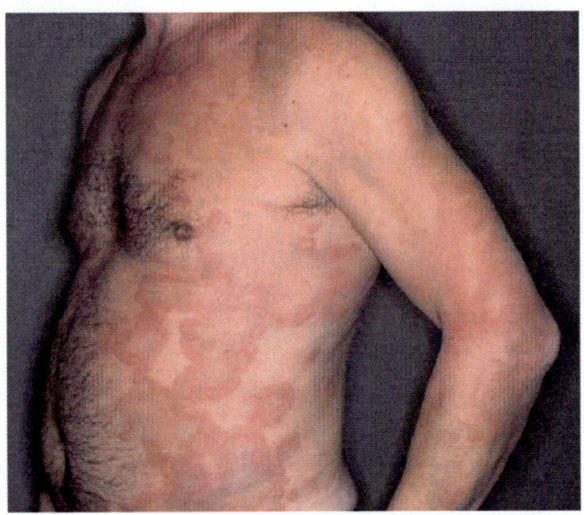

**Fig. 16.1** Typical clinical feature of wheals defined by pale centers surrounded by a red flare in a patient with chronic urticaria

perivascular and interstitial infiltrate presented by CD4+ T lymphocytes, monocytes, basophil, neutrophil and eosinophil granulocytes surrounding small venules within the superficial and deep venular plexus.[8] The number of accumulating eosinophil granulocytes varies in urticaria skin lesions, due to their degranulation, assessed by the remaining major basic protein.[9] The recruitment and activation of inflammatory cells is mediated via the increase of endothelial adhesion molecules together with the release of cytokines such as IL-4 and IL-5 in urticaria skin lesions.[10]

## 16.4 Urticaria Classification

According to the new European guidelines, urticaria subtypes can be grouped into spontaneous urticaria, which includes acute urticaria (AU) and CU, the physical urticarias and other urticaria disorders[11] (Table 16.1). Of note, two or more different subtypes of urticaria can coexist in one patient. To assess the disease activity classifying non-physical spontaneous urticaria, an urticaria activity score (UAS) including the number of wheals and the intensity of pruritus has been introduced by the current European guideline on the diagnosis of urticaria.[11] The lowest score 0 had been defined by no wheals and no pruritus, followed by score 1 = mild urticaria (<20

wheals/ 24 h, mild pruritus), score 2 = moderate urticaria (21–50 wheals/ 24 h, moderate pruritus) and score 3 = intense urticaria (>50 wheals/24 h or large confluent areas of wheals with intense pruritus). Recently, the use of this UAS has been proven for a positive correlation with UAS values and quality of life in CU patients, suggesting that this UAS is useful in daily practice for the classification of urticaria severity.[12]

## 16.5 Urticaria Diagnostic Workup

To assess urticaria and subtypes a detailed history of the patient considering potential triggering factors and a physical examination including a test for dermographism should be performed.[13] In case of positive history for physical triggering, standardized physical tests should be performed (Table 16.1). Laboratory tests should include at least the differential blood count, eryth-rocyte sedimentation rate or C-reactive protein, whereas specific analysis should be based on an individual basis to identify the suspected trigger factor. Reliable and successful diagnostic approaches in CU include *Helicobacter pylori* (HP) urea, breath or stool antigen test, serology for anti-DNAse B, antistreptolysin, antistaphylolysin, yersinia IgA/IgG antibodies and immunoblot, thyroidautoantibodies, (antinuclear antibodies), autologous-serum skin test (ASST) and in some cases diet low in pseudoallergens diet for 4 weeks.[14, 15]

## 16.6 Subtypes of Spontaneous Urticaria and Pathogenesis

### 16.6.1 Acute Urticaria

Viral infections of the upper respiratory tract and bacterial infections including cystitis and tonsillitis are regarded as most frequent causes in triggering AU.[16] In some patients, combinations of viral infections (increasing mast cell reactivity) and nonsteroidal anti-inflammatory drug (NSAID) intake (particularly of aspirin) elicit AU.[17] A specific diagnostic workup is not recommended for AU unless strongly suggested by the patient's history (Table 16.1).

**Table 16.1** Urticaria group, subtype, eliciting factors/characteristics and routine diagnostic tests

| Urticaria group | Urticaria subtype | Eliciting factors/characteristics | Routine diagnostic tests |
|---|---|---|---|
| Spontaneous urticaria | AU | Spontaneous/< 6 weeks | None[a] |
| | Chronic urticaria | Spontaneous/> 6 weeks | Differential blood count, ESR/CRP, avoidance of suspected drugs (NSAIDs) |
| Physical urticaria | Cold contact urticaria | Cold/air/water/wind/food/objects | Cold provocation and threshold test (ice cube, cold water, cold wind) |
| | Delayed pressure urticaria | Vertical pressure/wheals arising with a 3–8 h latency | Pressure test (0.2–1.5 kg/cm$^2$ for 10 and 20 min) |
| | Urticaria factitia/demographic urticaria | Mechanical shearing forces | Elicit dermographism |
| | Heat contact urticaria | Localized heat | Heat provocation and threshold test (warm water) |
| | Solar urticaria | Ultraviolet and/or visible light | Ultraviolet and visible light of different wave lengths |
| | Vibratory urticaria/angioedema | Vibratory forces | Test with vibratory device (e.g., for body massage or vibrator) |
| Other urticaria disorders | Aquagenic urticaria | Water | Wet compresses at body temperature applied for 20 min |
| | Cholinergic urticaria | Increase of body temperature, pinhead-sized wheals | Exercise and hot bath provocation |
| | Contact urticaria | Contact with urticariogenic substances | Prick/patch test, reading after 20 min |
| | Exercise-induced anaphylaxis/urticaria | Physical exercise | According to history, exercise test with/without food/drugs |

[a]Unless strongly suggested by the patient's history, e.g., allergy.

ESR, erythrocyte sedimentation rate; CRP, C-reactive protein; NSAID, nonsteroidal anti-inflammatory drugs.

## 16.6.2 Chronic Urticaria

The prevalence of CU has been described with 0.6% in an epidemiologic population-based study performed with 5,003 adults 2004 in Spain.[18] In addition, this study described a higher prevalence of CU in women than in men.[18] Even though CU is a self-limited disease, yet in 8.7% of cases CU lasts from 1–5 years and in 11.3% for more than 5 years, explaining why CU has a profound impact on health-related quality of life.[18, 19]

Infections are the most common causes of AU, and by definition all CU must have started as AU.[4] However, the underlying mechanism why and which patients develop CU is still unclear. One explanation may be a genetic predisposition, as major histocompatibility complex II associations have been found in CU.[20] Further, some patients with CU demonstrate a prior susceptibility to develop (transient) nonallergic hypersensitivity to NSAIDs, particularly aspirin, and/or food additives.[21, 22]

Patients with CU have no increased incidence of atopy. However, about 13% of patients with CU present autoantibodies to thyroid,[23] and about 30%

histamine releasing antibodies to the high-affinity IgE receptor (FcεRI) or to IgE.[24, 25] A positive ASST is found in a subgroup of patients but is not clearly correlated to the functional serum activity or the presence of autoantibodies.[26-28]

Viral infections (e.g., hepatitis B, C), bacterial infections such as streptococci and staphylococci of the nasopharynx or the dental area and HP infection of the gastrointestinal tract have been associated with CU.[4] With regard to HP infection, an appropriate antibiotic treatment (e.g., triple therapy with proton pump inhibitor, amoxicillin and clarithromycin) as well as a careful reassessment of the success of eradication treatment is necessary, as patients may need two or more treatment courses.[29, 30]

Parasitic infections are seldom found in CU in Northern Europe, whereas this seems to be more frequent in other countries in the South.[31] In the past, it had been described that patients with CU are twice as often affected with candida infections compared to control patients.[32] However, there is no recent evidence supporting a role for candida in CU.

In addition to infections, noninfectious chronic inflammatory processes, e.g., gastritis, reflux oesophagitis, inflammation of the bile duct or gland, neoplasia and rarely autoimmune disorders such as systemic lupus erythematosus have been described in some cases of CU.

Interestingly, two or more different trigger factors, e.g., nonallergic hypersensitivity, autoreactivity, and several infections can be identified in CU. Of note, the frequency and relevance of infectious and noninfectious diseases vary between different patient groups depending on geographic background. This explains why some infections have been identified as triggering factors in some regions whereas in others they are uncommon.

The exact prevalence of infections in CU is unknown. However, several studies demonstrate a benefit after eradication of infectious processes such as HP,[30, 33, 34] suggesting that it is worthwhile following the diagnostic workup and therapy of the identified cause.

## 16.7 Physical Urticaria and Subtypes

Physical urticarias are different types of urticaria and should be excluded by appropriate physical tests as shown in Table 16.1.

Cold contact urticaria represents 3–5% of all physical urticarias.[35] It affects mainly young adults, is more frequent in women than in men and has a mean duration of $7.9 \pm 5.8$ years.[36] While it has long been suggested that cold contact urticaria is idiopathic, it is also possible that infections are important trigger factors, as antibiotic treatment, e.g., with penicillin, can lead to a complete remission of the disease.[37]

Dermographic urticaria affects mainly young adults and represents the most frequent subtype of physical urticarias with an incidence of 7–17% of all urticarias.[35] It is induced by shearing forces on the skin, which induce a rapid occurrence of wheals associated with intense pruritus.

Delayed pressure urticaria is characterized by deep and sometimes painful swellings 4–8 h after exposure to static or vertical pressure, which can last upto 48 h. Therefore, especially the soles are often affected by delayed pressure urticaria. The average age of onset is approximately 30 years, with men being two times more often affected than women, with a mean duration of approximately 6–9 years.[38]

Heat contact urticaria is induced by temperature ranges from 38°C to more than 50°C. In solar urticaria, wavelengths of 280–760 nm can elicit urticaria symptomatology. Interestingly, those areas of the skin that are constantly exposed to sunlight are not frequently involved because of photohardening. Vibratory angioedema represents a very rare subtype of physical urticaria. So far, it has only been described as case reports revealing vibrating mechanical forces as induction factors.

## 16.8 Other Subtypes of Urticaria

Cholinergic urticaria is induced by an increase of the body core temperature, due to hot bath, sweating, physical exercise and emotional stress. Spicy food or alcoholic beverages may also induce a small rise in body core temperature leading to cholinergic urticaria.[17] Cholinergic urticaria comprises up to 7% of all urticarias, and the wheals are typically of pinhead size.[35] Also, exercise induced anaphylaxis/urticaria is induced by physical exercise but not by the passive increase of the body temperature via bathing. Contact urticaria occurs at contact sites of the eliciting factor such as food, plants, drugs, cosmetics, etc., but can also occur generalized due to IgE-mediated allergic sensitization. By contrast, aquagenic urticaria is not mediated by the contact of water itself but possibly due to the delivery of soluble allergens from the skin. It affects young adults, with women five times more frequently affected than men.

### 16.8.1 Angioedema

At least half of the patients with CU also suffer from agnioedema, mostly affecting the eyelids, lips, tongue, pharynx, genitals and extremities, whereas 15–20% develop recurrent angioedema without wheals.[14] Angioedema subtypes include allergic angioedema (which usually occurs within 1–2 h after allergen exposure and lasts from 1 to 3 days), bradykinin-induced angioedema due to C1-esterase inhibitor deficiency or dysfunction, angioedema induced by drug intake (e.g., ACE inhibitors), cytokine-mediated angioedema associated with eosinophilia (Gleich's syndrome), physically induced angioedema and idiopathic angioedema.[39]

Especially, angioedema of the tongue or laryngopharynx can be caused pharmacologically by ACE inhibitors and less frequently by angiotensin-II blockers (sartans). Therefore, in recurrent angioedema, as well as in cases of CU, ACE inhibitors and sartans as well as nonsteroidal antirheumatic agents should be avoided.[14] Of note, angioedema my occur several years later after start of ACE inhibitor intake and can still occur for several weeks after discontinuation of this antihypertensive therapy.

Management of hereditary angioedema (HAE), which is a rare but life-threatening condition with acute attacks of facial, laryngeal, genital, or peripheral swelling or abdominal pain secondary to intra-abdominal edema, is challenging and includes (I) the treatment of acute attacks, and (II) long- and (III) short-term prophylaxis.[40] Untreated HAE is associated with a high mortality due to laryngeal angioedema, which does not respond to corticosteroid and epinephrine treatment. Therefore, the treatment of choice for recurrent life-threatening attacks includes infusions of C1 esterase inhibitor concentrate. Long-term prophylaxis includes attenuated androgens and antifibrinolytic agents in HAE, whereas short-term prophylaxis is recommended to prevent angioedema episodes during dental or endoscopic manipulations.[39]

Acquired angioedema (AAE) is a rare disorder that has been categorized into two forms: AAE-I associated with other diseases, most commonly B-cell lymphoproliferative disorders; and AAE-II defined by autoantibody production directed against the C1-inhibitor molecule. Severe acute attacks can be treated by plasma-derived C1 inhibitor in AAE; however, due to rapid catabolism, large quantities may be needed in case of an acute attack.[39] For the AAE II type immunosuppressive therapy, decreasing autoantibody production aside from the management of acute attacks with C1 inhibitor concentrate represents the only effective therapeutic approach.[41]

## 16.9 Treatment of Urticaria

The treatment of urticaria is based on specific principles including (I) avoidance of the triggering factor, (II) treatment of the identifiable cause, and (III) inhibition of mast cell mediators.[13] Further, explanation and information, a good physician–patient relationship and patient diaries are helpful in the management of patients with CU.

First, every identifiable trigger factor should be eradicated or avoided, including NSAIDs and acetylsalicylic acid, which can trigger urticaria in 10–30% of patients. In the case of angioedema, an early recognition and discontinuation of ACE inhibitor should be made, and angitiotentsin-II receptor antagonist intake should be avoided.

Chronic infections as identifiable cause of urticaria including persistent, chronic and usually subclinical infections with streptococci, staphylococci or yersinia should be eradicated.[4] For the therapy of HP infections it is important to note that triple therapy has best evidence for remission, which also leads to a more likely remission of urticaria.[42] The success of the treatment for all infectious trigger factors should be monitored by adequate methods accordingly, as therapeutic failures may occur.

Due to the high burden of pruritus, the recommended first-line therapy for urticaria treatment consists of nonsedating H1 antihistamines which represent the only licensed therapy so far.[14] In this regard, a dosage increased up to fourfold over the recommended doses (off-label use) of modern antihistamines may be necessary considering possible side effects.[13] The use of the higher doses may be explained by the fact that antihistamines have originally been developed for the treatment of allergic rhinitis, which affects a much smaller organ than the skin. Sedating anthihistamines are not more effective than modern antihistamines but cause more frequent adverse reactions including sedation and anticholinergic effects. Therefore, sedating antihistamines are not recommended as first-line therapy. The best evidence for the treatment of urticaria exists for nonsedating modern H1 antihistamines, including azelastine, cetirizine, desloratadine, ebastine, fexofenadine, levocetirizine, loratadine and mizolastine (in alphabetical order).[14]

There is no therapeutic rationale for administering an H2 blocker along with a nonsedating H1 antihistamine. Leukotriene receptor antagonists seem to be effective in certain subgroups of patients with CU including those with a positive ASST. However, so far it has not been possible to determine whether the positive effects of leukotriene receptor antagonists differ in mono- or in combined therapy with antihistamines.[14] A subset of urticaria patients with associated autoimmune thyroiditis may respond to the administration of thyroxine, even though controlled trials are lacking.[43]

Glucocorticosterids which have potent anti-inflammatory activity should be used with caution as a short-term second-line treatment for severe AU and exacerbations of CU. However, in specific cases, such as delayed pressure urticaria, the use of low doses of glucocorticosteroids may be helpful. For severe CU, immunosuppressive drugs including cyclosporine A represent an additional therapeutic alternative taking into account a careful benefit-risk analysis.[14, 39, 39] Antidepressants (doxepin), mast cell stabilizers (ketotifen), sympathomimetics (terbutaline), calcium channel blockers (nifedipine), warfarin and stanozol cannot be recommended for urticaria therapy, based on the high rates of side effects and limited benefit according to trials of low quality.[14] Dapsone and (hydroxyl-)chloroquine, which have a relatively good profile of adverse effects, represent other second-line anti-inflammatory drugs which have been found to be effective especially in CU patients with positive ASSt and for dapsone also for pressure urticaria.[5, 14] The clinical efficacies of biologicals including rituximab (a monoclonal humanized antibody directed against the B-cell-specific cell surface antigen CD20) and omalizumab (a recombinant humanized monoclonal antibody that targets free-serum IgE antibodies) are currently under clinical observation. In contrast to rituximab, which lacked a therapeutic effect in a case report of a patient with severe CU,[44] omalizumab seems to be a promising drug for the treatment of CU as presented in several case reports,[45, 46] but controlled trials are needed.

# References

1. Yosipovitch G, Ansari N, Goon A, et al. Clinical characteristics of pruritus in chronic idiopathic urticaria. *Br J Dermatol*. 2002;147:32–36.
2. Yosipovitch G, Goon A, Wee J, et al. The prevalence and clinical characteristics of pruritus among patients with extensive psoriasis. *Br J Dermatol*. 2000;143:969–973.
3. Cooper KD. Urticaria and angioedema: diagnosis and evaluation. *J Am Acad Dermatol*. 1991;25:166–174.
4. Wedi B, Raap U, Kapp A. Chronic urticaria and infections. *Curr Opin Allergy Clin Immunol*. 2004;4:387–396.
5. Raap U, Liekenbrocker T, Wieczorek D, et al. New therapeutic strategies for the different subtypes of urticaria. *Hautarzt* 2004;55:361–366.
6. Raap U, Gieler U, Schmid-Ott G. Urticaria. *Dermatol Psychosom*. 2004;5:203–205.
7. Wedi B, Kapp A. Urticaria and angioedema. In: Mahmoudi M, ed. *Allergy: Practical Diagnosis and Management*. New York: Mc Graw Hill; 2008:84–94.
8. Elias J, Boss E, Kaplan AP. Studies of the cellular infiltrate of chronic idiopathic urticaria: prominence of T-lymphocytes, monocytes, and mast cells. *J Allergy Clin Immunol*. 1986;78:914–918.
9. Sabroe RA, Poon E, Orchard GE, et al. Cutaneous inflammatory cell infiltrate in chronic idiopathic urticaria: comparison of patients with and without anti-FcepsilonRI or anti-IgE autoantibodies. *J Allergy Clin Immunol*. 1999;103:484–493.
10. Caproni M, Giomi B, Melani L, et al. Cellular infiltrate and related cytokines, chemokines, chemokine receptors and adhesion molecules in chronic autoimmune urticaria: comparison between spontaneous and autologous serum skin test induced wheal. *Int J Immunopathol Pharmacol*. 2006;19:507–515.
11. Zuberbier T, Bindslev-Jensen C, Canonica W, et al. EAACI/GA2LEN/EDF guideline: definition, classification and diagnosis of urticaria. *Allergy*. 2006;61:316–320.
12. Mlynek A, Zalewska-Janowska A, Martus P, et al. How to assess disease activity in patients with chronic urticaria? *Allergy*. 2008;63:777–780.
13. Zuberbier T, Bindslev-Jensen C, Canonica W, et al. EAACI/GA2LEN/EDF guideline: management of urticaria. *Allergy*. 2006;61:321–331.
14. Wedi B, Kapp A. Evidence-based therapy of chronic urticaria. *J Dtsch Dermatol Ges*. 2007;5:146–157.
15. Zuberbier T, Chantraine-Hess S, Hartmann K, Czarnetzki BM. Pseudoallergen-free diet in the treatment of chronic urticaria. A prospective study. *Acta Derm Venereol*. 1995;75:484–487.
16. Sackesen C, Sekerel BE, Orhan F, et al. The etiology of different forms of urticaria in childhood. *Pediatr Dermatol*. 2004;21:102–108.
17. Zuberbier T, Maurer M. Urticaria: current opinions about etiology, diagnosis and therapy. *Acta Derm Venereol*. 2007;87:196–205.
18. Gaig P, Olona M, Munoz LD, et al. Epidemiology of urticaria in Spain. *J Invest Allergol Clin Immunol*. 2004;14:214–220.
19. O'Donnell BF, Lawlor F, Simpson J, et al. The impact of chronic urticaria on the quality of life. *Br J Dermatol*. 1997;136:197–201.
20. O'Donnell BF, O'Neill CM, Francis DM, et al. Human leucocyte antigen class II associations in chronic idiopathic urticaria. *Br J Dermatol*. 1999;140:853–858.
21. Zuberbier T, Chantraine-Hess S, Hartmann K, Czarnetzki BM. Pseudoallergen-free diet in the treatment of chronic urticaria. A prospective study [see comments]. *Acta Derm Venereol*. 1995;75:484–487.
22. Wedi B, Kapp A. Aspirin induced adverse skin reactions: new pathophysiological aspects. *Thorax*. 2000;55(suppl 2):S70–S71.
23. Leznoff A, Sussman GL. Syndrome of idiopathic chronic urticaria and angioedema with thyroid autoimmunity: a study of 90 patients. *J Allergy Clin Immunol*. 1989;84:66–71.
24. Hide M, Francis DM, Grattan CE, et al. Autoantibodies against the high-affinity IgE receptor as a cause of histamine release in chronic urticaria [see comments]. *N Engl J Med*. 1993;328:1599–1604.
25. Marone G, Spadaro G, Palumbo C, Condorelli G. The anti-IgE/anti-FcεRIα autoantibody network in allergic and autoimmune diseases. *Clin Exp Allergy*. 1999;29:17–27.
26. Grattan CEH, Hamon CGB, Cowan MA, Leeming RJ. Preliminary identification of a low molecular weight serological medicator in chronic idiopathic urticaria. *Br J Dermatol*. 1988;119:179–184.

27. Kikuchi Y, Kaplan AP. Mechanisms of autoimmune activation of basophils in chronic urticaria. *J Allergy Clin Immunol*. 2001; 107:1056–1062.

28. Wedi B, Novacovic V, Koerner M, Kapp A. Chronic urticaria serum induces histamine release, leukotriene production and basophil CD63 surface expression – inhibitory effects of anti-inflammatory drugs. *J Allergy Clin Immunol*. 2000;105:552–560.

29. Wedi B, Wagner S, Werfel T, et al. Prevalence of *Helicobacter pylori* associated gastritis in chronic urticaria. *Int Arch Allergy Immunol*. 1998;116:288–294.

30. Shiotani A, Okada K, Yanaoka K, et al. Beneficial effect of *Helicobacter pylori* eradication in dermatologic diseases. *Helicobacter* 2001;6:60–65.

31. Daschner A, Vega dl O, Pascual CY. Allergy and parasites reevaluated: wide-scale induction of chronic urticaria by the ubiquitous fish-nematode Anisakis simplex in an endemic region. *Allergol Immunopathol (Madr)*. 2005;33:31–37.

32. Henseler T. Mucocutaneous candidiasis in patients with skin diseases. *Mycoses*. 1995;38(suppl 1):7–13.

33. Federman DG, Kirsner RS, Moriarty JP, Concato J. The effect of antibiotic therapy for patients infected with *Helicobacter pylori* who have chronic urticaria. *J Am Acad Dermatol*. 2003;49:861–864.

34. Wedi B, Wagner S, Werfel T, et al. Prevalence of *Helicobacter pylori*-associated gastritis in chronic urticaria. *Int Arch Allergy Immunol*. 1998;116:288–294.

35. Kontou-Fili K, Borici-Mazi R, Kapp A, et al. Physical urticaria: classification and diagnostic guidelines. An EAACI position paper. *Allergy*. 1997;52:504–513.

36. Moller A, Henning M, Zuberbier T, Czarnetzki-Henz BM. Epidemiology and clinical aspects of cold urticaria. *Hautarzt*. 1996;47:510–514.

37. Liebeskind H, Schwarze G. Penicillin therapy in cold contact urticaria. *Hautarzt*. 1974;25:482–485.

38. Zuberbier T, Grabbe J. *Urticaria*. Springer Verlag; Berlin 1996.

39. Borzova E, Grattan CE. Urticaria: current future treatments. *Expert Rev Dermatol*. 2007;2(3):317–334.

40. Agostoni A, Aygoren-Pursun E, Binkley KE, et al. Hereditary and acquired angioedema: problems and progress: proceedings of the third C1 esterase inhibitor deficiency workshop and beyond. *J Allergy Clin Immunol*. 2004;114:S51–S131.

41. Kaplan AP, Greaves MW. Angioedema. *J Am Acad Dermatol*. 2005;53:373–388.

42. Federman DG, Kirsner RS, Moriarty JP, Concato J. The effect of antibiotic therapy for patients infected with *Helicobacter pylori* who have chronic urticaria. *J Am Acad Dermatol*. 2003;49:861–864.

43. Dreskin SC, Andrews KY. The thyroid and urticaria. *Curr Opin Allergy Clin Immunol*. 2005;5:408–412.

44. Mallipeddi R, Grattan CE. Lack of response of severe steroid-dependent chronic urticaria to rituximab. *Clin Exp Dermatol*. 2007;32:333–334.

45. Metz M, Bergmann P, Zuberbier T, Maurer M. Successful treatment of cholinergic urticaria with anti-immunoglobulin E therapy. *Allergy*. 2008;63:247–249.

46. Spector SL, Tan RA. Effect of omalizumab on patients with chronic urticaria. *Ann Allergy Asthma Immunol*. 2007;99:190–193.

# Chapter 17
# Pruritic Skin Diseases in Travellers

Eric Caumes

## 17.1 Introduction

Pruritus is a leading cause of skin complaints in travelers who may present with either localized or generalized pruritus, which may be acute or chronic (>6 weeks).[1,2] Pruritic skin diseases include infections of exotic or cosmopolitan origin as well as environmental skin diseases (Table 17.1).

From a clinician's point of view, the distinction between localized and generalized pruritus is of outstanding interest. While the latter may be observed in some parasitic diseases (scabies, invasive phase of helminthic diseases) and some viral infections, the former is usually linked to infestations by arthropods, localized parasitic diseases and, to a lesser extent, fungal diseases. The travel history with focus on possible epidemiologic exposures (e.g., risky behavior, country visited) and the clinical examination with focus on the morphologic characteristics of associated cutaneous lesions together with the distribution of the lesions (i.e., generalized or localized, limited to a specific anatomic location) provide the best additional diagnostic clues. Whatever the skin disease, specific cutaneous lesions have to be distinguished from skin changes secondary to pruritus (i.e., excoriation, lichenification, impetiginization). For travelers in tropical moist areas, the predominant complication is cutaneous bacterial infection. Further diagnostic procedures such as blood tests, serologies, skin biopsy, polymerase chain reaction (PCR), cultures and imaging techniques may be warranted according to the results of clinical examination.

## 17.2 Epidemiological Data

Dermatoses are considered as one of the three most common causes of health problems in travelers, with diarrhea and respiratory tract infections during and after travel.[3]

Whatever the method of the epidemiological study (questionnaire-based survey, cohort study of specific groups of travelers, observational study) and the place of the study (on site, returning travelers), the most common travel-associated dermatoses are related to insect bites or stings, sun exposure, dermatophytes, contact allergy and superficial injuries (including those due to contact with marine creatures) as well as bacterial, viral and parasite infections.

The part occupied by imported exotic diseases within the spectrum of dermatoses diagnosed in returning travelers varies from 35 to 53% according to the study, but whatever the nature of the study, the main dermatologic symptom in this setting is pruritus.[1,2]

## 17.3 Infestations by Arthropods

### 17.3.1 Scabies

Scabies, the infestation by the mite *Sarcoptes scabiei*, is the commonest cause of diffuse pruritic skin disease diagnosed in travelers returning from the tropics.[1,2] Patients usually complain of generalized and intense itching, worsening at night and usually sparing the face and head, that occurs within 1 month after return in case of primary exposure and within a few days in travelers with a history of previous scabies exposure.[4] The most specific skin findings include 5–10 mm burrows, vesiculopustules and papulonodular genital lesions. The classic distribution sites of lesions are the interdigital web spaces, flexor surfaces of the wrists,

**Table 17.1** Causes of pruritus in travelers

| Localized Pruritus | Generalized Pruritus |
|---|---|
| Arthropods: myiasis, lice | Scabies |
| Helminthic infections: HrCLMs, enterobiasis (perianal), gnathostomiasis, loiasis, strongyloidiasis (larva currens), onchocerciasis-associated limb swelling | Invasive phase of helminthic diseases (in association with urticarial rash (see Table 17.3), cercarial dermatitis, onchocerciasis loiasis Viral infection: varicella, dengue, chikungunya Noninfectious causes: ciguatera fish poisoning, adverse drug reactions, atopic dermatitis exacerbation |
| Noninfectious causes: arthropod bite reaction, contact dermatitis, irritant dermatitis, seabather's eruption | |

the elbows, the axillae, the buttocks, genitalia in men and breasts in women. A family history of pruritus is a classic clue to the diagnosis ("itching in the marital bed is scabies"). Diagnosis is confirmed by the microscopic identification of the female mite, eggs, or fecal pellets on skin scrapings of a cutaneous lesion.

## 17.3.2 Furuncular Myiasis

Human myiasis is the infestation of human tissues by larvae (or maggots) of various flies (*Diptera*). According to the results of series of imported cases in Western countries, the most common form of human myiasis reported in travelers is furuncular myiasis which is usually caused by *Cordylobia anthropophaga* (the Tumbu fly) acquired in sub-Saharan Africa and *Dermatobia hominis* (the human botfly) acquired in Central and South America.[1,5,6]

Depending on which fly is involved, the presentation of myiasis differs by the way of infestation, place of acquisition, duration of maturation, number of cutaneous lesions, anatomic location, and the ability to manually extract the larvae. *C. anthropophaga* larvae penetrate the skin after hatching from eggs deposited on moist soil or clothing and bed linen hung to dry outdoors and which have not been ironed. The infestation by *D. hominis* larvae develops from fly eggs and is carried to humans through a mosquito bite. In both cases, the larvae develop by successive molts. The incubation period varies from 7 days to 6 weeks (7–10 days for the Tumbu fly and 15–45 days for the botfly).

The cutaneous lesion is a 1–2-cm furuncle-like lesion with a central punctum through which serosanguineous or purulent fluid discharges. Importantly, the patient complains more of a crawling sensation within

the lesion than of pruritus. Movements of the larvae may be seen within the central punctum. *C. anthropophaga* lesions are more commonly multiple, whereas *D. hominis* lesions usually number from one to three.[6] *C. anthropophaga* lesions are usually located on areas of the body covered by clothing (such as the trunk), whereas *D. hominis* lesions are commonly located on areas of the body (such as the scalp, face, forearms and legs) exposed to insect bites. The largest number of lesions ever reported was 94 in a child from Ghana infected by *C. anthropophaga*.[7]

The diagnosis of myiasis is made by the identification of the larva from the lesion.

The treatment is the removal of the larvae by paying attention not to break the larvae because incomplete removal may result in a hypersensitivity or foreign body reaction to the larvae. In the case of *C. anthropophaga*, manual pressure to the lateral aspects of the lesion easily allows the expression of the maggot. In the case of *D. hominis*, extraction is facilitated by first placing an occlusive agent (e.g., paraffin, petrolatum, pork fat, toothpaste cap) onto the lesion.[8]

## 17.4 Helminthic Diseases

### 17.4.1 Hookworm-Related Cutaneous Larva Migrans

Hookworm-related cutaneous larva migrans (HrCLM) is one of the most frequent travel-associated skin disease of tropical origin.[9] HrCLM is caused by the penetration of the human skin by cat or dog hookworm's larvae usually while landing or walking on the beaches in hot seaside areas of tropical and subtropical countries worldwide.

The incubation period of HrCLM is usually a few days and rarely goes beyond 1 month. In series of HrCLM diagnosed in returning travelers, the cutaneous lesions appeared on return in approximately half the patients whereas in the remaining patients the mean time of onset after return was usually less than 1 month. However, some extremely long incubation periods have been reported.[9]

The striking symptom of HrCLM is pruritus localized at the site of the eruption and reported in all patients. The most frequent and characteristic sign of HrCLM is "creeping dermatitis," a clinical sign defined as an erythematous, subcutaneous linear or serpiginous track (Fig. 17.1) that is approximately 3 mm wide and may be upto 15–20 cm in length, which may extend by a few millimeters to a few centimeters daily.[9] The mean number of lesions per person commonly varies from one to three. Other clinical signs are local swelling, reported in 6–17%, and vesiculobullous lesions, reported in 4–40% of returning travelers.[9] The most frequent anatomic locations of HrCLM lesions are the feet, followed by buttocks and thighs. Without any treatment, the eruption usually lasts between 2 and 8 weeks but it may be almost 2 years. Hookworm folliculitis is a particular form of HrCLM, consisting of pruritic folliculitis-like lesions associated with numerous relatively short tracks, generally arising from follicular lesions and located on the buttocks.[10]

HrCLM is usually diagnosed clinically based on the typical clinical presentation in the context of recent travel to a tropical country and beach exposure. Differential diagnosis includes the other dermatoses that give rise to creeping eruption and the other causes of cutaneous larva migrans syndrome.[11] In any case,

**Table 17.2** Causes of creeping eruption in travelers (adapted from ref. 11)

| |
|---|
| **Nematode's larvae** |
| Animal hookworms (HrCLM), *Pelodera strongyloides*, zoonotic *Strongyloides* spp. |
| Gnathostomiasis (*Gnathostoma* spp.) |
| *Spirurina* spp. |
| Larva currens |
|     *Strongyloides stercoralis* |
| **Trematode's larvae** |
| Fascioliasis (*Fasciola gigantica*) |
| **Adult nematodes** |
| Loiasis (*Loa loa*) |
| Dracunculiasis (*Dracunculus medinensis*) |
| **Fly's maggot** |
| Migratory myiasis (*Gasterophilus* spp.) |
| **Arthropod** |
| Scabies (*Sarcoptes scabiei*) |

pruritus may be associated with the subcutaneous migrations of a nematode's or a trematode's larvae, adult nematode, fly maggot or mite (Table 17.2).

Where still available, thiabendazole ointment remains the first-choice treatment (15% thiabendazole). A single dose of ivermectin and a three-day course of albendazole are the first-line oral treatments. Albendazole ointment is an alternative treatment.[9]

### 17.4.2 Cutaneous Gnathostomiasis

Gnathostomiasis is a foodborne parasitic zoonosis infection caused by ingestion of uncooked food infected with the third-stage nematode larvae of the helminth *Gnathostoma* spp. (mainly *G. spinigerum*).[12] Typical implicated foods include raw freshwater fish and also shrimp, crab, crayfish, frog or chicken. Gnathostomiasis is endemic in Southeast Asia (particularly Thailand) and Latin America (particularly in Mexico). Gnathostomiasis cases have been reported in travelers returning from these areas and more recently from western Zambia.[12,13]

The most common clinical presentation of gnathostomiasis is cutaneous gnathostomiasis. Typical cutaneous manifestations are recurrent subcutaneous swelling (Fig. 17.2), creeping eruption and edema of the extremities, all being more or less pruritic. In a series of five travelers, cutaneous lesions appeared within a mean period of 62 days (range 10–150 days) after return and consisted of four different clinical forms: creeping

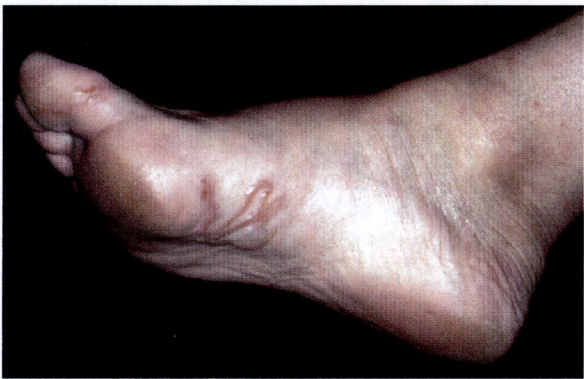

**Fig. 17.1** Creeping eruption of the foot due to hookworm-related cutaneous larva migrans

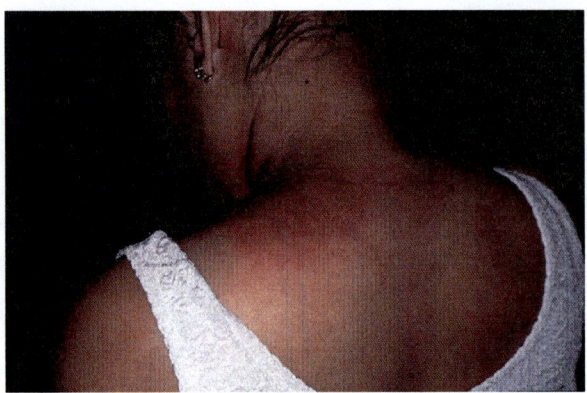

**Fig. 17.2** Panniculitis revealing cutaneous gnathostomiasis

**Table 17.3** Causes of urticaria in travelers

Helminthic infection: invasive phase of schistosomiasis, ascariasis, hookworm, anisakiasis, trichinellosis, strongyloidiasis, fascioliasis, toxocariasis, gnathostomiasis and rupture of cyst during hydatid disease; chronic phase of visceral larva migrans syndrome (toxocariasis)

Viral infection: Hepatitis A infection

Noninfectious causes: adverse drug reaction

before cure because approximately half of the travelers may require at least one other course of treatment.[13]

### 17.4.3 Invasive Phase of Helminthic Infections

Helminthic infections may give rise to acute urticaria during the invasive phase of the helminthic cycle, whereas chronic helminthic infections may be associated with chronic urticaria, both being pruritic (Table 17.3). The acute phase of schistosomiasis has been the most extensively described in travelers.

#### 17.4.3.1 Schistosomiasis

Pruritic wheals of acute urticaria are a typical skin manifestation of acute schistosomiasis (or invasive schistosomiasis) (Fig. 17.3). It can be observed 2–6 weeks after exposure to infested freshwater in endemic areas.[16] As an example, among 18 nonimmune travelers who acquired schistosomiasis after swimming in freshwater pools in Mali, 10 (36%) had complained of pruritic cercarial-like dermatitis just after the bath and 15 (54%) further presented with signs of invasive schistosomiasis (fever, urticaria, cough, headaches).

Diagnosis should thus be systematically considered for any febrile traveler with acute urticaria and a history of exposure to freshwater in an area of endemicity. The diagnosis relies on serology and eosinophilia, which are often negative and within normal limits at the beginning of the invasive phase and must be repeated.

Clinician should be aware of the risk of acute neuroschistosomiasis, which needs early treatment with corticosteroids to prevent irreversible damage.[17] In addition, praziquantel, which only kills adult worms and is associated with worsening in 40% in cases of acute schistosomiasis, should not be given during the acute phase of the disease.[16,17]

eruption in three patients (in addition one also had papules, one had nodules) and migratory swellings in two patients.[13] Of the three patients who presented with a pruritic creeping eruption, two were initially misdiagnosed with HrCLM. For the two patients with recurrent and migratory plaques with pruritus, subsequent episodes of subcutaneous edema lasted for 1–4 weeks each and occurred in different areas. Symptoms are intermittent but recurrent, which explains why the delay in diagnosis may be especially prolonged in areas where the disease is not endemic. Indeed, in a series of 16 travelers with imported gnathostomiasis diagnosed in London, the median time from onset of symptoms to diagnosis was 12 months.[12] Severe neurologic complications have been reported.[14] Thus, the diagnosis of cutaneous gnathostomiasis allows early treatment before the onset of neurological involvement.[13]

Diagnosis of cutaneous gnathostomiasis usually relies on the association of recurrent dermatological manifestations, history of ingestion of uncooked meat of animal hosts in endemic area, hypereosinophilia (common but not constant) and results of serological tests to be repeated in case of negativity.[13] Some authors report definitive confirmation of cases by isolation of the nematode's larva in a biopsy specimen.[13] Nevertheless, the biopsy is frequently unsuccessful, and subsequent blind biopsies are not recommended.[12,13]

The reported efficacy of albendazole in the treatment of gnathostomiasis in Thailand is >90%. Ivermectin 0.2 mg/kg for 2 days is as effective as albendazole (400 mg twice daily for 21 days) for treatment of cutaneous gnathostomiasis in Thailand.[15] However, a prolonged period of follow-up is necessary

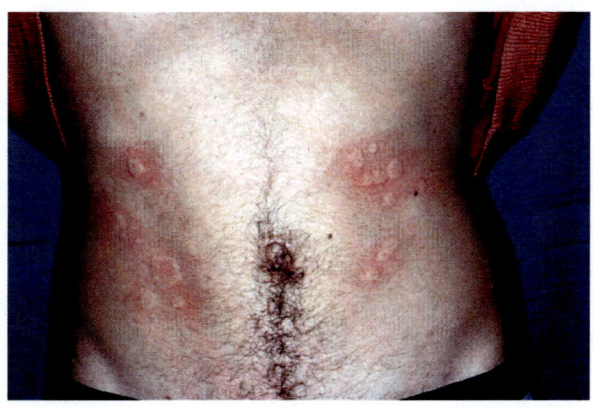

**Fig. 17.3** Acute urticaria during the invasive phase of schistosomiasis

### 17.4.3.2  Other Helminthic Infections

Other helminthic infections may be associated with pruritic wheals of acute urticaria during their invasive phase or chronic urticaria during the visceral larva migrans syndrome (Table 17.3).

## 17.4.4  Cercarial Dermatitis

Cercarial dermatitis results from penetration of the skin by nonhuman schistosomal cercariae while bathing in freshwater or coastal water. Those schistosomes are usual hosts of birds and small mammals and the cercariae penetrate intact human skin of swimmers in endemic areas of all continents. Identified risk factors in the United States (Michigan lake) and Switzerland (Leman lake) are bathing in shallow waters and in areas with onshore winds, prolonged lake use, previous history of cercarial dermatitis, time spent in the water, hour of the day and climatic conditions while bathing.[18,19]

A significant outbreak that occurred in Annecy's lake in France during a unique exposure (a swimming race) provided a good description of the disease.[20] The time from exposure to onset of symptoms varied from a few minutes to a maximum of 24 h after exposure. A prickling sensation during or shortly after exposure to infested water was reported. Typically, and approximately 1 h later, the eruption began with numerous pruritic macular erythematous cutaneous lesions that progressed to a papular, papulovesicular or urticarial eruption. The eruption usually involved exposed parts of the skin but also the parts covered by the bathing costume in approximately 20% of cases.[19,20] The eruption peaked in 1–3 days and lasted 1–3 weeks.[20] The diagnosis was made by history of water exposure and the characteristic dermatological findings. Cercarial dermatitis is self-limited and treatment is only symptomatic; oral antihistamines and topical steroids reduce the symptoms.

## 17.4.5  Filariasis

Cases of filariasis such as loiasis and onchocerciasis have been reported in travelers, mostly expatriates and migrants returning from Africa, and may be associated with pruritic skin manifestations.

### 17.4.5.1  Onchocerciasis

Onchocerciasis due to *Onchocerca volvulus* is transmitted by bites of blackflies mainly in tropical Africa. On one hand endemic onchocerciasis is seen in migrants originating from sub-Saharan Africa and returning from visiting friends and relatives in their country of origin, but these migrants are more likely to have acquired this infection after long-term exposure during their childhood rather than during their last travel.[2] On the other hand, (non-migrant) travelers who are exposed for brief periods are more often diagnosed with onchocerciasis-associated limb swelling after return from central Africa.[21,22] This is a particular epidemiological and clinical form of onchocerciasis, a fact underlined more than 20 years ago. This particular form of onchocerciasis is characterized by its epidemiology (contamination in a forested area whereas onchocerciasis is usually a disease of the savanas, and incubation time), its clinical presentation (limb swelling) and its diagnosis (skin snip in the affected area). In a series of five such cases, pruritic and inflammatory limb edema located on one arm occurred from 5 months to 2 years after travel to forested areas of Cameroon or Ivory Coast. Blood eosinophilia above 2000/mm$^3$ was present in four patients. The diagnosis was confirmed by detection on the skin of microfilariae of *O. volvulus*. Patients were cured with ivermectin and/or diethylcarbamazine.[21] Today, patients are treated by a single dose of ivermectin, in association with doxycycline.[23]

### 17.4.5.2 Loiasis

Loiasis (*Loa loa*) is exclusively endemic in West and Central Africa. Cutaneous manifestations are pruritus migratory angioedema (Calabar swelling), subcutaneous (creeping dermatitis) and subconjunctival passage of the adult worm. They are more likely to be seen in migrants originating from endemic countries rather than in short-term travelers such as tourists and business travelers.[2] In 26 Moroccan patients who had visited Equatorial Guinea, transient and migratory edema with pruritus were described in all cases, a history of eyeworm was reported in 13 patients and subcutaneous migration of adult *Loa loa* in 19 patients.[24]

Diagnosis is based on positive microfilariae (to be quantified before initiating treatment), filarial serology and eosinophil count. Recommended antiparasitic treatments are diethylcarbamazine and ivermectin.

## 17.5 Mycoses

Dermatophytosis and candidosis are worldwide cutaneous infections but their incidence is higher in the tropics.[25] It ranks among the most common skin diseases observed after travel abroad.[1,2] Pityriasis versicolor is probably the most common fungal disease in travelers but is not particularly pruritic. Tinea corporis is a fungal infection of the glabrous skin located on the nonhairy parts of the body with the exception of the axillae, groins, hands and feet. The characteristic lesion is a well-defined round or oval erythematous plaque with a vesicular border and central clearing. Tinea cruris and axillaris may be common in travelers due to the excessive perspiration and friction of the major intertriginous areas, such as groins and axillae, respectively. Tinea pedis (athlete's foot) is common in travelers who go barefoot or wear sandals. Tinea capitis is a common variety of dermatophytosis in children coming back from visiting friends and relatives, or who are adopted, in Africa.[26]

## 17.6 Viroses

The most frequent viroses that may give rise to a pruritic disseminated cutaneous eruption in travelers are varicella, dengue and chikungunya infection. The latter two infections are transmitted to humans by arthropods, whereas the former disease is transmitted between humans. Nonetheless, varicella is less likely to occur in travelers given its high prevalence in Western countries compared to most of the developing countries.

### 17.6.1 Dengue

Dengue is the most common cause of arboviral disease in the world, one of the most frequent specific causes of systemic febrile illness among travelers and the most frequent arbovirose reported after travel to tropical and subtropical countries.[27] Dengue virus belongs to the family *Flaviviridae* and is transmitted by mosquitoes *Aedes aegypti* and *A. albopictus*. Dengue is widely reported in tropical and subtropical countries and Dengue hemorrhagic fever has been reported in travelers returning from Southeast Asia, South Pacific Islands, the Caribbean and Latin America.

Typical presentation of classic dengue fever include the sudden onset of fever, headache, retro-orbital pain, fatigue, musculoskeletal symptoms (arthralgia and myalgia) and a rash which usually appears near the time of defervescence. The rash is typically macular or maculopapular, confluent with the sparing of small islands of normal skin. Other dermatological signs include pruritus, flushed facies and hemorrhagic manifestations such as petechiae and purpura. Most patients present with classic dengue fever and have benign febrile illness but dengue hemorrhagic fever and dengue shock syndrome must be systematically clinically and biologically evaluated.

### 17.6.2 Chikungunya

Since the chikungunya virus was first isolated in Tanzania in 1953, outbreaks have been reported in Africa and Asia and more recently in the Indian Ocean region. Transmission to humans occurs through bites of *Aedes* (mainly *Aedes aegypti* and *A. albopictus*) mosquitoes. Since 2005, chikungunya cases have been reported in travelers returning from known outbreak areas to Europe (especially in France), Canada and the United States.[28,29]

Skin manifestations of chikungunya infection in travelers seem to be very similar to those described for classic dengue fever infection, with a pruritic, macular or a maculopapular rash in which small islands of normal skin are spared.[28] Chikungunya and dengue skin manifestations are difficult to differentiate clinically.

## 17.7  Environmental Skin Diseases

### 17.7.1  Arthropod-Related Dermatoses

Arthropod-related dermatoses are very common in travelers.[1–3] Identification of the implicated arthropod on clinical grounds is difficult because arthropods of different species may give rise to similar dermatologic manifestations, whereas a given arthropod may give rise to multiple dermatologic manifestations. The best diagnostic clues for identifying the culprit arthropod are the circumstances of appearance together with the distribution of the lesions on the body. However, this has no significant consequence, the treatment being usually the same with oral antihistamines and topical corticosteroids.

The predominant feature of the arthropod reaction is prurigo (Fig. 17.4), an eruption of intensely pruritic erythematous and excoriated papules. This reaction is considered to be an evolutive stage of papular urticaria related to a hypersensitivity reaction to the bites of insects such as fleas, bedbugs and, less commonly, mosquitoes, chiggers, ants and mites.[30] Arthropod bites may also result in vesiculobullous lesions.

Bacterial skin infections are one of the most common complications of arthropod bites and stings in travelers.[3] It acts as a portal of entry for bacteria either through the bite or secondary to scratching. The clinical spectrum ranges from impetigo and ecthyma to erysipelas, abscess and necrotizing cellulites. Lesions usually appear while the patient is still abroad, but are also a leading cause of consultation in returning travelers.[1–3] In one series of 19 returning travelers with impetigo (*S. aureus* and *S. pyogenes* being identified in 80% of the 15 available swab samples), 63% were secondary to an insect bite.[1] In another series of 21 infectious cellulites in returning travelers, 28% were secondary to insect bites.[2] Last in the largest series to date, insect bites, with or without

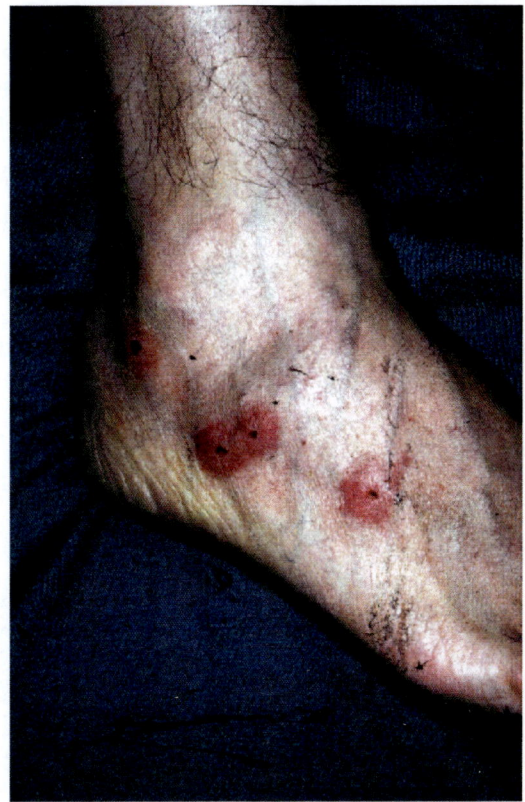

**Fig. 17.4**  Acute prurigo after walking accidentally on an anthill

superinfection, were the first etiologic diagnosis in 2947 travelers with dermatologic disorder.[3]

### 17.7.2  Contact Dermatitis

Contact dermatitis is a major cause of noninfectious dermatoses among travelers but is more often seen during travel than in returning travelers.[31] It may be related to exposure to plants, insects and marine creatures.

Allergic contact dermatitis has been widely reported after contacts with plants in the *Anacardiaceae* family which include the cashew tree, poison ivy/oak, mango, and pistachio.[32] Travelers with a history of poison ivy sensitivity should be informed of this immunological cross-reactivity. Poison ivy dermatitis clears by itself in absence of renewed exposure to the allergen. Local treatment is indicated in mild to moderate cases to promote healing of active lesions and suppress itching, whereas systemic corticosteroids should be considered in more severe cases.

*Paederus* dermatitis (also called blister beetle dermatitis) has been widely reported. One recent outbreak concerned 191 U.S. personnel deployed to Pakistan, and staphylinid (rove) beetles were implicated.[33] It occurs when nocturnal beetles of the genus *Paederus* (rove beetles) are crushed on the skin, releasing the vesicant pederin and resulting in linear, geographic, erythematous pruritic plaques with the presence of vesicles or pustules 1 or 2 days after contact with the insect. Skin manifestations commonly involve uncovered areas such as the neck, face and arms. As for irritant contact dermatitis, one should remove the irritant by washing the implicated area and using a topical steroid and antibiotic, if secondarily infected.

Dermatoses related to insect exposure have been also reported among travelers after contact with moths in Mexico and presenting with pruritic papular eruption.[34]

Dermatoses associated with contact with a marine creature are one of the most frequent causes of disease in travelers to tropical islands. Cnidarians such as jellyfish, anemones and corals use venom application devices (so-called nematocysts) for hunting and self-defense, which are responsible of severe envenomations in travelers to tropical or subtropical area, inducing a stinging sensation that varies from a slight burning sensation to excruciating pain and may include pruritus.[35,36] The cutaneous lesions appear at the site of exposition within a few minutes, begin as macules and papules, and may progress to vesicles, bulles and ulceration. Episodes of flare-up reactions can also occur and subside several weeks with persistent pruritic lesions at sites of previous contact.[37] The other marine creatures that may induce pruritic dermatitis include sea urchins and other echinoderms, and produce sea leech burns and coral cuts and scratches.

### 17.7.3 Ciguatera

Ciguatera is a significant cause of pruritus which may last for months after the initial event. This fish poisoning is acquired by the ingestion of fish containing the toxins produced by the dinoflagellate *Gambierdiscus toxicus*, which is frequently found in damaged coral reef systems in tropical and subtropical regions. These lipid-soluble, thermostable toxins accumulate in predatory carnivorous fish that consume contaminated herbivorous reef fish.

Ciguatera is characterized by gastrointestinal effects (nausea, vomiting, diarrhoea and abdominal cramps) and neurological effects (myalgia, paraesthesia, cold allodynia, ataxia and pruritus).[38] The diagnosis relies on history of fish consumption, other cases among travelers sharing the same food habit, a short incubation period (2–30 h) and the association initially to gastrointestinal and cardiac signs then to neurological signs such as fatigue, myalgias (particularly of the lower extremities), pruritus, and neurosensory manifestations (perioral and distal extremity paresthesias). Patients typically experience paradoxical reversal of temperature perception with tingling, burning, "dry ice-like," smarting and "electric" sensations. The reversal of the temperature sensation (i.e., cold beverages and objects are described as feeling hot) is unique to ciguatera. Whereas gastrointestinal symptoms resolve in a few hours, myalgias, pruritus and neurosensory symptoms last longer. In a series of 13 Italian travelers returning from the Caribbean, the incubation period varied between 2 and 9 h, nearly all patients had initial gastrointestinal symptoms and itching occurred in 8 patients but cold-to-hot reversal of temperature sensation occurred in only two patients.[39] The duration of symptoms varied from 1 to 16 months.

Because there are no antidotes, treatment is essentially supportive. Although IV mannitol is considered the treatment of choice for ciguatera, a prospective clinical study of 50 patients with ciguatera on Rarotonga, Cook Islands, reported that mannitol was not superior to normal saline in relieving symptoms of ciguatera at 24 h but had more side effects.[40]

### 17.7.4 Seabather's Eruption

Seabather's eruption (also called sea lice) is a highly pruritic eruption generally confined to the skin under swimwear that occurs after bathing in the ocean. It is caused by larval forms of sea anemones (e.g., *Edwardsiella lineata*) and jellyfish (e.g., *Linuche unguiculata*) that become trapped under swimwear.[41] Seabather's eruption has been widely reported on the Atlantic coast of the United States, the Caribbean, Central and South America, and in Southeast Asia.

The time from exposure to onset of symptoms is usually a few minutes to 24 h. Individuals with a history of previous exposures may develop a prickling or stinging sensation or urticarial lesions while in the water. The clinical features include pruritic, erythematous macules that progresses to papules, vesicles and urticarial lesions. The anatomic distribution typically includes skin surfaces covered by swimwear and uncovered skin surfaces where there is friction (e.g., axillae, medial thighs, surfer's chest). The eruption can last from 3 days to 3 weeks. The average duration of the eruption and pruritus was 12.5 days in 70 patients in southeast Florida.[42] A prospective cohort study conducted in Palm Beach County, Florida, concluded that children, people with a history of seabather's eruption and surfers were at greatest risk for seabather's eruption.[43]

The diagnosis is made by the characteristic clinical findings and history of exposure. The differential diagnosis include cercarial dermatitis, contact dermatitis (secondary to marine life inhabitants) and insect bites. Seabather's eruption resolves spontaneously within 1–3 weeks, and therapy is symptomatic but often ineffective. Oral antihistamines and topical steroids may reduce the symptoms.

## 17.8 Other Cosmopolitan Pruritic Dermatoses of Interest for Travelers

Pruritus of unknown origin (PUO) was the third cause of consultation in one study of returning travelers with skin disease.[2] It was significantly associated with older age and immigrant status, most of the cases being seen among immigrants originating from Africa. Pruritus predominates on the anterior surface of the lower limbs. PUO in this setting could be due to acclimatization. In addition, Africans are used to bathing frequently and using detergents. In doing so, they defat their skin and that leads to xerosis and itching. Moreover the in-house and in-office climate in Europe is often dry, increasing the problem.[2]

Hypersensitivity to drugs, not only daily medications but prophylaxis, must always be considered in the differential diagnosis of urticaria and exanthema in travelers.[44]

Exacerbation of chronic pruritic diseases such as atopic dermatitis may occur. Other dermatoses of interest include miliaria rubra, which is usually associated with particular climatic conditions.

## 17.9 Conclusion

Regarding pruritic skin diseases, travelers must be specifically instructed to avoid arthropod bites. They should be informed of the risk of walking barefoot and advised to avoid itching in case of pruritus. Travel first-aid kits should include antibiotics effective against bacterial skin infection, oral antihistamines and corticosteroid ointments.

## References

1. Caumes E, Carriere J, Guermonprez G, Bricaire F, Danis M, Gentilini M. Dermatoses associated with travel to tropical countries: a prospective study of the diagnosis and management of 269 patients presenting to a tropical disease unit. *Clin Infect Dis*. 1995;20:542–548.
2. Ansart S, Perez L, Jaureguiberry S, Danis M, Bricaire F, Caumes E. Spectrum of dermatoses in 165 travelers returning from the tropics with skin diseases. *Am J Trop Med Hyg*. 2007;76:184–186.
3. Freedman DO, Weld LH, Kozarsky PE, et al. Spectrum of disease and relation to place of exposure among ill returned travelers. *N Engl J Med*. 2006;354:119–130.
4. Chosidow O. Clinical practices scabies. *N Engl J Med*. 2006;354:1718–1727.
5. McGarry JW, McCall PJ, Welby S. Arthropod dermatoses acquired in the UK and overseas. *Lancet*. 2001;357: 2105–2106.
6. Jelinek T, Nothdurft HD, Rieder N, Loscher T. Cutaneous myiasis: review of 13 cases in travelers returning from tropical countries. *Int J Dermatol*. 1995;34:624–626.
7. Biggar RJ, Morrow H, Morrow RH. Extensive myiasis from tumbu fly larvae in Ghana, West Africa. *Clin Pediatr (Phila)*. 1980;19:231–232.
8. Brewer TF, Wilson ME, Gonzalez E, Felsenstein D. Bacon therapy and furuncular myiasis. *JAMA*. 1993;270:2087–2088.
9. Hochedez P, Caumes E. Hookworm related cutaneous larva migrans. *J Travel Med*. 2007;14:326–333.
10. Caumes E, Ly F, Bricaire F. Cutaneous larva migrans with folliculitis: report of seven cases and review of the literature. *Br J Dermatol*. 2002;146:314–316.
11. Caumes E. It's time to distinguish the sign "creeping eruption" from the syndrome "cutaneous larva migrans". *Dermatology*. 2006;213:179–181.
12. Moore DA, McCroddan J, Dekumyoy P, Chiodini PL. Gnathostomiasis: an emerging imported disease. *Emerg Infect Dis*. 2003;9:647–650.
13. Menard A, Dos Santos G, Dekumyoy P, et al. Imported cutaneous gnathostomiasis: report of five cases. *Trans R Soc Trop Med Hyg*. 2003;97:200–202.
14. Gorgolas M, Santos-O'Connor F, Unzu AL, et al. Cutaneous and medullar gnathostomiasis in travelers to Mexico and Thailand. *J Travel Med*. 2003;10:358–361.

15. Nontasut P, Claesson BA, Dekumyoy P, Pakdee W, Chullawichit S. Double-dose ivermectin vs albendazole for the treatment of gnathostomiasis. *Southeast Asian J Trop Med Public Health*. 2005;36:650–652.

16. Grandiere-Perez L, Ansart S, Paris L, et al. Efficacy of praziquantel during the incubation and invasive phase of Schistosoma haematobium schistosomiasis in 18 travelers. *Am J Trop Med Hyg*. 2006;74:814–818.

17. Jaureguiberry S, Ansart S, Perez L, Danis M, Bricaire F, Caumes E. Acute neuroschistosomiasis: two cases associated with cerebral vasculitis. *Am J Trop Med Hyg*. 2007;76: 964–966.

18. Verbrugge LM, Rainey JJ, Reimink RL, Blankespoor HD. Swimmer's itch: incidence and risk factors. *Am J Public Health*. 2004;94:738–741.

19. Chamot E, Toscani L, Rougemont A. Public health importance and risk factors for cercarial dermatitis associated with swimming in Lake Leman at Geneva. *Switzerland. Epidemiol Infect*. 1998;120:305–314.

20. Caumes E, Felder-Moinet S, Couzigou C, Darras-Joly C, Latour P, Leger N. Failure of an ointment based on IR3535 (ethyl butylacetylaminopropionate) to prevent an outbreak of cercarial dermatitis during swimming races across Lake Annecy, France. *Ann Trop Med Parasitol*. 2003;97:157–163.

21. Nozais JP, Caumes E, Datry A, Bricaire F, Danis M, Gentilini M. Apropos of 5 new cases of onchocerciasis edema. *Bull Soc Pathol Exot*. 1997;90:335–338.

22. Wolfe MS, Petersen JL, Neafie RC, Connor DH, Purtilo DT. Onchocerciasis presenting with limb swelling. *Am J Trop Med Hyg*. 1974;23:361–368.

23. Ezzedine K, Malvy D, Dhaussy I, et al. Onchocerciasis-associated limb swelling in a traveler returning from Cameroon. *J Travel Med*. 2006;13:50–53.

24. El Haouri M, Erragragui Y, Sbai M, et al. Cutaneous filariasis *Loa loa*: 26 moroccan cases of importation. *Ann Dermatol Venereol*. 2001;128:899–902.

25. Panackal AA, Hajjeh RA, Cetron MS, Warnock DW. Fungal infections among returning travelers. *Clin Infect Dis*. 2002;35:1088–1095.

26. Markey RJ, Staat MA, Gerrety MJ, Lucky AW. Tinea capitis due to Trichophyton soudanense in Cincinnati, Ohio, in internationally adopted children from Liberia. *Pediatr Dermatol*. 2003;20:408–410.

27. Jelinek T, Muhlberger N, Harms G, et al. Epidemiology and clinical features of imported dengue fever in Europe: sentinel surveillance data from TropNetEurop. *Clin Infect Dis*. 2002;35:1047–1052.

28. Hochedez P, Jaureguiberry S, Debruyne M, et al. Chikungunya infection in travelers. *Emerg Infect Dis*. 2006; 12:1565–1567.

29. Simon F, Parola P, Grandadam M, et al. Chikungunya infection; an emerging rheumatism among travelers returning from Indian Ocean islands. Report of 47 cases. *Medicine*. 2007;86:123–137.

30. Steen CJ, Carbonaro PA, Schwartz RA. Arthropods in dermatology. *J Am Acad Dermatol*. 2004;50:819–842.

31. Caumes E, Le Bris V, Couzigou C, Menard A, Janier M, Flahault A. Dermatoses associated with travel to Burkina Faso and diagnosed by means of teledermatology. *Br J Dermatol*. 2004;150:312–316.

32. Maje HA, Freedman DO. Cashew nut dermatitis in a returned traveler. *J Travel Med*. 2001;8:213–215.

33. Dursteler BB, Nyquist RA. Outbreak of rove beetle (Staphylinid) pustular contact dermatitis in Pakistan among deployed U.S. personnel. *Mil Med*. 2004;169:57–60.

34. Jamieson F, Keystone JS, From L, Rosen C. Moth-associated dermatitis in Canadian travellers returning from Mexico. *CMAJ*. 1991;145:1119–1121.

35. Fenner PJ. Dangers in the ocean: the traveler and marine envenomation. I. jellyfish. *J Travel Med*. 1998;5:135–141.

36. Fenner PJ. Dangers in the ocean: the traveler and marine envenomation. II. Marine vertebrates. *J Travel Med*. 1998;5:213–216.

37. Ohtaki N, Satoh A, Azuma H, Nakajima T. Delayed flare-up reactions caused by jellyfish. *Dermatologica*. 1986;172:98–103.

38. Isbister GK, Kiernan MC. Neurotoxic marine poisoning. *Lancet Neurol*. 2005;4:219–228.

39. Bavastrelli M, Bertucci P, Midulla M, Giardini O, Sanguigni S. Ciguatera fish poisoning: an emerging syndrome in Italian travelers. *J Travel Med*. 2001;8:139–142.

40. Schnorf H, Taurarii M, Cundy T. Ciguatera fish poisoning: a double-blind randomized trial of mannitol therapy. *Neurology*. 2002;58:873–880.

41. Freudenthal AR, Joseph PR. Seabather's eruption. *N Engl J Med*. 1993;329:542–544.

42. Wong DE, Meinking TL, Rosen LB, Taplin D, Hogan DJ, Burnett JW. Seabather's eruption. Clinical, histologic, and immunologic features. *J Am Acad Dermatol*. 1994; 30:399–406.

43. Kumar S, Hlady WG, Malecki JM. Risk factors for seabather's eruption: a prospective cohort study. *Public Health Rep*. 1997;112:59–62.

44. Schlagenhauf P, Tschopp A, Johnson R, et al. Tolerability of malaria chemoprophylaxis in non-immune travellers to sub-Saharan Africa: multicentre, randomised, double blind, four arm study. *BMJ*. 2003;327:1078–1083.

# Chapter 18
# Pruritus in Cutaneous T-cell Lymphoma

Tobias Görge and Meinhard Schiller

Cutaneous T-cell lymphomas (CTCL) account for about 80% of skin lymphomas. CTCL encompasses a diverse group of diseases that are characterized by malignant T lymphocytes that initially home to the skin.[1] Within the CTCL, mykosis fungoides (MF) is the most common variant.[2] The classical form of MF is characterized by erythematous flat patches in early stages, which may progress to palpable reddish-brown infiltrated plaques. In late stages of MF, the patients show a combination of patches, plaques and tumor lesions or may present as generalized diffuse erythema. A prolonged natural history is one of the remarkable clinical features of MF.[3] By contrast, Sezary syndrome (SS) is a rare disease characterized by erythroderma, generalized lymphadenopathy and the presence of atypical convoluted Sézary T cells in the blood count.

A characteristic hallmark of CTCL, especially SS, is pruritus, the sensation of itch which is repeatedly observed in various CTCL types.[4–10] Despite great advances in recent pruritus research, it is still unknown how T-cell lymphoma mediates the itch sensation, and, especially, the molecular mechanisms involved remain to be elucidated.[11] In the present chapter we review the literature on CTCL and itch. We particularly focus on the concept that pruritus might be a good diagnostic tool for assessment of CTCL activity and we evaluate current treatment options for pruritus in CTCL. This is of special interest, as the clinician needs to be aware of the fact that pruritus can also be an unwanted side effect of therapies intended to treat the CTCL (secondary to treatment). According to the state of the art, we conclude that further intensive research is needed to gain more insight into pruritus in CTCL.

In an outpatient setting, approximately one-third of the patients with the diagnosis of CTCL complain of itch that accompanies the disease. This observation points to the importance of a detailed history of itch in patients with CTCL. Clinical reports suggest that pruritus is particularly elevated in the follicular type of MF.[5] What is more, in some cases pruritus was the only symptom in a patient leading to the diagnosis of a CTCL.[10,12,13] For instance, one patient had no cutaneous skin lesions but presented with persistent generalized pruritus.[12,13] A skin biopsy of visually unaltered but pruritic skin then revealed the diagnosis of a monoclonal T-cell infiltration in the characteristic pattern of MFs. This example further illustrates the importance of measuring the itch intensity (e.g., by the visual analog scale, VAS) as a tool for monitoring disease activity in patients with lymphoma. Pruritus as a symptom is almost invariably present in CTCL progressing into generalized erythrodermic MF (Fig. 18.1) and Sézary syndrome. Both are characterized by erythroderma (a state of skin vasodilatation involving the whole or most of the body). It may be speculated that T cells homing to the skin provoke the release of inflammatory cytokines, but the precise molecular mechanism of how pruritus is evoked in CTCL is, however, still unknown. In addition, mast cells were shown to be increased in MF skin biopsies, and IgE levels were massively elevated (>1,400 U/ml) in late stage CTCL.[14]

Treatment modalities of CTCL aim at reducing the inflammatory activity of T cells in the skin. Standard treatments include topical steroids, radiation with UV light (mostly psoralen and ultraviolet A, PUVA) and radiation with electrons, as well as systemic treatments with interferon, bexaroten and extracorporal photopheresis. There is well-documented evidence that all these therapies not only reduce lymphatic infiltration but also diminish the pruritus in patients with CTCL

L. Misery and S. Ständer (eds.), *Pruritus*,
DOI 10.1007/978-1-84882-322-8_18, © Springer-Verlag London Limited 2010

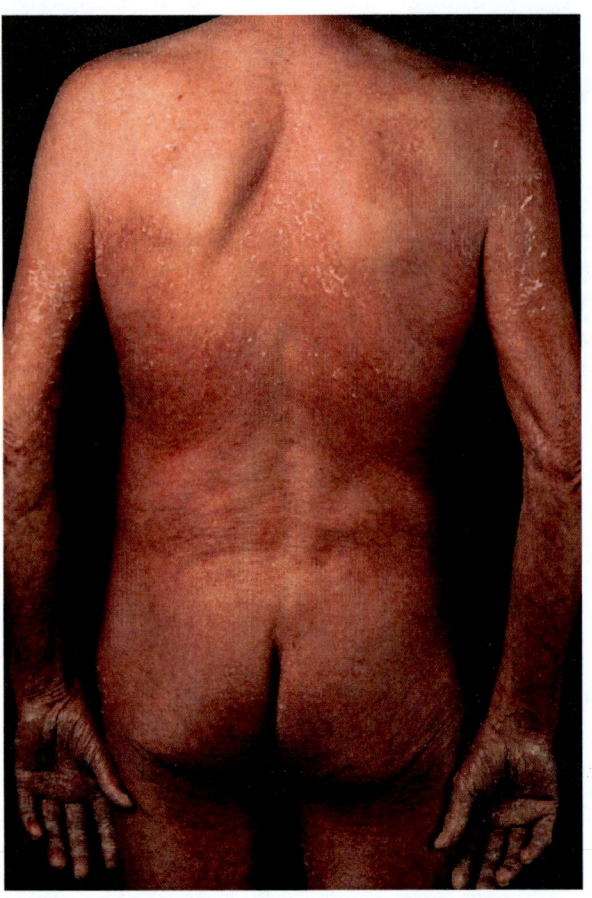

(Table 18.1). Especially, extracorporeal photopheresis[15] and emerging drugs with novel therapeutic targets for the treatment of CTCL, i.e., Denileukin difitox, Alemtuzumab, an anti-CD52 monoclonal antibody, and Vorinostat, a histone deacetylase inhibitor, have been shown to reduce pruritus in patients with the advanced stage of MF or SS (Table 18.1).[3,15–20] As different treatment options independently lead to reduction of inflammatory activity and pruritus, it may be assumed that the pruritogenic effect of CTCL is derived from the T-cell infiltration. Despite clear evidence that the above-mentioned treatment modalities positively affect pruritus, there is also published evidence that some patients with pruritus respond to these treatments. As displayed in Table 18.2, Wilson et al. reported the development of pruritus under electron therapy,[22] and the same was found for bexarotene,[23,24] extracorporeal photochemotherapy (ECP)[25] and PUVA in other studies.[24,26] It may be argued that bexarotene and ECP are treatment modalities that are only broadly used in the later stages of CTCL and, therefore, pruritus occurred during disease onset independent of the treatment modality. Nevertheless, meticulous clinical observations are required to unravel predictive markers for the putative development of pruritus as an adverse side effect following treatment of the CTCL.

Treatment of iatrogen pruritus during CTCL treatment is challenging. The chosen therapy may be indispensable, and therefore anti-pruritus treatment requires special attention. While the general treatment of pruritus (emol-

**Fig. 18.1** Erythrodermic mykosis fungoides (MF): the patient presented with erythroderma, palmoplantar hyperkeratosis and intense pruritus

**Table 18.1** Improvement of CTCL-related pruritus due to lymphoma-directed treatment regimes

| Treatment concept | Documented impact on pruritus | References |
|---|---|---|
| Oral bexoraotene | Gradual improvement of pruritus (about 50%) in a patient with Sézary syndrome | (el Azhzry and Bouwhuis, 2005) |
| Oral bexoraotene | Improvement of pruritus from initial VAS 4 (mean grade of all patients) to VAS 1 (phase II–III trial with 94 patients in advanced stages (IIB–IVB) | (Duvic et al, 2001) |
| Prednisolone, cyclophosphamide and psoralen and ultraviolet A (PUVA) | Improvement of pruritus in a patient with Sézary syndrome (case report) | (Lowe et al, 1979) |
| 13-*cis*-Retinoic acid | Improvement of pruritus in three patients with refractory CTCL (tumor stage) | (Kesseler et al, 1983) |
| Denileukin difitox (ONTAK) | Improvement of pruritus from initially VAS $x$ (mean grade of all patients) to VAS $y$ (phase III trial with 71 patients with stage IB–IVA) | (Duvic et al, 2002) |
| Extracorporeal photopheresis | Improvement of pruritus (>50%) in 34 out of 55 patients with Sézary syndrome (single-center retrospective review) | (Bouwhuis et al, 2002) |
| Alemtuzumab (anti-CD52 monoclonal antibody) | Improvement of pruritus from initial VAS 8 (median of all patients) to VAS 2 (phase II trial in 22 patients with stage III-IV) | (Lundin et al, 2003) |

(continued)

**Table 18.1**  (continued)

| Treatment concept | Documented impact on pruritus | References |
|---|---|---|
| Vorinostat (suberoylanilide hydroxamic acid), a histone deacetylase inhibitor | Among study patients with baseline VAS > = 3 (*n* = 65), 32% had pruritus relief (decrease of VAS > 3 points) (phase IIB trial in 74 patients with stage IB–IVB) | (Olsen et al, 2007) |
| Vorinostat | Mean VAS decreased approx. 3 points (phase II trial in 31 patients with stage IB–IVB) | (Duvic et al, 2007) |

**Table 18.2**  CTCL treatment concepts with documented pruritus as an adverse event

| Treatment concept | Adverse event | References |
|---|---|---|
| Total skin electron beam therapy (TSEBT) (median dose 57 Gy) | 14 out of 14 patients developed pruritus either during or within 6 months of TSEBT; 1 out of 14 suffered from long-term pruitus | (Wilson et al, 1996) |
| Topical mechlorethamine hydrochloride (concentration 10 g/50 ml), daily or every other day for 3 months | 23 out of 43 patients developed cutaneous intolerance of mechlorethamine with intense local pruritus (in 12 patients mechlorethamine patch test was positive) | (Esteve et al, 1999) |
| Topical bexarotene | Several phase II to III studies, case series, case reports: pruritus w or w/o irritant dermatitis | (Heald et al, 2003) (Lowe and Plosker 2000) |
| Topical miltefosine (concentration 6% solution, daily for 8 weeks) | Phase II trial, local pruritus in 7 out of 12 patients | (Dumontet et al, 2006) |
| Extracorporeal photochemotherapy (ECP) | Case report, generalized pruritus 20 min after initiating ECP, allergic reaction to ethylene oxide (EtO) (IgE-mediated type I allergy | (Geogieva et al, 2004) |
| PUVA | Several studies report pruritus as the main adverse effects to PUVA treatment of various dermatoses | (Tran et al, 2001) |
| PUVA + systemic bexarotene | 4 out of 8 patients developed rash/pruritus (most common adverse event in study population | (Singh and Lebwohl, 2004) |

lients, topical steroids and anti-histamines) is discussed elsewhere in this book, it is worth mentioning that both gabapentin and mirtazapine have been reported to be helpful in therapy-resistant pruritus. Gabapentin binds to the alpha2delta subunit of the voltage-dependent calcium channel where it suppresses neuronal hyperexcitability, while mirtazapine is a dual serotonergic and noradrenergic antidepressant.[27] These substances are of particular interest in the treatment of pruritus related to SS.[27]

In summary, pruritus in CTCL seems to be both a blessing and a curse: ablessing in those patients in whom it may lead to early diagnosis, and a curse for those that are resistant to therapy. Further research is mandatory to unravel the molecular mechanisms to provide more specific treatment of pruritus in CTCL.

# References

1. Burg G, Kempf W, Cozzio A, et al. WHO/EORTC classification of cutaneous lymphomas 2005: histological and molecular aspects. *J Cutan Pathol.* 2005;32:647–674.
2. Willemze R, Jaffe ES, Burg G, et al. WHO-EORTC classification for cutaneous lymphomas. *Blood.* 2005;105:3768–3785.
3. Olsen E, Vonderheid E, Pimpinelli N, et al. Revisions to the staging and classification of mycosis fungoides and Sezary syndrome: a proposal of the International Society for Cutaneous Lymphomas (ISCL) and the cutaneous lymphoma task force of the European Organization of Research and Treatment of Cancer (EORTC). *Blood.* 2007;110:1713–1722.
4. Kotz EA, Anderson D, Thiers BH. Cutaneous T-cell lymphoma. *J Eur Acad Dermatol Venereol.* 2003;17:131–137.
5. van Doorn R, Scheffer E, Willemze R. Follicular mycosis fungoides, a distinct disease entity with or without associated follicular mucinosis: a clinicopathologic and follow-up study of 51 patients. *Arch Dermatol.* 2002;138:191–198.

6. Akhyani M, Ghodsi ZS, Toosi S, Dabbaghian H. Erythroderma: a clinical study of 97 cases. *BMC Dermatol.* 2005;5:5.

7. Green SB, Byar DP, Lamberg SI. Prognostic variables in mycosis fungoides. *Cancer.* 1981;47:2671–2677.

8. Ikai K, Uchiyama T, Maeda M, Takigawa M. Sezary-like syndrome in a 10-year-old girl with serologic evidence of human T-cell lymphotropic virus type I infection. *Arch Dermatol.* 1987;123:1351–1355.

9. Meister L, Duarte AM, Davis J, Perez JL, Schachner LA. Sezary syndrome in an 11-year-old girl. *J Am Acad Dermatol.* 1993;28:93–95.

10. Bowen GM, Stevens SR, Dubin HV, Siddiqui J, Cooper KD. Diagnosis of Sezary syndrome in a patient with generalized pruritus based on early molecular study and flow cytometry. *J Am Acad Dermatol.* 1995;33:678–680.

11. Ikoma A, Steinhoff M, Stander S, Yosipovitch G, Schmelz M. The neurobiology of itch. *Nat Rev Neurosci.* 2006;7:535–547.

12. Pujol RM, Gallardo F, Llistosella E, et al. Invisible mycosis fungoides: a diagnostic challenge. *J Am Acad Dermatol.* 2002;47:S168–S171.

13. Pujol RM, Gallardo F, Llistosella E, et al. Invisible mycosis fungoides: a diagnostic challenge. *J Am Acad Dermatol.* 2000;42:324–328.

14. Yamamoto T, Katayama I, Nishioka K. Role of mast cell and stem cell factor in hyperpigmented mycosis fungoides. *Blood.* 1997;90:1338–1340.

15. Bouwhuis SA, el Azhary RA, Gibson LE, McEvoy MT, Pittelkow MR. Effect of insulin-dependent diabetes mellitus on response to extracorporeal photopheresis in patients with Sezary syndrome. *J Am Acad Dermatol.* 2002;47:63–67.

16. Duvic M, Hymes K, Heald P, et al. Bexarotene is effective and safe for treatment of refractory advanced-stage cutaneous T-cell lymphoma: multinational phase II-III trial results. *J Clin Oncol.* 2001;19:2456–2471.

17. Duvic M, Kuzel TM, Olsen EA, et al. Quality-of-life improvements in cutaneous T-cell lymphoma patients treated with denileukin diftitox (ONTAK). *Clin Lymphoma.* 2002;2:222–228.

18. Lundin J, Hagberg H, Repp R, et al. Phase 2 study of alemtuzumab (anti-CD52 monoclonal antibody) in patients with advanced mycosis fungoides/Sezary syndrome. *Blood.* 2003;101:4267–4272.

19. Duvic M, Talpur R, Ni X, et al. Phase 2 trial of oral vorinostat (suberoylanilide hydroxamic acid, SAHA) for refractory cutaneous T-cell lymphoma (CTCL). *Blood.* 2007;109:31–39.

20. Mann BS, Johnson JR, He K, et al. Vorinostat for treatment of cutaneous manifestations of advanced primary cutaneous T-cell lymphoma. *Clin Cancer Res.* 2007;13:2318–2322.

21. Olsen EA, Kim YH, Kuzel TM, et al. Phase IIb multicenter trial of vorinostat in patients with persistent, progressive, or treatment refractory cutaneous T-cell lymphoma. *J Clin Oncol.* 2007;25:3109–3115.

22. Wilson LD, Quiros PA, Kolenik SA, et al. Additional courses of total skin electron beam therapy in the treatment of patients with recurrent cutaneous T-cell lymphoma. *J Am Acad Dermatol.* 1996;35:69–73.

23. Lowe MN, Plosker GL. Bexarotene. *Am J Clin Dermatol.* 2000;1:245–250.

24. Singh F, Lebwohl MG. Cutaneous T-cell lymphoma treatment using bexarotene and PUVA: a case series. *J Am Acad Dermatol.* 2004;51:570–573.

25. Georgieva J, Steinhoff M, Orfanos CE, Treudler R. Ethylene-oxide-induced pruritus associated with extracorporeal photochemotherapy. *Transfusion.* 2004;44:1532–1533.

26. Tran D, Kwok YK, Goh CL. A retrospective review of PUVA therapy at the National Skin Centre of Singapore. *Photodermatol Photoimmunol Photomed.* 2001;17:164–67.

27. Demierre MF, Taverna J. Mirtazapine and gabapentin for reducing pruritus in cutaneous T-cell lymphoma. *J Am Acad Dermatol.* 2006;55:543–544.

28. el Azhary RA, Bouwhuis SA. Oral bexarotene in a therapy-resistant Sezary syndrome patient: observations on Sezary cell compartmentalization. *Int J Dermatol.* 2005;44:25–28.

29. Lowe NJ, Cripps DJ, Dufton PA, Vickers CF. Photochemotherapy for mycosis fungoides: a clinical and histological study. *Arch Dermatol.* 1979;115:50–53.

30. Kessler JF, Meyskens FL, Jr., Levine N, Lynch PJ, Jones SE. Treatment of cutaneous T-cell lymphoma (mycosis fungoides) with 13-cis-retinoic acid. *Lancet.* 1983;1:1345–1347.

31. Esteve E, Bagot M, Joly P, et al. A prospective study of cutaneous intolerance to topical mechlorethamine therapy in patients with cutaneous T-cell lymphomas. French Study Group of Cutaneous Lymphomas. *Arch Dermatol.* 1999;135:1349–1353.

32. Heald P, Mehlmauer M, Martin AG, Crowley CA, Yocum RC, Reich SD. Topical bexarotene therapy for patients with refractory or persistent early-stage cutaneous T-cell lymphoma: results of the phase III clinical trial. *J Am Acad Dermatol.* 2003;49:801–815.

33. Dumontet C, Thomas L, Berard F, Gimonet JF, Coiffier B. A phase II trial of miltefosine in patients with cutaneous T-cell lymphoma. *Bull Cancer.* 2006;93:E115–E118.

# Chapter 19
# Anal Pruritus

Sylvia Proske and Wolfgang Hartschuh

## 19.1 Introduction

Anal itching presents a major challenge in the procto-logical office. It is the most frequent accompanying symptom of different dermatological, proctological and microbiological disorders of the anal region – more often than bleeding, pain, redness and others. As in the case of other locations, therefore, anal pruritus has been divided into acute and chronic as well as into the two subtypes: secondary to underlying diseases and "of unknown origin." In secondary pruritus, the main diagnosis is anal eczema, which must be differentiated into atopic, irritant and allergic contact dermatitis.

Obese patients and patients with a funnel anus are at increased risk for irritant contact dermatitis because of the skin-to-skin contact with sweat and moist occlusion as contributing factors.[1,2] Heat and the sitting posture probably exacerbate the problem. A local reaction to contact with feces, especially feces of softer consistency, has been implicated, probably because of the different contents of soft feces with higher amounts of acids. Feces in contact with the perianal skin causes irritation because moisture from sweat or mucus softens the skin and the chemicals produced by the fecal bacteria irritate, although there is no evidence that the microbial content of soft feces is different.

The itching leads to scratching. Consequently, this breaks the skin surface and encourages more softening. Because of the loss of cutaneous integrity, a vicious circle of skin damage and inflammation is set up, which is often difficult to break.

If fecal incontinence is left untreated, the effects can range from mild (superficial skin irritation) to profound (severe perianal dermatitis). A host of dermatological complications can occur, including contact dermatitis and intertrigo, all leading to pruritus.

In most cases, fungal or yeast organisms are not the primary cause of pruritus ani. But in cases of extensive candidiasis intestinalis, the yeast infection may be relevant for the pruritus. Nutritive factors such as intake of citrus fruits or spicy foods may aggravate pruritus caused probably by the acids in citrus fruits or capsaicin contained in chilli peppers. Consuming certain beverages – possibly milk or coffeinated drinks – may cause some people to experience diarrhea followed by anal itch.

A history of atopy may be relevant, since at least 25% of anal eczema cases are atopic, and many patients with atopic dermatitis are especially affected in the anal region. In these patients, even small amounts of fecal contamination or secretion caused by low-grade hemorrhoids may be responsible for anal itching. Atopic diathesis is likely to be an important contributing factor but so far has not been adequately estimated in the literature.

Pruritus may occur as a severe and therapy-refractory symptom of various underlying dermatological and systemic diseases. Malignancies must be ruled out as well (see Table 19.1). The chronic, severe pruritus induces chronic rubbing, scratching or pinching, which all lead to secondary skin lesions such as erosions, excoriations, crusts, hyperpigmentation or hypopigmentation and lichenification.[3,4]

## 19.2 Diagnostic Procedures

Proctologic diagnostic procedures are often complicated because the symptoms are uniform and can be in the context of several diseases. Further, proctological disorders are associated with a taboo area, and therefore the patients put the symptoms under taboo as well. Anal itch is associated with similar symptoms in and

L. Misery and S. Ständer (eds.), *Pruritus*,
DOI 10.1007/978-1-84882-322-8_19, © Springer-Verlag London Limited 2010

**Table 19.1** Differential diagnosis to clarify pruritus analis

*Inflammatory dermatoses*
  Atopic anal eczema
  Perianal irritant contact dermatitis
  Perianal allergic contact dermatitis
  Seborrhoic dermatitis
  Fixed drug eruption
  Baboon syndrome
  Inverse psoriasis
  Lichen sclerosus (see Fig. 19.3)
  Lichen planus (see Fig. 19.2)
  Porokeratosis of the natal clefts
*Bacterial diseases*
  Erythrasma
  Perianal streptococcal dermatitis
*Fungal diseases*
  Candidiasis
  Tinea perianalis
*Infestation*
  Scabies, pinworms
*Hereditary akantholytic diseases*
  Darier disease, Hailey–Hailey disease
*Viral diseases*
  Herpes simplex infection
  Human papilloma virus infections
*Malignancies*
  Extramammary Paget's disease
  Bowenoid papulosis
  Inflammatory bowel disease
  Squamous cell carcinoma of the anal margin
  Basal cell carcinoma
  Langerhans cell histiocytosis
  Hodgkin's disease
*Pruritus caused by internal diseases*
  Uremic pruritus in hemodialysis patients
  Pruritus of cholestasis
  Diabetes mellitus
*Pruritus of unknown origin*
  Neuropathic pruritus
  Pruritus due to compression of nerve fibers[10]
*Psychogenic pruritus*

around the anus, including burning and soreness. The irritation can be a temporary condition, or it may be a persistent and bothersome problem. It can be so intense that the urge to scratch is irresistible. The history to clarify pruritus analis should include the onset of the pruritus, intermittent or persistent, history of defecation with bowel movements, stool consistency and frequency, blood, pain, atopic diathesis as well as the use and quantity of toilet paper, hemorrhoid creams or ointments and different medications.

For the inspection of the anal region, the nates must be straddled. Erythema, erosions, excoriations, crusts, lichenification, fissuring, large anal tags, fistula or anal fissures can be observed. The complete proctologic examination includes a rectal digital examination, proctoscopy, sigmoidoscopy and perhaps colonoscopy. An examination of the entire integument and mucous membranes is necessary to clarify anal pruritus, searching for an underlying mucocutaneous disorder. Generalized dermatoses such as seborrheic dermatitis,[5] psoriasis and atopic dermatitis may present with perianal features alone, but history and full skin exam should reveal some other signs of these conditions.

Depending on the individual case, additional diagnostic procedures should include patch testing to rule out perianal allergic contact dermatitis, wood light examination to rule out erythrasma, tape test to demonstrate pinworms, differential blood count, checking for eosinophilia, and rarely bacteriological and fungal cultures (not in routine diagnostics!).

Altered skin which is resistant to treatment must be biopsied for histological investigation.

## 19.3  Differential Diagnosis

Differential diagnoses that must be considered to clarify anal itching are listed in Table 19.1.

The main complaint that leads the patient to the proctologist is the anal eczema. But it must be differentiated into more detail as mentioned above (irritant, atopic, contact allergic dermatitis), as the irritant anal eczema can be the consequence of a number of different dermatological and proctological diseases that need different therapies.

Figures 19.1–19.3 show examples of perianal diseases that go along with excessive pruritus.

## 19.4  Conservative Treatment

The first priority is the identification and correction of any underlying dermatosis or irritation. Once these have been excluded, both general and specific measures must be initiated.[6–8]

General measures for relieving symptoms of pruritus are aimed at limiting exacerbating factors such as sweat,

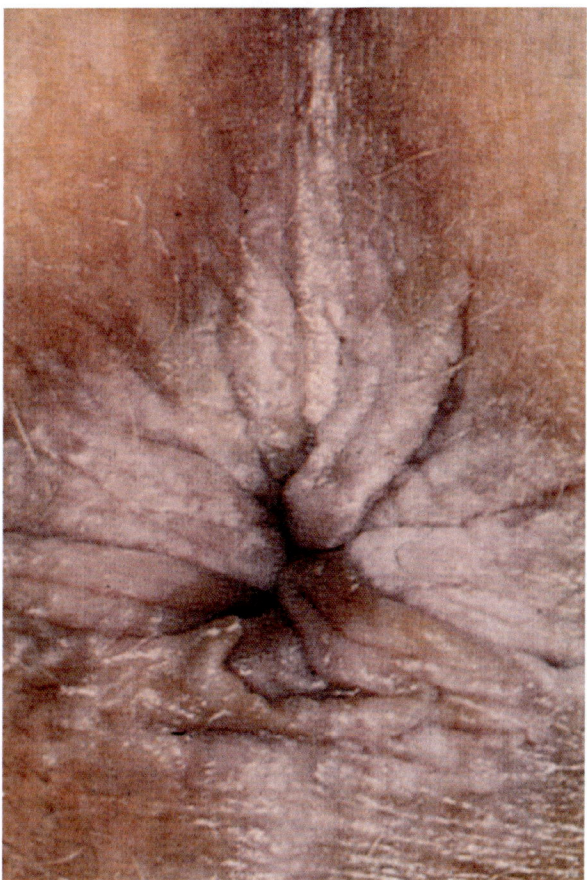

**Fig. 19.1** Lichen simplex chronicus as the chronic form of perianal atopic dermatitis: excessive lichenification

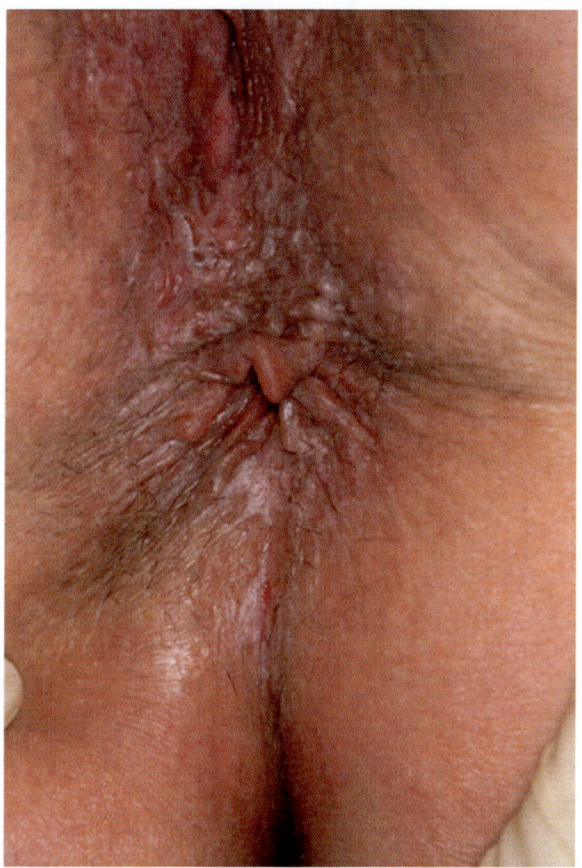

**Fig. 19.2** Lichen ruber perianalis: very pruritic inflammatory dermatosis with white striae, the so-called Whickham striae

occlusion and improper cleansing habits. Therefore easing constipation and limiting diarrhea appropriately with either a high-fiber diet or stool softeners should be initiated. Patients must reduce excessive cleaning, especially excessive wiping with dry, harsh toilet paper or excessive scrubbing, and avoid tight-fitting pants (which restricts air circulation). Certain laundry soaps, colognes, douches and birth control products contain chemicals that can irritate skin. During menses, tampons are a better alternative than pads. Concerning the choice of underwear, comfortable absorptive cotton underwear materials are preferable to synthetic materials.

In the anal region, topical treatment with an antipruritic effect can include cooling agents, e.g., 3% menthol, 3% urea or 2% polidocanol in basic lotion. Camphor gel, capsaicin cream 0.025% and cannabinoid agonists are also used. For short-term treatment, topical steroids such as hydrocortisone 0.1% may be necessary[9]; higher percentages of topical steroid should be avoided, and,

when necessary, should be used only under critical observation. Calcineurin inhibitors (pimecrolimus, tacrolimus) now offer a useful tool to treat chronic atopic dermatitis of the anogenital region (lichen simplex chronicus, see Fig. 19.1; lichen planus, see Fig. 19.2; or lichen sclerosus; see Fig. 19.3). The use of UVA radiation is limited in the anal region because of the topography, especially in a funnel anus.

Systemic treatment may include antihistamines, internal steroids, oral opioid receptor antagonist naltrexone and, additionally, bedtime sedation, in order to provide relief from scratching

## 19.5 Surgical Treatment

Surgery to "tidy up" the anus (anal tags) is not helpful. Attempts to treat intractable pruritus ani of unknown origin may include perianal injection of anesthetics,

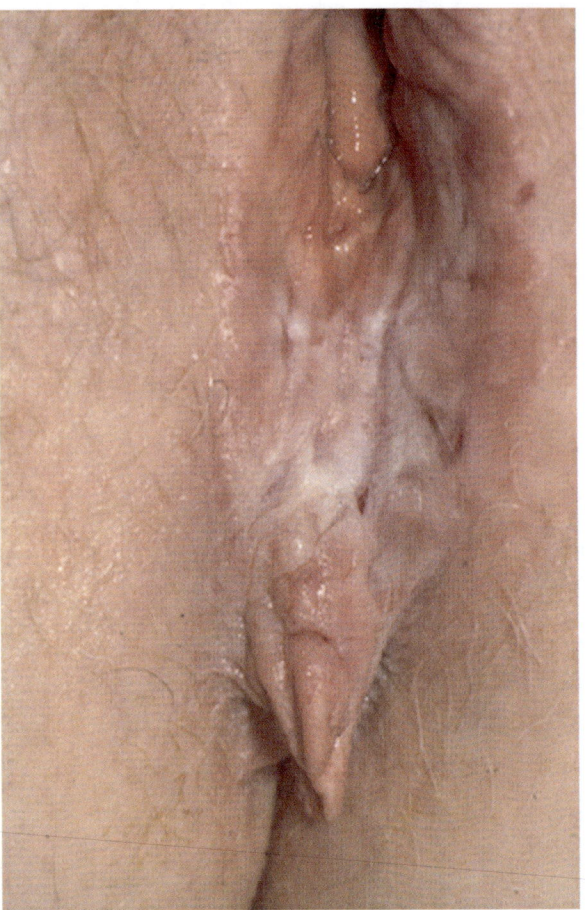

**Fig. 19.3** Lichen sclerosus: very pruritic connective tissue disease with sclerosis, atrophy and follicular hyperkeratosis

surgical disruption of the sensory nerve supply to the perianal area, cryotherapy and, very rarely, intradermal methylene blue injection (to destroy dermal nerve endings).

## 19.6 Prognostic Considerations

Prognostic considerations of anal itch depend very much on the underlying disease. Management of acute anogenital pruritus depends upon the clinician identifying the etiology of the symptoms. However, when the etiology is clarified appropriately, therapy should lead to prompt resolution of symptoms. Chronic pruritus ani can be very recalcitrant. In cases of severe pruritus ani without underlying dermatosis, therapy by a specialist psychiatrist may be necessary.

## References

1. Daniel GL, Longo WE, Vernava AM. Pruritus ani: causes and concerns. *Dis Colon Rectum*. 1994;37:670–674.
2. Harrington CI, Lewis FM, McDonagh AJ, Gawkrodger DJ. Dermatological causes of pruritus ani. *BMJ*. 1992;305:955.
3. Heard S. Pruritus ani. *Aust Fam Physician*. 2004;33:511–513.
4. Bernhard JD. Medical pearl: pruritus ani and seborrheic dermatitis. *J Am Acad Dermatol*. 2005;52:895.
5. Kränke B, Trummer M, Brabek E, Komericki P, Turek TD, Aberer W. Etiologic and causative factors in perianal dermatitis: results of a prospective study in 126 patients. *Wien Klin Wochenschr*. 2006;118:90–94.
6. Dasan S, Neill SM, Donaldson DR, Scott HJ. Treatment of persistent pruritus ani in a combined colorectal and dermatological clinic. *Br J Surg*. 1999;86:1337–1340.
7. Weichert GE. An approach to the treatment of anogenital pruritus. *Derm Ther*. 2004;17:129–133.
8. Zuccati G, Lotti T, Mastrolorenzo A, Rapaccini A, Tiradritti L. Pruritus ani. *Dermatol Ther*. 2005;18:355–362.
9. Al-Ghnaniem R, Short K, Pullen A, Fuller LC, Rennie JA, Leather AJ. 1% hydrocortisone ointment is an effective treatment of pruritus ani: a pilot randomized controlled crossover trial. *Int J Colorectal Dis*. 2007;22:1463–1467.
10. Cohen AD, Vander T, Medvendovsky E, et al. Neuropathic scrotal pruritus: anogenital pruritus is a symptom of lumbosacral radiculopathy. *J Am Acad Dermatol*. 2005 Jan;52(1):61–66.

# Chapter 20
# Secondary Reactive Conditions in Pruritic Skin

Joanna Wallengren

The definition of itch as an unpleasant sensation that elicits an urge or desire to scratch describes the close relationship between the feeling and the response. The physiological role of scratching in response to acute itch is to remove harmful agents from the skin. In the short term, mild scratching relieves itching. With more fierce and prolonged scratching in chronic pruritus, the skin becomes damaged and the changes induced intensify itch, setting up a vicious circle. In pruritus due to an underlying internal disease, these reactive skin conditions occur in normal skin, whereas in inflammatory skin disease they may be superimposed on the primary skin lesions. This chapter will summarize elicitation of scratching as well as different clinical patterns it induces, such as excoriations, lichen simplex chronicus, lichen amyloidosus and prurigo.

## 20.1 Elicitation of Scratching

Pruritogenic agents or physical factors such as thermal stimuli activate histamine-sensitive C-fibers with low conduction velocity and large innervation territories.[1] The orthodromic nerve transmission of these nerve fibers is conducted through the spinal ganglia to the superficial region of the dorsal horn of the spinal cord. Here, neurons selectively sensitive to histamine, "itch specific neurons," have been identified.[2] These neurons with slow conduction velocities cross over the spinal cord to the contralateral spinothalamic tract and pass the midbrain. The supraspinal processing of itch and scratching response has recently been investigated by functional positron emission tomography (PET) and functional magnetic resonance imaging (fMRI).[3–5]

Based on these studies, neuronal pathways have been shown to project to two sites in thalamus and thereafter to diverge to the primary and secondary somatosensory cortices, to the insular cortex or to the anterior cingulate cortex.[6,7] Involvement of the motor cortex explains the planning of the volunteer scratch response contingent to the perception of unpleasant itch. Activation of thalamus induces emotional processing including pleasure and reward.[6] Both insula and anterior cingulum are involved in obsessive compulsive disorders,[8] which may contribute to the compulsive component of itch and scratching. Although the exact pathways are not known, these circuits project to the frontal brain areas, such as prefrontal and orbitofrontal cortices, which are also involved in obsessive compulsive disorders.[6–9] That explains the pleasure that may accompany violent scratching of itchy skin and the uncontrollable itch–scratch cycles.[7,10,11] However, these hedonic aspects do not explain all forms of scratching in severe itchy patients who may spend about 10% of the night scratching.[12] Studies have revealed that scratching occurs throughout the night, and increased severity of itch is accompanied by an increase in the number of bouts of itch and not in their duration in an individual patient.[12,13] Nocturnal scratching occurs during all stages of sleep, even during orthodox sleep.[13,14] However, although the frequency of the bouts of scratching is the same during wakefulness as during sleep, the bouts of scratching last significantly longer when the patients are awake (approximately 14 s vs. 10 s).[13] While in nonprimates (cats and turtles)[15,16] scratching can be elicited as a spinal reflex, it requires some awareness in humans.[13] This is the background for the loss of control scratching patients are often accused of, which makes their suffering even harder.

L. Misery and S. Ständer (eds.), *Pruritus*
DOI 10.1007/978-1-84882-322-8_20, © Springer-Verlag London Limited 2010

## 20.2 General Morphological Alterations in Pruritic Skin

### 20.2.1 Induced by Scratching or Rubbing

Scratching is only one of many measures that patients take to alleviate pruritus. Rubbing, squeezing, kneading, pinching, scraping, scrubbing with brush, digging with fingernails and scratching until the skin bleeds are quite common.[17] The kind of trauma induced by the different behaviors has an impact on the pattern of the skin response. Scratching can induce inflammation, with a great number of pruritogenic inflammatory mediators set free. As long as the inflammation lasts, the inflammatory mediators will be continuously produced, fuelling the firing of sensory nerve fibers conducting itch.[18] However, in lichenified lesions the inflammatory infiltrate usually is minor and may be absent.[19] When the skin is already itchy, fierce attacks of itching may be triggered by nonspecific stimuli, such as rough clothes, excercise or alcohol, due to vasodilation.

Prolonged scratching, kneading, scrubbing with brush or rubbing may mechanically induce epidermal proliferation with increased number of keratinocytes that normally produce interleukins (ILs). The concentration of IL-20 will increase and potentiate the proliferation of keratinocytes with epidermal hyperplasia,[20] while IL-31, which has been shown to be significantly overexpressed in prurigo, contributes to itch.[21]

The most impressive and pathognomonic finding of prurigo is the presence of thick nerve fiber bundles and fine, reticularly arranged terminal nerve fibers.[19] These subepidermal and intraepidermal nerve fibers have been shown to contain neuropeptides.[22] That means that increased concentrations of neuropeptides will be released upon stimulation of these pruritoceptive nerve fibers. Substance P and calcitonin gene-related peptide have been shown to stimulate in vitro proliferation of keratinocytes, which contributes to the lichenification process.[23,24]

Hyperpigmentation seen in most chronic pruritic conditions in predisposed individuals is due to the amount of melanin, which is increased within the epidermis and present in macrophages of the upper part of the dermis.[25]

Another component of lichenification is proliferation of bundles of collagen in the papillary dermis.[24] Proliferation of substance P and calcitonin gene-related peptide nerve fibers have been shown in patients with hypertophic human scars with densely packed collagen fibers.[26]

As many dermatologists observe, primary diseases of mast cells such as urticaria and mastocytosis never present with scratch marks or lichenification. One reason may be that "pure histaminergic itch" is not met by scraping but rather by stroking of the skin, which does not cause trauma. In addition, scratching at one place is never prolonged since the lesions are short lived.

The skin manifestations that will be discussed below, such as lichen simplex chronicus and prurigo, occur frequently in patients with atopic dermatitis, a disorder where pruritus is one of the major criteria.[27] Here it is often very difficult to determine which lesions are primary and which occur after scratching. In addition, patients with atopic dermatitis display low threshold for pruritus (central sensitization)[28] and are more prone to scratch than nonatopic patients. However, no correlation between the duration of scratch and serum IgE levels was found in patients with atopic dermatitis.[14]

While lichen simplex chronicus is localized to one or a few single areas, prurigo lesions are scattered over extremities and upper back where generalized itch is severe. The pattern and degree of hyperkeratosis, as well as the extent of hyperpigmentation in the reactive conditions, vary with ethnicity and skin color (see below).

## 20.3 Excoriations

Generalized itch in noninflamed skin is common in elderly but may also be a prominent feature of systemic disease due to cholestasis, chronic renal disease, adverse drug reactions or HIV.[29,30] Linear excoriations may be the only sign of the suffering the patients present to the physician. More vigorous scratching may result in erosions that are typically a few millimeters in diameter, weeping or crusted. In chronic cases, scarring with hypopigmentation or hyperpigmentation will appear. The lesions occur predominantly at sites that are easily reached to scratch. The so-called "butterfly sign" was first described in patients with chronic jaundice and primary biliary cirrhosis (Fig. 20.1).[31,32] The "butterfly" refers to the shape of the normal-looking skin at the mid-upper back that is spared from scratching and secondary hyperpigmentation. However, this sign has also been described in Japanese patients with atopic dermatitis.[33] In addition, some patients exhibited also "ballon" and "umbrella" shaped unreachable area

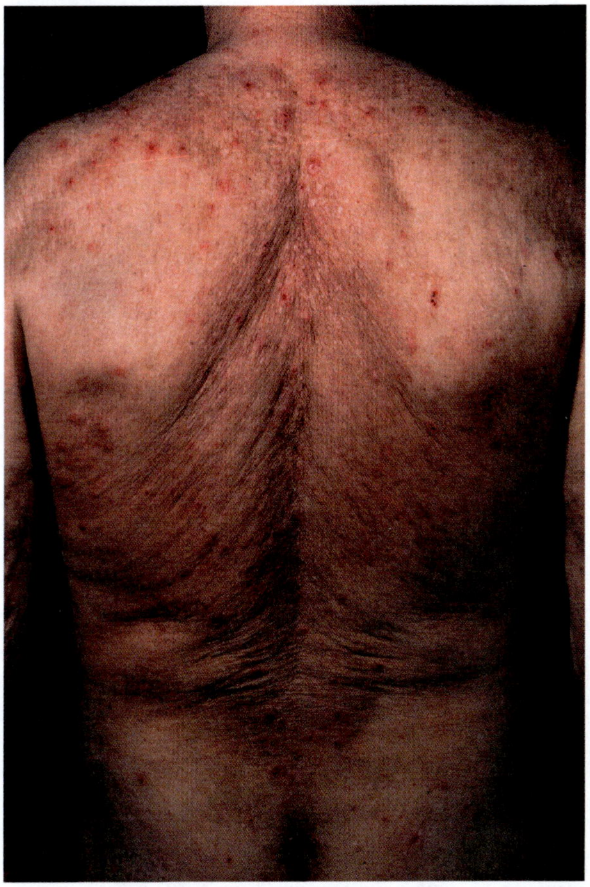

**Fig. 20.1** Patient's back showing excoriations sparing the characteristic unreachable "butterfly" area

of the backs surrounded by pigmentation, lichenification or prurigo nodules. Whatever the shape, this sign shows the significance of scratching in producing the symptoms.

## 20.4 Histopathology

Excoriations are punctuate ulcerations lined by necrotic superficial papillary dermis, fibrin and neutrophils.[18]

## 20.5 Differential Diagnosis

In some patients there is no underlying systemic or cutaneous disease to explain pruritus. In such cases, excoriations are not associated with itch and reflect an underlying psychiatric disorder, including psychosis,

obsessive–compulsive disorder, depression or anxiety.[34] Picking behavior may function to modulate emotions.[35] A 10-item skin picking impact scale (SPIS) has been developed to discriminate individuals with self-injurious skin picking from noninjurious skin pickers.[35] Here the scores correlated with the duration of daily skin picking, satisfaction during picking and the subsequent shame, as well as with Beck Depression and Anxiety Inventory scores.[35] This type of psychogenic excoriations typically runs a chronic course. In addition to symptomatic dermatologic treatments for the self-inflicted excoriations and secondary pruritus, the treatment for this disorder is primarily psychiatric.[34]

## 20.6 Lichenification

Lichenification is a term used to describe a leathery thickening of the skin induced by scratching and rubbing. The normal markings of the skin become exaggerated, producing a mosaic composed of flat-topped, shiny, smooth rhomboid facets. In primary lichenification, the changes are produced in structurally normal skin. In secondary lichenification, the changes are produced in skin with a pre-existing disease such as eczema.

Rubbing may also result in tumor-like growths with a warty surface, which is called giant lichenification. It has been described in the scalp following an attack of herpes zoster at the same site[36] and in vulva.[37]

An interesting question is which factors are essential to develop lichenification. That scratching alone is not responsible for lichenification is evident by the numerous examples of both local and general pruritus in which scratching is liberally practised without lichenification. There must therefore be some other factor or cutaneous susceptibility that induces the thickening and other changes when traumatized. Goldblum and Piper constructed a scratching machine with lead weights of varying sizes attached by a screw to a scratching arm to produce a constant pressure.[38] This pressure was applied for 1 h daily for 5–95 days to a demarcated skin area on the left side of the back about 5 cm below the inferior costal margin on the normal appearing skin of three patients with eczema and one with pityriasis rubra pilaris. Lichenification was produced in all patients in 60–90 h of scratching with a pressure of 75 g with a minimum of 140,000 scratches. The authors concluded that it was a result of both inflammation and pressure. It would be interesting to test whether such a scratching machine is able to induce lichenification in patients with no previous history of eczema.

## 20.7 Histopathology

The epidermis shows hyperplasia with hypergranulosis and compact orthokeratosis. Coarse collagen boundless in vertical streaks and perivascular lymphohistiocytic infiltration are found in the papillary dermis.[25,39]

## 20.8 Differential Diagnosis

Lichenification may develop on skin that is the site of another disease, such as atopic or allergic contact dermatitis or tinea.

## 20.9 Lichen Simplex Chronicus

Lichen simplex chronicus presents with a circumscribed, chronic, inflammatory, severely pruritic thickened skin complicating prolonged and severe scratching in patients with no underlying dermatological condition. It was first described by Willan in 1808, and Brocq coined the synonymous term "neurodermatitis" circumsripta in 1891.[40]

The disease usually remains limited to a single area; rarely two or three lesions are observed. In women the nape of the neck is a preferred site. Further sites of predilection are extensor aspects of the forearm, the median aspects of the thigh and the anogenital region involving scrotum or vulva.

The clinical morphology is that of a lichenoid disease. The basic lesion is a solid round papule with a flat surface, and the color is red or brownish red.[39] These papules aggregate into plaques which appear rounded or linear. Often, a typical three-zone structure can be found[39]: the central part consisting of a flat lichenification surrounded by lichenoid papules with hyperpigmented border. Sometimes a hypopigmentation (leukoderma) can occur within the lesion instead.[39]

Very severe itching is typical, being especially troublesome at night. It is still unresolved whether itching and scratching cause the lichenified lesions, or whether it is the lichenoid papule itself that itches so severely. Experimental studies with a "scratching machine" demonstrated that lichenification can be caused by chronic mechanical stress.[39]

## 20.10 Histopathology

The most prominent histopathologic feature of lichen simplex chronicus is extensive compact orthokeratosis that resembles the normal stratum corneum on a palm or sole.[25] This finding serves as a valuable clue to diagnosis of lichen simplex chronicus on sites other than on volar skin, namely, "hairy palm skin." When a corified layer like that of a palm or sole is seen on an anatomic site that surely is not palm or sole, as is obvious by the presence of follicular and/or sebaceous units, the diagnosis must be lichen simplex chronicus.

Sometimes erosions occur if scratching accompanies rubbing.[25] Papillary dermis is thickened by coarse bundles of collagen in vertical streaks with loss of elastic fibers as a result of many bouts of mechanical injury and repair.[25] Inflammatory infiltrate usually is minor and may be absent.[25]

## 20.11 Differential Diagnosis

Lichenified manifestations in atopic dermatitis are symmetrical, affecting flexures (elbows, popliteal fossae, flexor aspects of the wrist) and nape of the neck but the individual lesions can look very much like lichen simplex chronicus. Typical lichen simplex chronicus lesions show the three-zoned structure described above,[39] while lichenified chronic eczemas present more inflammatory changes.[25] The differentiation of a flat lichen planus lesion can be difficult but the lesions are polygonal.

Because of rubbing, lichen simplex chronicus can sometimes resemble a verruca, which is called verrucous lichen simplex. Such verrucous lesions may cover squamous cell carcinomas, which may be discovered only by a deep biopsy.[40]

## 20.12 Lichen Amyloidosus

Lichen amyloidosus is considered to be a variant of lichen simplex chronicus and presents as groups of extremely pruritic, small (2–3 mm in diameter) waxy brownish firm papules mainly on the extensor part of the extremities, especially on the extensor surface of the legs and less often on the arms.[41] Some papules have a thickened scaly surface due to prolonged and severe scratching. The patients have no underlying dermatological condition and no visceral involvement. Lichen amyloidosus generally follows a chronic course with intractable pruritus.

The name lichen amyloidosus refers to amyloid deposits in the skin. The term "amyloid" (starch-like) was coined in 1854 by Virchow, who was convinced by its resemblance to starch or cellulose.[42] In lichen amyloidosus, amyloid originates from keratinocytes (so-called amyloid K) that become necrotic due to scratching and descend from epidermis to papillary dermis where they are coated by fibrocytes – the result being the globules of amyloid.[43]

While unusual in Caucasians, lichen amyloidosus is a relatively common skin disorder among Chinese and affects men more than women.[41–45] In a study on 30 patients with lichen amyloidosus in South India, pruritus was the presenting symptom in 90% of the patients and 20% reported a family history of lichen amyloidosus suggesting a genetic predisposition.[42] In addition, 60% of the patients in this study gave a history of using a nylon wire brush scrub while bathing for more than 2 years, suggesting a role of friction in lichen amyloidosus.

## 20.13 Histopathology

In addition to the common histopathological signs of rubbing such as epithelial hyperplasia with hypergranulosis, compact orthokeratosis, and coarse collagen in vertical streaks in the stratum papillare, amyloid deposits are found in the papillary layer.[25] The presence of amyloid deposits can be detected by light microscopy with haematoxylin and eosin staining and confirmed by special stains such as Congo red or Crystal violet.[25,41] IgM and C3 can be found within the foci of the amyloid. In addition, immunoperoxidase stains positive for cytokeratinesis in globules of amyloid, thereby confirming their keratinocytic nature.[25]

## 20.14 Differential Diagnosis

Macular cutaneous amyloidosis has mostly been described in more pigmented patients, in Central and South America, Middle East, China and India.[46–49] It is more common in women and is usually localized between the shoulder blades. The main characteristics are moderate itch and hyperpigmentation. Often there are only very minor amyloid deposits in the papillary dermis.[39]

Another entity confined to the interscapular region is notalgia paresthetica, a form of localized neuropathy, described by Astwazaturow in1934 as a focal, burning itch on the medial border of the scapula.[50] One explanation is that the thoracic nerves at the level of T2 to T6 penetrate the spinal muscle at right angles, which predisposes them for injury from mild insults.[50] Another explanation that has been suggested is an impingement of the nerve root as confirmed by MRI.[50] In addition, Springall et al. have found an increased number of dermal sensory nerve fibers in notalgia paresthetica, whereas Weber found necrotic keratinocytes in the epidermis.[50,51] While some authors regard macular amyloidosis and notalgia paresthetica as overlapping conditions, Bernhard has suggested that macular amyloidosis may be a consequence of notalgia paresthetica with prolonged scratching behavior that leads to deposition of amyloid in dermis.[52,53]

Yet others have suggested that macular amyloidisis may transform gradually over the years into lichen amyloidosis as a result of chronic irritation of the skin from scratching.[54]

## 20.15 Prurigo Simplex Chronica

This is a disseminated, chronic, inflammatory, severely pruritic skin disease with reddened, flattened, slightly keratotic papules, usually 0.4–1.0 cm in diameter (Fig. 20.2). The lesions occur mainly on the extremities and upper back secondary to prolonged and severe scratching in patients with no underlying dermatological condition. The term prurigo, originating from Latin pruire – to itch – was coined by Ferdinand von Hebra in the mid-nineteenth century to characterize intensely itching papules and nodules occurring mainly on the arms and legs.[55] At that time, prurigo was one of the most frequent forms of skin disease in Europe, being

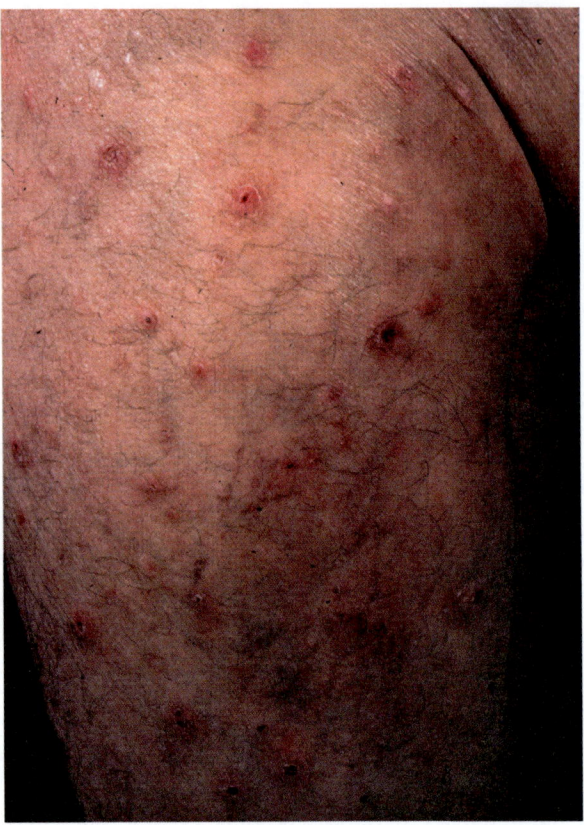

**Fig. 20.2** Patient's arm showing the characteristic papules and small nodules of prurigo secondary to scratching

associated with stings of parasites, especially fleas and mites. Today, prurigo strophulus can still be provoked by stings of fleas, mosquitos, ticks or dog parasites but has come to designate an acute form of prurigo.

Immunosuppressed patients such as patients with HIV infection are more susceptible to parasitic and helminthic infections, and the pruriginous lesions are often more persistant and chronic, such as in Norwegian scabies.[55]

Itch associated with several internal diseases such as renal failure or various collagen diseases may involve chronic prurigo.[56,55] Also, itch in patients with anorexia nervosa or malabsorption may result in prurigo.[55] Prurigo may also complicate severe pruritus in patients with T-cell lymphoma and visceral neoplasia in the esophagus, the ventricle, the rectum, the liver and the bile duct.[55] Prurigo of the lymphoma may precede symptoms of malignancy. The occurrence of prurigo can also be a warning signal for malignant transformation in patients with tumors previously diagnosed as being benign.[55]

Squamous cell carcinoma may occasionally complicate chronic prurigo nodules of long duration.

As shown in a clinical study of 46 patients with chronic prurigo by Rowland Payne et al., 72% of the patients felt that psychosocial problems were of relevance to their skin disease. Fifty percent of the patients were found to be suffering from depression, anxiety or some other psychological disorder requiring medical intervention.[57] The explanation for such an association is probably that neurotransmitters of mood such as dopamine, serotonin or opioid peptides modulate sensory perception. Around 65–80% of the patients in this study were atopic.[57] In addition, potential metabolic causes of pruritus, such as anemia, hepatic dysfunction, uremia and myxoedema, were present in 50% of the patients.[57]

## 20.16 Histopathology

The most prominent histopathologic feature of prurigo is irregular marked accanthosis, hyperkeratosis and parakeratosis.[39] Perivascular lymphohistiocytic reaction occur in papillary dermis, which becomes thickened by coarse bundles of collagen in vertical streaks.[25,39]

## 20.17 Differential Diagnosis

Primary forms of prurigo elicited by external factors, such as insect stings, parasites, UV light, contact allergy or drugs, are often easy to exclude because of the more acute course.[55]

The most important differential diagnosis causing much confusion in the prurigo literature is prurigo nodularis, described originally by Hyde in 1909. It is an endogenous form of primary chronic prurigo associated often with atopy.[39] The lesions are larger and nodular compared to secondary prurigo and may be as much as 3 cm in diameter. They are mainly located on extensor surfaces of the extremities, although the trunk, face and even the palms can likewise be affected.[39] During the nineteenth century, there was much discussion among leading dermatologists about whether the prurigo nodularis lesion appears first and produces an urge to scratch or, instead, its appearance is only secondary to scratching.[55] According to Hebra, the prurigo papule appears first. Already in 1899, Johnston wrote in the *Archives of Dermatology* that the number of hypertrophic nerve fibers in prurigo lesions is increased. The nerve fibres in the lesional skin of prurigo nodularis show immunoreactivity for sensory neuropeptides, such as calcitonin gene-related peptide and substance P, that act as transmitters of itch both in the peripheral and in the central nervous system.[55] This finding would support the theory of itch being elicited from the prurigo lesion.

However, occlusion with elastic bandages for 4 weeks improves the clinical picture of prurigo, and no enlarged nerve fibers or neurinoma-like structures are visible any longer. Such an involution of prurigo nodules would favor the theory of scratching being the triggering factor of prurigo.

In conclusion, it seems that there are some conditions that predispose for the prurigo pattern of skin changes due to rubbing. One is susceptibility of the skin such as atopy. Others are not yet identified circulating factors that occur in renal failure, malabsorption or malignancies, which can be associated with pruritus and prurigo.

## 20.18  Treatment

As chronic scratching seems to be the cause and not the result of the skin reactions described in this chapter, treatment should be directed at the amelioration of pruritus. Ways of minimizing the damage from scratching play also a big part in the treatment of secondary reactive conditions. For example, rough clothing should be avoided, gloves may be worn at night, nails should be cut short and adhesive films may be used to cover small lichenified areas. Psychocutaneous interventions aimed at reducing tension and stress may also be helpful because of the psychologic causes and concomitants in secondary reactive conditions.[58] In milder forms of pruritus and prurigo, topical treatment may suffice, but generalized therapy-resistant cases require often combined sequential treatments tailored to the exacerbations. I agree with the unknown author of a ballad written 50 years ago:

> And before I throw all my tars away
> Put a *couch* in the place of my old *grenz ray*,
> Before I discard *hydrocortisone creams*,

> And just quiz my patients about their *dreams*,
> Before I accept that it's *lack of embraces*
> Which makes the skin pop in the *cubital spaces*,
> Before I grant that when wanting to *cry*
> The *skin must weep* if the *eyes stay dry!*
> A lot more proof I shall have to see
> And a lot more cures by *psychiatree*.

## References

1. Schmelz M, Schmidt R, Bickel A, et al. Specific C-receptors for itch in human skin. *J Neurosci.* 1997;17(20):8003–8008.
2. Andrew D, Craig AD. Spinothalamic lamina I neurons selectively sensitive to histamine: a central neural pathway for itch. *Nat Neurosci.* 2001;4(1):72–77.
3. Hsieh JC, Hägermark O, Ståhle-Bäckdahl M, et al. Urge to scratch represented in the human cerebral cortex during itch. *J Neurophysiol.* 1994;72(6):3004–3008.
4. Drzezga A, Darsow U, Treede RD, et al. Central activation by histamine-induced itch: analogies to pain processing: a correlational analysis of O-15 H$_2$O positron emission tomography studies. *Pain.* 2001;92(1–2):295–305.
5. Mochizuki H, Tashiro M, Kano M, et al. Imaging of central itch modulation in the human brain using positron emission tomography. *Pain.* 2003;105(1–2):339–346.
6. Paus R, Schmelz M, Bíró T, Steinhoff M. Frontiers in pruritus research: scratching the brain for more effective itch therapy. *J Clin Invest.* 2006;116(5):1174–1186.
7. Ikoma A, Steinhoff M, Ständer S, et al. The neurobiology of itch. *Nat Rev Neurosci.* 2006;7(7):535–547.
8. Chamberlain SR, Blackwell AD, Fineberg NA, et al. The neuropsychology of obsessive compulsive disorder: the importance of failures in cognitive and behavioural inhibition as candidate endophenotypic markers. *Neurosci Biobehav Rev.* 2005;29(3):399–419.
9. Hendler T, Goshen E, Tzila Zwas S, et al. Brain reactivity to specific symptom provocation indicates prospective therapeutic outcome in OCD. *Psychiatry Res.* 2003;124(2): 87–103.
10. Leknes SG, Bantick S, Willis CM, et al. Itch and motivation to scratch: an investigation of the central and peripheral correlates of allergen- and histamine-induced itch in humans. *J Neurophysiol.* 2007;97(1):415–422.
11. Bishop GH. The skin as an organ of senses with special reference to the itching sensation. *J Invest Derm.* 1948;11: 143–154.
12. Felix R, Shuster S. A new method for the measurement of itch and the response to treatment. *Br J Dermatol.* 1975;93(3): 303–312.
13. Savin JA, Paterson WD, Oswald I, et al. Further studies of scratching during sleep. *Br J Dermatol.* 1975;93(3):297–302.
14. Aoki T, Kushimoto H, Hisikawa Y, et al. Nocturnal scratching and its relationship to the disturbed sleep of itchy subjects. *Clin Exp Dermatol.* 1991;16(4):268–272.
15. Burke RE. The use of state-dependent modulation of spinal reflexes as a tool to investigate the organization of spinal interneurons. *Exp Brain Res.* 1999;128(3): 263–277.

16. Berkowitz A. Spinal interneurons that are selectively activated during fictive flexion reflex. *J Neurosci*. 2007;27(17): 4634–4641.

17. Darsow U, Scharein E, Simon D, et al. New aspects of itch pathophysiology: component analysis of atopic itch using the "Eppendorf Itch Questionnaire". *Int Arch Allergy Immunol*. 2001;124(1–3): 326–331.

18. Wallengren J. Vasoactive peptides in the skin. *JID Symp Proc*. 1997;2:49–55.

19. Pinkus H, Mehregan AH. *A Guide to Dermatohistopathology*. London: Butterworths; 1969.

20. Sa SM, Valdez PA, Wu J, et al. The effects of IL-20 subfamily cytokines on reconstituted human epidermis suggest potential roles in cutaneous innate defense and pathogenic adaptive immunity in psoriasis. *J Immunol*. 2007;178(4):2229–2240.

21. Sonkoly E, Muller A, Lauerma AI, et al. IL-31: a new link between T cells and pruritus in atopic skin inflammation. *J Allergy Clin Immunol*. 2006;117(2):411–417.

22. Vaalasti A, Suomalainen H, Rechardt L. Calcitonin gene-related peptide immunoreactivity in prurigo nodularis: a comparative study with neurodermatitis circumscripta. *Br J Dermatol*. 1989;120(5):619–623.

23. Benrath J, Zimmermann M, Gillardon F. Substance P and nitric oxide mediate would healing of ultraviolet photodamaged rat skin: evidence for an effect of nitric oxide on keratinocyte proliferation. *Neurosci Lett*. 1995;200(1):17–20.

24. Seike M, Ikeda M, Morimoto A, et al. Increased synthesis of calcitonin gene-related peptide stimulates keratinocyte proliferation in murine UVB-irradiated skin. *J Dermatol Sci*. 2002;28(2):135–143.

25. Ackerman AB, Chongchitnant N, Sanches J, et al. *Histologic Diagnosis of Inflammatory Skin Diseases. An Algorithmic Method Based on Pattern Analysis*. 2 ed. Baltimore: Williams@Wilkins; 1997.

26. Crowe R, Parkhouse N, McGrouther D, et al. Neuropeptide-containing nerves in painful hypertrophic human scar tissue. *Br J Dermatol*. 1994;130(4):444–452.

27. Rajka G, Langeland T. Grading of the severity of atopic dermatitis. *Acta Derm Venereol Suppl (Stockh)*. 1989;144:13–14.

28. Ikoma A, Rukwied R, Ständer S, et al. Neuronal sensitization for histamine-induced itch in lesional skin of patients with atopic dermatitis. *Arch Dermatol*. 2003;139(11):1455–1458.

29. Greaves MW. Itch in systemic disease: therapeutic options. *Dermatol Ther*. 2005;18(4):323–327.

30. Freytes DM, Arroyo-Novoa CM, Fiqueroa-Ramos MI. Skin disease in HIV-positive persons living in Puerto Rico. *Adv Skin Wound Care*. 2007;20(3):149–150, 152–156.

31. Reynolds TB. The "butterfly" sign in patients with chronic jaundice and pruritus. *Ann Intern Med*. 1973;78(4):545–546.

32. Venencie PY, Cuny M, Samuel D, et al. The "butterfly" sign in patients with primary biliary cirrhosis. *J Am Acad Dermatol*. 1988;19(3):571–572.

33. Kimura T, Miyazawa H. The "butterfly" sign in patients with atopic dermatitis: evidence for the role of scratching in the development of skin manifestations. *J Am Acad Dermatol*. 1989;21:579–580.

34. Gupta MA, Gupta AK, Haberman HF. Neurotic excoriations: a review and some new perspectives. *Compr Psychiatry*. 1986;27(4):381–386.

35. Keuthen NJ, Deckersbach T, Wilhelm S, et al. The skin picking impact scale (SPIS): scale development and psychometric analyses. *Psychosomatics*. 2001;42(5):397–403.

36. Arseculeratne G, Altmann P, Millard PR, et al. Giant lichenification of the scalp. *Clin Exp Dermatol*. 2003;28(3): 257–259.

37. Goldstein RK, Bastian BC, Elsner P, et al. Giant lichenification of the vulva with marked ulcerations. A case report. *J Reprod Med*. 1991;36(4):309–311.

38. Goldblum RW, Piper WN. Artificial lichenification produced by a scratching machine. *J Invest Dermatol*. 1954;22(5): 405–415.

39. Braun-Falco O, Plewig G, Wolff HH, et al. *Dermatology*. 2nd ed. Berlin: Springer; 2000.

40. Resnik KS. Verrucous – but is it a verruca? *Am J Dermatopathol*. 2003;25(4):347–348.

41. Tay CH, Dacosta JL. Lichen amyloidosis. Clinical study of 40 cases. *Br J Dermatol*. 1970;82(2):129–136.

42. Salim T, Shenoi SD, Balachandran C, et al. Lichen amyloidosus: a study of clinical, histopathologic and immunofluorescence findings in 30 cases. *Indian J Dermatol Venereol Leprol*. 2005;71(3):166–169.

43. Weyers W, Weyers I, Bonczkowitz M, et al. Lichen amyloidosus: a consequence of scratching. *J Am Acad Dermatol*. 1997;37(6):923–928.

44. Wong CK. Lichen amyloidosus. A relatively common skin disorder in Taiwan. *Arch Dermatol*. 1974;110(3):438–440.

45. Looi LM. Primary localised cutaneous amyloidosis in Malaysians. *Australas J Dermatol*. 1991;32(1):439–449.

46. Leonforte JF. Origin of macular amyloidosis. Apropos of 160 cases. *Ann Dermatol Venereol*. 1987;114(6–7): 801–806.

47. Kibbi AG, Rubeiz NG, Zaynoun ST, Primary localized cutaneous amyloidosis. *Int J Dermatol*. 1992;31(2):95–98.

48. Wang WJ, Chang YT, Huang CY, Lee DD. Clinical and histopathological characteristics of primary cutaneous amyloidosis in 794 Chinese patients. *Zhonghua Yi Xue Za Zhi (Taipei)*. 2001;64(2):101–107.

49. Eswaramoorthy V, Kaur I, Das A, Kumar B. Macular amyloidosis: etiological factors. *J Dermatol*. 1999;26(5): 305–310.

50. Wallengren J. Neuroanatomy and neurophysiology of itch. *Dermatol Ther*. 2005;18:292–303.

51. Weber PJ, Poulos EG. Notalgia paresthetica. Case reports and histologic appraisal. *J Am Acad Dermatol*. 1988;18(1 pt 1):25–30.

52. Westermark P, Ridderström E, Vahlquist A. Macular posterior pigmentary incontinence: its relation to macular amyloidosis and notalgia paresthetica. *Acta Derm Venereol*. 1996; 76(4):302–304.

53. Bernhard JD. Notalgia paresthetica, macular posterior pigmentary incontinence, macular amyloidosis and pruritus. *Acta Derm Venereol*. 1997;77(2):164.

54. Bedi TR, Datta BN. Diffuse biphasic cutaneous amyloidosis. *Dermatologica*. 1979;158(6):433–437.

55. Wallengren J. Prurigo: Diagnosis and management. *Am J Clin Dermatol*. 2004;5;1–11.

56. Murphy M, Carmichael AJ. Renal itch. *Clin Exp Dermatol*. 2000;25(2):103–106.

57. Rowland Payne CM, Wilkinson JD, McKee PH et al. Nodular prurigo – a clinicopathological study of 46 patients. *Br J Dermatol*. 1985;113:431–439.

58. Fried RG, Fried S. Picking apart the picker: a clinician's guide for management of the patient presenting with excoriations. *Cutis*. 2003;71(4):291–298.

# Chapter 21
# Aquadynia and Aquagenic Pruritus

Laurent Misery

## 21.1 Definitions

Aquagenic pruritus is pruritus that appears to be induced by contact with water and is not associated with apparent skin lesions. It has to be differentiated from aquadynia, which is water-related cutaneous pain without skin lesion, or aquagenic urticaria (see Chapter 16 of Section 2 of this part), which is water-related urticaria.[1]

## 21.2 Aquagenic Pruritus

### 21.2.1 Clinical and Epidemiological Aspects

Because of its vague definition, the frequency of discussion on aquagenic pruritus is limited. Pruritus evoked by contact with water at any temperature without observable skin change may be a trivial condition, which could be observed with a prevalence of 45% of the general population.[2] But cases that lead to a dermatological consultation are of a severe disabling disorder.

Aquagenic pruritus is especially induced in circumstances where the whole body is in contact with water: shower, swimming pool, sea, etc. Sometimes sweating is enough to induce itch. Sensations begin from 2 to 15 min after water exposure and last for 10 to 120 min. The sparing of palms, soles and scalp is usual. Mucosa are not involved. The main (and often first) location is legs. Pruritus is not the sole sensation, and many patients describe prickings, burnings, stingings or swarmings.

Usually, the first occurrence is before the age of 30 but they also occur in many elderly patients. Men are more affected than women (sex ratio = 1.4). The mean age of occurrence is 40 years.[3] Familial occurrence might be observed in one-third of cases.[4]

### 21.2.2 Pathogenesis

Pathogenesis of aquagenic pruritus remains mysterious. Increased levels of histamine in blood, as well as cutaneous mast cell degranulation prior to water exposure and increasing with water exposure, have been shown.[5] Nonetheless, the role of histamine is probably not important because antihistamines are ineffective, and the absence of wheal and flare suggests that histamine is not clearly involved. A role of acetylcholine is suggested by the enhancement of cholinesterasic activity after water application in comparison to healthy subjects, and by the efficacy of topical application of scopolamine.[6]

A new hypothesis is that sensory proteins on keratinocytes could be directly activated (see Chapter 3 of Part I), and then an "itch message" could be transmitted to the nervous system. Aquagenic pruritus could be a particular type of sensitive skin syndrome that does not affect the face.[7] Because of their sensitivity to the application of a hypotonic solution, volume-regulated anion channels (VRACs) could be involved.[8]

### 21.2.3 Associations

Aquagenic pruritus has been reported to be associated with the use of bupropion or antimalarials in patients with lupus[9] and familial lactose intolerance.[10] In some cases, aquagenic pruritus is secondary to, or associated with, other diseases, such as

L. Misery and S. Ständer (eds.), *Pruritus*,
DOI 10.1007/978-1-84882-322-8_21, © Springer-Verlag London Limited 2010

- metastatic cervical squamous cell carcinoma
- juvenile xanthogranuloma
- acute lymphoblastic leukemia
- hemochromatosis
- hypereosinophilic syndrome
- myelodysplatic syndrome
- essential thrombocythemia
- polycythemia vera

Among these conditions, the frequency of polycythema vera justifies a blood count for all patients consulting for polycythemia vera. Other exams do not seem to be necessary in the absence of other clinical arguments.

About 50% of patients with polycythemia vera suffer from aquagenic pruritus, but it can be present several years before the diagnosis of a hematological disease. A very interesting recent study has shown that aquagenic pruritus is more frequent in patients with polycythema vera when they have a mutation of the janus tyrosine kinase 2 (JAK2) and are JAK2V617F homozygous, suggesting a role for this tyrosine kinase.[11] These patients are also at risk of developing myelodysplastic syndrome since constitutive JAK activation is present due to the mutation-induced cell transformation. This association was not found in patients with essential thrombocythemia.

## 21.2.4 Treatment

Numerous treatments have been proposed but none has proved efficacious in a comparative randomized study. They include

- Sodium bicarbonate (200–500 g) in bathwater
- Rapid showers
- Hydrophobic emollients
- Topical capsaicin
- Oral anthistamines and anti-cholinergics
- Ultraviolet B (UVB), psoralen and ultraviolet A (PUVA)
- Aspirin
- Propanolol, clonidine
- Fluoxetine
- Interferon
- Steroids
- Naltrexone

Only water alkalinization,[4] UVB[12] and antihistamines were used in more than ten published cases. UVB could be efficient in 50% of patients, with a delay of 4 weeks.

Antihistamines are not more efficient than the usual effect of placebo against itch. An etiological treatment is useful when aquagenic pruritus is secondary.

## 21.3 Aquadynia

Aquadynia appears very rare and has been reported only in three papers,[13–15] but it is probably more frequent. It could be a complication of aquagenic pruritus, which, however, is discussed. The clinical presentation is identical, but itch is replaced by pain. Treatments with propanolol, clonidine or topical capsaicin have been proposed.

The activation of adrenergic nerve endings is suggested by the evidenced dramatic release of vasoactive intestinal peptide (VIP) in the epidermis.[13–15]

## References

1. Greaves MW, Black AK, Eady RAJ, Coutts A. Aquagenic pruritus. *Br Med J.* 1981;282:2008–2010.
2. Potasman I, Heinrich I, Bassan HM. Aquagenic pruritus: prevalence and clinical characteristics. *Isr J Med Sci.* 1990;26:499–503.
3. Bircher AJ. Water-induced itching. *Br J Dermatol Dermatologica.* 1990;181:83–87.
4. Bayrou O, Leynadier F. Prurit aquagénique. *Ann Dermatol Venereol.* 1999;126:76–80.
5. Steinman HK, Greaves MW. Aquagenic pruritus. *J Am Acad Dermatol.* 1985;13:91–96.
6. Bircher AJ, Meier-Ruge W. Aquagenic pruritus. Water-induced activation of acetylcholinesterase. *Arch Dermatol.* 1988;124:84–89.
7. Saint-Martory C, Roguedas-Contios AM, Sibaud V, Degouy A, Schmitt AM, Misery L. Sensitive skin syndrome is not limited to the face. *Br J Dermatol.* 2008;158:130–133.
8. Raoux M, Colomban C, Delmas P, Crest M. The amine-containing cutaneous irritant heptylamine inhibits the volume-regulated anion channel and mobilizes intracellular calcium in normal human epidermal keratinocytes. *Mol Pharmacol.* 2007;71:1685–1694.
9. Jimenez-Alonso J, Tercedor J, Jaimez L, Garcia-Lora E. Antimalarial drug-induced aquagenic-type pruritus in patients with lupus. *Arthritis Rheum.* 1998;41:744–745.
10. Treudler R, Tebbe B, Steinhoff M, Orfanos CE. Familial aquagenic urticaria associated with familial lactose intolerance. *J Am Acad Dermatol.* 2002;47:611–613.
11. Vannucchi AM, Antonioli E, Guglielmelli P, et al. Clinical profile of homozygous JAK2 617V > F mutation in patients with polycythemia vera or essential thrombocythemia. *Blood.* 2007;110:840–846.

12. Greaves MW, Handfield-Jones SE. Aquagenic pruritus: pharmacological findings and treatment. *Eur J Dermatol.* 1992;2:482–484.

13. Misery L, Bonnetblanc JM, Staniek V, Gaudillère A, Schmitt D, Claudy A. Localized pains following contact with liquids. *Br J Dermatol.* 1997;136:980–981.

14. Shelley WB, Shelley ED. Aquadynia: noradrenergic pain induced by bathing and responsive to clonidine. *J Am Acad Dermatol.* 1998;38:357–358.

15. Misery L, Meyronet D, Pichon M, Brutin JL, Pestre P, Cambazard F. Aquadynie : rôle du VIP? *Ann Dermatol Venereol.* 2003;130:195–198.

# Chapter 22
# Sensitive Skin

Laurent Misery and Sonja Ständer

## 22.1 What Is Sensitive Skin?

Sensitive skin (or reactive, hypereactive, intolerant or irritable skin) is defined[1,3,5,13,19] by the onset of erythema and/or pruritus, prickling, burning or tingling sensations (sometimes pain) due to various factors, which may be physical (UV radiation, heat, cold, wind), chemical (cosmetics, soap, water, pollution), psychological (stress) or hormonal (menstrual cycle). Sensitive skin was initially described on the face, but other locations are possible, mainly the scalp and the hands.[12,15]

Pathophysiogeny of sensitive skin is poorly understood.[4,17] There is a decrease in the "skin's tolerance threshold" which is not directly related to any immunological or allergic mechanism. An impaired skin barrier function, together with an increase in transepidermal water loss, which could increase exposure to irritants, has been reported.[16] The presence of abnormal sensations and vasodilatation demonstrates the involvement of the skin's nervous system.[9] Neurogenic inflammation probably results from the release of neurotransmitters such as substance P, calcitonin gene-related peptide (CGRP) and vasoactive intestinal peptide (VIP), which induce vasodilatation and mast cell degranulation. Neurotrophins probably act as modulators of neuropeptide release. Nonspecific inflammation may also be associated with the release of IL-1, IL-8, PgE2, PgF2 and TNFα.[14] The only proteins that can be activated by both chemical and physical factors belong to the transient receptor potential (TRP) family, such as TRPV1, but also TRPV2, TRPV3, TRPV4, TRPM8 or TRPA1. These sensory receptors are expressed not only on nerve endings but also on keratinocytes.[2] Endothelin (ET) and its receptors may also be involved in the symptoms of sensitive skin. ET-1, -2 and -3 produced by endothelial cells and mast cells induce neurogenic inflammation associated with a burning pruritus.[8]

Sensitive skin is a frequent occurrence. Several epidemiological studies have been conducted in the United Kingdom,[20] the United States,[7] France[6,11] and eight other European countries.[16] These studies showed that about one-half of the population in these countries is affected (approximately 60% women and 40% men). The quality of life is adversely affected, mainly through the mental component,[11] although it does not induce depression.[10] Sensitive skin and very sensitive skin are more frequently observed in summer than in winter.[10]

## 22.2 Pruritus in Sensitive Skin

For many people, it is very difficult to differentiate itch from burnings or prickings or other sensations. Itch was reported in 61.5% of subjects with sensitive skin in any location.[6] Itchings were reported by 37.61% of people with scalp sensitivity versus 15.71% of people with no scalp sensitivity or slight scalp sensitivity.[7] Some ethnic variations have been noted[13]: itching is more frequent among Asians than Euro-Americans, Hispanics or Afro-Americans with sensitive skin.

The experimental induction of itching may be used for diagnosis of skin reactivity[18] because the dimensions of the wheals do not correlate with pruritus or stinging after histamine application. In a study comparing the cumulative lactic acid sting scores with the histamine itch scores,[19] all the subjects who were stingers were also moderate to intense itchers, whereas 50% of the itchers showed little or no stinging response.

L. Misery and S. Ständer (eds.), *Pruritus*,
DOI 10.1007/978-1-84882-322-8_22, © Springer-Verlag London Limited 2010

## 22.3 Treatments

Because the mechanisms of skin reactivity are poorly understood, treatments remain a challenge and are not standardized. It has been proposed to have adequate hygiene and moisturizing but to avoid the use of cosmetics! Cosmetics with low concentrations of detergents, tension actives and irritant substances should be preferred. A curative treatment with cosmetics with upraising substances might be possible. A few new products have recently arrived on the market. It is probable that cosmetics with low irritating potential and those containing substances with effects on sensory endings and the epidermis as a sensory organ[20] would provide the best response to pruritus in the course of skin reactivity.[18]

## References

1. Berardesca E, Fluhr JW, Maibach HI. What is sensitive skin? In: Berardesca E, Fluhr JW, Maibach HI, eds. *Sensitive skin syndrome*. New York: Taylor & Francis; 2006:1–6.
2. Boulais N, Misery L. The epidermis: a sensory tissue. *Eur J Dermatol*. 2008;18:119–127.
3. Slodownik D, Williams J, Lee A, Tate B, Nixon R. Controversies regarding the sensitive skin syndrome. *Expert Rev Dermatol*. 2007;2:579–584.
4. Farage MA, Katsarou A, Maibach HI. Sensory, clinical and physiological factors in sensitive skin: a review. *Contact Dermatitis*. 2006;55:1–14.
5. Frosch PJ, Kligman AM. A method of appraising the stinging capacity of topically applied substances. *J Soc Cosmet Chem*. 1977;28:197–209.
6. Guinot C, Malvy D, Mauger E, et al. Self-reported skin sensitivity in a general adult population in France: data of the SU.VI.MAX cohort. *J Eur Acad Dermatol Venereol*. 2006;20:380–390.
7. Jourdain R, de Lacharrière O, Bastien P, Maibach H. Ethnic variations in self-perceived sensitive skin: epidemiological survey. *Contact Dermatitis*. 2002;46:162–169.
8. Katugampola R, Church M, Clough G. The neurogenic vasodilator response to endothelin-1: a study in human skin in vivo. *Exp Physiol*. 2000;85:839–846.
9. Misery L. Les nerfs à fleur de peau. *Int J Cosmet Sci*. 2002;24:111–116.
10. Misery L, Myon E, Martin N, et al. Sensitive skin: psychological effects and seasonal changes. *J Eur Acad Dermatol Venereol*. 2007;21:620–628.
11. Misery L, Myon E, Martin N, Verriere F, Nocera T, Taieb C. Sensitive skin in France: an epidemiological approach. *Ann Dermatol Venereol*. 2005;132:425–429.
12. Misery L, Sibaud V, Ambronati M, Macy G, Boussetta S, Taieb C. Sensitive scalp: does this condition exist ? An epidemiological study. *Contact Dermatitis*. 2008;58:234–238.
13. Muizzuddin N, Marenus KD, Maes DH. Factors defining sensitive skin and its treatment. *Am J Contact Dermat*. 1998;9:170–175.
14. Reilly DM, Parslew R, Sharpe GR, Powell S, Green MR. Inflammatory mediators in normal, sensitive and diseased skin types. *Acta Dermato-Venereologica*. 2000;80:171–174.
15. Saint-Martory C, Roguedas AM, Sibaud V, Degouy A, Schmitt AM, Misery L. Sensitive skin is not limited to the face. *Br J Dermatol*. 2008;158:130–133.
16. Seidenari S, Francomano M, Mantavoni L. Baseline biophysical parameters in subjects with sensitive skin. *Contact Dermatitis*. 1998;38:311–315.
17. Ständer S, Schneider SW, Weishaupt C, Luger TA, Misery L. Putative neuronal mechanisms of sensitive skin. *Exp Dermatol*. 2009;18:417–423.
18. Ständer S, Weisshaar E, Luger T. Neurophysiological and neurochemical basis of modern pruritus treatment. *Exper Dermatol*. 2008;17:161–169.
19. Thiers H. Peau sensible. In: Thiers H ed. *Les Cosmétiques (2ème édition)*. Paris: Masson; 1986:266–268.
20. Willis CM, Shaw S, de Lacharrière O, et al. Sensitive skin: an epidemiological study. *Br J Dermatol*. 2001;145:258–263.

# Chapter 23
# Neurogenic Pruritus with Cerebral and/or Medullary Abnormalities

Camille Fleuret and Laurent Misery

Medullary or cerebral lesions that cause a pruritus are care.

## 23.1 Medullary Lesions

Several types of medullary lesions responsible for pruritic sensations are described in the literature. Neurogenic factors infrequently cause pruritus, but must be considered each time the pruritus follows a metameric distribution with impairment of one or several dermatomes. In the majority of pruritus cases with a neurological cause, hypo- or hyperaesthesia accompanies the pruritus in the zone affected; this clinical characteristic allows the clinician to distinguish these cases of neurogenic pruritus.

### 23.1.1 Spinal Cord (SC) Tumors

Andreev et al.[1] studied cutaneous signs combined with SC tumors. Thirteen of their 77 patients complained of pruritus, six of whom had pruritus topographically limited to the nostrils. We can distinguish different nosological entities according to the tumor aetiologies.

#### 23.1.1.1 Ependymoma

Ependymoma is a benign tumor, more frequent in children. The aetiology is unknown. It represents ten percent of children's central nervous system (CNS) tumors, and it most often develops in the posterior cranial fossa. Clinical symptoms depend on the location of the tumor: they are signs of intracranial hypertension (IH) for tumors of the posterior cranial fossa; behavioral disorders and pyramidal signs for supratentorial tumors; or dysaesthesias for topographically medullary tumors.[2]

Two cases of brachioradial pruritus (BRP) revealing an ependymoma were reported in the literature:

• The first case of ependymoma revealed by a BRP was reported in 2002.[3]

A young woman 36 years of age presented a bilateral BRP down to the thenar regions. For a year she complained of itching in these regions of the body and of neck pains. Physiotherapy was ineffective.

This BRP was combined with neurological signs in the examination:

– Hypohidrosis localized in the same areas Signs of pyramidal irritation
– Positive bilateral Hoffman (H-) reflex
– Slight dyskinesias of interosseous muscles
– And in particular a *hyperaesthesia* localized in the left C5-C6 dermatomes

Magnetic resonance imaging (MRI) with T1 and T2 incidences showed a voluminous, intramedullary tumor.

• A second case of an ependymoma revealed by a BRP was reported quite recently.[4]

This involved a 53-year-old man who had presented a unilateral pruritus on the upper left extremity for 7 years. Neck pains appeared secondarily and were also combined with neurological disorders: dysaesthesias of the two upper extremities, searing pains, and even paresis in the left ulnar territory. Here also

L. Misery and S. Ständer (eds.), *Pruritus*,
DOI 10.1007/978-1-84882-322-8_23, © Springer-Verlag London Limited 2010

the MRI, supplemented by the medullary angiography (to eliminate a cavernous angioma), made it possible to diagnose an ependymoma - a diagnosis confirmed histologically through the anatomopathological examination of the piece surgically excised.

### 23.1.1.2 Syringomyelia

Syringomyelia is a medullary ailment characterized [5]

*Anatomically*, by the existence of a relatively wide cavity next to the canal of the ependyma, most often in the cervical spinal cord, that seems due to a disorder in medullary development;

*Clinicaly*, by the combination of a spastic paraplegia and symptoms localized to the upper extremities, the neck and the thorax, called "suspended"; muscular atrophy, elimination of sensitivity to pain and temperature, with preservation of tactile sensitivity; and trophic disorders.

A case of BRP (the first case of BRP described), revea-ling a syringomyelia and an intramedullary tumor, was reported in 1992.[6] The telltale signs were a pruritus localized to the left C5 dermatome, combined with a chronic lichenoid rash, probably secondary to the scratching.

These two types of medullary tumors cited above are sometimes revealed by a localized pruritus, BRP, described in an earlier chapter. BRP is rare. It involves a unilateral or bilateral pruritus, confined to the arms and shoulders of a single side, sometimes extending to the hemithorax and to the entire upper extremity. It affects both sexes. Cervical arthrosis (posterior cervical arthrosis) or the existence of a surplus cervical rib is currently recognized as causative factors of BRP. Alongside these two most frequent aetiologies, other neurological causes may arise, each time causing cervical nerve compression. BRP reveals the neurological abnormality in the majority of cases.

### 23.1.1.3 Medullary Tumors Combined with Neurofibromatoses

A case of localized pruritus was reported in 2000[7] in a 15-year-old, revealing an intramedullary tumor, and allowing a retrospective diagnosis of neurofibromatosis. The case involved a young adolescent 15 years of age who presented a pruritus localized to the C6 and C7 dermatomes circling her waist (bilateral),

starting at the age of 4 months. The itch was so intense that she suffered from insomnia. The examination revealed multiple excoriations and a T6-T7 topographical zone of postinflammatory hypopigmentation circling the abdomen, as well as eight café-au-lait spots 0.5–3 cm in diameter. No axillary lentigo or neurofibroma was observed. The complete neurological examination did not reveal other abnormalities. However, a medullary MRI showed an intramedullary tumor extending from T4 to T8. A subtotal resection (90%) of the tumor was performed. The anatomopathological examination of the excised piece revealed a pilocytic astrocytoma. The pruritus completely and immediately improved after the operation.

While brain tumors remain asymptomatic for years, SC tumors become symptomatic early on with signs and symptoms that reflect their topography.

In the case of this young 15-year-old girl, the symmetrical pruritus localized on the dermatomes corresponding to the intramedullary level of the astrocytoma was the initial symptom, and was therefore revealing.

Mautner et al.[8] reported the cases of nine children suffering from NF 2, who presented outward signs revealing intramedullary tumors. The initial symptoms were tetraplegia or paraplegia.[9]

NF 2 represents a wide-ranging spectrum of possible clinical signs. Cutaneous manifestations are less frequent than in NF 1; in particular, there are rarely more than 5 café-au-lait spots.[10] On the other hand, intramedullary and brain tumors are frequent in NF 2 (astrocytomas in 4% of cases and intramedullary tumors in 25% of cases).[8,10]

In recent publications, NF that presented both a loca-lized and a generalized pruritus cases had been reported. These cases of generalized pruritus described, in the context of NF, are then probably not neurogenic pruritus.

Monk et al.[11] described two cases of patients with NF who complained of generalized pruritus, in whom an unexplained biological cholestasis was found. Similar descriptions showed that this cholestasis

> Any localized pruritus in patients suffering from NF should therefore indicate, as a priority, to doctors to look for a brain or intramedullary tumor, most often involving malignant tumors, the prognosis of which remains doubtful.

was linked to a neurofibroma obstructing the ampulla of Vater.

In the same way, several cases of localized pruritus, combined with neurofibromas, have been described since 1956,[12] although not neurogenic ones, since they were probably related to an abundance of granular cells around the neurofibromas, including the mast cells.[13]

### 23.1.2 Medullary Abscesses

Infectious medullary lesions[14] may lead to a pruritic symptomatology, the topography of which always matches the anatomic location of the medullary lesion.

### 23.1.3 Multiple Sclerosis (MS)

A paroxysmal pruritus was described in three Japanese patients suffering from MS.[15] This symptom is rare, but may represent the first and only symptom of a developing MS.

### 23.1.4 Transverse Myelitis

Transverse myelitis is usually revealed by a bilateral debility of the lower limbs, a sensitive deficiency with metameric topography and urinary retention.

The first case of neurogenic pruritus induced by a transverse myelitis was reported in 2003.[16] It involved a 43-year-old patient who initially presented with pains and paraesthesias in her legs. Three weeks following the appearance of this initial symptomatology, she complained of severe pruritus and a hyperaesthesia in a clearly defined zone of her upper limbs combined with dysuria. She reported no notable history of multiple sclerosis or known medullary tumor. There was also no recent history of upper respiratory infections or infections from vaccination, which would have allowed a Guillain-Barré syndrome to be suspected. The clinical exam revealed a hyperpigmentation of lichenoid plaques with excoriations in a clearly defined and symmetrical area of her arms. The impairment had a C3-C5 metameric distribution. The neurological examination found a marked hyperaesthesia and an allodynia on this same lichenoid area, while the motor

examination proved to be normal. The biological and immunological examinations, as well as the electromyogram were all normal. The MRI permitted a diagnosis by showing a hyperintense zone in the T2 sequence extending from C2-3 to C5-6. This involved a transverse myelitis of the spinal cord. The pruritus and allodynia improved when the myelitis was cured.

### 23.1.2 Cerebral Lesions

Cerebral lesions may be responsible for localized pruritus, which are always unilateral and sometimes paroxysmal in nature.[17–19] This is one of the arguments in favor of the cerebral representation of pruritus.

### 23.1.2.1 Aneurysms of the Basilar Artery[17–19]

There are clinical descriptions of unilateral and localized pruritus for which a link with the aneurysms of the basilar artery have been found in these patients.

### 23.2.2 Cerebrovascular Accidents (CVA)[17–19]

While the pain after a CVA is a well-known phenomenon, pruritus itself is generally under-diagnosed. More than a dozen cases of post-CVA pruritus have been reported in the literature.

For illustration, we will describe two of these cases:[20]

- A 74-year-old woman with a history of arterial hypertension (AHT) and dyslipemia developed a pruritus several weeks after a right thalamic CVA. The pruritus was paroxysmal and affected varying, but always localized, zones on the left side of the trunk and the left limbs. The right half of the body was left alone. The patient had no history of kidney, liver, endocrine, or haematological disease that could explain the pruritus; the results of the biological examinations performed confirmed the absence of abnormality. The clinical examination found scratching injuries on the left side of the body, with clear respect for the right side.
- A 69-year-old man with a history of AHT developed an intense pruritus at the level of his left thigh several days after a cerebral ischaemia by occlusion of a

right middle cerebral artery. The pruritus was localized and intermittent, sometimes not allowing him to sleep. Also, the patient had no history of kidney, liver, endocrine, or haematological disease, and all examinations were normal. The clinical examination found a left hemiparesis and scratching injuries on the front side of his left thigh.

It is important that doctors know how to recognise a post-CVA pruritus to avoid any unnecessary aetiological investigation, and to be able to inform patients suffering from CVA of the possibility of developing such pruritic symptoms. The syndrome consists in a topographically limited or a generalized pruritus, always contralateral to the brain injury. As with post-CVA pain, post-CVA pruritus arises several days, even weeks, after the cerebral accident.

## 23.1.3 Physiopathogenesis of Neurogenic Pruritus

The physiopathological (neuroanatomical and neurophysiological) bases of neurogenic pruritus have not yet been completely elucidated.[20,21]. Much research and observation suggests that this type of pruritus could be a "submodality" of pain. In the event of brain or medullary lesions, pruritic perceptions use the same neural paths as painful sensations. The sensations of neurogenic pruritus would therefore originate from the nerve endings of the A delta myelinated fibres and the unmyelinated C fibres near the basement membrane. While physiologically the pruritic sensations are transmitted only by the A delta rapid conduction fibres, pain is transmitted by the slow conduction C (unmyelinated) fibres.

Consequently, neurogenic pruritus is probably not caused by the usual peripheral mediators such as histamine and endopeptidases, but rather through a brain or medullary pathological process.

The exact mechanisms through which some patients suffering from brain or medullary lesions develop a pruritus remain poorly understood.

The currently accepted hypothesis is that, following an impairment of the CNS, the pruritus would be linked to the interruption of a still-undefined neural path, which is capable of modulating sensations of pruritus and pain.

## 23.1.4 Treatment of Neurogenic Pruritus

This is based above all on *AETIOLOGICAL* treatment, when it is possible.

### 23.1.4.1 Aetiological Treatment

In the two cases of ependymoma revealed through BRP[3,4] described previously, 1 of the 2 (the 53-year-old patient) was given surgical treatment for the tumor, which remains the benchmark treatment for this type of tumor.

The 36-year-old patient refused the procedure.

Four months after the operation, the patient complained of residual pains (requiring oral treatment by class-2 analgesics and gabapentin), but no longer had pruritus or motor impairment.

In the young girl who presented a BRP revealing an astrocytoma,[7] and in the context of neurofibromatosis, surgery by laminectomy and subtotal resection (90%) of the tumor allowed complete and immediate improvement of the pruritus.[19]

In the patient suffering from transverse myelitis,[16] the pruritus and the allodynia improved after the myelitis was cured.

As to the post-CVA pruritus treatments,[19,20] the majority are still exclusively symptomatic cases.

### 23.1.4.2 Symptomatic Treatment

Symptomatic treatment, in some cases representing the only possible treatment, remains very difficult.

• *Individual case of BRP:*

The usual treatments for BRP[22–24] can only have moderate and transitory effectiveness in the event of a medullary lesion.

Anticonvulsant-class medications, such as gabapentin and more recently pregabalin can prove significant[25] (see below).

• *Neurogenic pruritus, of any kind:*

The symptoms often respond quite well to gabapentin[25] or pregabalin; carbamazepine works as well, but it is being used less and less due to the adverse, and sometimes very serious, reactions of the Drug Hypersensitivity Syndrome (DRESS) variety.

Belonging to the class of anticonvulsants, these two medications appear to allow clear improvement. They are currently used in post therapeutic pains and in the majority of neuropathic pains. Gabapentin and pregabalin, by potentiating the GABAergic system, could therefore be useful in cases of neuropathic pruritus.

The main side effects described with these products are the risks of dizziness and drowsiness. These effects can add to that of deteriorating cognitive functions by opioids, which sometimes have already been prescribed when introducing these treatments to patients who are often polymedicated.

## 23.1.5 Conclusion

Although they are rare, neurological causes of pruritus exist. Medullary causes are dominated by intramedullary tumors, and cerebral causes by CVA. A careful neurological examination is important.

The distinctive feature of this type of pruritus is based on the limited nature of the pruritic area, in connection with the topography of the neurological impairment within the CNS. The pruritus is homolateral to the lesion in the event of medullary impairment, while it is always contralateral to the CNS injury in the event of a cerebral impairment.

Its physiopathogenesis is only hypothetical at present.

The key to its treatment is handling the aetiology. When this is impossible or insufficient, a symptomatic approach is considered.

## References

1. Andreev VC, Petkov I. Skin manifestations associated with tumors of the brain. *Br J Dermatol.* 1975;92:675–678.
2. Hasselblatt M. Ependymal tumors. *Recent Results Cancer Res* 2009;171:51–66.
3. Kavak A, Dosoglu M. Can a spinal cord tumor cause brachioradial pruritus? *J Am Acad Dermatol.* 2002;46(3): 437–440.
4. Fleuret C, Misery L. Prurit brachio-radial révélant un épendymome. *Annales de Dermatologie* 2009;136:435–437.
5. Synder P. Chiari Malformation and Syringomyélie Radiol Technol 2008;79:555–558.
6. Kinsella LJ, Carney-Godley K, Feldmann E. Lichen simplex chronicus as the initial manifestation of intramedullary neoplasm and syringomyelia. *Neurosurgery.* 1992;30(3): 418–421.
7. Johnson RE, Kanigsberg ND, Jimenez CL. Localized pruritus: a presenting symptom of a spinal cord tumor in a child with features of neurofibromatosis. *J Am Acad Dermatol.* 2000;43(5 pt 2):958–961.
8. Mautner VF, Tatagiba M, Guthoff R, Samii M, Pulst SM. Neurofibromatosis 2 in the pediatric age group. *Neurosurgery.* 1993;33(1):92–96.
9. Lewis RA, Gerson LP, Axelson KA, Riccardi VM, Whitford RP. von Recklinghausen neurofibromatosis. II. Incidence of optic gliomata. *Ophthalmology.* 1984;91(8):929–935.
10. Monk BE, Pembroke AC, du Vivier A. Neurofibromatosis, generalized pruritus and cholestatic liver dysfunction - report of two cases. *Clin Exp Dermatol.* 1985;10(6):590–591.
11. Cross FW, Schull WJ, Neel JV. A clinical, pathological and genetic study of multiple neurofibromes. Springfield: Charles C. Thomas Publishers; 1956:3–181.
12. Greggio, H. Les cellules granuleuses (mast zellen) dans les tissues normaux et dans certaines maladies chirurgicales. *Arch Med Exp.* 1911;23:323.
13. Sullivan MJ, Drake ME Jr. Unilateral pruritus and Nocardia brain abscess. *Neurology.* 1984;34(6):828–829.
14. Yamamoto M, Yabuki S, Hayabara T, Otsuki S. Paroxysmal itching in multiple sclerosis: a report of three cases. *J Neurol Neurosurg Psychiatry.* 1981;44(1):19–22.
15. Bond LD, Keough GC. Neurogenic pruritus: a case of pruritus induced by transverse myelitis. *Br J Dermatol.* 2003;149:193–227.
16. King CA, Huff FJ, Jorizzo JL. Unilateral neurogenic pruritus: paroxysmal itching associated with central nervous system lesions. *Ann Intern Med.* 1982;97(2):222–223.
17. Massey EW. Unilateral neurogenic pruritus following stroke. *Stroke.* 1984;15(5):901–903.
18. Shapiro PE, Braun CW. Unilateral pruritus after a stroke. *Arch Dermatol.* 1987;123(11):1527–1530.
19. Kimyai-Asadi, Hossein C. Poststroke pruritus. *Stroke*; 1993;30:692–695.
20. Wallengren J. Neuroanatomy and neurophysiology of itch. *Dermatol Ther.* 2005;18:292–303.
21. Knight TE, Hayashi T. Solar (brachioradial) pruritus - response to capsaicin cream. *Int J Dermatol.* 1994;33(3):206–209.
22. Bernhard JD, Bordeaux JS. Medical pearl: the ice-pack sign in brachioradial pruritus. *J Am Acad Dermatol.* 2005;52(6): 1073.
23. Bernhard JD. Neurogenic pruritus and strange skin sensations. In: Bernhard JD, ed. *Itch, Mechanisms and Management of Pruritus.* New York: McGraw-Hill; 1994:185–201.
24. Tait CP, Grigg E, Quirk CJ. Brachioradial pruritus and cervical spine manipulation. *Australas J Dermatol.* 1998;39(3): 168–170.
25. Kanitakis J. Brachioradial pruritus: report of a new case responding to gabapentin. *Eur J Dermatol.* 2006;16(3): 311–312.

# Chapter 24
# Localized Neuropathic Pruritus

Martin Marziniak, Esther Pogatzki-Zahn, and Stefan Evers

Localized neuropathic pruritus is a matter of mutual interest for dermatologists, neurologists, and pain specialists. Many patients report a mixture of different sensations including localized itch, burning, and tingling. The predominant sensation, either pruritus or paresthesias or dysesthesias, will decide whether the patient consults a dermatologist or a neurologist. The most common localized pruritus syndrome is postherpetic neuralgia. Notalgia paresthetica (NP) and brachioradial pruritus (see Chapter 25) are other circumscribed itch syndromes.

## 24.1 Postherpetic Neuralgia and Postherpetic Itch

**Epidemiology:** Herpes zoster occurs in up to 30% of the whole population during lifetime and in as many as 50% of those living until 85 years of age. The most important risk factor for postherpetic neuralgia (PHN) is old age. Thirty to fifty eight percent of patients with PHN report itch as a symptom.[1] A minority of patients (7%) with recent shingles classified the complaints as postherpetic itch without pain. In 109 patients with PHN from Seattle, itch was reported in 23% as mild, in 22% as moderate, and in 13% as severe, whereas 42% did not describe itch as a disturbing symptom. There were no significant differences between subjects with PHN and (with or without) itch with respect to age, gender, or smoking habits.[1] Subjects whose shingles affected the head, face, and neck were more likely to experience postherpetic itch than those whose shingles affected the body.[1]

**Clinical picture:** Herpes zoster is usually diagnosed according to the following characteristics[1]: the presence of a prodromal pain (sometimes itch) before the appearance of the rash (75% of the patients),[2] a unilateral dermatomal rash,[3] grouped vesicles or papules,[4] pain and allodynia in the area of the rash. In 10% of clinically suspected herpes zoster a recurrence of herpes simplex is the differential diagnosis, especially if a history of a rash in the same dermatome is reported. Other differentials are contact dermatitis and rash caused by plant exposure.

Three phases of pain have been described to distinguish acute pain from PHN[1]: herpes zoster acute pain is defined as pain that occurs within 30 days after rash onset;[2] subacute herpetic neuralgia is a pain that persists longer than 30 days and resolves before 120 days; and[3] PHN is defined as pain that persist longer than 120 days after the occurrence of the rash.[2] The quality of pain in PHN can be divided into stimulus-independent intermittent pain, stimulus-evoked pain, especially brush-evoked dynamic allodynia, and paresthesias, dysesthesias, and itching.[3] In 10–15%, shingles affect the first division of the trigeminal nerve called herpes zoster ophthalmicus with the painful zoster rash on the forehead, periocular region, and nose. Ocular complications including keratitis, iritis, and in severe cases neuritis of the optic nerve are the most dreaded complications.[4]

**Pathogenesis:** Herpes zoster is caused by the reactivation of a latent varicella zoster virus in the sensory ganglia. Histological examination of nerves and ganglia affected by PHN shows chronic neuronal loss and quiescent scarring without signs of inflammation.[5] In punch biopsies of the affected skin a correlation between the presence of PHN and the severity of persistent distal nociceptive axonal loss has been described.[6] Autoptic studies underlined the importance of central changes within the spinal cord and showed a segmental atrophy of the dorsal horn in correlation with pain persistence.[7] Postherpetic itch seems to be

L. Misery and S. Ständer (eds.), *Pruritus*,
DOI 10.1007/978-1-84882-322-8_24, © Springer-Verlag London Limited 2010

caused by unprovoked firing of the peripheral and central neurons that mediate itch. Dysregulation of the skin function (pH changes, trauma, disrupted barrier function, inflammation, and infection) can directly or indirectly stimulate sensory nerve endings and thereby induce itch.[8] In a subpopulation of patients who had herpes zoster associated neuropathic itch the skin is desensitized for other sensory qualities. In these patients it is discussed whether cutaneous itch fibres from adjacent unaffected dermatomes may be the cause of postherpetic itch because these fibres have extraordinary, large innervation territories (up to 8.5 cm diameter) overlapping one single dermatome.[9] In some patients it can lead to a self-injury from scratching desensitized skin.[10]

**Diagnostics:** The features of herpes zoster are typical that a diagnosis is based on just the presence of prodromal pain and/or itching and the rash (Fig. 24.1). The prodromal period with pain, itch, or dysesthesias may

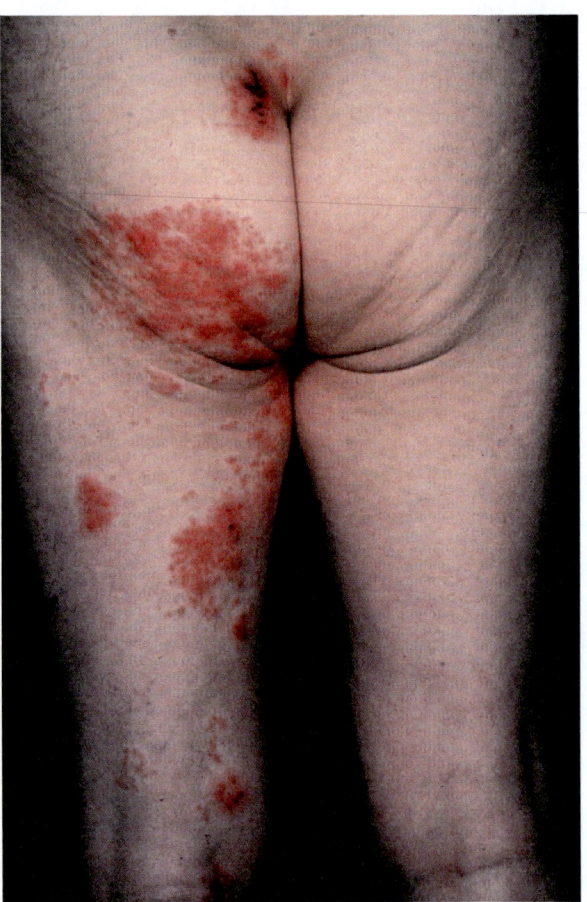

**Fig. 24.1** Patient with herpes zoster affecting the S2 and S3 dermatome of the left leg

require differentiation from trauma, myocardial ischemia, renal colic, gallbladder disease, or dental pain depending on the body region involved.[11] Atypical lesions may require a laboratory work-up including direct immunofluorescence assays or real-time polymerase chain reaction testing of samples from skin lesions.[12] The most important differential diagnosis is a herpes simplex viral infection that mimics herpes zoster. Risk factors such as immunocompromised state, immunosuppressive drugs, HIV infection, bone-marrow or organ transplantation, cancer, chronic steroid therapy, and psychological stress or a trauma have to be considered.[13]

**Therapy:** A review of the antiviral therapy of herpes zoster is beyond the scope of this chapter. The herpes zoster vaccine seems to have an effect in reducing a patient's risk for developing herpes zoster and PHN,[14] whereas corticosteroids seem to be ineffective for preventing PHN.[15] Recent guidelines of evidence-based treatment of neuropathic pain (including PHN) consider tricyclic antidepressants (TCAs), gabapentin and pregabalin, and topical lidocaine as first-line analgesics for PHN. Opioids and tramadol are recommended as second-line treatment and topical capsaicin and valproate as third-line therapy.[16–18] Up to now, special guidelines about the treatment of postherpetic itch do not exist; therefore drugs for neuropathic pain are frequently used.

TCAs inhibit norepinephrine and serotonin reuptake and have peripheral effects on sodium channel-blockade. Amitriptyline (65–100 mg/day), nortriptyline (75–100 mg/day), and desipramine (about 70 mg/day) are effective in PHN on the basis of class I–II placebo-controlled trials with a combined number needed to treat (NNT) of 2.6 (95% confidence interval (CI) 2.1–3.5).[19,20] Maprotiline has been found slightly less effective than amitriptyline[21] and nortriptyline as effective as amitriptyline but better tolerated.[22] There are no randomized, controlled trails on the efficacy of selective serotonin reuptake inhibitors in PHN. Palpitations, QT prolongation, orthostatic hypotension, dizziness, and sedation are the limiting therapeutic factors of TCAs especially in the elderly. For TCAs, the number needed to cause minor harm is 5.7 (95% CI 3.3–18.6), and that for major harm 16.9 (95% CI 8.9–178).[20,23]

Gabapentin and pregabalin are the two antiepileptic drugs most often used in the treatment of neuropathic pain including PHN and itch. The mechanism of the analgesic action is the inhibition of the release of excitatory neurotransmitters such as glutamate from the central terminal of primary afferent fibers in the spinal cord.[24] Gabapentin 1,800–3,600 mg/day[25,26] and pregabalin 150–600 mg/day[27,28] have consistently shown efficacy in PHN with a NNT of 4.4 (95% CI 3.3–6.1) for gabapentin and 4.9 (95% CI 3.7–7.6) for pregabalin.[20] Encouraging results have recently been reported for 1,000 mg valproate in one study with an NNT of 2.1 (95% CI 1.4–4.2).[29] Dizziness, somnolence, and peripheral edema are the most frequently reported side effects of pregabaline and gabapentin in the elderly. The number needed to cause minor harm has been reported as 4.1 (95% CI 3.2–5.7), and that for major harm as 17.3 (95% CI 7.7–30.9).[20]

Topical application is an alternative treatment option. Repeated application of lidocaine patches (5%) has shown efficacy in PHN patients with allodynia in three placebo-controlled studies.[30–32] Due to excellent tolerance, application of lidocaine patches may be preferred in the elderly, particularly in patients with allodynia, and with a small area of itch or pain. Topical capsaicin 0.075% has been found effective, though to a small degree, in two parallel group randomized control trials but has a reduced compliance due to burning sensations in most subjects.[33,34]

Tramadol (average dosage 275 mg/day up to 400 mg/day) was shown moderately effective only on some measures of spontaneous pain intensity in PHN with an NNT of 4.8 (95% CI 2.6–26.9).[35] Oxycodone, morphine, and methadone have shown efficacy on PHN in two crossover placebo-controlled randomized trials.[36,37] The combined NNT for strong opioids in PHN is 2.7 (95% CI 2.1–3.7).[20] In one trial comparing slow-release morphine (91 mg/day, range 15 to 225mg/day) and methadone (15 mg/day) with TCAs and placebo, pain relief was significantly greater with morphine than with nortriptyline, whereas the analgesic efficacy of methadone was comparable with that of TCAs.[37]

## 24.2 Notalgia Paresthetica

NP as an uni- or bilateral syndrome of paresthesias, burning pain, or itching in a restricted interscapular region was first defined by Astwazaturow in 1934 as a sensory neuropathy involving the dorsal spinal nerves[38] and was specified in more detail by Pleet and Massey in the late seventies.[39–41]

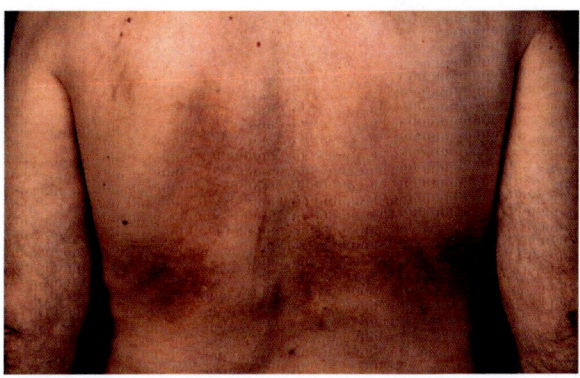

**Fig. 24.2** Patient with notalgia paresthetica and corresponding scratch lesions on the back (courtesy of S. Ständer)

**Epidemiology:** Although the condition is not believed to be rare, NP is not frequently reported and data about prevalence and incidence rates are missing.

**Clinical picture:** The main symptom is pruritus on the back with a characteristic hyperpigmented patch within the dermatomes T2–T6 (Fig. 24.2).[42–44] In the largest study of 43 patients with NP,[45] 30% complained of episodic pain which was limited to the pruritic area and did not radiate, 28% described paresthesias, and 12% complained of hyperesthesia, both of an intermittent character. None of these symptoms were reported to be severe enough to cause sleep deprivation or interfere with daily activities. No patient described any specific factor that would aggravate the pruritus. Family history was negative in all cases. Orthopedic history and physical examination of the spine and extremities for an evaluation of motor and sensory functions did not reveal any abnormalities. No patient showed any muscle weakness, spasticity, changes in reflexes, bowel and/or bladder dysfunction, or sensory abnormalities other than that of the symptoms at the localization of NP.[45]

The dermatological finding of a circumscribed hyperpigmented patch is thought to be secondary to the chronic rubbing and scratching due to pruritus.[46–49]

**Pathogenesis:** NP is thought to be a sensory neuropathy. The exact pathomechanisms of NP are still under discussion, and only a few investigational studies on its pathogenesis exist.[43,46,49,50] The most widely excepted explanation is that NP may be due to compression of posterior rami of the spinal nerves of the T2 to T6 segments.[43,51] Degenerative changes are often but not always observed in the vertebrae or vertebral discs corresponding to the dermatome of cutaneous lesions and the described pruritus.[49,52] A radiographic evaluation (anteroposterior and lateral radiographs, magnet resonance imaging (MRI) of the entire vertebral column) of 43 patients with NP revealed various vertebral pathologies (79%) such as degenerative changes (58%) or a herniated nucleus pulposus (40%).[45] In 65% of the patients, these changes were most prominent in the vertebrae which corresponded to the dermatome(s) of at least one of the cutaneous lesions present on that patient and thus were labelled as "relevant." Because the spinal nerves emerge through the multifidus spinae muscle at right angles, Massey and Fleet[40] have suggested that the spinal nerves are prone to be injured by trauma or entrapment. Additionally, Eisenberg et al.[53] reported a single NP case in whom nerve root impingement precisely correlated with the clinical findings, and a case report describing the onset of NP after neuralgic amyotrophy discusses a transient entrapment of thoracic roots further distally, where they pass through the long spine erector muscles.[54]

At the moment, results are inconsistent because degenerative changes in the spinal column are not rare especially among the elderly. Nevertheless, the explanation for NP by the entrapment hypothesis is the one with the best evidence to date. Successful physiotherapy[52] or paravertebral local anesthetic blocks[55] strengthens this hypothesis.

Skin biopsies appear to be normal and the described dermatological changes have been interpreted by dermatologists as a result of the chronic rubbing and scratching. A study on 14 patients described a normal epidermis and only very mild inflammatory infiltrates, including a moderate number of diffusely spread melanophages, in the papillary dermis. Amyloid deposits and gross alterations of the cutaneous nerves could not be found.[49,56] Additional immunohistochemical staining with antibodies for S-100, vasoactive-intestinal-polypeptide, substance P and protein gene product 9.5 (PGP 9.5), as a panaxonal marker, did not reveal significant differences between the affected and unaffected skin.[56] A second study investigated 12 cases of NP and revealed no significant differences in the presence, distribution, or density of immunoreactive fibers in lesional and contralateral unaffected skin.[57] While discussing the article by Şavk et al.[56], it is worth mentioning that the staining methods have been improved and that the number of stained nerve fibers is not described in the paper. Another pitfall of this paper might be the very high number of skin biopsies which did not show any staining, especially of the immunohistochemistry with PGP 9.5 in both the patients and in the healthy controls. Therefore, more studies are warranted to investigate this topic according to the current guidelines of staining skin biopsies in neuropathy.[58] In this context, it is worth mentioning the article by Springall et al. that showed an increased dermal innervation in the affected skin of patients with NP.[46] Furthermore, the effectiveness of topical capsaicin suggests an involvement of cutaneous nerve endings in the generation of itch in NP patients.[47]

Due to chronic rubbing, keratinocytes may become necrotic. As a consequence, amyloid may be present in the papillary dermis, and macular amyloidosis presents with brown patches.[50,59]

**Diagnostics:** In patients who are susceptive for NP, a skin and histological investigation should rule out any other possible underlying dermatosis. Accordingly, laboratory investigation should exclude other underlying diseases (diabetes mellitus, uremia). To rule out spinal compression, an MRI scan of the cervical and thoracic spinal column is recommended. If pathological changes are observed upon MRI, a detailed neurological examination, including electroneurography and if necessary electromyography is advisable. Association of notalgia with MEN II syndrome (multiple endocrine neoplasia) has been described. Therefore, patients should be investigated clinically to rule out MEN II.

**Therapy:** Due to the low number of publications there are only single case reports or studies with a very small number of patients, and therapeutic recommendations beyond the general therapy of pruritus (antihistamines and topicals) are therefore limited. In a vehicle-controlled, double blind, crossover study, topical capsaicin was successful in treating the clinical symptoms of NP.[47] An open pilot study with oxcarbazepine showed a promising therapeutic effect,[60] but double blind placebo controlled studies have not been published yet in a peer-reviewed journal. Gabapentin was successfully prescribed in one patient with NP,[61] and it is also used in brachioradial pruritus.[62] Alternatively, botulinum toxin type A injections were successful in a patient with NP.[63]

Transcutaneous electrical nerve stimulation (TENS) was reported to offer partial relief in a group of 15 patients with NP and "relevant spinal pathology." Ten out of the fifteen patients described a sufficient relief, and the average pruritus score of all patients was reduced from 10 to 6.8 after ten sessions of TENS.[64]

Physiotherapy was successful in four out of six patients in one study[52] and in a few in another study.[65] Goulden et al. reported successful paravertebral local anesthetic blocks in a patient with NP.[55]

In the dermatological literature some of the classical entrapment neuropathies are connected to localized neuropathic pruritus syndromes,[66] although pruritus is not often mentioned in the literature and paresthesias are the main complaint: *Meralgia paresthetica* is characterized by burning, tingling, and numbness on the anterolateral thigh due to a compression of the femoral cutaneous nerve by a fibrous band or external compressors (very tight trousers). Obesity, pregnancy, and backpacks are predisposing factors.[67] Tarsal tunnel syndrome is a lesion of the posterior tibial nerve caused by repetitive dorsiflexion of the ankle. It is common among runners and mountain climbers.[68] Lesions of the central nervous system as cause of pruritus and brachioradial pruritus are described in separate chapters of this book.

In summary, searching for an underlying abnormality in the skeletal system, nervous system, or both may be warranted in a localized pruritus syndrome without recognizable dermatosis.

## References

1. Oaklander Al, Bowsher D, Galer B, et al. Herpes zoster itch: preliminary epidemiologic data. *J Pain.* 2003;6:338–343.
2. Arami RB, Soong SJ, Weiss HL, et al. Phase specific analysis of herpes zoster associated pain data: a new statistical approach. *Stat Med.* 2001;20:2429–2439.
3. Dworkin RH, Gnann JW, Oaklander AW, et al. Diagnosis and assessment of pain associated with herpes zoster and postherpetic neuralgia. *J Pain.* 2008;9(suppl 1):S37–S44.
4. Gnann JW Jr, Whitley RJ. Clinical practice: herpes zoster. *N Engl J Med.* 2002;347:340–346.
5. Oaklander AL. Mechanisms of pain and itch caused by herpes zoster (shingles). *J Pain.* 2008;9(suppl 1):S10–S18.
6. Oaklander AL. The density of remaining nerve endings in human skin with and without Postherpetic neuralgia after shingles. *Pain.* 2001;92:139–145.
7. Watson CP, Deck JH, Morshead C, et al. Post-herpetic neuralgia: further post-mortem studies of cases with and without pain. *Pain.* 1991;44:105–117.
8. Steinhoff M, Bienenstock J, Schmelz M, et al. Neurophysiological, neuroimmunological, and neuroendocrine basis of pruritus. *J Invest Dermatol.* 2006;126:1705–1718.
9. Schmelz M, Schmidt R, Bickel A, et al. Specific C-receptors for itch in human skin. *J Neurosci.* 1997;17:8003–8008.
10. Oaklander AL, Cohen SP, Raju SVY. Intractable postherpetic itch and cutaneous deafferentation after facial shingles. *Pain.* 2002;96:9–12.
11. Weinberg JM. Herpes zoster: epidemiology, natural history, and common complications. *J Am Acad Dermatol.* 2007;57:S130–S135.
12. Schmutzhard J, Riedel HM, Wirgartz BZ, et al. Detection of herpes simplex virus type 1, herpes simplex virus type 2 and varicella-zoster virus in skin lesions: comparison of real-time PCR, nested PCR and virus isolation. *J Clin Virol.* 2004;29:120–126.
13. Arvin AM. Varicella-zoster virus. *Clin Microbiol Rev.* 1996;9:361–381.
14. Gnann JW Jr. Vaccination to prevent herpes zoster in older adults. *J Pain.* 2008;9(suppl 1):S31–S36.
15. He L, Zhang D, Zhou M, et al. Corticosteroids for preventing postherpetic neuralgia. *Cochrane Database Syst Rev.* 2008;1:CD005582.
16. Attal N, Cruccu G, Haanpää M, et al. EFNS guidelines on pharmacological treatment of neuropathic pain. *Eur J Neurol.* 2006;13:1153–1169.
17. Dworkin RH, O'Connor AB; Backonja M, et al. Pharmacologic management of neuropathic pain: evidence-based recommendations. *Pain.* 2007;132:237–251.
18. Moulin DE, Clark AJ, Gilran I, et al. Pharmacological management of chronic neuropathic pain – consensus statement and guidelines from the Canadian Pain Society. *Pain Res Manag.* 2007;12:13–21.
19. Dubinsky RM, Kabbani H, El-Chami Z, et al. Quality Standards Subcommittee of the American Academy of Neurology. Practice parameter: treatment of postherpetic neuralgia: an evidence-based report of the Quality Standards Subcommittee of the American Academy of Neurology. *Neurology.* 2004;63:959–965.
20. Hempenstall K, Nurmikko TJ, Johnson RW, et al. Analgesic therapy in postherpetic neuralgia: a quantitative systematic review. *PLoS Med.* 2005;2:628–644.
21. Watson CP, Chipman M, Reed K, et al. Amitriptyline versus maprotiline in postherpetic neuralgia: a randomized, double-blind, crossover trial. *Pain.* 1992;48:29–36.
22. Watson CP, Vernich L, Chipman M, et al. Nortriptyline versus amitriptyline in postherpetic neuralgia: a randomized trial. *Neurology.* 1998;51:1166–1171.
23. Saarto T, Wiffen PJ. Antidepressants for neuropathic pain. Cochrane Database Syst Rev. 2007;4:CD005454.
24. Maneuf YP, Gonzalez MI, Sutton KS, et al. Cellular and molecular action of the putative GABA-mimetic, gabapentin. *Cell Mol Life Sci.* 2003;60:742–750.
25. Rowbotham MC, Harden N, Stacey B, et al. Gabapentin for treatment of postherpetic neuralgia. *JAMA.* 1998;280:1837–1843.
26. Rice ASC, Maton S. Post Herpetic Neuralgia Study Group. Gabapentin in postherpetic neuralgia; a randomised, double-blind, controlled study. *Pain.* 2001;94:215–224.
27. Dworkin RH, Corbin AE, Young JP Jr, et al. Pregabalin for the treatment of postherpetic neuralgia: a randomized, placebo-controlled trial. *Neurology.* 2003;60:1274–1283.
28. Sabatowski R, Galvez R, Cherry DA, et al. Pregabalin reduces pain and improves sleep and mood disturbances in patients with post-herpetic neuralgia: results of a randomised, placebo-controlled clinical trial. *Pain.* 2004;109:26–35.

29. Kochar DK, Garg P, Bumb RA, et al. Divalproex sodium in the management of post-herpetic neuralgia: a randomized double-blind placebo-controlled study. *QJM*. 2005;98:29–34.

30. Galer BS, Rowbotham MC, Perander J, et al. Topical lidocaine patch relieves postherpetic neuralgia more effectively than a vehicle topical patch: results of an enriched enrolment study. *Pain*. 1999;80:533–538.

31. Galer BS, Jensen MP, Ma T, et al. The lidocaine patch 5% effectively treats all neuropathic pain qualities: results of a randomized, double-blind, vehicle-controlled, 3-week efficacy study with use of the neuropathic pain scale. *Clin J Pain*. 2002;5:297–301.

32. Wasner G, Kleinert A, Binder A, et al. Postherpetic neuralgia: topical lidocaine is effective in nociceptor-deprived skin. *J Neurol*. 2005;252:677–686.

33. Bernstein JE, Korman NJ, Bickers DR, et al. Topical capsaicin treatment of chronic postherpetic neuralgia. *J Am Acad Dermatol*. 1989;21:265–270.

34. Watson CP, Tyler KL, Bickers DR, et al. A randomized vehicle-controlled trial of topical capsaicin in the treatment of postherpetic neuralgia. *Clin Ther*. 1993;15:510–526.

35. Boureau F, Legallicier P, Kabir-Ahmadi M. Tramadol in post-herpetic neuralgia: a randomized, double-blind, placebo-controlled trial. *Pain*. 2003;104:323–331.

36. Watson CP, Babul N. Efficacy of oxycodone in neuropathic pain: a randomized trial in postherpetic neuralgia. *Neurology*. 1998;50:1837–1841.

37. Raja SN, Haythornwaite JA, Pappagallo M, et al. Opioids versus antidepressants in postherpetic neuralgia. *Neurology*. 2002;59:1015–1021.

38. Astwazaturow M. Über paresthetische Neuralgien und eine besondere Form derselben-Notalgia paresthetica. *Nervenarzt*. 1934;133:188–196.

39. Pleet AB, Massey EW. Notalgia paresthetica. *Neurology*. 1978;28:1310–1312.

40. Massey EW, Pleet AB. Localized pruritus – notalgia paresthetica. *Arch Dermatol*. 1979;115:982–983.

41. Massey EW, Pleet AB. Notalgia paresthetica. *JAMA*. 1979;214:1464.

42. Weber P, Paulos EG. Notalgia paresthetica, case reports and histologic appraisal. *J Am Acad Dermatol*. 1988;18:25–30.

43. Massey EW, Pleet AB. Electromyographic evaluation of notalgia paresthetica. *Neurology*. 1981;31:642.

44. Wallengren J. Treatment of notalgia paresthetica with topical capsaicin. *J Am Acad Dermatol*. 1991;24:286–288.

45. Şavk O, Şavk E. Investigation of spinal pathology in notalgia paresthetica. *J Am Acad Dermatol*. 2005;52:1085–1087.

46. Springall DR, Karanth SS, Kirkham N, *et al*. Symptoms of notalgia paresthetica may be explained by increased dermal innervation. *J Invest Dermatol*. 1991;97:555–561.

47. Wallengren J, Klinker M. Successful treatment of notalgia paresthetica with topical capsaicin: vehicle controlled, double blind, crossover study. *J Am Acad Dermatol*. 1995;32:287–289.

48. Marcusson, JA, Lundh B, Siden A, et al. Notalgia paresthetica – puzzling posterior pigmented pruritic patch. *Acta Derm Venereol*. 1990;70:452–454.

49. Şavk E, Şavk Ö, Bolukbasi N, et al. Notalgia paresthetica: a study on pathogenesis. *Int J Dermatol*. 2000;39:754–760.

50. Bernhard, JD. Notalgia paresthetica, macular posterior pigmentary incontinence, macular amyloidosis and Pruritus. *Acta Derm Venereol*. 1997;77:164.

51. Streib EW, Sun SF. Notalgia paresthetica owing to compression neuropathy: case presentation including electrodiagnostic studies. *Eur Neurol*. 1981;20:64–67.

52. Raison-Peyron N, Meunier L, Acevedo M, et al. Notalgia paresthetica: clinical, physiopathological and therapeutic aspects. A study of 12 cases. *J Eur Acad Dermatol Venereol*. 1999;12:215–221.

53. Eisenberg E, Barmeir E, Bergman R. Notalgia paresthetica associated with nerve root impingement. *J Am Acad Dermatol*. 1997;37:998–1000.

54. Tacconi P, Manca D, Tamburini G, et al. Notalgia paresthetica following neuralgic amyotrophy: a case report. *Neurol Sci*. 2004;25:27–29.

55. Goulden V, Toomey PJ, Highet AS. Successful treatment of notalgia paresthetica: a study on pathogenesis. *J Am Acad Dermatol*. 1998;38:114–116.

56. Şavk E, Dikicioglu E, Cullaci N, et al. Immunohistochemical findings in notalgia paresthetica. *Dermatology*. 2002;204:88–93.

57. Fantini F, Zorzi F, Rizzitelli G, et al. Notalgia paresthetica: clinical, pathological and immunohistochemical observations in 12 cases. *Eur J Dermatol*. 1994;4:649–653.

58. Lauria G, Cornblath DR, Johansson O, et al. EFNS guidelines on the use of skin biopsy in the diagnosis of peripheral neuropathy. *Eur J Neurol*. 2005;12:747–758.

59. Westermark P, Ridderström E, Vahlquist A. Macular posterior pigmentary incontinence. Its Relation to Macular Amyloidosis and Notalgia Paresthetica. *Acta Derm Venereol*. 1996;76:302–304.

60. Şavk E, Bölükba O, Akyol A, et al. Open pilot study on oxcarbazepine for the treatment of notalgia paresthetica. *J Am Acad Dermatol*. 2001;45:630–632.

61. Loosemore MP, Bordeaux JS, Bernhard JD. Gabapentin treatment for notalgia paresthetica, a common isolated peripheral sensory neuropathy. *J Eur Acad Dermatol Venereol*. 2007;21:1440–1441.

62. Winhoven SM, Coulson ICH, Bottomley WW. Brachioradial pruritus: response to treatment with gabapentin. *Br J Dermatol*. 2004;150:786–787.

63. Weinfeld PK. Successful treatment of notalgia paresthetica with botulinum toxin type A. *Arch Dermatol*. 2007;143:980–982.

64. Şavk E, Şavk O, Sendur F. Transcutaneous electrical nerve stimulation offers partial relief in notalgia paresthetica patients with a relevant spinal pathology. *J Dermatol*. 2007;34:315–319.

65. Şavk E, Şavk O. On brachioradial pruritus and nostalgia paresthetica. *J Am Acad Dermatol*. 2004;50:800–801.

66. Wallengren J. Neuroanatomy and neurophysiology of itch. *Dermatol Ther*. 2005;18:292–303.

67. Seror P, Seror R. Meralgia paresthetica: clinical and electrophysiological diagnosis in 120 cases. *Muscle Nerve*. 2006;33:650–654.

68. Hirose CB, McGarvey WC. Peripheral nerve entrapments. *Foot Ankle Clin*. 2004;9:255–269.

# Chapter 25
# Brachioradial Pruritus

Martin Marziniak and Sonja Ständer

Brachioradial pruritus (BRP) is a localized itch in the skin of the lateral aspects of the arms. It was first reported by Waisman in 1968, who termed it solar pruritus of the elbows, describing its occurrence in patients in Florida who showed a localized itch of the skin on the dorsolateral aspect of the arm.[1] In 1984, 14 patients were reported from South Africa[2] and a group of 110 Hawaiian patients with chronic intermittent pruritus has been described in two early reports.[3,4] All of the patients described earlier lived in the tropics or subtropics, therefore it was suggested that BRP is a photoneurological disorder caused by sun-induced damage to nerve endings that results in pruritus and altered sensation in susceptible individuals.[3,5] There has been some controversy about the origin of BRP and another theory favors cervical root impingement as the cause of BRP.[6]

**Epidemiology:** BRP is a rare form of pruritus. The prevalence of BRP seems to be higher in countries with a high sunlight exposure, but prevalence or incidence rates are not available. BRP could be found more often in females than in males and patients are between 39 and 72 years of age.[7] One report about familial BRP discussed an autosomal dominant transmission with a preferential expression in women,[8] but no other reports about inheritance are published in a peer-reviewed journal.

**Clinical picture:** BRP affects a circumscribed area of the lateral aspect of the arms (Fig. 25.1). It is often bilateral and covers classically the skin over the brachioradial muscle and is therefore named BRP. The area of pruritus can extend to the shoulders and the upper thorax and distally to the wrist, involving one or all of the C5–C8 cervical nerve root segments (Fig. 3.1). In the affected area allodynia and/or dysesthesias and paresthesias (tingling, burning) may be present. A deterioration of pruritus was reported during nights.[9]

Many patients notice that the disease had been progressive, the pruritus either more intense, involving increasing areas of skin or becoming more persistent. Usually BRP is not accompanied by primary dermatitis. Due to pruritus, many patients develop some kind of scratch lesions ranging from excoriations to prurigo nodularis in the affected area (Fig. 25.2).

**Pathogenesis:** There has been some controversy about the origin of BRP: on the one hand, a long-term exposure to UV-light has been described as a major trigger factor[10] and on the other hand, a second theory favors cervical root impingement as the cause of BRP.[6]

Seasonal variation of the occurrence of BRP was reported in regions with temperate climate.[11] A relapse of pruritus in summer with a peak at the end of summer was noticed, and pruritus was restricted to sun-exposed regions such as upper and lower arm, shoulders, neck, or upper thorax. This has lead to the hypothesis and its first name: solar pruritus.[10] The first patients with BRP have been reported from sunny countries such as Hawaii[4] and South Africa,[3] and a relapse of the BRP was not reported in those patients.

These observations suggest that long-term exposure to UV light induces local hyperexcitability of sensory nerve fibers in the skin. In high temperate climates the damage to the local nerve fibers and their functional impairment is probably reversible during winter times and new UV-exposure leads to an exacerbation during the next summer. Cutaneous innervation in 16 patients with BRP taken in early autumn showed a reduced (minus 23%) number of intraepidermal nerve fibers (IENFs) stained with the panaxonal marker protein gene product 9.5 (PGP 9.5), a reduced number of sensory, mainly intradermal, nerve fibers immunoreactive for calcitonin gene-related peptide (CGRP) and capsaicin-sensitive nerve fibers immunoreactive for the

L. Misery and S. Ständer (eds.), *Pruritus*
DOI 10.1007/978-1-84882-322-8_25, © Springer-Verlag London Limited 2010

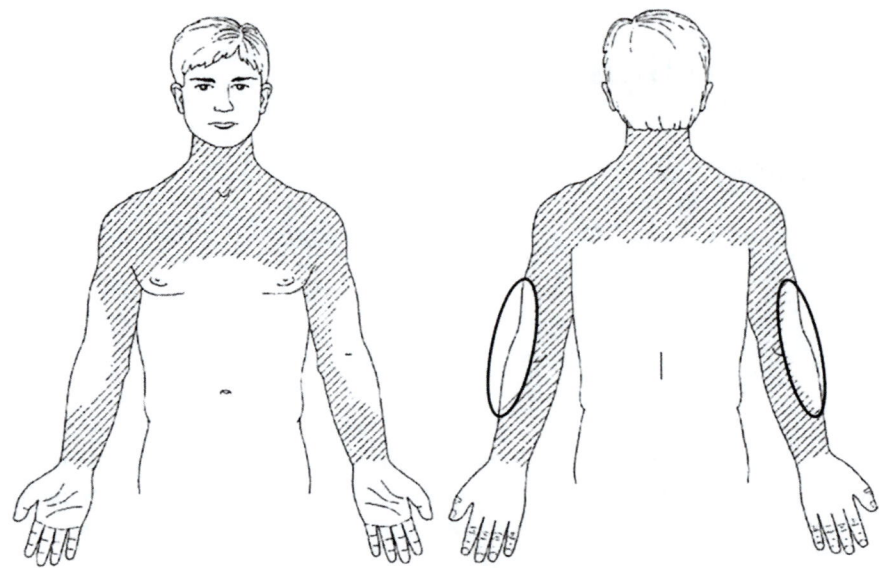

**Fig. 25.1** Skin areas which may be affected by BRP. In most patients, pruritus starts in the skin over the brachioradial muscle (circles). Pruritus may spread over the arms, the shoulders and the upper thorax and distally to the wrist (modified from ref.[7])

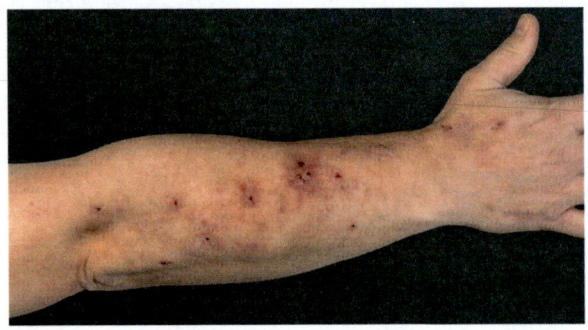

**Fig. 25.2** Patient with BRP and corresponding scratch lesions on the right arm

vanilloid-receptor (TRPV1).[5] Four patients of this group received another punch biopsy after disapperance of BRP during winter time and the number of IENFs normalized and was not significantly different from healthy controls.[5] The authors speculate that the cutaneous innervation resembles skin biopsies of patients after serial phototherapy.[12]

There are several unanswered questions concerning this hypothesis[6]:

1. The observations do not explain the complaints of patients with BRP around the whole year.

2. Most cases of dermatologically photosensitive diseases involve the arms and the hands, if not the face, and are sharply demarcated at the sleeves.
3. BRP, unlike all other sensitivity disorders, has not been reported in children.

Several articles suggest an association of cervical radiographic changes (spondylosis, foraminal narrowing, spurs, narrowing of disk space, cervical ribs) and BRP leading to cervical nerve root impingement, involving one (most common C6) or all of the C5–C8 cervical nerve root segments (Fig. 3.3).[2,6] The question, whether the radiographic changes are causal or coincidental, is not finally answered. The authenticity of the association may be emphasized by the fact, that comparable findings have been described in notalgia paresthetica, another localized pruritus disorder.

There is no article that compares the incidence and the patterns of radiographic cervical spine abnormalities in patients with BRP to an age- and sex-matched control group. Gore et al.[13] investigated radiographic changes of the cervical spine in 200 asymptomatic men and women to determine the effect of aging on the cervical spine and re-evaluated a subgroup of 159 people 10 years later.[14] Of those, 35% had radiographic changes of the cervical spine by the age of 45, and

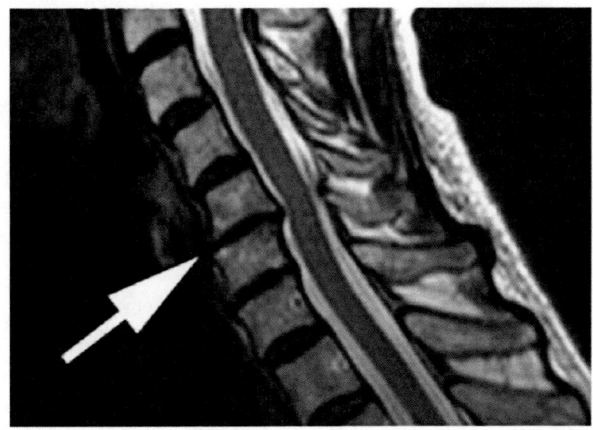

**Fig. 25.3** Magnetic resonance image of a patient with BRP Osteophyte at vertrebral bodies C5/C6 (arrow) leading to moderate compression of spinal nerve structures (modified from **ref**.[30])

70% of women and 95% of men had these changes by the age of 65.[13] Interestingly 10 years later, only 15% of the participants had developed pain, although in 44% of the participants the degeneration showed progression and 19% showed an initial degeneration on the second roentgenogram.[14] In comparison to these data, 100% of radiographically examined patients with BRP had abnormalities of the cervical spine in a study by Goodkin et al.[7] Therefore, data suggest a higher prevalence of cervical radiographic changes in patients with BRP than in asymptomatic controls. The hypothesis of cervical damage of nerve fibers is supported by electrophysiological studies in BRP describing hints for cervical radiculopathy,[15] although these data have to be confirmed in a larger population.

Additionally, case reports about a patient who was able to trigger symptoms of BRP by changes in the neck position,[16] about a patient with a cervical rib and hypertrophic transverse process of C7 and the remission of BRP after an operation,[17] and about two patients who developed BRP after a motor vehicle accident with whiplash injury[2,18] suggest a possible role of spinal traumata as a cause of BRP. Other case reports describe a spinal ependymoma as a cause of BRP[19,20] or a spinal cavernous hemangioma leading to itch and dysesthesias of the inner side of one arm.[21] Therefore spinal pathological changes may lead to a spinal hyperexcitability by interfering with the descending inhibitory pathways.

There are several unanswered questions concerning this hypothesis[22]:

1. Cervical spine disease alone does not explain the exacerbation of the symptoms during summer time.
2. There are a high number of patients (between 5% and 77%) with BRP without any hints of cervical or spinal pathological changes.[3,15]

In summary, it is believed that both cervical spine disease and sun-induced cutaneous nerve injury are important contributors of variable degrees in patients with BRP leading to a damage of afferent nerve fibers with accentuation of the itch signalling fibers.[23]

**Diagnostics:** In patients who are susceptive for BRP, a skin and histological investigation should rule out any other possible underlying dermatosis. Other underlying diseases such as porphyria cutanea tarda may induce, next to pruritus of the hands, pruritus and excoriations at the lower arms also. Accordingly, laboratory investigation should rule out other underlying diseases. Some authors report on association between diabetes mellitus, polyneuropathy and brachiradial pruritus.[23] Therefore, a laboratory testing for yet unidentified diabetes mellitus is advisable. To rule out spinal compression, a magnetic resonance imaging (MRI) scan of the cervical and thoracic spinal column is recommended. If pathological changes are observed upon MRI, a detailed neurological examination, including electroneurography and if necessary electromyography is advisable.

**Therapy:** Many patients with BRP report using ice packs or cold or wet towels to relieve their itch, especially during nights. Some authors have discussed whether this sign is pathognomonic for BRP and have called it "the ice-pack sign."[7,24] Protection of the affected area from sun exposure with clothing has been reported as giving relief.[25]

Medical treatment of BRP seems to be difficult. Controlled double blind studies fulfilling the international criteria do not exist. Topical capsaicin is described as beneficial in several case reports, but many patients did not tolerate the initial burning and therefore the compliance is reduced.[4,26,27] Furthermore, in the only small double blind placebo controlled study, 13 patients with BRP and symmetric, bilateral symptoms received two identical tubes with either capsaicin 0.025% or vehicle cream and had to apply randomized cream to the right and left arm each at the same time. There was no benefit for capsaicin in comparison to placebo, although 12 out of 13 patients reported a reduction of the itch of about 65% on both sides.[10] There is a significant drawback of the study: due to the simultaneous bilateral application systemic and central nervous system effects could not be subtracted from the placebo effect.

Besides the topical application, anticonvulsants and antidepressants, also used for the treatment of neuropathic pain, lead to an improvement or regression of BRP. The number of published articles is very low: gabapentin in the dose between 900–1,800 mg was successfully used in four patients,[28–30] amitryptyline 25 mg/day in two patients,[26] carbamazepine and lamotrigine in one patient each.[9,31] The authors have used gabapentin (900–2,700 mg) and pregabalin (300–450 mg) with success in a large number of patients (Marziniak and Ständer, personal observation).

There are several reports about nondrug treatment:

After a single cervical spine manipulation six patients with BRP and a history of neck problems reported complete resolution of the pruritus for 2 days (one patient) to several weeks (two patients) to months (two patients) to permanent relief (one patient). The same patients again had relief after a second manipulation.[9] Additionally, four out of eight patients with BRP without a history of cervical neck pain had a longstanding (permanent: two patients; several years: one patient; several months: onepatient) relief of BRP after cervical spine manipulations, the four patients who did not benefit refused a second treatment.[9] Acupuncture of the paravertebral muscles lead to a total resolution of pruritus in 75% of the patients with a 37% relapse rate within 1–12 months following treatment.[32]

Taken together, a combined therapy of sun avoidance, intermittent cooling and an anticonvulsant drug seems to be a promising therapy for BRP, until better evidence based studies and treating guidelines come into existence.

# References

1. Waisman M. Solar pruritus of the elbows (Brachioradial summer pruritus). *Arch Dermatol.* 1968;98:481–485.
2. Heyl T. Brachioradial pruritus. *Arch Dermatol.* 1983; 119:115–116.
3. Walcyk PJ, Elpern DJ. Brachioradial pruritus: a tropical dermopathy. *Br J Dermatol.* 1986;115:177–180.
4. Knight TE, Hayashi T. Solar (brachioradial) pruritus – response to capsaicin cream. *Int J Dermatol.* 1994;33: 206–209.
5. Wallengren J, Sundler F. Brachioradial pruritus is associated with a reduction in cutaneous innervation that normalizes during the symptom-free remissions. *J Am Acad Dermatol.* 2005;52:142–145.
6. Fisher DA. Brachioradial pruritus: a recurrent solar dermopathy. *J Am Acad Dermatol.* 1999;42:656–657.
7. Goodkin R, Wingard E, Bernhard JD. Brachioradial pruritus: cervical spine disease and neurogenic/neuropathic pruritus. *J Am Acad Dermatol.* 2003;48:521–524.
8. Wallengren J, Dahlbäck K. Familial brachioradial pruritus. *Br J Dermatol.* 2005;153:1016–1018.
9. Tait CP, Grigg E, Quirk CJ. Brachioradial pruritus and cervical spine manipulation. *Australas J Dermatol.* 1998;39:168–170.
10. Wallengren J. Brachioradial pruritus: a recurrent solar dermopathy. *J Am Acad Dermatol.* 1998;39:803–806.
11. Veien NK, Hattel T, Laurberg G, et al. Brachioradial pruritus. *J Am Acad Dermatol.* 2001;44:704–705.
12. Wallengren J, Sundler F. Phototherapy induces loss of epidermal and dermal nerve fibers. *Acta Derm Venerol.* 2004;84:111–115.
13. Gore DR, Sepic SB, Gardner GM. Roentgenographic fndings of the cervical spine in asymptomatic people. *Spine.* 1986;11:521–524.
14. Gore DR. Roentgenographic findings in the cervical spine in asymptomatic persons: a ten-year follow-up. *Spine.* 2001;26: 2463–2466.
15. Cohen AD, Masalha R, Medvedovsky E, et al. Brachioradial pruritus: a symptom of neuropathy. *J Am Acad Dermatol.* 2003;48:825–828.
16. Abbott LG. Neuropathic pruritus. *Australas J Dermatol.* 1998;39:803–806.
17. Rongioletti F. Pruritus as presenting sign of cervical rib. *Lancet.* 1992;339:55.
18. Fisher DA. Brachioradial pruritus wanted: a sure cause (and cure) for brachioradial pruritus. *Int J Dermatol.* 1997;36: 817–818.
19. Kavak A, Dosoglu M. Can a spinal cord tumor cause brachioradial pruritus? *J Am Acad Dermatol.* 2002;46:437–440.
20. Wiesner T, Leinweber B, Quasthoff S, et al. Itch, skin lesions – and a stiff neck. *Lancet.* 2007;370:290.
21. Vuadens Ph, Regli F, Uske A. Segmental pruritus and intramedullary vascular malformation. *Schweiz Arch Neurol Psychiatr.* 1994;145:14–16.
22. Wallengren J. Brachioradial pruritus: a recurrent solar dermopathy. *J Am Acad Dermatol.* 1999;41:657–658.
23. Bernhard JD. Brachioradial pruritus: a recurrent solar dermopathy. *J Am Acad Dermatol.* 1999;41:658.
24. Bernhard JD, Bordeaux JS. Medical pearl: the ice-pack sign in brachioradial pruritus. *J Am Acad Dermatol.* 2005;52:1073.
25. Orton DI, Wakelin SH, George SA. Brachioradial photopruritus – a rare chronic photodermatosis in Europe. *Br J Dermatol.* 1996;135:486–487.
26. Barry R, Roger S. Brachioradial pruritus – an enigmatic entity. *Clin Exp Dermatol.* 2004;29:637–638.
27. Goodless DR, Eaglstein WH. Brachioradial pruritus: treatment with topical capsaicin. *J Am Acad Dermatol.* 1993;29:783–784.
28. Bueller HA, Bernhard JD, Dubroff LM. Gabapentin treatment for brachioradial pruritus. *J Eur Acad Dermatol Venereol.* 1999;13:227–230.

29. Winhoven SM, Coulson ICH, Bottomley WW. Brachioradial pruritus: response to treatment with gabapentin. *Br J Dermatol*. 2004;150:786–787.

30. Schürmeyer-Horst F, Fischbach R, Nabavi D, et al. Brachioradialer pruritus. *Hautarzt*. 2006;57:523–527.

31. Crevitis L. Brachioradial pruritus – a peculiar neuropathic disorder. *Clin Neurol Neurosurg*. 2006;108:803–805.

32. Stellon A. Neurogenic pruritus. An unrecognised problem? A retrospective case series of treatment by acupuncture. *Acupunct Med*. 2002;20:186–190.

# Chapter 26
# Other Neurological Causes of Itch

Martin Marziniak, Esther Pogatzki-Zahn, and Stefan Evers

Lesions of the central nervous system are another rare cause of neuropathic pruritus. The most extensive review describes 27 cases.[1] Diseases that may cause localized pruritus include stroke, brain tumors, brain abscesses, and transverse myelitis. Most of these patients report additional sensory disturbances leading to hyper- or hypoesthesia. These additional symptoms may help the clinician to distinguish cases of central neurogenic pruritus from others of different causes.

Brain regions that are involved in central itch processing are the posterior part of the ventromedial thalamic nucleus and the dorsal insular cortex, a region involved in different sensory modalities such as thermoregulation, visceral sensations, thirst, and hunger.[2] Pruritus induced by histamine injections leads to a coactivation of the anterior cingulate cortex, supplementary motor area, and inferior parietal lobe predominantly in the left hemisphere.[3] Neurological disorders leading to lesions of these brain regions may provoke itch phenomena.

Anticonvulsants (gabapentin, pregabaline) and tricyclic antidepressants seem to be the drugs of choice in neurogenic pruritus due to lesions of the central nervous system, although randomized placebo controlled studies are not available.

Neuropathic pruritus following *stroke* is probably an under-recognized poststroke symptom.[4] The largest case series described four patients after an ischemic stroke in the middle cerebral artery territory and five patients with an impairment of the internal capsule (two with cerebral hemorrhage and three with an ischemic stroke); they all had pruritus contralateral to the cerebral lesion. The authors discuss an involvement of thalamic structures that lead to the itch phenomena.[5] Additionally, one report described unilateral pruritus after a cerebral infarction of the parietal lobe.[6] Another study reported *trigeminal trophic syndrome* after brain stem infarction.[7] Trigeminal trophic

syndrome includes laceration of the ipsilateral nostrils, delayed wound healing, deep facial ulcerations caused by itch that urged patients to scratch these areas. It has also been described as a rare complication after local anesthetic injection into the Gasserian ganglion for trigeminal neuralgia therapy.[8]

Furthermore, pruritus is described in *infectious diseases* with primarily central nervous system affection. Severe generalized pruritus was reported as the first symptom in three patients with *Creutzfeld-Jakob disease* in a case series of 26 patients.[9] All three patients underwent an extensive work-up for pruritus without a result and therapy with antihistamines was not successful. The authors speculated that the origin of the pruritus is due to lesions in the central nervous system in the brainstem.[9] Unilateral pruritus was reported after a *Nocardia* brain abscess in the central region with a contralateral sensorimotor hemiparesis.[10]

Andreev et al. studied skin manifestations associated with *brain tumours*, and 13 out of 77 patients reported pruritus. Seven complained of general pruritus and six of pruritus of the nostrils. Interestingly, two out of the seven patients with generalized pruritus reported a resolution of itch after the treatment of their tumor.[11] Two children were reported with severe, episodic, unilateral facial itch due to brainstem gliomas and disappearance of the pruritus after the resection of the tumor.[12]

Paroxysmal itching has been described in *multiple sclerosis* (MS).[13–15] Seventeen out of 377 MS patients reported pruritus in different parts of their body and in diverse intensities.[16] These attacks last from several seconds to a few minutes and may occur several times a day. The very short form of paroxysmal itching shows similarities with the Lhermitte's sign, which is a sudden, transient, electric-like shock extending down

L. Misery and S. Ständer (eds.), *Pruritus*,
DOI 10.1007/978-1-84882-322-8_26, © Springer-Verlag London Limited 2010

the arms, trunk, or legs on bending the head forward, and which is due to demyelinating cervical spinal lesions in MS. The localized, sometimes symmetric and paroxysmal pattern of this pruritus supports an origin in the central nervous system, and it is conceivable that demyelinating spinal cord lesions affect itch-selective neurons in lamina I of the spinal cord or their corresponding inhibitory interneurons.[17] Furthermore, paroxysmal itching is described in coincidence with the neurological recovery of spinal symptoms[15] and may be a rare symptom of spinal reorganization.

Other spinal cord lesions may also provoke pruritus: a 43 year old black woman reported severe pruritus and allodynia due to *transverse myelitis* without motor weakness,[18] another patient sought treatment for pruritus and lichen simplex chronicus unilateral in the C5 dermatome due to *syringomyelia*[19] and three patients suffered from severe localized pruritus provoked by *spinal cavernous hemangioma*.[20–22] Other reports of spinal tumors provoking pruritus are described in a separate chapter of this book.

*Polyneuropathy* of the large fibers as a cause of pruritus is often mentioned in reviews. However, itch as a cause of polyneuropathy is seen in pruritus patients with comorbidities like uremia or diabetes. Studies and reports on patients with polyneuropathy and pruritus but without a metabolic disease could rarely be found in an extensive Medline research. One cohort study of 703 patients with neurofibromatosis type 1 reported itching in 19.3% of the patients and described an association between the presence of pruritus and mortality among children.[23] A second study with eight patients mentioned an association between nodular prurigo and subclinical peripheral neuropathy.[24] In summary, the association between polyneuropathy and pruritus has not been finally proven yet.

# References

1. Canavero S, Bonicalzi V, Massa-Micon B. Central neurogenic pruritus: a literature review. *Acta Neurol Belg.* 1997;97:244–247.
2. Steinhoff M, Bienenstock J, Schmelz M, et al. Neurophysiological, neuroimmunological, and neuroendocrine basis of pruritus. *J Invest Dermatol.* 2006;126:1705–1718.
3. Mochizuki H, Tashiro M, Kano M, et al. Imaging of central itch modulation in the human brain using positron emission tomography. *Pain.* 2003;105:339–346.
4. Kimyai-Asadi A, Nousari HC, Kimyai-Asadi T, et al. Poststroke pruritus. *Stroke.* 1999;30:692–693.
5. Massey EW. Unilateral neurogenic pruritus following stroke. *Stroke.* 1984;15:901–903.
6. Shapiro PE, Braun CW. Unilateral pruritus after a stroke. *Arch Dermatol.* 1987;123:1527–1530.
7. Fitzek S, Baumgärtner U, Marx J, et al. Pain and itch in Wallenberg`s syndrome: anatomical-functional correlations. *Suppl Clin Neurophysiol.* 2006;58:187–194.
8. Rashid RM, Khachemoune A. Trigeminal trophic syndrome. *J Eur Acad Dermatol Venereol.* 2007;21:725–731.
9. Shabtai H, Nisipeanu P, Chapman J, et al. Pruritus in Creutzfeld-Jakob disease. *Neurology.* 1996;46:940–941.
10. Sullivan MJ, Drake ME. Unilateral pruritus and Nocardia abscess. *Neurology.* 1984;34:828–829.
11. Andreev VC, Petkov I. Skin manifestations associated with tumours of the brain. *Br J Dermatol.* 1975;92:675–678.
12. Summers CG, MacDonald JT. Paroxysmal facial itch: a presenting sign of childhood brainstem glioma. *J Child Neurol.* 1988;3:189–192.
13. King CA, Huff J, Jorizzo JL. Unilateral neurogenic pruritus: paroxysmal itching associated with central nervous system lesions. *Ann Intern Med.* 1982;97:222–223.
14. Koeppel MC, Bramont C, Ceccaldi M, et al. Paroxysmal pruritus in multiple sclerosis. *Br J Dermatol.* 1993;129:597–598.
15. Sandyk R. Paroxysmal itching in multiple sclerosis during treatment with external magnetic fields. *Int J Neurosci.* 1994;75:65–71.
16. Matthews WB, Comston A, Allen IV, et al. McAlpine's multiple sclerosis. Edinburgh: Churchill Livingstone; 1991:68.
17. Andrew D, Craig AD. Spinothalamic lamina I neurons selectively sensitive to histamine: a central neural pathway for itch. *Nat Neurosci.* 2001;4:72–77.
18. Bond LD, Keough GC. Neurogenic pruritus: a case of pruritus induced by transverse myelitis. *Br J Dermatol.* 2003;149:204–205.
19. Kinsella LJ, Carney-Godley K, Feldman E. Lichen simplex chronicus as the initial manifestation of intramedullary neoplasm and syringomyelia. *Neurosurgery.* 1992;30:418–420.
20. Vuadens P, Regli F, Dolivo M, et al. Segmental pruritus and intramedullary vascular malformation. *Schweiz Arch Neurol Psychiatr.* 1994;145:13–16.
21. Sandroni P. Central neuropathic itch: a new treatment option? *Neurology.* 2002;59:778–779.
22. Dey DD, Landrum O, Oaklander AL. Central neuropathic itch from spinal-cord cavernous hemangioma: a human case, a possible animal model, and hypotheses about pathogenesis. *Pain.* 2005;113:233–237.
23. Khosrotehrani K, Bastuji-Garin S, Riccardi VM, et al. Subcutaneous neurofibromas are associated with mortality in neurofibromatosis 1: a cohort study of 703 patients. *Am J Med Genet A.* 2005;132:49–53.
24. Bharati A, Wilson NJ. Peripheral neuropathy associated with nodular prurigo. *Clin Exp Dermatol.* 2007;32:67–70.

# Chapter 27
# Chronic Kidney Disease-Associated Pruritus

Thomas Mettang

## 27.1 Introduction

Chronic kidney disease-associated pruritus (CKD-associated pruritus, formerly named "uraemic pruritus") remains a frequent and sometimes tormenting problem in patients with advanced or end-stage renal disease.[1] Many attempts have been made to relieve this bothersome symptom in affected patients, but with limited success in general. After a new treatment option is reported to be effective, only a little time elapses before conflicting results concerning CKD-associated pruritus are published. In the meantime patients' and physicians' mood changes from euphoria to disillusionment. This happened with erythropoetin[2, 3] and naltrexone[4, 5] as the last propagated treatment modalities in this respect.

The main obstacle in the effort to create effective treatment modalities is the incomplete knowledge of the underlying pathophysiological mechanisms. Furthermore, given the great clinical heterogeneity of CKD-associated pruritus, systematic studies are hard to obtain and therefore sparse.

## 27.2 Clinical Features of CKD-Associated Pruritus

Intensity and spatial distribution of pruritus vary significantly over time and some patients with renal disease are affected to varying degrees throughout the duration of their disease. The intensity of CKD-associated pruritus ranges from sporadic discomfort to complete restlessness during day and night. Initially, patients with CKD-associated pruritus do not show any changes in skin appearance, except for common changes in skin color and a frequently observed xerosis. Excoriation by scratching with or without impetigo can occur as secondary phenomenon, and occasionally prurigo nodularis is observed (Fig. 1.1a–c). There are interindividual differences in the spatial distribution of CKD-associated pruritus: 25–50% of patients with CKD-associated pruritus complain about generalized pruritus.[6, 7] In the remaining patients CKD-associated pruritus seems to affect the back, the face, and the shunt arm predominantly.[8] In about 25% of patients with CKD-associated pruritus, it is most severe during or immediately after dialysis.[8]

## 27.3 Prevalence of CKD-Associated Pruritus

While in the initial days of dialysis treatment CKD-associated pruritus was a very common problem, it appears that its incidence has declined over the past 20 years. In the early 1970s Young and coworkers reported that about 85%[9] of patients were affected by CKD-associated pruritus. This number decreased to 50–60% in the late 1980s.[10] In one of our studies performed in Germany, only 22% of all patients undergoing dialysis complained about pruritus at the time they were questioned.[5] However, in the past 5 years several studies have been published showing a higher prevalence of CKD-associated pruritus. Duque and coworkers, e.g., found CKD-associated pruritus to be present in 58% of younger patients on hemodialysis.[11] Similarly, Narita et al. could demonstrate that nearly 70% of patients undergoing hemodialysis were suffering from CKD-associated pruritus. Furthermore, in their study CKD-associated pruritus seemed to be an independent risk factor for all-cause mortality.[12] Data from the DOPPS (Dialysis outcome and practice patterns study) study in a very large cohort of patients on dialysis revealed that ~45% of patients were suffering from CKD-associated pruritus.[13] Some of the representative studies are shown in Table 27.1.

L. Misery and S. Ständer (ed.), *Pruritus*
DOI 10.1007/978-1-84882-322-8_27, © Springer-Verlag London Limited 2010

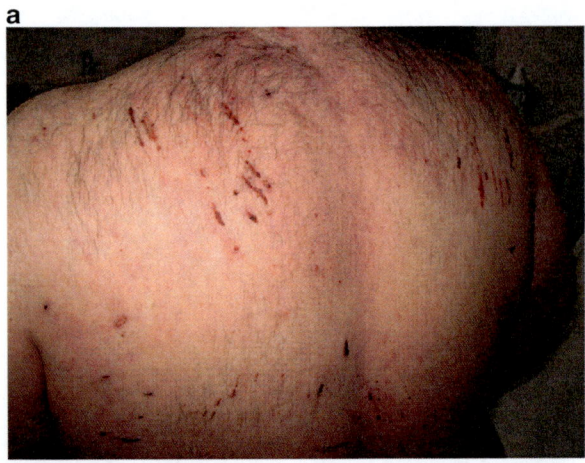

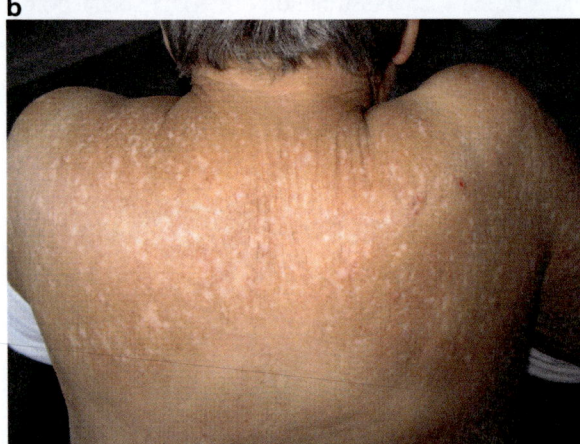

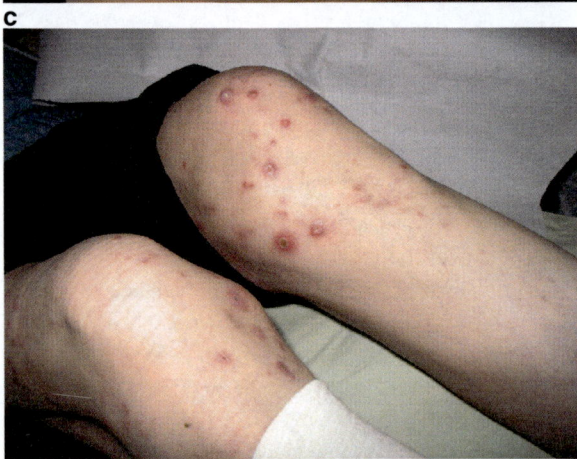

**Fig. 27.1** Skin conditions observed in patients with CKD-associated pruritus: **a**: scratches on the arm hosting the fistula. **b**: deep scars on the shoulders and at the back of a woman on hemodialysis. **c**: prurigo nodularis with excoreations and superinfection on the forearm of a patient on peritoneal dialysis

Interestingly, severe pruritus is very rare in pediatric patients on dialysis. In a systematic review of all German pediatric dialysis centers involving 199 children, only 9.1% of the children on dialysis complained about pruritus. Moreover, the intensity reported was not very severe in the affected patients[14] (Fig. 27.2).

## 27.4 Pathophysiological Concepts of CKD-Associated Pruritus

In the past 20 years different hypotheses on the pathophysiology of CKD-associated pruritus have been made. The most prominent concept focused on parathyroid hormone (PTH) as a culprit compound because CKD-associated pruritus seemed to be most severe in patients with marked hyperparathyroidism and resolved after parathyroidektomy.[15, 16] However, subsequent data could not confirm this theory.[17] Similarly, the concept of precipitated calcium phosphate crystals in the setting of elevated serum calcium and phosphate levels as the responsible event in CKD-associated pruritus[18] could not be sustained. Recently, it was discussed, though controversially, whether histamine secreted by proliferated mast cells might cause CKD-associated pruritus.[19] However, like the theories mentioned above, the "histamine story" ceased because of conflicting results.[10, 20, 21] It is still not clear as to what extent alterations in skin structure do contribute to the pathophysiology of CKD-associated pruritus.[22]

Xerosis is a frequent symptom in patients on dialysis, afflicting between 50 and 100% patients.[23] Most frequently, the lower extremities and the forearms are affected. It has been reported that CKD-associated pruritus is more prevalent and more severe in patients with xerosis, suggesting that xerosis might be an aggravating factor.

The newer concepts of CKD-associated pruritus are presented in detail in the following.

## 27.5 The "Immuno-Hypothesis"

In the light of several observations and information from other studies, there is increasing evidence that CKD-associated pruritus is rather a systemic than an

**Table 27.1**  Prevalence of CKD-associated pruritus reported in the literature*

| Author (Year) | Prevalence % (n) | | Anamnestic UP % (n) | | Statistical relevance |
|---|---|---|---|---|---|
| | HD | CAPD | HD | CAPD | |
| Young (1973) | 86 (86) | | | | |
| Altmeyer (1982) | 78 (28) | | | | |
| Gilchrest (1982) | 37 (237) | | | 41 (237) | |
| Bencini (1985) | 41 (54) | 16 (19) | | | HD > CAPD |
| Matsumoto (1985) | 57 (51) | | | | |
| Parfrey (1988) | 49 | 50 (97) | | | n.s. |
| Bäckdahl (1988) | 66 (29) | | | | |
| Mettang (1990) | 64 (28) | 50 (26) | 17 (28) | 21 (26) | n.s. |
| Albert (1991) | 54 (71) | 48 (79) | | | n.s. |
| Balaskas (1993) | 54 (76) | 62 | | | n.s. |
| Pauli-Magnus (1999) | 22 (378) | 43 (44) | | | CAPD>HD |
| Pisoni (2005) | 46% (3690) | | | | |
| Duque (2006) | 58% (105) | | | | |
| Narita (2005) | 70% (1773) | | | | |

*Homodialysis = HD, Chronic ambulatory pnitoneal dialysis = CAPD, UP = Uraemic Pruritu, N.S. = Not significant

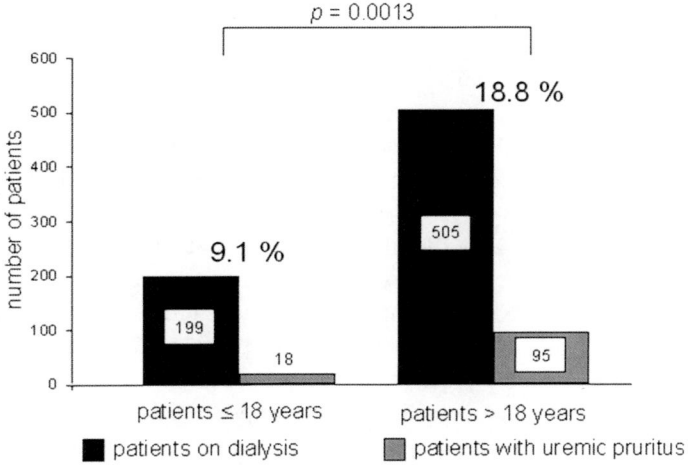

**Fig. 27.2**  Prevalence of CKD-associated pruritus in children on dialysis (18 years or younger) and in adult dialysis patients (older than 18 years). Prevalence of uremic pruritus in children is significantly lower than in adult patients (chi-square test[11])

isolated skin disease and that derangements of the immune system with a proinflammatory pattern may be involved in the pathogenesis of CKD-associated pruritus. This hypothesis is confirmed by several lines of evidence.

Gilchrest et al. showed that tanning patients with ultraviolet B (UVB) light led to relief of CKD-associated pruritus in a considerable number of patients.[24] This effect could be demonstrated even when only one-half of the body was irradiated. This observation led to the conclusion that there must be a systemic effect of UVB radiation. Interestingly, UVB

exposure was shown to be a pronounced modulator of Th1 and Th2 lymphocyte differentiation and an attenuator of Th1 expression.[25]

Some studies have shown that increasing the dose of dialysis led to an improvement of CKD-associated pruritus.[26] Consequently, the lower incidence of CKD-associated pruritus over the last decades has been attributed to the improvements in dialysis modalities. Increasing concerns about adequate dialysis dosage and the wide use of Kt/V- or creatinine- clearance-guided dialysis regimens might have contributed to the decreased incidence of CKD-associated pruritus. In addition, dialysis efficacy has increased following the use of high-flux dialysis membranes with larger surfaces and improved biocompatibility with the introduction of synthetic fibers, such as polysulfone or polyacrylnitrile. These new materials activate the complement system and leukocytes to a much lower degree than conventional, less biocompatible materials, such as cuprophane, generating less proinflammatory cytokines.[27]

It has been shown that thalidomide and tacrolimus (as ointment) are effective in the therapy of CKD-associated pruritus, at least to a certain degree.[28, 29] Thalidomide, which is currently used as an immunomodulator to treat graft-versus-host reactions, suppresses tumor necrosis factor alpha (TNF-$\alpha$) production and leads to a predominant differentiation of Th2 lymphocytes with suppression of interleukin-2 (IL-2)-producing Th1 cells.[30] A similar effect can be observed with tacrolimus, which also suppresses differentiation of Th1-lymphocytes and the ensuing IL-2 production.[31]

After kidney transplantation, patients almost never complain of CKD-associated pruritus as long as immunosuppressive therapy including cyclosporine is administered, even when a substantial loss of transplant function has occurred.[32]

The bottom line of all these observations is that they point to a substantial role of the immunological mechanisms in the pathogenesis of CKD-associated pruritus. Numerous factors are probably involved, including IL-2 and IL-6, both secreted by activated Th1 lymphocytes. In line with this hypothesis, patients receiving IL-2 for the treatment of malignant diseases frequently report tormenting pruritus.[33] Additionally, it has been shown that intradermally applied IL-2 had a rapid, although weak, pruritogenic effect.[34] In a study of Virga et al., it could be demonstrated that patients on hemodialysis with CKD-associated pruritus had significantly higher C-reactive protein (CRP) levels than those without CKD-associated pruritus.[35]

Results of a multicenter study initiated by our group revealed that patients with CKD-associated pruritus exhibited a more pronounced Th1 differentiation than patients without CKD-associated pruritus, as determined by measuring intracytoplasmatic TNF-$\alpha$ in CD4 cells (Fig. 27.3). Additionally CRP and IL levels in the blood of patients with CKD-associated pruritus were significantly increased.[36] These results may support the hypothesis that an inflammatory state conveys CKD-associated pruritus.

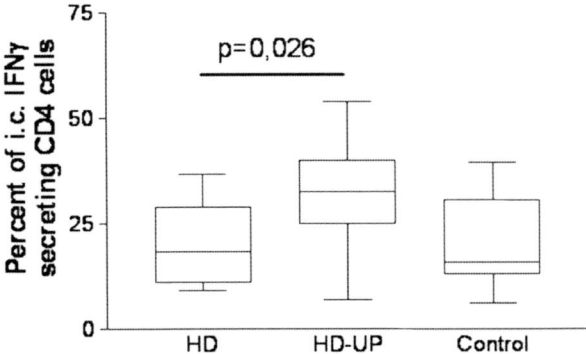

**Fig. 27.3** Differences in i.c. IFN-secreting CD4 cells (TH1) in patients with and without CKD-associated pruritus[10]

## 27.6 The "Opioid Hypothesis"

This pathogenetical concept that changes in the opiodergic system might be involved in the pathophysiology of pruritus was first developed for cholestatic pruritus and supported by different lines of evidence. First, several $\mu$-receptor agonistic drugs are known to induce pruritus, particularly after central administration.[37, 38] Second, it could be demonstrated in animal studies that cholestasis is associated with an increased opioidergic tone.[39, 40] Third, the administration of opiate antagonists was successful in the treatment of cholestatic pruritus.[41, 42] It was suggested that cholestatic pruritus may be mediated by pathological changes in the central nervous system. This hypothesis was supported by the findings that a global downregulation of $\mu$-receptors occurred in the brain of cholestatic rats[43] and that in patients with chronic cholestasis an opiate withdrawal-like syndrome was precipitated by the administration of an oral opiate antagonist.[44]

In 1985, there was a first case report describing the successful treatment of CKD- associated pruritus by intravenous administration of the opiate antagonist naloxone.[45] The therapeutic use of opiate antagonists in patients with CKD-associated pruritus was based on the assumption that endogenous opiate peptides may also be involved in the pathogenesis of CKD- associated pruritus. A subsequent placebo-controlled clinical trial by Peer et al. showed that administration of the oral $\mu$-receptor antagonist naltrexone was associated with a significant decrease in pruritus perception in all of the treated patients with severe CKD-associated pruritus.[4] However, the number of patients studied was small and the treatment period (1 week) was short.

When trying to confirm the data from Peer et al. in a larger cohort (23 patients with moderate to severe CKD-associated pruritus) treated for a longer time period (4 weeks), we failed to obtain any statistically significant response to naltrexone.[5]

Recently, Kumagai developed the hypothesis that the activation of κ-receptors expressed by dermal cells and lymphocytes might lead to the suppression of pruritus sensation. Therefore, when these receptors are not adequately stimulated or μ-receptors are overexpressed, patients may experience more severe itching. (Kumagai, personal communication). In line with this hypothesis, it was tested whether κ-receptor agonists (nalfurafine) were able to reduce CKD-associated pruritus (see therapeutic options). Considering the conflicting results mentioned above, it remains to be established whether the opioidergic system plays a significant role in the pathophysiology of CKD-associated pruritus.

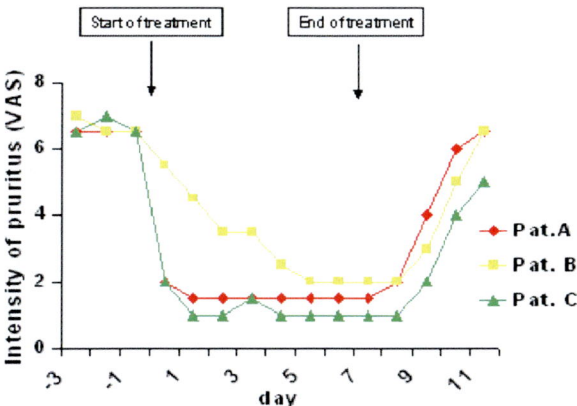

**Fig. 27.4**  Treatment of CKD-associated pruritus with tacrolimus ointment in three patients with otherwise refractory pruritus (adapted from ref. [29])

## 27.7  Therapeutic Options

As stated above, therapeutic options are sparse in CKD-associated pruritus. Most of the success stories turned into failure reports later. Based on the aforementioned pathophysiological concepts, we will focus on the following modalities:

1. Topical treatment with different ointments
2. Systemic treatment with μ-receptor antagonists and κ-agonists
3. Treatment with gabapentin and anti-inflammatory agents
4. Phototherapy

## 27.8  Topical Treatment with Tacrolimus and Gamma Linolenic Ointment

Being helpless with some severely tormented patients with CKD-associated pruritus, we decided to take a new approach.

It has been shown previously that administering tacrolimus ointment to the skin of patients with atopic dermatitis led to complete or partial resolution of illness-related symptoms.[46] In a preliminary study we reported on three patients undergoing peritoneal dialysis with severe CKD-associated pruritus. Patients who applied a 0.03% tacrolimus ointment twice daily to the most affected areas for a period of 7 days showed a dramatic improvement of CKD-associated pruritus (Fig. 27.4).[29] In a proof-of-concept study, Kuypers and colleagues treated 25 patients with tacrolimus ointment for a period of 6 weeks with great success.[47] Tacrolimus ointment seems to be a safe and highly effective short-term treatment option for patients suffering from severe CKD-associated pruritus.

In a recent study by Chen et al., a cream containing high concentrations of γ-linolenic acid and essential fatty acids was able to reduce itch in 17 patients suffering from severe CKD-associated pruritus.[48] The authors speculated that the effect of this treatment was conveyed by the anti-inflammatory properties of γ-linolenic acid as a precursor of the prostaglandin system.

## 27.9  Systemic Treatment with Naltrexone, a μ-Receptor Antagonist

We undertook a placebo-controlled, double-blind, crossover study in patients on hemodialysis or peritoneal dialysis with persistent, treatment-resistant pruritus. Of 422 patients, 93 suffered from pruritus and 23 were eligible for the study. Patients started either with a 4-week naltrexone sequence (50 mg/day) or matched placebo. Pruritus intensity was scored daily by the visual analog scale (VAS) and weekly by a detailed score.

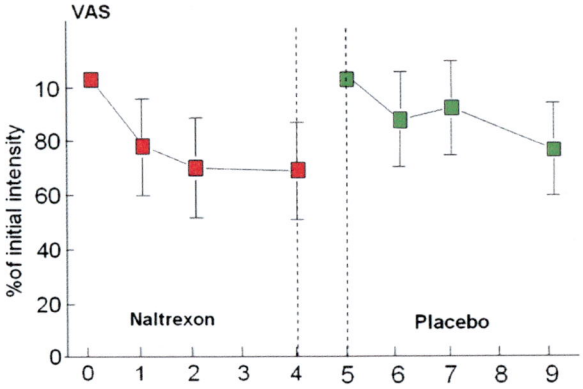

**Fig. 27.5** Response of CKD-associated pruritus in 23 patients with refractory pruritus during treatment with either 50 mg naltrexone or placebo for 4 weeks. There was no statistically significant difference between the two treatment phases[5]

Sixteen of 23 patients completed the study. During treatment with naltrexone, pruritus decreased by 29.2% on VAS and by 17.6% on the detailed score. In comparison, pruritus decreased by 16.9% on VAS and by 22.3% during the placebo period. The difference between the naltrexone and the placebo treatment period was not statistically significant (Fig. 27.5). Nine of 23 patients complained about adverse gastrointestinal events during the naltrexone treatment period, in comparison to only 1 of 23 patients during the placebo period ($p < 0.005$).[5]

The results of Peer and coworkers[4] are in sharp contrast to the results of our study and cannot be explained by differences in patient compliance, naltrexone dose, or study design, as both studies were randomized, placebo-controlled, double-blind crossover trials.

The pathogenesis of CKD-associated pruritus may be influenced by differences in the management of patients on dialysis and by the regional differences in life and eating habits in different parts of the world. In the study of Peer et al., no details have been given on the dialysis modalities. Possibly, the involvement of such additional pathogenetic factors led to a higher incidence of severe pruritus and to differences in naltrexone response.

## 27.10 Treatment with κ-Receptor-Agonists

As mentioned above, it was speculated that a derangement of the μ- and κ-opiod system might lead to CKD-associated pruritus. In a meta-analysis of two randomized controlled studies, Wikstrom and colleagues could show that treatment with nalfurafine (a potent κ-receptor agonist) could reduce itch in patients on hemodialysis although the effect was not a very dramatic one.[49]

Whether or not butorphenol, a drug with both κ-agonistic and μ-antagonistic properties, is effective in CKD-associated pruritus remains to be elucidated. Dwan and Yosipovitch had used this drug in patients with "intractable itch," with promising results.[50]

## 27.11 Treatment with Gabapentin and Pentoxyfilline

In recent years, gabapentin, which is a γ-aminobutyric acid originally developed as an anticonvulsant, had proven its efficacy as a pain-modulating drug in patients with diabetic neuropathy. In a controlled randomized trial in 25 patients on hemodialysis, Gunal and coworkers could prove its effectiveness in lowering itch in these patients.[51] Given the various other positive observations in the treatment with this compound and its good tolerability, this drug will become an important tool in the treatment of CKD-associated pruritus.

Recently we treated seven patients on hemodialysis with treatment-refractory CKD-associated pruritus with an i.v. series of pentoxyfilline. In those patients who tolerated the drug, pruritus almost disappeared for a long period (even after the drug was discontinued). However, in four patients the therapy had to be discontinued because of side effects.[52]

## 27.12 Phototherapy

A series of studies have dealt with the effectiveness of phototherapy in CKD-associated pruritus, especially radiation with broad-band UVB. According to a meta-analysis of Tan and coworkers, the most promising therapy is UVB radiation, whereas UVA does not seem to be effective.[53]

Newer data seem to indicate that narrow-band UVB attenuates CKD-associated pruritus with fewer side effects.[54] The associated risk for skin malignancies following UVB irradiation as well as the long-term topical immunosuppression is still a matter of debate.[55, 56]

An approach to therapy in CKD-associated pruritus is depicted in Fig. 27.6.

In conclusion, CKD-associated pruritus remains a clinically important problem in patients on dialysis. The pathogenesis of this bothersome and sometimes tormenting symptom is still obscure. There are hints that derangements of either the opioidergic and/or the immune system are involved. A unifying concept probably would suggest that inflammatory stimuli, conveyed by uraemia and/or dialysis, would lead to both an augmented differentiation of Th1 lymphocytes and subsequently a suppression of itch-reducing κ-receptors or

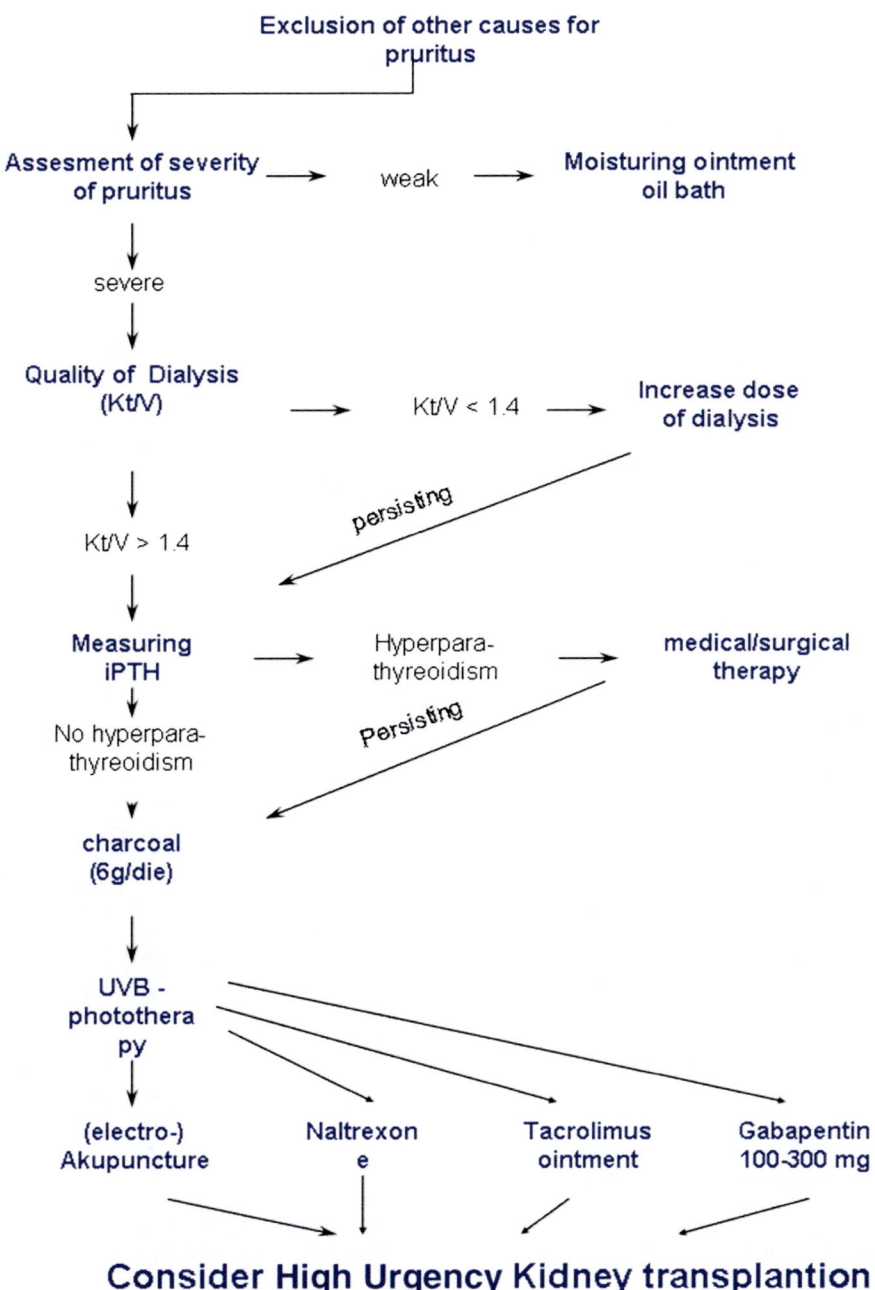

**Consider High Urgency Kidney transplantion**

**Fig. 27.6** Therapeutic approach to CKD-associated pruritus. IPTH, intact parathyreoid hormone; Kt/V, urea clearance by dialysis

an increase of μ-receptors in the skin of patients on dialysis. However, this hypothesis remains unproven at present, and safe and effective therapeutic modalities are lacking. Probably, immunomodulatory and κ-receptor agonistic drugs may prove helpful in the most severe cases.

# References

1. Mettang T, Fischer FP, Kuhlmann U. Urämischer pruritus – pathophysiologische und therapeutische konzepte. *Dtsch Med Wschr*. 1996;121:1025–1031.
2. De Marchi S, Cecchin E, Villalta D, Sepiacci G, Santini G, Bartoli E. Relief of pruritus and decreases in plasma histamine concentrations during erythropoietin therapy in patients with uremia. *N Engl J Med*. 1992;326:969–974.
3. Balaskas EV, Uldall RP. Erytropoietin does not improve uremic pruritus. *Perit Dial Int*. 1992;12:330–331.
4. Peer G, Kivity S, Agami O, et al. Randomised crossover trial of naltrexone in uraemic pruritus. *Lancet*. 1996;348: 1552–1554.
5. Pauli-Magnus C, Mikus G, Alscher DM, et al. Naltrexone does not relieve uremic pruritus: results of a randomized, placebo-controlled crossover-study. *J Am Soc Nephrol*. 2000;11:514–519.
6. Morvay M, Marghescu S. Hautveränderungen bei Haemodialysepatienten. *Med Klin*. 1988;83:507–510.
7. Ponticelli C, Bencini PL. Uremic pruritus: a review. *Nephron*. 1992;60:1–5.
8. Gilchrest GA, Stern RS, Steinman TI, Brown RS, Arndt KA, Anderson WW. Clinical features of pruritus among patients undergoing maintenance hemodialysis. *Arch Dermatol*. 1982;118:154–156.
9. Young AW, Sweeney EW, David DS, et al. Dermatologic evaluation of pruritus in patients on hemodialysis. *N.Y. St. J. Med*. 1973;73:2670–2674.
10. Mettang T, Fritz P, Weber J, Machleidt C, Hübel E, Kuhlmann U. Uremic pruritus in patients on hemodialysis or Continuous Ambulatory Peritoneal Dialysis (CAPD). The role of plasma histamine and skin mast cells. *Clin Neprol*. 1990;34:136–141.
11. Duque MI, Thevarajah S, Chan YH, Tuttle AB, Freedman BI, Yosipovitch G. Uremic pruritus is associated with higher kt/V and serum calcium concentration. *Clin Nephrol*. 2006;66:184–191.
12. Narita I, Alchi B, Omori K, et al. Etiology and prognostic significance of severe uremic pruritus in chronic hemodialysis patients. *Kidney Int*. 2006;69:1626–1632.
13. Pisoni RL, Wikström B, Elder SJ, et al. Pruritus in haemodialysis patients: international results from the Dialysis Outcomes and Practice Patterns Study (DOPPS). *Nephrol Dial Transplant*. 2006;21:3495–3505.
14. Schwab M, Mikus G, Mettang T, Pauli-Magnus C, Kuhlmann U. Arbeitsgemeinschaft für Pädiatrische Nephrologie: Urämischer Pruritus im Kindes- und Jugendalter. *Z Kinderheilkd*. 1999;147:232.

15. Massry S, Popovzer MM, Coburn JM, Mokoff DL, Maxwell MH, Kleeman CR. 1968 Interactable pruritus as a manifestation of secondary hyperparathyroidism in uremia. *N Engl J Med*. 1968;279:697–700.
16. Hampers CL, Katz AI, Wilson RE, Merrill JP. Disappearance of uremic itching after subtotal parathyreoidectomy. *NEJM*. 1968;279:695–697.
17. Stahle-Bäckdahl M, Hägermark O, Lins LE, Törring O, Hilliges M, Johansson O. Experimental and immunohistochemical studies on the possible role of parathyroid hormone in uremic pruritus. *J. Intern. Med*. 1989;225:411–415.
18. Blachley JD, Blankenship DM, Menter A, Parker TF III, Knochel JP. Uremic pruritus: skin divalent ion content and response to ultraviolet phototherapy. *Am J Kidney Dis*. 1985;5:237–241.
19. Stockenhuber F, Kurz RW, Sertl K, Grimm G, Balcke P. Increased plasma histamine in uremic pruritus. *Clin Sci*. 1990;79/5:477–482.
20. Hiroshige K, Kabashima N, Takasugi M, Kuroiwa A. Optimal dialysis improves uremic pruritus. *Am J Kidney Dis*. 1995;25:413–419.
21. Dimkovic N, Djukanovic L, Radmilovic A, Bojic P, Juloski T. Uremic pruritus and skin mast cells. *Nephron*. 1992;61:5–9.
22. Yosipovitch G, Duque MI, Patel TS, et al. . Skin barrier structure and function and their relationship to pruritus in end-stage renal disease. *Nephrol Dial Transplant*. 2007;22:3268–3272.
23. Szepietowski JC, Reich A, Schwartz RA. Uraemic xerosis. *Nephrol Dial Transplant*. 2004;19:2709–2712.
24. Gilchrest BA, Rowe JW, Brown RS, Steinman TI, Arndt KA. Ultraviolet phototherapy of uremic pruritus. Long-term results and possible mechanisms of action. *Ann Intern Med*. 1979;91:17–21.
25. Garssen J, Vandebriel RJ, DeGruijl FR, et al. UVB exposure-induced systemic modulation of Th1- and Th2-mediated immune responses. *Immunology*. 1999;97:506–514.
26. Hiroshige K, Kabashima N, Takasugi M, Kuroiwa A. Optimal dialysis improves uremic pruritus. *Am J Kidney Dis*. 1995;25:413–419.
27. Rousseau Y, Haeffner-Cavaillon N, Poignet JL, Meyrier A. Carreno: in vivo intracellular cytokine production by leukocytes during hemodialysis. *Cytokine*. 2000;12:506–517.
28. Silva SRB, Viana PCF, Lugon NV, Hoette M, Ruzany F, Lugon JR. Thalidomide for the treatment of uremic pruritus: a crossover randomized double-blind trial. *Nephron*. 1994;67:270–273.
29. Pauli-Magnus C, Klumpp S, Alscher D, Kuhlmann U, Mettang T. Short-term efficacy of tacrolimus ointment in severe uremic pruritus. *Perit Dial Int*. 2000;6:802–803.
30. McHugh SM, Rifkin IR, Deigghton J, et al. The immunosuppressive drug thalidomide induces T helper cell type 2 (Th2) and concomitantly inhibits Th1 cytokine production in mitogen- and antigen-stimulated human peripheral blood mononuclear cell cultures. *Clin Exp Immunol*. 1995;99:160–167.
31. Suthanthiran M, Strom TB. Renal transplantation. *N Engl J Med*. 1994;331:365–376.
32. Altmeyer P, Kachel HG, Schäfer G, Faßbinder W. Normalisierung der urämischen Hautveränderungen nach Nierentransplantation. *Hautarzt*. 1986;37:217–221.
33. Call TG, Creagan ET, Frytak S, et al. Phase I trial of combined interleukin-2 with lev in patients with advanced malignant disease. *Am J Clin Oncol*. 1994;17:344–347.

34. Darsow U, Scharein E, Bromm B, Ring J. Skin testing of the pruritogenic activity of histamine and cytokines (interleukin-2 and tumour necrosis factor-alpha) at the dermo-epidermal junction. *Br J Dermatol*. 1997;137:415–417.

35. Virga G, Visentin I, La MV, Bonadonna A. Inflammation and pruritus in haemodialysis patients. *Nephrol Dial Transplant*. 2002;17:2164–2169.

36. Kimmel M, Alscher DM, Dunst R, et al. The role of microinflammation in the pathogenesis of uraemic pruritus in haemodialysis patients. *Nephrol Dial Transplant*. 2006;21: 749–755.

37. Reiz S, Westberg M. Side effects of epidural morphine. *Lancet*. 1980;2:203–204.

38. Cousins MJ, Mather LE. Intrathecal and epidural administration of opioids. *Anesthesiology*. 1984;62:276–310.

39. Bergasa NV, Jones EA. The pruritus of cholestasis: potential pathogenic and therapeutic implications of opioids. *Gastroenterology*. 1995;108:1582–8.

40. Bergasa NV, Alling DW, Vergalla J, Jones EA. Cholestasis in the male rat is associated with naloxone-reversible antinociception. *J Hepatol*. 1994;20:85–90.

41. Bergasa NV, Alling DW, Talbot TL, et al. Effects of naloxone infusion in patients with the pruritus of cholestasis: a double-blind randomised controls trial. *Ann Intern Med*. 1995;123:161–167.

42. Bergasa NV, Schmitt JM, Talbot TL, et al. Open-label trial of oral nalmefene therapy for the pruritus of cholestasis. *Hepatology*. 1998;27:679–684.

43. Bergasa NV, Rothman RB, Vergalla J, Xu H, Swain MG, Jones EA. Central mu-opioid-receptors are down-regulated in a rat model of acute cholestasis. *J Hepatol*. 1992;15:220–224.

44. Thornton JR, Losowsky MS. Opioid peptides and primary biliary cirrhosis. *Br Med J*. 1988;297:1501–1504.

45. Andersen LW, Friedberg M, Lokkegaard N. Naloxone in treatment of uremic pruritus: a case history. *Clin Nephrol*. 1984;21:355–356.

46. Gianni LM, Sulli MM. Topical tacrolimus in the treatment of atopic dermatitis. *Ann Pharmacother*. 2001;35:943–946.

47. Kuypers DR, Claes K, Evenepoel P, Maes B, Vanrenterghem Y. A prospective proof of concept study of the efficacy of tacrolimus ointment on uraemic pruritus (UP) in patients on chronic dialysis therapy. *Nephrol Dial Transplant*. 2004;19:1895–1901.

48. Chen YC, Chiu WT, Wu MS. Therapeutic effect of topical gamma-linolenic acid on refractory uremic pruritus. *Am J Kidney Dis*. 2006;48:69–76.

49. Wikström B, Gellert R, Ladefoged SD, et al. Kappa-opioid system in uremic pruritus: multicenter, randomized, double-blind, placebo-controlled clinical studies. *J Am Soc Nephrol*. 2005;16:3742–3747.

50. Dawn AG, Yosipovitch G. Butorphanol for treatment of intractable pruritus. *Am Acad Dermatol*. 2006;54:527–531.

51. Gunal AI, Ozalp G, Yoldas TK, Gunal SY, Kirciman E, Celiker H. Gabapentin therapy for pruritus in haemodialysis patients: a randomized, placebo-controlled, double-blind trial. *Nephrol Dial Transplant*. 2004;19:3137–3139.

52. Mettang T, Krumme B, Bohler J, Roeckel A. Pentoxifylline as treatment for uraemic pruritus - an addition to the weak armentarium for a common clinical symptom? *Nephrol Dial Transplant*. 2007;22:2727–2728.

53. Tan JKL, Haberman HF, Coldman AJ. Identifying effective treatments for uremic pruritus. *J Amer Acad Dermatol*. 1991;25:811–818.

54. Baldo A, Sammarco E, Plaitano R, Martinelli V. Monfrecola. Narrowband (TL-01) ultraviolet B phototherapy for pruritus in polycythaemia vera. *Br J Dermatol*. 2002;147:979–981.

55. Lee E, Koo J. Berger: UVB phototherapy and skin cancer risk: a review of the literature. *Int J Dermatol*. 2005;44:355–360.

56. Ulrich C, Stockfleth E. Azathioprine, UV light, and skin cancer in organ transplant patients - do we have an answer? *Nephrol Dial Transplant*. 2007;22:1027–1029.

# Chapter 28
# Pruritus in Patients with Hepatobiliary Diseases

Andreas E. Kremer, Ronald P.J. Oude-Elferink, and Ulrich Beuers

## 28.1 Introduction

Pruritus can be caused by numerous diseases and has recently been classified into six different categories: (1) dermatological itch, which is associated with primary skin disorders; (2) systemic itch, which is caused by systemic diseases, pregnancy, tumors and infectious diseases; (3) neurological itch, which is induced by anatomical lesions of the peripheral or central nervous system; (4) psychogenic itch, which may occur in different psychiatric diseases such as schizophrenia, depression, and tactile hallucinosis; (5) mixed forms of itch in case of coexistence of diseases; and finally (6) other forms of itch the origin of which cannot be determined.[1] Here, we focus on systemic itch caused by hepatobiliary diseases.

Pruritus is a common symptom of various, mainly cholestatic, hepatobiliary diseases. Both, intra- and extrahepatic cholestasis may cause pruritus. Intrahepatic cholestasis may be induced by pure hepatocyte secretory failure as observed in intrahepatic cholestasis of pregnancy (ICP), viral hepatitis, certain forms of drug-induced cholestasis, progressive familial intrahepatic cholestasis (PFIC), and benign recurrent intrahepatic cholestasis (BRIC), but also by intrahepatic bile duct damage and secondary hepatocyte secretory failure as observed in primary biliary cirrhosis (PBC), primary sclerosing cholangitis (PSC), and pediatric cholestatic syndromes such as the Alagille syndrome. Extrahepatic cholestatic syndromes are less frequently associated with pruritus and are caused by various kinds of extrahepatic biliary obstructions (Table 28.1).

Cholestatic liver disease should be considered as a cause of chronic pruritus in any patient who does not show obvious signs of a dermatological disease. Patients with cholestatic liver disease frequently report most intense itching sensations on the palms and soles, but itch may also be generalized. Pruritus in cholestasis undergoes diurnal variations and is reported by most patients to be most intense in the late evening and early night hours. Specific skin lesions are not observed, but scratching-induced excoriations and prurigo nodularis are common.[2] Severity of pruritus can range from mild, in which normal activities of life are limited, moderate in which sleep is disturbed, to severe when normal daily activities become impossible. Extreme itch may even lead to suicidal tendencies and may become an indication for liver transplantation.[3, 4] Clinical signs of chronic liver diseases such as jaundice, spider angioma, palmar erythema, Dupuytren's contractures, leuconychia (white nails), gynecomastia and testicular atrophy in men, abdominal collateral veins, or splenomegaly are found only in a minority of patients with hepatobiliary disease who suffer from pruritus, as pruritus is frequently observed in early stages of liver disease. Thus, serum liver tests including alkaline phosphatase and $\gamma$-glutamyl transferase should always be included in the work-up of patients with pruritus of unknown origin. Medical and interventional treatment of cholestatic pruritus (see below) alleviates itch in most, but not all, patients, highlighting the fact that the pathogenesis of this symptom is still poorly understood.

### 28.1.1 Pathogenesis

Itch perception depends on a complex interplay of receptors, peripheral nerve fibers, intraspinal and cerebral neural pathways, as well as cerebral processing in thalamic nuclei and cortical areas that have been unraveled during the recent 2–3 decades.[5-7] It is well established

L. Misery and S. Ständer (eds.), *Pruritus*,
DOI 10.1007/978-1-84882-322-8_28, © Springer-Verlag London Limited 2010

**Table 28.1** Hepatobiliary diseases associated with pruritus

|  | Diseases |
| --- | --- |
| Intrahepatic cholestasis | ICP |
| a. Hepatocellular | BRIC |
|    secretory failure | Drug-induced cholestasis |
|  | Alcoholic hepatopathy |
|  | Chronic hepatitis B infection |
|  | Chronic hepatitis C infection |
| b. Bile ductular damage | PBC |
|    and hepatocellular | PSC |
|    secretory failure | Pediatric cholestatic syndromes |
| Extrahepatic | PSC |
|    cholestasis | Cholangiocellular carcinoma (CCC) |
|  | Hilar lymphadenopathy |
|  | Metastases/tumours causing biliary obstruction |

that itch and pain perception are closely intertwined processes. The previous assumption that itch signals are transmitted via pain-sensitive nerve fibers either by low-level nociceptor activation or itch-specific patterns of action potentials[8] has been overthrown recently by the finding that itch and pain signals are transduced by different subgroups of unmyelinated C-fibers. Thus, itch perception is induced by stimulation of an itch-specific subgroup of mechano-insensitive C-nociceptors located in cutis and subcutis.[9]

Interestingly, pain (e.g., scratching the skin) represses itch sensation, and antinociception (e.g., intrathecally applied μ-opioid receptor agonists or anesthetics) can cause itch[10] as outlined in detail elsewhere in this book. The antagonistic synaptic linkage between pain and itch neurons was identified at the spinal level leading to the impairment of itch signals by pain perception.[11] Recordings of single neurons revealed that those neurons transmitting pruritic stimuli are not spontaneously active in contrast to pain-transmitting neurons.[12] Thus, itch perception seems to be under the tonic inhibitory control of mechano-sensitive neurons. This may explain why pharmacological inhibition of pain processing may lead to itch as demonstrated by induction of segmental analgesia as well as segmental itch by spinally or epidurally administered opioids and anesthetics.

Itch-specific unmyelinated C-fibres transmit their signals from the skin through the dorsal root ganglia to a second neuron in the dorsal horn of the spinal cord, crossing to the contralateral side and projecting via the spinothalamic tract to the ventromedial nucleus of the thalamus. These neurons, which are sensitive to histamine but insensitive to mechanical stimulation, have been first identified in cats.[13] In humans, the supraspinal processing of pruritus and its corresponding scratch response have been visualized by positron emission tomography (PET).[14] Itch was induced by intradermal histamine injections and revealed an activation of the primary sensory cortex, supplementary motor area, anterior cingulate cortex, and inferior parietal lobe predominantly in the left hemisphere.[15] Coactivation of the pre-motor cortical areas may explain why itch is linked to the desire to scratch. Interestingly, multiple sites in brain are activated by histamine-induced itch perception and show a wide overlap with those areas being activated by pain sensations.[16] However, a different sensitivity of the posterior cingulate cortex, the posterior insula, and the thalamus, in particular, may be responsible for the perceptual difference between itch and pain sensations as indicated by functional magnetic resonance imaging.[17] Inhibition of histamine-induced itch by painful cold stimuli revealed an activation of the periaquaeductal gray as visualized by PET.[15]

Thus, a selective pathway for itch perception could be unraveled for histamine-induced itch in humans. But why do patients with cholestatic liver diseases suffer from itch? The pathogenesis of pruritus in cholestasis appears to be histamine-independent and remains poorly understood. The pruritogens in cholestasis are not yet defined. Treatment responses (see below) to the anion exchange resin cholestyramine, to the enzyme inducers rifampicin and phenobarbital, to the opioid antagonists naloxone and naltrexone, to the serotonin reuptake inhibitor sertraline, and to biliary diversion allow the conclusion that pruritogens in cholestasis (1) are biotransformed in liver (and intestine?), (2) are secreted into bile, (3) undergo an enterohepatic circulation, and (4) interact with the endogenous opioid and serotoninergic systems. Accumulation of bile salts, progesterone metabolites, histamine, and endogenous opioids in cholestasis have all been found responsible for induction of pruritus in the past.[18]

### 28.1.1.1 Bile Salts as Pruritogens?

Bile salts accumulate in the organism during cholestasis. Bile salts injected into the skin of healthy individuals induced itch,[19] and anion exchange resins, which bind bile salts inside the intestinal lumen, ameliorate pruritus.[20] Pruritus subsided rapidly (within hours) in patients with intractable pruritus after dilating a major bile duct stenosis or after nasobiliary drainage of bile.

Thus, it was claimed that cholestatic pruritus might be caused by enhanced concentrations of bile salts in the systemic circulation and peripheral tissues.[21] However, a number of observations are not consistent with a key role of bile salts for the induction of pruritus: (1) Not every patient with cholestatic liver disease and elevated plasma concentrations of bile salts develops itch;[22] (2) The development of itch in PBC, the most frequent chronic cholestatic liver disease associated with itch in up to 70% of patients, is independent of the degree of cholestasis and the stage of the disease and even diminishes in patients with end-stage disease when bile salts reach the highest levels in serum and peripheral tissues; (3) Pruritus ameliorates despite ongoing cholestasis and persistently elevated levels of bile salts in cholestatic disorders;[2,22] (4) No correlation between the severity of itch and the concentrations of bile salts in circulation and in skin could be demonstrated;[23–25] (5) After nasobiliary drainage, serum levels of major bile salts remained largely unchanged while pruritus improved dramatically in PBC patients with otherwise therapy-resistant pruritus;[26] (6) Anion exchange resins such as cholestyramine and colestipol improve itch sensations not only in patients with cholestatic liver disease but also in patients with chronic renal failure and polycythemia rubra vera, conditions which are not associated with elevation of bile salts in serum and peripheral tissues. Still, it cannot be excluded that a certain subgroup of bile salt metabolites may directly or indirectly induce itch and that the concentrations of these metabolites do not correlate with the extent of cholestasis and total bile salts. In summary, however, the evidence for a key role of bile salts in the induction of pruritus in cholestasis is weak at best.

### 28.1.1.2  Progesterone Metabolites as Pruritogens?

In ICP, a cholestatic disorder specific to pregnancy, pruritus develops in the 2nd and 3rd trimenon of pregnancy in parallel with an increase in progesterone metabolites and bile salts.[27] Interestingly, only urinary levels of disulfated progesterone metabolites were associated with the intensity of pruritus in patients with ICP before and after start of ursodeoxycholic acid (UDCA), and none of the analysed bile salt metabolites showed a similar correlation.[28] Thus, at least in ICP, progesterone disulfates should be further studied as potential inducers of pruritus.

### 28.1.1.3  Histamine as Pruritogen?

Histamine, a key mediator and potent pruritogen of allergic reactions, has been discussed as a mediator of cholestatic pruritus in the past, because levels of histamine have been shown to be elevated in sera of cholestatic patients[29] and bile salts are capable of releasing histamine from mast cells albeit at quite high concentrations.[30] However, antihistamines are mostly ineffective in pruritus associated with cholestasis.[21] In addition, typical histamine-induced skin lesions such as urticaria are not observed in patients with cholestatic pruritus. Thus, histamine appears highly unlikely to play a role in pruritus of cholestasis.

### 28.1.1.4  Endogenous Opioids as Pruritogens?

Endogenous opioids may play an important role in the pathogenesis of cholestatic pruritus.[5] Opioids that bind to the μ-opioid receptor induce pruritus in normal individuals presumably by a central mode of action.[31] Interestingly, elevated serum levels of endogenous opioids have been found in cholestatic PBC patients (although enkephalin levels did not correlate with the intensity of itch)[32] as well as in rats made cholestatic by bile duct resection.[33] The increased levels of endogenous opioids could be due to an enhanced synthesis or a reduced elimination.[18, 34, 35] Various studies showed a therapeutic effect of the μ-opioid receptor antagonists naloxone, naltrexone, and nalmefene in patients with cholestatic pruritus. These antagonists alleviated itch in up to 50% of the patients.[36–43] Opioid agonist centrally administered induced dose dependently facial scratching in monkeys.[44] Similar facial scratching appeared after injection of plasma extracts from cholestatic patients with pruritus into the medullary dorsal horn of monkeys. In contrast, plasma extracts from cholestatic patients without pruritus did not lead to enhanced scratching behavior.[45] While μ-opioid receptor antagonists attenuate pruritus, κ-opioid receptor antagonists enhanced itch in rats.[46] In line with these results, the new κ-opioid receptor agonist nalfurafine improved pruritus in patients with uremic pruritus[47] and the κ-opioid receptor agonist TRK-820 reduced itch in mice.[48] Thus, μ-opioid and κ-opioid receptor agonists act synergistically regarding their analgesic properties but inversely regarding their pruritic properties. Thus, μ-opioid receptor agonists participate in perception of pruritus associated with cholestasis and may play a key role in the induction of pruritus of cholestasis.

### 28.1.1.5 Serotonine as Pruritogen?

The serotoninergic system modulates nociception and may play a role in the perception of itch. Subcutaneously injected 5-hydroxytryptamine (5-HT$_3$ = serotonine) causes pruritus[49] putatively via unmyelinated C-fibres. Several clinical studies investigated the antipruritic effect of the 5-HT$_3$-receptor antagonist ondansentrone in cholestatic patients with equivocal results.[50, 51] Most recently, the serotonine reuptake inhibitor sertraline was shown to partly relieve pruritus in cholestatic patients.[52] Thus, serotonine may be involved in perception of pruritus in cholestasis, but is not likely to represent a key pruritogen in cholestasis.

### 28.1.1.6 Other Receptor Ligands as Pruritogens?

Cholestasis leads to antinociceptive effects in animal studies.[53, 54] Although pain and itch signals are transmitted via different unmyelinated C-fibres, the signal transduction pathways involved show remarkable similarities. Ligands of several receptors are capable of initiating or modulating pain as well as itch perception albeit not to the same extent. Relevant transmitters of both sensations are bradykinin, histamine, serotonine, prostaglandin E$_2$, endogenous opioids, endocannabinoids, and endovanilloids. Interestingly, various signaling pathways confluence in the activation of the nonspecific cation channel TRPV1 (transient receptor potential vanilloid 1), also known as the capsaicin receptor. Bradykinin induces activation of the G-protein-coupled bradykinin-2 receptor which stimulates intracellular phospholipase A$_2$ and gives rise to 12-lipoxygenase metabolites which in turn activate the TRPV1 channel.[55] Similarly, histamine activates TRPV1 in sensory neurons through the phospholipase A$_2$/lipooxygenase pathway.[56] Interestingly, expression of TRPV1 was dramatically increased in epidermal keratinocytes and nerve fibres of patients with prurigo nodularis and normalized after successful treatment of these pruritic lesions with topical capsaicin.[57] Hence, the vanilloid receptor TRPV1 can be regarded as a molecular integrator of several nociceptive and pruriceptive stimuli.

Besides neurons, keratinocytes may play a major role in itch (and pain) perception. Keratinocytes located around nerve endings in the stratum granulosum of the rat epidermis have been shown to release β-endorphins. This release was induced via (endo)cannabinoids, which bind to cannabinoid-2 receptors on β-endorphin-expressing keratinocytes. After release, β-endorphins bound to μ-opioid receptors of unmyelinated C-fibres and inhibited nociception in the rats under study.[58] Moreover, endocannabinoids such as anandamide have been shown to sensitize TRPV1, demonstrating the complex role of cannabinoids in the modulation of pruritus and pain.[59]

Gastrin-releasing peptide (GRP) and its receptor (GRPR) have recently been demonstrated to play a role in mediating pruritic stimuli of different origin within the spinal cord. Scratching behavior of GRPR mutant mice after intradermal application of different itch inducers was significantly reduced in comparison to wild-type mice. Furthermore, scratching could be induced by intrathecal injection of GRP and inhibited by co-administration of a GRPR blocker. Interestingly, pain sensation was not altered in GRPR mutant mice, indicating no relevant role of GRP and its receptor in pain perception.[60]

Thus, a number of receptor ligands including GRP, bradykinin, and endocannabinoids and their effects on keratinocytes and sensitive neurons deserve further study to unravel their role in the induction of pruritus in cholestasis.

## 28.1.2 Treatment

Therapeutic efforts to alleviate pruritus associated with cholestasis should include an adequate therapy of the underlying hepatobiliary disease, which may result in relief of pruritus. In extrahepatic malignant biliary obstruction, stenting, nasobiliary or transcutaneous drainage, or surgical biliodigestive anastomoses are usually effective in eliminating pruritus.[21] In intrahepatic cholestasis, a number of therapeutic approaches have been evaluated to alleviate or relieve pruritus (Table 28.2). These will be discussed in detail below.

Pruritus – like pain – is a subjective symptom being difficult to quantify in an objective way. It is a common experience that the intensity of pruritus may be

**Table 28.2** Therapeutic recommendations for pruritus in cholestasis

|  | Drug/therapy | Dosage | Evidence |
|---|---|---|---|
| First choice | UDCA* | 10–15 mg/kg/d | I A-II C* |
|  | Cholestyramine | 4–16 g/d | I B-II C* |
| Second choice | Rifampicin | 300–600 mg/d | I A |
| Third choice | Naltrexone | 25–50 mg/d | I A |
|  | Naloxone | 0.2 µg/kg/min | I B |
| Fourth choice | SSRI (e.g., Sertraline) | 75–100 mg/d | IIa B |
| Experimental | 5-HT$_3$-antagonists, e.g., Ondansentron | 12–24 mg/d | II A |
|  | Cannabinoids, e.g., Dronabinol | 2.5–5 mg/d | IIb C |
|  | Plasmapheresis |  | IIa C |
|  | Albumin dialysis (e.g., MARS) |  |  |
|  | Plasma separation/anion absorption |  |  |
|  | Nasobiliary drainage |  |  |
|  | Biliary diversion |  |  |
| Ultima ratio | Liver transplantation |  | I C |

Recommendation grades:

I. Condition for which there is evidence and/or general agreement that a treatment is beneficial, useful and effective.

II. Condition for which there is conflicting evidence and/or a divergence of opinion about the usefulness/efficacy of a treatment.

IIa. Weight of evidence is in favor of usefulness/efficacy.

IIb. Usefulness/efficacy is less well established.

III. Condition for which there is evidence and/or general agreement that a treatment is not useful/effective and in some cases may be harmful.

Evidence grades:

A. Multiple randomized clinical trials or meta-analyses.

B. Single randomized trial or non-randomized studies.

C. Only consensus opinion of experts, case studies or standard-of-care opinion.

* Recommendation and evidence grade vary depending on the underlying disease (e.g., ICP, PBC, PSC).

temporarily affected by parenteral or oral application of a placebo. Therefore, randomized, placebo-controlled, and double-blinded trials are required for reliable validation of antipruritic treatment strategies. To adequately evaluate and quantify the intensity of itch, behavioral methodologies, such as the scratching activity monitoring system (SAMS), have been applied successfully. This "pruritometer" uses piezoelectric crystals that are attached to a fingernail and records every scratching movement.[61, 62]

### 28.1.2.1  Ursodeoxycholic Acid (UDCA)

The bile acid UDCA (Ursodiol) forms up to 3% of the human bile pool. When orally administered as a drug, UDCA changes the bile pool to a more hydrophilic mix.[63,64] For the most common chronic cholestatic liver disease PBC, UDCA represents the only approved medical treatment so far. It improves serum liver tests and, in particular cholestasis, reduces progression to

fibrosis and cirrhosis, diminishes the frequency of complications, normalizes life expectancy in early-stage disease, and may prolong transplant-free survival in the PBC cohort. Due to its anticholestatic effect, UDCA is also used in a number of other cholestatic disorders such as PSC, ICP, cystic fibrosis-associated liver disease, and a number of pediatric disorders. The beneficial effect of UDCA has mainly been attributed to post-translational stimulation of synthesis, targeting, and insertion of key transporters into the apical membrane of hepatocytes, detoxification of bile, anti-apoptotic effects in hepatocytes and cholangiocytes, and stimulation of cholangiocyte secretion.[65] Interestingly, UDCA has not been convincingly shown to reduce pruritus in patients with PBC or PSC compared to placebo.[66,67] However, no adequate trials focusing on the effect of UDCA in pruritus of cholestasis have been performed in PBC or PSC. In women with ICP, UDCA is a safe and effective therapy, showing not only improvement of pruritus[28, 68, 69] but also of maternal liver enzymes and duration of pregnancy.

### 28.1.2.2  Anion Exchange Resins

The anion exchange resins cholestyramine and colestipol are non-reabsorbable alkaline macromolecules that bind anions and amphipathic substances including bile salts in the gut lumen and prevent their reuptake in the terminal ileum. Cholestyramine (alternatively colestipol) is an effective first-line therapy in the management of cholestatic pruritus.[70,71] The starting dose is 4 g daily, which can be extended to 16 g. As pruritogens presumably accumulate in the gallbladder overnight, efficacy might be increased by administering a 4-g dose before and after breakfast. As anion exchange resins interfere with the absorption of several drugs such as UDCA, digoxin, warfarin, propranolol, and oral contraceptive hormones as well as fat-soluble vitamins, they have to be taken at least 4 h prior to any other medication. The compliance might be diminished by the relatively unpalatable taste of resins and their side effects including constipation and abdominal discomfort.

### 28.1.2.3  Rifampicin

Rifampicin is a semisynthetic compound derived from *Amycolatopsis rifamycinica*, which is used to treat mycobacterial infections. Beside its antibiotic property, rifampicin induces emzymes of the microsomal drug-oxidizing cytochrome $P_{450}$ system such as CYP3A4 and CYP2D6 and key membrane transporters such as the conjugate export pump MRP2 in the liver through the activation of the steroid and xenobiotic receptor.[72,73] Thereby, this drug accelerates the metabolism and excretion of numerous endogenous and exogenous compounds such as hormones, bile, and drugs. The antipruritic effect of rifampicin might, therefore, be due to an enhanced metabolism and secretion of pruritogenic compounds.[73]

Several early reports have demonstrated improvement of pruritus in cholestasis as assessed subjectively during rifampicin treatment with 300–600 mg/d[74,75] and 10 mg/kg/d.[76] Rifampicin was effective also in children with chronic cholestasis.[77] Recent meta-analyses of prospective randomized, controlled trials revealed that rifampicin is an effective and safe short-term treatment of pruritus.[78,79] During long-term administration, hepatotoxicity has been observed in up to 13% of patients after 2 months.[76] Therefore, serum transaminase levels should be monitored if rifampicin is prescribed.[80] In addition, patients should be informed that this drug changes the color of body fluids, such as urine and tears, to orange-red, a benign but sometimes frightening side effect.

### 28.1.2.4  Opioid Antagonists

Several clinical trials have proven the ameliorating effect of opioid antagonists in patients with cholestatic pruritus over the last 20 years.[79] This supports the hypothesis that endogenous opioids play a critical role in the pathogenesis of cholestatic pruritus. Opiate antagonists such as naloxone (given as an intravenous bolus of 0.4 mg followed by continuous infusion of 0.2 µg/kg/min),[37,38] nalmefene (60–120 mg/d orally)[36,41] and naltrexone (25–50 mg/d orally)[39,40,42,43] showed a significant reduction of itch perception and scratching behavior. Opioid antagonists are regarded as third-line therapy in patients with otherwise intractable pruritus. Parenterally administered naloxone is barely practical for long-term use and should be kept for emergency treatment. Two randomized, double-blind, placebo-controlled trials proved that naltrexone is more effective than placebo in reducing pruritus as well as in improving fatigue and depression.[40,42] Opioid antagonists are well tolerated during long-term treatment, but may lead to severe opiate withdrawal-like reactions during the first days of treatment putatively due to an enhanced opioidergic tone in cholestatic patients. Therefore, opioid antagonists should be started very carefully at low doses. Alternatively, opioid antagonists could be either co-administered with clonidine[36] or initiated with intravenous naloxone at subtherapeutical doses (e.g., 0.002 µg/kg/min), and then gradually increased until reaching therapeutic doses before switching to oral naltrexone.[81] In some patients undergoing opioid antagonist therapy, pruritus might recur after successful attenuation. This breakthrough phenomenon can be explained by drug-induced upregulation of µ-opioid receptors and may be prevented by interrupting treatment at 2 days of the week, e.g., Saturday and Sunday.[39]

### 28.1.2.5  Serotonin Antagonists (5-HT3-Antagonists)

Serotonin is known to mediate nociception.[82] Serotonin might also play a role in itch signaling because serotonergic receptors modulate the transmission of opioid pain-inhibitory signals in the brain.[83] Initial studies using subjective methodology reported that intravenous administration of the 5-HT$_3$ antagonist ondansentrone markedly reduced pruritus within hours in patients suffering from cholestatic liver diseases[50,84] and ICP.[85] Controversial results are reported for oral administration of 5-HT$_3$ antagonists. Only a minor benefit could be demonstrated in a study using the visual analog scale for evaluation of pruritus intensity,[86] but these results were not confirmed when the intensity of pruritus was analyzed by objective methodology using a piezoelectric crystal attached to the finger nail as a "pruritometer."[51] Thus, the effectiveness of 5-HT$_3$ antagonists for the treatment of pruritus in cholestasis remains questionable. In desperate cases in which the above-mentioned medications are ineffective or cannot be applied, experimental use of 5-HT$_3$ antagonists may be justified.

Interestingly, the serotonin-reuptake inhibitors (SSRI) sertraline[52,87] and paroxetine[88] have also been reported to improve pruritus in cholestasis and advanced cancer stages. It remains unclear whether the apparently paradoxical effect of these antidepressants is due to dichotomous effects of serotonin on the central versus the peripheral nervous system,[87] to downregulation of excitatory 5-HT$_3$ receptors, or to a modification of central opioid receptors.[88]

### 28.1.2.6 Dronabinol (Cannabis)

Dronabinol (Marinol) is the semisynthetic analog of $\Delta^9$-tetrahydrocannabinol (THC), the psychoactive compound of cannabis sativa (marijuana). In three patients with intractable cholestatic pruritus, 5 mg of dronabinol every 8 h reduced temporarily itch and improved sleep and depression.[89] Interestingly, topical application of the cannabinoid receptor agonist N-palmitoylethanolamine significantly reduced chronic pruritus in various diseases in an open application observation.[90] Amelioration of pruritus by dronabinol might be due to interactions of opioid and cannabinoid receptors on nerve fibres. Further investigations in randomized, double-blinded, placebo-controlled clinical trials are needed to validate these preliminary observations.

### 28.1.2.7 Others

A number of other therapeutic approaches have been evaluated in small numbers of patients and are briefly summarized.

*Immunosuppressive drugs in PBC:* A prospective observational study compared the effects of methotrexate and colchicine on serum liver tests, symptoms like pruritus, and histology in naïve patients with PBC and elevated alkaline phosphatase levels at least two times above normal over a period of up to 2 years. Interestingly, methotrexate improved not only serum liver tests and some histological features but also pruritus as evaluated by a subjective score in this observational study.[91] Methotrexate is not beneficial when added to standard treatment with UDCA in PBC,[92] but anti-inflammatory treatment with budesonide in addition to UDCA is considered as a future treatment strategy[93–95] in those PBC patients who do not completely respond to UDCA alone. A randomized, placebo-controlled trial will be able to disclose whether this strategy may be beneficial in affecting pruritus intensity in this subgroup of PBC patients.

*Inducers of hepatic and intestinal biotransformation:* The barbiturate phenobarbital is a ligand of the nuclear receptor CAR (constitutive audrostaue receptor) and induces isoenzymes of the cytochrome P$_{450}$ family like rifampicin. Phenobarbital has been reported to relieve pruritus in cholestasis, but it was clearly inferior to rifampicin in a randomized, controlled, cross-over study.[96] In small case series, other hepatic enzyme inducers such as flumecinol[97] and the androgen stanozolol[98] have been reported to attenuate pruritus in cholestasis. However, stanozolol worsened cholestasis, limiting the use of this drug.

*Anesthetics:* The anesthetic drug propofol relieved cholestatic pruritus in 10 patients in a cross-over, placebo-controlled trial at subhypnotic doses via intravenous infusion.[99] Propofol presumably inhibits ventral and dorsal spinal nerve roots which are modulated by endogenous opioid-like ligands, rather than being anti-pruritic via sedation. Furthermore, intravenous infusion of the anesthetic lidocaine (100 mg) ameliorated pruritus and fatigue in a small number of PBC patients compared to placebo.[100]

*Phototherapy:* Phototherapy with ultraviolet light B (UVB) on the skin[101,102] and bright light directed towards the eyes[103] decreased the intensity of pruritus in some cholestatic patients. The mechanisms are unknown, but modifications of pruritogens in the skin or alteration in skin sensitivity to pruritogens have been discussed.

*Pruritogen elimination*: A beneficial effect of therapeutic procedures such as plasmapheresis,[104] molecular adsorbent recirculating system (MARS) therapy,[105,106] plasma separation and anion absorption,[107] partial external diversion of bile,[108] ileal diversion in children,[109] and nasobiliary drainage in children[110] and adults[26] with otherwise intractable pruritus has been reported in cases series. The rationale for these mostly invasive interventions was to remove pruritogens from plasma and bile. Their apparent (temporary) success is in line with the view that putative pruritogens in cholestasis accumulate in cholestatic plasma and undergo an enterohepatic circulation. However, all these reports have to be interpreted with some caution as they were not placebo-controlled. As all these techniques are more or less invasive, very elaborate, and too expensive for routine use, they are reserved for otherwise intractable pruritus in mostly desperate patients.

In patients in whom severe pruritus is refractory to the above-mentioned treatments, liver transplantation is considered as an ultimate option.[4] A successful transplantation cures the underlying disease and resolves pruritus immediately.

A step-by-step recommendation of therapeutic approaches is provided in Table 2.2 and summarizes the validated and experimental treatments for pruritus in cholestatic patients.

# References

1. Ständer S, Weisshaar E, Thomas M, et al. Clinical classification of itch: a position paper of the International Forum for the Study of Itch. *Acta Derm Venerol*. 2007;87:291–294.
2. Swain MG. Pruritus and lethargy in the primary biliary cirrhosis patient. In: Neuberger J, ed. *Primary Biliary Cirrhosis*. Eastbourne: West End Studios; 1999:75–81.
3. Elias E, Burra P. Primary biliary cirrhosis: symptomatic treatment. *J Gastroenterol Hepatol*. 1991;6:570–573.
4. Neuberger J, Jones EA. Liver transplantation for intractable pruritus is contraindicated before an adequate trial of opiate antagonist therapy. *Eur J Gastroenterol Hepatol*. 2001;13:1393–1394.
5. Bergasa NV. The pruritus of cholestasis. *J Hepatol*. 2005;43:1078–1088.
6. Steinhoff M, Bienenstock J, Schmelz M, et al. Neurophysiological, neuroimmunological, and neuroendocrine basis of pruritus. *J Invest Dermatol*. 2006;126:1705–1718.
7. Paus R, Schmelz M, Bíró T, et al. Frontiers in pruritus research: scratching the brain for more effective itch therapy. *J Clin Invest*. 2006;116:1174–1186.
8. Greaves MW, Wall PD. Pathophysiology of itching. *Lancet*. 1996;384:938–940.
9. Schmelz M, Schmidt R, Bickel A, et al. Specific C-receptors for itch in human skin. *J Neurosci*. 1997;17:8003–8008.
10. Atanassoff PG, Brull SJ, Zhang J, et al. Enhancement of experimental pruritus and mechanically evoked dysesthesiae with local anesthesia. *Somatosens Mot Res*. 1999;16:291–298.
11. Schmelz M. Itch - mediators and mechanisms. *J Dermatol Sci*. 2002;28:91–96.
12. Ikoma A, Rukwied R, Ständer S, et al. Neurophysiology of pruritus: interaction of itch and pain. *Arch Dermatol*. 2003;139:1475–1478.
13. Andrew D, Craig AD. Spinothalamic lamina I neurons selectively sensitive to histamine: a central neural pathway for itch. *Nat Neurosci*. 2001;4:72–77.
14. Darsow U, Drzezga A, Frisch M, et al. Processing of histamine-induced itch in the human cerebral cortex: a correlation analysis with dermal reactions. *J Invest Dermatol*. 2000;115:1029–1033.
15. Mochizuki H, Tashiro M, Kano M, et al. Imaging of central itch modulation in the human brain using positron emission tomography. *Pain*. 2003;105:339–346.
16. Drzezga A, Darsow U, Treede RD, et al. Central activation by histamine-induced itch: analogies to pain processing: a correlational analysis of O-15 $H_2O$ positron emission tomography studies. *Pain*. 2001;92:295–305.
17. Mochizuki H, Sadato N, Saito DN, et al. Neural correlates of perceptual difference between itching and pain: a human fmri study. *Neuroimage*. 2007;36:706–717.
18. Jones EA, Bergasa NV. The pruritus of cholestasis: from bile acids to opiate agonists. *Hepatology*. 1990;11:884–887.
19. Kirby J, Heaton KW, Burton JL. Pruritic effect of bile salts. *Br Med J*. 1974;4:693–695.
20. Datta DV, Sherlock S. Cholestyramine for long term relief in jaundiced patients fed a bile acid sequestering resin. *Gastroenterology*. 1966;50:323–332.
21. Jones EA, Bergasa NV. Evolving concepts of the pathogenesis and treatment of the pruritus of cholestasis. *Can J Gastroenterol*. 2000;14:33–40.
22. Murphy GM, Ross A, Billing BH. Serum bile acids in primary biliary cirrhosis. *Gut*. 1972;13:201–206
23. Ghent CN, Bloomer JR, Klatskin G. Elevations in skin tissue levels of bile acids in human cholestasis: relation to serum levels and to pruritus. *Gastroenterology*. 1977;73:1125–1130.
24. Freedman MR, Holzbach RT, Ferguson DR. Pruritus in cholestasis: no direct causative role for bile acid retention. *Am J Med*. 1981;70:1011–1016.
25. Bartholomew TC, Summerfield JA, Billing BH, et al. Bile acid profiles of human serum and skin interstitial fluid and their relationship to pruritus studied by gas chromatography-mass spectrometry. *Clin Sci (Lond)*. 1982;63:65–73.
26. Beuers U, Gerken G, Pusl T. Biliary drainage transiently relieves intractable pruritus in primary biliary cirrhosis. *Hepatology*. 2006;44:280–281.
27. Reyes H, Sjövall J. Bile acids and progesterone metabolites in intrahepatic cholestasis of pregnancy. *Ann Med*. 2000;32:94–106.
28. Glantz A, Reilly SJ, Benthin L, et al. Intrahepatic cholestasis of pregnancy: amelioration of pruritus by UDCA is associated with decreased progesterone disulphates in urine. *Hepatology*. 2008;47:544–551.
29. Gittlen SD, Schulman ES, Maddrey WC. Raised histamine concentrations in chronic cholestatic liver disease. *Gut*. 1990;31:96–99.

30. Quist RG, Ton-Nu HT, Lillienau J, et al. Activation of mast cells by bile acids. *Gastroenterology.* 1991;101:446–456.
31. Ballantyne JC, Loach AB, Carr DB. Itching after epidural and spinal opiates. *Pain.* 1988;33:149–160.
32. Spivey JR, Jorgensen RA, Gores GJ, et al. Methionine-enkephalin concentrations correlate with stage of disease but not pruritus in patients with primary biliary cirrhosis. *Am J Gastroenterol.* 1994;89:2028–2032.
33. Swain MG, Rothman RB, Xu H, et al. Endogenous opioids accumulate in plasma in a rat model of acute cholestasis. *Gastroenterology.* 1992;103:630–635.
34. Jones EA, Bergasa NV. The pruritus of cholestasis and the opioid system. *JAMA.* 1992;268:3359–3362.
35. Jones A, Bergasa NV. The pruritus of cholestasis. *Hepatology.* 1999;29:1003–1006.
36. Thornton JR, Losowsky MS. Opioid peptides and primary biliary cirrhosis. *Br Med J.* 1988;297:1501–1504.
37. Bergasa NV, Talbot TL, Alling DW, et al. A controlled trial of naloxone infusions for the pruritus of chronic cholestasis. *Gastroenterology.* 1992;102:544–549.
38. Bergasa NV, Alling DW, Talbot TL, et al. Effects of naloxone infusions in patients with the pruritus of cholestasis. A double-blind, randomized, controlled trial. *Ann Intern Med.* 1995;123:167–167.
39. Carson KL, Tran TT, Cotton P, et al. Pilot study of the use of naltrexone to treat the severe pruritus of cholestatic liver disease. *Am J Gastroenterol.* 1996;91:1022–1023.
40. Wolfhagen FH, Sternieri E, Hop WC, et al. Oral naltrexone treatment for cholestatic pruritus: a double-blind, placebo-controlled study. *Gastroenterology.* 1997;113:1264–1269.
41. Bergasa NV, Schmitt JM, Talbot TL, et al. Open-label trial of oral nalmefene therapy for the pruritus of cholestasis. *Hepatology.* 1998;27:679–684.
42. Terg R, Coronel E, Sordá J, et al. Efficacy and safety of oral naltrexone treatment for pruritus of cholestasis, a crossover, double blind, placebo-controlled study. *J Hepatol.* 2002;37:717–722.
43. Mansour-Ghanaei F, Taheri A, Froutan H, et al. Effect of oral naltrexone on pruritus in cholestatic patients. *World J Gastroenterol.* 2006;12:1125–1128.
44. Thomas DA, Williams GM, Iwata K, et al. Effects of central administration of opioids on facial scratching in monkeys. *Brain Res.* 1992;585:315–317.
45. Bergasa NV, Thomas DA, Vergalla J, et al. Plasma from patients with the pruritus of cholestasis induces opioid receptor-mediated scratching in monkeys. *Life Sci.* 1993;53:1253–1257.
46. Kamei J, Nagase H. Norbinaltorphimine, a selective kappa-opioid receptor antagonist, induces an itch-associated response in mice. *Eur J Pharmacol.* 2001;418:141–145.
47. Wikström B, Gellert R, Ladefoged SD, et al. Kappa-opioid system in uremic pruritus: multicenter, randomized, double-blind, placebo-controlled clinical studies. *J Am Soc Nephrol.* 2005;16:3742–3747.
48. Togashi Y, Umeuchi H, Okano K, et al. Antipruritic activity of the kappa-opioid receptor agonist, TRK-820. *Eur J Pharmacol.* 2002;435:259–264.
49. Weisshaar E, Ziethen B, Gollnick H. Can serotonin type 3 (5-HT$_3$) receptor antagonists reduce experimentally induced itch? *Inflamm Res.* 1997;46:412–416.
50. Schwörer H, Hartmann H, Ramadori G. Relief of cholestatic pruritus by a novel class of drugs: 5-hydroxytryptamine type 3 (5-HT$_3$) receptor antagonists: effectiveness of ondansetron. *Pain.* 1995;61:33–37.
51. O'Donohue JW, Pereira SP, Ashdown AC, et al. A controlled trial of ondansetron in the pruritus of cholestasis. *Aliment Pharmacol Ther.* 2005;21:1041–1045.
52. Mayo MJ, Handem I, Saldana S, et al. Sertraline as a first-line treatment for cholestatic pruritus. *Hepatology.* 2007;45:666–674.
53. Bergasa NV, Alling DW, Vergalla J, et al. Cholestasis in the male rat is associated with naloxone-reversible antinociception. *J Hepatol.* 1994;20:85–90.
54. Nelson L, Vergnolle N, D'Mello C, et al. Endogenous opioid-mediated antinociception in cholestatic mice is peripherally, not centrally, mediated. *J Hepatol.* 2006;44:1141–1149.
55. Shin J, Cho H, Hwang SW, et al. Bradykinin-12-lipoxygenase-VR1 signaling pathway for inflammatory hyperalgesia. *Proc Natl Acad Sci USA.* 2002;99:10150–10155.
56. Kim BM, Lee SH, Shim WS, et al. Histamine-induced Ca(2+) influx via the PLA(2)/lipoxygenase/TRPV1 pathway in rat sensory neurons. *Neurosci Lett.* 2004;361:159–162.
57. Ständer S, Moormann C, Schumacher M, et al. Expression of vanilloid receptor subtype 1 in cutaneous sensory nerve fibers, mast cells, and epithelial cells of appendage structures. *Exp Dermatol.* 2004;13:129–139.
58. Ibrahim MM, Porreca F, Lai J, et al. CB2 cannabinoid receptor activation produces antinociception by stimulating peripheral release of endogenous opioids. *Proc Natl Acad Sci USA.* 2005;102:3093–3098.
59. Hermann H, De Petrocellis L, Bisogno T, et al. Dual effect of cannabinoid CB1 receptor stimulation on a vanilloid VR1 receptor-mediated response. *Cell Mol Life Sci.* 2003;60:607–613.
60. Sun YG, Chen ZF. A gastrin-releasing peptide receptor mediates the itch sensation in the spinal cord. *Nature.* 2007;448:700–703.
61. Stein H, Bijak M, Heerd E, et al. Pruritometer 1: portable measuring system for quantifying scratching as an objective measure of cholestatic pruritus. *Biomed Tech.* 1996;41:248–252.
62. Bijak M, Mayr W, Rafolt D, et al. Pruritometer 2: portable recording system for the quantification of scratching as objective criterion for the pruritus. *Biomed Tech.* 2001;46:137–141.
63. Batta AK, Salen G, Mirchandani R, et al. Effect of long-term treatment with ursodiol on clinical and biochemical features and biliary bile acid metabolism in patients with primary biliary cirrhosis. *Am J Gastroenterol.* 1993;88:691–700.
64. Poupon RE, Chrétien Y, Poupon R, et al. Serum bile acids in primary biliary cirrhosis: effect of ursodeoxycholic acid therapy. *Hepatology.* 1993;17:599–604.
65. Beuers U. Drug insight: mechanisms and sites of action of ursodeoxycholic acid in cholestasis. *Nat Clin Pract Gastroenterol Hepatol.* 2006;3:318–328.
66. Lindor KD. Ursodiol for primary sclerosing cholangitis. Mayo Primary Sclerosing Cholangitis-Ursodeoxycholic Acid Study Group. *N Engl J Med.* 1997;336:691–695.

67. Talwalkar JA, Souto E, Jorgensen RA, et al. Natural history of pruritus in primary biliary cirrhosis. *Clin Gastroenterol Hepatol.* 2003;1:297–302.

68. Palma J, Reyes H, Ribalta J, et al. Ursodeoxycholic acid in the treatment of cholestasis of pregnancy: a randomized, double-blind study controlled with placebo. *J Hepatol.* 1997;27:1022–1028.

69. Kondrackiene J, Beuers U, Kupcinskas L. Efficacy and safety of ursodeoxycholic acid versus cholestyramine in intrahepatic cholestasis of pregnancy. *Gastroenterology.* 2005;129:894–901.

70. Datta DV, Sherlock S. Treatment of pruritus of obstructive jaundice with cholestyramine. *Br J Med.* 1963;1:216–219.

71. Pusl T, Beuers U. Extrahepatic manifestations of cholestatic liver diseases: pathogenesis and therapy. *Clin Rev Allergy Immunol.* 2005;28:147–157.

72. LeCluyse EL. Pregnane X receptor: molecular basis for species differences in CYP3A induction by xenobiotics. *Chem Biol Interact.* 2001;134:283–289.

73. Marschall HU, Wagner M, Zollner G, et al. Complementary stimulation of hepatobiliary transport and detoxification systems by rifampicin and ursodeoxycholic acid in humans. *Gastroenterology.* 2005;129:476–485.

74. Ghent CN, Carruthers SG. Treatment of pruritus in primary biliary cirrhosis with rifampin. Results of a double-blind, crossover, randomized trial. *Gastroenterology.* 1988;94:488–493.

75. Podesta A, Lopez P, Terg R, et al. Treatment of pruritus of primary biliary cirrhosis with rifampin. *Dig Dis Sci.* 1991;36:216–220.

76. Bachs L, Parés A, Elena M, et al. Effects of long-term rifampicin administration in primary biliary cirrhosis. *Gastroenterology.* 1992;102:2077–2080.

77. Cynamon HA, Andres JM, Iafrate RP. Rifampin relieves pruritus in children with cholestatic liver disease. *Gastroenterology.* 1990;98:1013–1016.

78. Khurana S, Singh P. Rifampin is safe for treatment of pruritus due to chronic cholestasis: a meta-analysis of prospective randomized-controlled trials. *Liver Int.* 2006;26:943–948.

79. Tandon P, Rowe BH, Vandermeer B, et al. The efficacy and safety of bile Acid binding agents, opioid antagonists, or rifampin in the treatment of cholestasis-associated pruritus. *Am J Gastroenterol.* 2007;102:1528–1536.

80. Prince MI, Burt AD, Jones DE. Hepatitis and liver dysfunction with rifampicin therapy for pruritus in primary biliary cirrhosis. *Gut.* 2002;50:436–439.

81. Jones EA, Neuberger J, Bergasa NV. Opiate antagonist therapy for the pruritus of cholestasis: the avoidance of opioid withdrawal-like reactions. *QJM.* 2002;95:547–552.

82. Richardson BP. Serotonin and nociception. *Ann N Y Acad Sci.* 1990;600:511–520.

83. Kiefel JM, Cooper ML, Bodnar RJ. Serotonin receptor subtype antagonists in the medial ventral medulla inhibit mesencephalic opiate analgesia. *Brain Res.* 1992;597:331–338.

84. Schwörer H, Ramadori G. Improvement of cholestatic pruritus by ondansentron. *Lancet.* 1993;341:1277.

85. Schumann R, Hudcova J. Cholestasis of pregnancy, pruritus and 5-hydroxytryptamine 3 receptor antagonists. *Acta Obstet Gynecol Scand.* 2004;83:861–862.

86. Müller C, Pongratz S, Pidlich J, et al. Treatment of pruritus in chronic liver disease with the 5-hydroxytryptamine receptor type 3 antagonist ondansetron: a randomized, placebo-controlled, double-blind cross-over trial. *Eur J Gastroenterol Hepatol.* 1998;10:865–870.

87. Browning J, Combes B, Mayo MJ. Long-term efficacy of sertraline as a treatment for cholestatic pruritus in patients with primary biliary cirrhosis. *Am J Gastroenterol.* 2003;98:2736–2741.

88. Zylicz Z, Krajnik M, Sorge AA, et al. Paroxetine in the treatment of severe non-dermatological pruritus: a randomized, controlled trial. *J Pain Symptom Manage.* 2003;26:1105–1112.

89. Neff GW, O'Brien CB, Reddy KR, et al. Preliminary observation with dronabinol in patients with intractable pruritus secondary to cholestatic liver disease. *Am J Gastroenterol.* 2002;97:2117–2119.

90. Ständer S, Reinhardt HW, Luger TA. Topical cannabinoid agonists. An effective new possibility for treating chronic pruritus. *Hautarzt.* 2006;57:801–807.

91. Kaplan MM, Schmid C, Provenzale D, et al. A prospective trial of colchicine and methotrexate in the treatment of primary biliary cirrhosis. *Gastroenterology.* 1999;117:1173–1180.

92. Combes B. Reflections on therapeutic trials in primary biliary cirrhosis. *Hepatology.* 2005;42:1184–93.

93. Leuschner M, Maier KP, Schlichting J, et al. Oral budesonide and ursodeoxycholic acid for treatment of primary biliary cirrhosis: results of a prospective double-blind trial. *Gastroenterology.* 1999;117:918–925.

94. Hempfling W, Grunhage F, Dilger K et al. Pharmacokinetics and pharmacodynamic action of budesonide in early- and late-stage primary biliary cirrhosis. *Hepatology.* 2003;38:196–202.

95. Rautiainen H, Kärkkäinen P, Karvonen AL, et al. Budesonide combined with UDCA to improve liver histology in primary biliary cirrhosis: a three-year randomized trial. *Hepatology.* 2005;41:747–752.

96. Bachs L, Parés A, Elena M, et al. Comparison of rifampicin with phenobarbitone for treatment of pruritus in biliary cirrhosis. *Lancet.* 1989;18:574–576.

97. Turner IB, Rawlins MD, Wood P, et al. Flumecinol for the treatment of pruritus associated with primary biliary cirrhosis. *Aliment Pharmacol Ther.* 1994;8:337–342.

98. Walt RP, Daneshmend TK, Fellows IW, et al. Effect of stanozolol on itching in primary biliary cirrhosis. *Br Med J (Clin Res Ed).* 1988;296:607.

99. Borgeat A, Wilder-Smith OH, Mentha G, et al. Subhypnotic doses of propofol relieve pruritus associated with liver disease. *Gastroenterology.* 1993;104:244–247.

100. Villamil AG, Bandi JC, Galdame OA, et al. Efficacy of lidocaine in the treatment of pruritus in patients with chronic cholestatic liver diseases. *Am J Med.* 2005;118:1160–1163.

101. Hanid MA, Levi AJ. Phototherapy for pruritus in primary biliary cirrhosis. *Lancet.* 1980;2:530.

102. Cerio R, Murphy GM, Sladen GE, et al. A combination of phototherapy and cholestyramine for the relief of pruritus in primary biliary cirrhosis. *Br J Dermatol.* 1987;116:265–267.

103. Bergasa NV, Link MJ, Keogh M, et al. Pilot study of bright-light therapy reflected toward the eyes for the pruritus of chronic liver disease. *Am J Gastroenterol.* 2001;96:1563–1570.

104. Cohen LB, Ambinder EP, Wolke AM, et al. Role of plasmapheresis in primary biliary cirrhosis. *Gut.* 1985;26:291–294.

105. Macia M, Avilés J, Navarro J, et al. Efficacy of molecular adsorbent recirculating system for the treatment of intractable pruritus in cholestasis. *Am J Med*. 2003;114:62–64.

106. Parés A, Cisneros L, Salmeron JM, et al. Extracorporeal albumin dialysis: a procedure for prolonged relief of intractable pruritus in patients with primary biliary cirrhosis. *Am J Gastroenterol*. 2004;99:1105–1110.

107. Pusl T, Denk GU, Parhofer KG, et al. Plasma separation and anion adsorption transiently relieve intractable pruritus in primary biliary cirrhosis. *J Hepatol*. 2006;45: 887–891.

108. Emerick KM, Whitington PF. Partial external biliary diversion for intractable pruritus and xanthomas in Alagille syndrome. *Hepatology*. 2002;35:1501–1506.

109. Ng VL, Ryckman FC, Porta G, et al. Long-term outcome after partial external biliary diversion for intractable pruritus in patients with intrahepatic cholestasis. *J Pediatric Gastroenterol Nutr*. 2000;30:152–156.

110. Stapelbroek JM, van Erpecum KJ, Klomp LW, et al. Nasobiliary drainage induces long-lasting remission in benign recurrent intrahepatic cholestasis. *Hepatology*. 2006;43:51–53.

# Chapter 29
# Endocrine Diseases

Elke Weisshaar

## 29.1 Diabetes Mellitus

Diabetes mellitus is the most common endocrine disease characterized by various dermatological diseases and cutaneous manifestations in up to 70% of patients.[1] Diabetic patients are prone to skin diseases accompanied by pruritus such as mycosis (tinea, candidosis) and bacterial infections, e.g., folliculitis. Generalized pruritus as a presenting symptom of diabetes may occur, but is not significantly more frequent than in nondiabetic patients. It was found to affect 2.7% of the diabetic population.[2] Localized pruritus, especially in the genital and perianal areas, is significantly more common in diabetic women and mostly associated with poor diabetes control.[2] Pruritus vulvae was found to be significantly more common in diabetic women (18.4%) than in controls (5.6%).[2] In some cases this may be due to predisposition to candidiasis or dermatophyte infections. A study from Kuwait described pruritus as the second most common manifestation seen in 49% of diabetic patients.[3] There was no description included in distinguishing between local and generalized pruritus. Pruritus confined to the scalp was reported to be caused by diabetes, and all patients experienced complete relief when control of the underlying diabetes was achieved.[4] The mechanism of pruritus induction in diabetes is not known. Diabetic neuropathy presenting as distal symmetrical polyneuropathy is more characteristically associated with pain, burning or prickling sensation, and sensorimotor deficits, although pruritic sensations have been described as well. An investigation of the expression of cannabinoid CB1 receptors in models of diabetic neuropathy suggests that high glucose concentrations are associated with decreased expression of CB1 receptors in nerve cells.[5] This decline may account for the neurodegenerative process observed in diabetes.

## 29.2 Thyroid Diseases

Severe generalized pruritus may be a presenting symptom in hyperthyroidism, especially in thyrotoxicosis.[6,7] The cause is not known but is most likely explained by thyroid hormones' effects on the skin. Chronic urticaria may be caused by thyroid autoimmunity. Localized or generalized pruritus may be seen in hypothyroidism but is not reported as a frequent complication. It needs to be considered that the skin in hypothyroidism is dry which can lead to asteatotic eczema accompanied by pruritus.

### 29.2.1 Parathyroid Diseases

#### 29.2.1.1 Hyperparathyroidism

Parathyroid gland activity is frequently increased in chronic renal failure, and most patients with end-stage renal failure develop secondary hyperparathyroidism (see Chapter 27 of this section). This has been suggested to be a cause of renal pruritus. Complete or partial relief of pruritus after parathyroidectomy was observed in patients,[8–10] but the circulating parathyroid hormone (PTH) level alone does not explain pruritus. Pruritus is not always present in renal or uremic patients with hyperparathyroidism. It reoccurred in patients after an operation when they were made hypercalcemic by therapy with calcium and vitamin D.[8] Others showed that pruritus can be reduced by parathyroidectomy and that the only factor that seems to affect the postoperative extent of pruritus is a high-level product of calcium and phosphate.[10] It was shown that levels of PTH did not correlate with pruritus[11,12]

L. Misery and S. Ständer (eds.), *Pruritus*,
DOI 10.1007/978-1-84882-322-8_29, © Springer-Verlag London Limited 2010

and not all patients with pruritus had elevated PTH activity. Others found significantly higher serum levels of PTH in patients with pruritus compared to patients without pruritus.[13] Intradermal injection of PTH failed to evoke any acute or delayed cutaneous reactions in patients and controls.[13] Immunohistochemical investigations using several different antibodies against PTH were negative.[13] In summary, there is no clear evidence for any role of PTH in different forms of pruritus such as renal pruritus.

### 29.2.1.2 Premenstrual or Perimenstrual Pruritus

Premenstrual pruritus related to recurrent cholestasis induced by oral contraceptives or other hormonal treatment is well recognized.[14] Generalized pruritus related to menses and sensitivity to intradermal estrogen has been described.[15] Episodic pruritus is an occasional symptom in perimenopausal women and can be treated by hormone replacement therapy.

### 29.2.1.3 Carcinoid Syndrome

The carcinoid syndrome is usually characterized by flushing and erythema of the head and neck caused by a serotonin-producing tumor of the intestine. This may lead to generalized pruritus with or without rash.[6]

### 29.2.1.4 Multiple Endocrine Neoplasia Type 2A (MEN 2A)

Localized pruritus of the mid upper-back or scapular area has been reported in association with MEN 2A but differential diagnosis may include lichen amyloidosis and notalgia paresthetica. One report describes a family with localized pruritus occurring symmetrically on the back or crossing the midline. In all affected family members, pruritus had been present long before the clinical or biochemical diagnosis was made.[16]

## References

1. Yosipovitch G, Hodak E, Vardi P, et al. The prevalence of cutaneous manifestations in IDDM patients and their association with diabetes risk factors and microvasculature complications. *Diabetes Care.* 1998;21:506–509.
2. Neilly JB, Martin A, Simpson N, et al. Pruritus in diabetes mellitus: investigation of prevalence and correlation with diabetes control. *Diabetes Care.* 1986;9:273–275.
3. Al-Mutari N, Zaki A, Sharma AK, et al. Cutaneous manifestations of diabetes mellitus. *Med Princ Pract.* 2006;15: 427–430.
4. Scribner M. Diabetes and pruritus of the scalp. *JAMA.* 1977;237:1559.
5. Zhang F, Hong S, Stone V, et al. Expression of cannabinoid CB1 receptors in models of diabetic neuropathy. *Am Pharmacol Exp Ther.* 2007;Aug 16 (epub).
6. Weisshaar E, Kucenic MJ, Fleischer AB. Pruritus: a review. *Acta Derm Venereol.* 2003;213(suppl.):5–32.
7. Mullin GE, Eastern JS. Cutaneous signs of thyroid disease. *Am Fam Physicians.* 1986;34:93–98.
8. Hampers CL, Katz AI, Wilson RE, et al. Disappearance of "Uremic" itching after subtotal parathyreoidectomy. *N Engl Med J Med.* 1968;279:695–697.
9. Massry SG, Popovtzer MM, Coburn JW, et al. Intractable pruritus as a manifestation of secondary hyperparathyroidism in uremia. Disappearance of itching after subtotal parathyroidectomy. *N Engl J Med.* 1968;279:697–700.
10. Chou FF, Ho JC, Huang SC, et al. A study on pruritus after parathyreoidectomy for secondary hyperparathyreoidism. *J Am Coll Surg.* 2000;190:65–70.
11. Carmichael AJ, Mc Hugh MM, Martin AM, et al. Serological markers of renal itch in patients receiving long term haemodialysis. *Br med J.* 1988;296:1575.
12. Cho YL, Liu HN, Huang TP, et al. Uremic pruritus: roles of parathyroid hormone activity and substance P. *J Am Acad Dermatol.* 1997;36:538–543.
13. Stahle-Bäckdahl M, Hägermark Ö, Lins LE, et al. Experimental and immunohistochemical studies on the possible role of parathyroid hormone in uraemic pruritus. *J Int Med.* 1989;225:411–415.
14. Dahl M. Premenstrual pruritus dues to recurrent cholestasis. *Trans St Johns Hosp Dermatol Soc 1970.* 1970;56:11.
15. Leylek OA, Unlü S, Oztürkcan S, et al. Estrogen dermatitis. *Eur J Obstr Gynecol.* 1997;72:97–103.
16. Bugalho MJGM, Limbert E, Sobrinho LG, et al. A kindred with multiple endocrine neoplasia Type 2A associated with pruritic skin lesions. *Cancer.* 1992;70:2664–2667.

# Chapter 30
# Pruritus in the Course of Malignancy

Zbigniew Zylicz and Malgorzata Krajnik

## 30.1 Introduction

Most patients who suffer from pruritus in the course of malignant diseases wish they had pain rather than itch. This recalcitrant symptom, although rare in most malignant diseases, is difficult to treat. The reason for this is that we know hardly anything about its etiology and treatment. Most therapeutic methods have been derived from empirical and serendipitous observations, rather than targeted research. In solid tumors (cancers) the incidence of severe itch is less than 1%.[1] One of the authors (ZZ) interested in paraneoplastic itch has seen 32 cases in 15 years, treating more than 4,500 patients with advanced diseases during this time. In hematological malignancies, which are relatively rare in themselves, pruritus is much more common. In polycythemia vera up to 50%[2] and in some rare cutaneous lymphomas as much as 100%[3] of patients suffer from itch. On the other hand, chronic pruritus of unknown origin is thought to be associated with malignancies. Among 95 patients with this condition, a neoplasm was found in eight cases: seven hematological malignancies (three myeloma, two Hodgkin's disease, and two myeloproliferative syndromes) and one solid cancer (pulmonary adenocarcinoma).[4] This is in accordance with another study in which a thorough follow-up of 125 patients over 6 years with pruritus of unknown origin revealed no increased risk of cancer but a higher risk of lymphoma ($p < 0.01$).[5]

Clinically, there are several different syndromes which will be described here in more detail.

## 30.2 Pruritus Associated with a Malignant Process Infiltrating the Skin

Pruritus may be the first symptom of malignant involvement of the skin. A good example of this syndrome is basal cell carcinoma of the vulva, which usually starts as chronic vulvar pruritus, sometimes unrecognized for many weeks or months, and treated with all kinds of topical anti-inflammatory and antifungal agents.[6] Another example is the intracutaneous growth of breast cancer.[7] Itch is very much localized and limited to the altered skin. This type of itch is frequently seen in the early stages of the disease and may represent an alarm symptom. The changes can be identified as malignant by performing a skin biopsy, and removal of the skin tumor relieves the itch.

## 30.3 Pruritus Associated with Cancer Growing in a Remote Part of the Body/Organ

This type is known as paraneoplastic itch. Some of these cases may manifest themselves as paraneoplastic dermatoses.[8] The following dermatoses are seen as paraneoplastic: acanthosis nigricans, tripe palms, dermatitis herpetiformis, dermatomyositis, extramammary Paget's disease, hypertrophic pulmonary osteoarthropathy,

L. Misery and S. Ständer (eds.), *Pruritus*,
DOI 10.1007/978-1-84882-322-8_30, © Springer-Verlag London Limited 2010

pemphigus vulgaris, pyoderma gangrenosum, Sweet's syndrome, and reactive erythemas.[9] Most of them can be accompanied by itch. However, paraneoplastic itch may present without any primary skin involvement.[10] Itch may precede the diagnosis of cancer by months and even years. Paraneoplastic sensorimotor neuropathy occurs in association with many different types of cancer, especially breast cancer.[11] According to Cormia,[10] itch without skin involvement (formerly known as "pruritus sine materia") as a complication of cancer is usually moderate and is rarely generalized. It usually develops on the pretibial area, the inner aspect of the thigh, upper thorax and shoulders, and extensor surfaces. Paraneoplastic itch of this type has been described in lung, breast, prostate, stomach, and pharyngeal tumors.[10] The etiology of paraneoplastic pruritus is unknown. It is also not known whether all cases of paraneoplastic itch are related to sensimotor polyneuropathy. This type of itch does not respond to topical and systemic antipruritic agents, including antihistamines.[12,13] Pruritus may disappear when a tumor is in remission, but its reappearance may herald a recurrence. This type of itch was found to be especially susceptible to treatment with paroxetine.[14,35]

## 30.4  Pruritus Associated with Invasion of the Vital Organs

Tumor growth may disturb the normal function of the vital organs. The best example of this type can be tumor growth in certain areas of the brain.[15] However, tumor invasion of the liver may also induce the itch of cholestasis.[16] This type of itch is often associated with the increased synthesis of endogenous opioids in the liver, and opioid antagonists are a recognized form of treatment.[17,18] However, treatment of itch with opioid antagonists is much more difficult or even impossible in advanced cancer, where itch would immediately be exchanged for more pain. For this kind of situation, we proposed treatment with buprenorphine patches[19,20] and/or paroxetine.[14] Buprenorphine has a high affinity for opioid receptors and precludes their binding with endogenous opioids. In this way, buprenorphine acts as an opioid antagonist without evoking an abstinence response. On rare occasions, tumor invasion may cause uremia and uremic itch. However, patients usually die from their tumor before they develop uremic itch.

Shotani et al.[21] analyzed 134 patients with pruritic skin diseases who were positive for *Helicobacter pylori*. These cases included 55 cases of cutaneous pruritus, 21 cases of prurigo chronica multiforme, 15 cases of nummular dermatitis, and 43 cases of chronic urticaria. Early gastric cancer was detected in 2/36 patients with cutaneous pruritus and 3/16 with prurigo chronica multiforme. The prevalence of early gastric cancer was 5.6%, which was much higher than that among patients undergoing general endoscopic screening for gastric cancer.

Localized itch may result from invasion of the regional nerves. Vulval pruritus has been reported in patients with cancer of the cervix. Persistent pruritus of the scrotum may be the first manifestation of prostate cancer. Perianal pruritus may accompany rectal or sigmoid cancer, and patients with these symptoms should be assessed to exclude the possibility of these tumors. In 109 patients with perianal pruritus, rectal carcinoma was found in 11%, anal carcinoma in 6%, adenomateous polyps in 4%, and colon or sigmoid cancer in 2%.[22]

## 30.5  Pruritus Associated with Hematological Diseases

Itch is a common feature in some hematological disorders. Itch usually accompanies diseases such as polycythemia vera (in 50% of cases), Hodgkin's lymphoma (30%), Sezary's syndrome, some forms of leukemia, multiple myeloma, Waldenstrom's macroglobulinemia, and mycosis fungoides. The last condition, although rare, is invariably accompanied by itch (100% of patients).[3] Patients with Hodgkin's lymphoma complicated by itch have a poorer prognosis.[23] In some, but certainly not in all, cases, itch may be related to liver invasion and inflammation (see pruritus of cholestasis). In Hodgkin's lymphoma, lymphatic leukemia, and other lymphomas, itch is invariably severe, sometimes with excruciating burning sensations, more frequently generalized, with less tendency to jump from place to place, and excoriations or dermatoses are more common.[24] A specific syndrome of itch around the involved lymph nodes has been described in patients with Hodgkin's disease after alcohol consumption.[25] There are no specific treatments for this kind of itch and, again, causal treatment is most important. Although serotonin-specific reuptake inhibitors

(SSRIs) have been found to be effective in many cases of polycythemia vera,[26,27] these drugs are probably ineffective for Hodgkin's lymphoma.[14,35] In the case of itch during the course of lymphoma, steroids are frequently used. Although this therapy is undoubtedly effective in some cases, there is no mention of it in the evidence-based literature. In some cases of lymphoma, $H_2$ anitihistamines such as cimetidine were found to be useful.[28,29]

## 30.6  Pruritus Associated with Antitumor Treatment

Most of the known antineoplastic drugs (alkylating agents, antimetabolites, antibiotics, plant alkaloids, nitrosoureas, and enzymes) are capable of inducing skin reactions, including pruritus. Patients treated with these drugs frequently report dry skin, scaling, and itchiness. Many problems are self-limiting and require no active treatment. Certain others can be prevented more easily than treated.

Hypersensitivity to antineoplastic agents can manifest as pruritus, edema, urticaria, and erythema. Hypersensitivity may be related to the quality and quantity (dose) of the administered drug and may be more frequent in patients with a history of allergy. The most frequently seen itchy allergic reactions are related to the following: doxorubicin, daunorubicin, cytarabine, L-asparaginase, paclitaxel, and cisplatin. In many cases the itchy reaction is limited to the site of vascular access.

Different cytotoxic drugs may cause neuropathy, which might be accompanied by pain and/or itching. In addition, chemotherapy for some hematological malignancies is invariably accompanied by the induction of the herpes zoster infection. At least some of this infection may result in post-herpetic pruralgia.[30,31]

Dry and desquamating skin is frequently seen after radiotherapy. Dryness of the skin is seen with accumulated doses of 2,000–2,800 cGy,[32,33] and it is probable that dry skin is caused by obliteration of the sebaceous glands. Irradiated skin loses basal cells with each fraction of radiation. Other basal cells undergo keratinization and are shed at an increased rate. Subsequent peeling of the dead cells is called dry desquamation. Itching is experienced especially where the skin is dry. Scratching of irradiated skin may induce injury, necro-

sis, and poorly healing wounds. When desquamation is moist, the skin is prone to infections and pain. Not infrequently, skin changes necessitate interruption or even discontinuation of the treatment, thus compromising treatment efficacy. This effect may be even more pronounced where radiotherapy is combined with chemotherapy. Homeopathic treatment of radiation-induced pruritus has been tried and found to be effective in more than 80% of cases.[34]

Pruritus is a known side effect of several biological response modifiers. Interferons are notorious for this, which is ironic because they have been successful in the treatment of the itching which complicates various hematological disorders.

## References

1. Cormia FE, Domonkos AN. Cutaneous reactions to internal malignancy. *Med Clin North Am*. 1965;49:655–680.
2. Mesa RA, Niblack J, Wadleigh M, et al. The burden of fatigue and quality of life in myeloproliferative disorders (mpds): an international Internet-based survey of 1179 MPD patients. *Cancer*. 2007;109:68–76.
3. Krajnik M, Zylicz Z. Understanding pruritus in systemic disease. *J Pain Symptom Manage*. 2001;21:151–168.
4. Afifi Y, Aubin F, Puzenat E, et al. Pruritus sine materia: a prospective study of 95 patients. *Rev Med Interne*. 2004;25: 490–493.
5. Paul R, Jansen CT. Itch and malignancy prognosis in generalized pruritus: a 6-year follow-up of 125 patients. *J Am Acad Dermatol*. 1987;16:1179–1182.
6. Feakins RM, Lowe DG. Basal cell carcinoma of the vulva: a clinicopathologic study of 45 cases. *Int J Gynecol Pathol*. 1997;16:319–324.
7. Twycross RG. Pruritus and pain in en cuirass breast cancer. *Lancet*. 1981;2:696.
8. Cohen PR. Cutaneous paraneoplastic syndromes. *Am Fam Physician*. 1994;50:1273–1282.
9. Cohen PR. Paraneoplastic dermatopathology: cutaneous paraneoplastic syndromes. *Adv Dermatol*. 1996;11:215–252; discussion 53.
10. Cormia FE. Pruritus, an uncommon but important symptom of systemic carcinoma. *Arch Dermatol*. 1965;92:36–39.
11. Peterson K, Forsyth PA, Posner JB. Paraneoplastic sensorimotor neuropathy associated with breast cancer. *J Neurooncol*. 1994;21:159–170.
12. Bosonnet L. Pruritis: scratching the surface. *Eur J Cancer Care (Engl)*. 2003;12:162–165.
13. Krajnik M, Zylicz Z. Pruritus accompanying solid tumors. In: Zylicz Z, Twycross R, Jones EA, eds. *Pruritus in Advanced Disease*. Oxford: Oxford University Press; 2004:97–106.
14. Zylicz Z, Krajnik M, Sorge AA, Costantini M. Paroxetine in the treatment of severe non-dermatological pruritus:

a randomized, controlled trial. *J Pain Symptom Manage.* 2003;26:1105–1112.

15. Adreev VC, Petkov I. Skin manifestations associated with tumours of the brain. *Br J Dermatol.* 1975;92:675–678.

16. Twycross R, Greaves MW, Handwerker H, et al. Itch: scratching more than the surface. *QJM.* 2003;96:7–26.

17. Jones EA, Bergasa NV. The pruritus of cholestasis and the opioid system. *JAMA.* 1992;268:3359–3362.

18. Bergasa NV. Update on the treatment of the pruritus of cholestasis. *Clin Liver Dis.* 2008;12:219–234.

19. Zylicz Z, Stork N, Krajnik M. Severe pruritus of cholestasis in disseminated cancer: developing a rational treatment strategy. A case report. *J Pain Symptom Manage.* 2005;29:100–103.

20. Reddy L, Krajnik M, Zylicz Z. Transdermal buprenorphine may be effective in the treatment of pruritus in primary biliary cirrhosis. *J Pain Symptom Manage.* 2007;34:455–456.

21. Shiotani A, Sakurane M, Furukawa F. Helicobacter pylori-positive patients with pruritic skin diseases are at increased risk for gastric cancer. *Aliment Pharmacol Ther.* 2004;20: (suppl 1):80–84.

22. Daniel GL, Longo WE, Vernava AM 3rd. Pruritus ani. Causes and concerns. *Dis Colon Rectum.* 1994;37:670–674.

23. Gobbi PG, Attardo-Parrinello G, Lattanzio G, Rizzo SC, Ascari E. Severe pruritus should be a B-symptom in Hodgkin's disease. *Cancer.* 1983;51:1934–1936.

24. Rubenstein M, Duvic M. Cutaneous manifestations of Hodgkin's disease. *Int J Dermatol.* 2006;45:251–256.

25. Stadie V, Marsch WC. Itching attacks with generalized hyperhydrosis as initial symptoms of Hodgkin's disease. *J Eur Acad Dermatol Venereol.* 2003;17:559–561.

26. Diehn F, Tefferi A. Pruritus in polycythaemia vera: prevalence, laboratory correlates and management. *Br J Haematol.* 2001; 115:619–621.

27. Tefferi A, Fonseca R. Selective serotonin reuptake inhibitors are effective in the treatment of polycythemia vera-associated pruritus. *Blood.* 2627;2002:99.

28. Easton P, Galbraith PR. Cimetidine treatment of pruritus in polycythemia vera. *N Engl J Med.* 1978;299:1134.

29. Roberts DL. Cimetidine for pruritis related to systemic disorders. *Br Med J.* 1980;280:405.

30. Oaklander AL, Bowsher D, Galer B, Haanpaa M, Jensen MP. Herpes zoster itch: preliminary epidemiologic data. *J Pain.* 2003;4:338–343.

31. Oaklander AL, Cohen SP, Raju SV. Intractable postherpetic itch and cutaneous deafferentation after facial shingles. *Pain.* 2002;96:9–12.

32. Hassey KM. Skin care for patients receiving radiation therapy for rectal cancer. *J Enterostomal Ther.* 1987;14:197–200.

33. Phillips TL, Fu KK. Quantification of combined radiation therapy and chemotherapy effects on critical normal tissues. *Cancer.* 1976;37:1186–1200.

34. Schlappack O. Homeopathic treatment of radiation-induced itching in breast cancer patients. A prospective observational study. *Homeopathy.* 2004;93:210–215.

# Chapter 31
# Drugs

Jacek C. Szepietowski and Adam Reich

## 31.1 Introduction

Pruritus is frequently recognized as a side effect of many systemically and topically administered drugs. Drug-induced pruritus may have localized as well as generalized character and may start with the first drug administration or be delayed in time for several weeks or even months.[1–4] However, the incidence and clinical manifestation of this treatment complication is difficult to establish for the vast majority of drugs, as no detailed studies evaluating this symptom have been carried out until now. Frequently the underlying mechanism is not fully known. Only a few drugs have been analyzed more carefully, mainly opioids, hydroxyethyl starch (HES), and vancomycin (see below). Very commonly, only case reports have been presented in the literature. Moreover, sometimes it is very difficult to distinguish between primary drug-induced pruritus and accompanying symptomatic pruritus secondary to e.g., drug-induced urticaria or lichenoid eruptions.[3–5] It is nearly impossible to mention all the drugs that could induce itching. Pruritus, secondary to drug-induced skin lesions was reported in case of antibiotics,[3,6–17] angiotensin converting enzyme (ACE)-inhibitors,[5] sartans,[4] β-adrenergic blockers,[18,19] diuretics,[20] minoxidil,[21] methyldopa,[22] statins,[23–25] allopurinol,[26] nonsteroidal anti-inflammatory drugs,[27–31] chlorambucil,[32] and fractionated heparins[33] (Table 31.1). Pruritus was also observed as a result of the use of cephalosporins,[34–39] quinolones,[40–44] rifampin,[45] thiamphenicol,[46] antimalarials,[47,48] amlodipine,[2] isradipine,[49] diltiazem,[50,51] gliclazide,[52] selective serotonine reuptake inhibitors,[53,54] anticonvulsives,[55–59] paclitaxel,[60] tamoxifen,[61] gemcitabine,[62] or granulocyte-macrophage colony-stimulating factor[63] (Table 31.1). In addition, pruritus may also accompany local skin or mucous membrane reaction after topical application of different medicines including clonidine,[64,65] ciprofloxacin,[66] or calcineurin inhibitors.[67]

One of the most commonly reported drug-induced pruritus is also pruritus concomitant to the liver damage provoked by drugs. Such kind of pruritus was reported after administration of estrogens and anabolic steroids,[68–71] antibiotics,[1,3,72–78] trimethoprim/sulfamethoxazole,[79] ACE-inhibitors,[80–85] β-adrenergic blokers,[86] sartans,[5,87] calcium channel blockers,[88,89] amiodarone,[90] ticlopidine,[91] biguanides,[92] thyreostatics,[93] antidepressants,[94] neuroleptics,[95–98] corticosteroids,[99] and nonsteroidal anti-inflammatory drugs[100] (Table 31.1). In case of liver dysfunction, pruritus usually appears several weeks after the commencement of the treatment,[1,74,91–93] although it was also reported after relatively short-term therapy periods.[75,77] Signs and symptoms of jaundice and pruritus may appear up to six weeks after stopping the therapy.[1] Pruritus may resolve shortly after drug discontinuation[89] or may persist even for several months or years after treatment withdrawal.[79,94,100] Cholestyramine or ursodeoxycholic acid seems to be the best choice for the treatment of drug-associated cholestasis with pruritus.[75,87] Rifampicin and opioid antagonists should be reserved for patients who fail first-line therapy.[87]

Another interesting group of drugs which may be responsible for itching are serotonine reuptake inhibitors.[53,54] These drugs are sometimes used as effective antipruritic agents due to their activity on the central nervous system. However, in some patients these drugs may lead to increased peripheral concentration of serotonine and thus induce itching in individuals who are very sensitive to increased serotonin concentrations, as it was shown that intradermally injected serotonine may provoke itching.[53,54]

L. Misery and S. Ständer (eds.), *Pruritus*,
DOI 10.1007/978-1-84882-322-8_31, © Springer-Verlag London Limited 2010

**Table 31.1** Medicines that are able to induce pruritus

| Medicine group | Examples |
| --- | --- |
| ACE inhibitors | Captopril, enalapril, fosinopril, lisinopril |
| Angiotensin II antagonists (sartans) | Candesartan, irbesartan |
| Beta-adrenergic blockers | Bupranolol, carvedilol, metoprolol, pindolol |
| Calcium channel blockers | Amlodipine, diltiazem, isradipine, verapamil |
| Other antihypertensive drugs | Clonidine, methyldopa |
| Antiarrhythmic drugs | Amiodarone |
| Antiplatelet agents | Ticlopidine |
| Biguanides | Metformin |
| Sulfonylurea derivates | Gliclazide |
| Statins | Lovastatin, simvastatin |
| Penicillins | Amoxycyline/clavulanate, ampicillin, penicillin g, piperacillin |
| Cephalosporins | Cefotaxime, cefepime, cefixime, ceftazidime |
| Macrolides | Erythromycin |
| Carbapenemes | Imipenem/cilastatin |
| Monobactams | Aztreonam |
| Quinolones | Amifloxacin, ciprofloxacin, lomefloxacin, ofloxacin, trovafloxacin |
| Tetracyclines | Tetracycline, minocycline |
| Lincosamides | Clindamycin |
| Glycopeptide antibiotics | Vancomycin, teicoplanin |
| Streptogramins | Quinupristin/dalfopristin |
| Other antibiotics and chemiotherapeutics | Metronidazole, rifampin, tiamphenicol, trimethoprim/sulfamethoxazole |
| Antimalarials | Amodiaquine, chloroquine, halofantrine, hydroxychloroquine |
| Antithyroid agents | Methimazole |
| Tricyclic antidepressants | Amitriptyline |
| Selective serotonine reuptake inhibitors | Citalopram, fluoxetine, paroxetine, sertraline |
| Neuroleptics | Chlorpromazine, phenothiazine, promazine, risperidone |
| Antiepileptics | Carbamazepine, fosphenytoin, oxcarbazepine, phenytoin, topiramat |
| Inhibitors of xanthine oxidase | Allopurinol |
| Corticosteroids | Methylprednisolone |
| Nonsteroidal anti-inflammatory drugs | Acetaminofen, aspirin, celecoxib, diclofenac, ibuprofen, sodium salicylate |
| Opioids | Codein, fentanyl, methadon, morphin, oxycodon, oxymorphon, sufentanil, tramadol |
| Sex hormones | Danazol, oral contraceptives |
| Cytostatics and anticancer drugs | Chlorambucil, gemcitabine, paclitaxel, tamoxifen |
| Fractionated heparins | Enoxaparin |
| Cytokines and growth factors | Granulocyte-macrophage colony-stimulating factor |
| Plasma volume expanders | Hydroxyethyl starch (HES) |

## 31.2 Vancomycin and "Red Man Syndrome"

Vancomycin is a glycopeptide antibiotic originally derived from *Streptomyces (Nocardia) orientalis*, which is widely used for severe Gram-positive bacterial infections, especially those of methicillin-resistant strains of *Staphylococcus* sp.[101] Vancomycin is rarely associated with serious toxicity. However, in some patients a so-called red man syndrome is observed during the administration of the drug, which is characterized by flushing of the upper body and pruritus, occasionally also accompanied by hypotension and bronchospasm.[102,103] Pruritus may be limited to the upper trunk or can be generalized.[104] This acute hypersensitivity reaction may start within a few minutes from the initiation of infusion and usually resolves over several hours after completion of the drug administration.[103,104] It is often mistaken for an allergic or anaphylactoid reaction, but patients usually tolerate subsequent doses, if the dilution and the period of infusion are increased.[102] The red man syndrome is believed to be a consequence of histamine release, as vancomycin possesses the ability to release histamine directly from mast cells by nonimmunological processes.[105] It was demonstrated that the severity of symptoms in healthy volunteers is strictly related to the level of histamine.

The most important factors influencing the incidence of this adverse reaction are the vancomycin infusion rate and dilution of the drug. While infusing 1 g vancomycin over 10 min to patients scheduled for elective prosthetic joint replacement, Renz et al.[106] observed rash and pruritus in about 90% of patients and significant hypotension in around 50%. During administration of 1 g vancomycin over 30 min to cardiac surgical patients, red man syndrome and hypotension was found in 25% of cases.[107] To reduce the risk of the side effects due to vancomycin infusion, it is recommended to infuse vancomycin over a period of 60 min.[104,108,109] In this schedule, the risk of red man syndrome is less than 5%.[104,110] If the drug has to be administered faster, then oral or intravenous antihistaminics should be given, which were shown to effectively reduce the occurrence of all the above-mentioned side effects.[106]

It was also demonstrated that pruritus occurrence during vancomycin administration can be considered as an alarm bell that indicates the presence of peripheral vasodilatation. It can help physicians to identify at an early stage those patients who are at risk for hypotension (e.g., hypovolemic patient) and to compensate for hypovolemia before continuing administration of vancomycin. This fact is of great importance, as hypotension for severely ill patients may be a life-threatening problem.

## 31.3 Pruritus Induced by Chloroquine and other Antimalarials

Chloroquine, a widely used antimalarial agent, was found to produce pruritus of unknown mechanism in up to 60–70% of Black Africans.[47,111–113] In nearly 60% of pruritic subjects pruritus could be considered very severe.[111–113] Interestingly, chloroquine-induced pruritus is uncommon in Caucasians or Asians.[114,115] In the study by Bussaratid et al.,[114] among Thailand population only 1.9% of 1,000 patients with malaria experienced pruritus due to chloroquine therapy. Regarding Black Africans, pruritus appeared mainly in young patients (<40), and the majority of patients had the onset of itching within 24 h of chloroquine ingestion.[113] In nearly half of the patients, pruritus lasted longer than 48 h after the last dose of chloroquine.[113] Pruritus may be limited to hands and feet, but some subjects may suffer from generalized pruritus.[113,114] Chloroquine-induced pruritus is the most common adverse drug reaction experienced by Black Africans, which significantly affects the compliance with therapy.[111] More than 10% of pregnant women avoided malaria chemoprophylaxis with chloroquine from fear of pruritus.[116]

The pathogenesis of chloroquine-induced pruritus remains unclear. Several mechanisms have been postulated. As it is observed mainly in Black Africans, genetic background seems to be a strong predisposing factor. Chloroquine has been shown to release histamine, and antihistamic drugs have been demonstrated to be effective in a subgroup of patients.[111,117,118] The severity of pruritus also correlated with the antecedent malaria parasite density in the blood.[117] In addition, it was suggested that subjects suffering from pruritus may present slower metabolism of chloroquine leading to higher plasma chloroquine concentration, although the overall pharmacokinetic patterns were comparable in both patients with pruritus and without.[119,120] Pruritus in patients with malaria may also be mediated by endogenous opioid peptides via the μ-opioid receptor.[111,121] Summarizing, it seems that chloroquine-induced pruritus should be considered as a multifactorial phenomenon.

The most commonly prescribed medications for chloroquine-induced pruritus are antihistaminics.[113,114] However, they are effective only partially.[118] Pruritus may also be reduced by the combined administration of chloroquine and a single oral dose of prednisolone (10 mg) or niacin (50 mg) with no negative influence on malaria parasite clearance or clinical amelioration.[47,122] The other interesting therapeutic option is naltrexone. Naltrexone therapy exerted at least a similar antipruritic effect in patients with chloroquine-induced itch as observed in the group treated with promethazine.[111]

Pruritus was also reported after other antimalarials, such as amodiaquine, halofantrine, and hydroxychloroquine, although less commonly and with lower intensity.[123–126] Frequently, aquagenic or post-wetness type of pruritus was observed, usually located on the lower extremities and back, without visible skin lesions.[126] It appeared about 1–3 weeks after initiation of treatment and developed mainly after a hot shower, beginning within minutes of water contact, persisting at a high intensity for several minutes and then remaining at low intensity for several hours.[126]

## 31.4 Opioid-Induced Pruritus

Opioids are frequently used for the treatment of acute and chronic pain. One of the common side effects due to opioid therapy is pruritus.[127] A wide variety of opioids has been identified as inducing itching.[128–133] Pruritus is recognized in 2–10% of patients treated systemically with this group of drugs, although its incidence depends on the opioid used and its mode of administration.[127,134] The risk is increased when opioids are administered epidurally or intraspinally, and the highest incidence (up to 100%) is associated with intrathecal morphine.[127,134–136] Parturients appear to be the most susceptible group.[135,136] The incidence of itching increases with increasing doses of opioids.[136] Facial areas innervated by the trigeminal nerve are mostly affected, probably due to the high concentration of opioid receptors in the spinal nucleus of the trigeminal nerve. Typically patients scratch the nose, perinasal area and upper part of the face.[134,135]

The postulated mechanism for opioid-induced pruritus is a centrally mediated process via the μ-opioid receptor.[137–140] Naloxon, a classic μ-receptor antagonist, is effective in preventing or treating intrathecal or epidural opioid-induced itching.[141] Medullary dorsal horn may be a critical site in the action of opioids in producing this symptom.[138,139] In monkeys, morphine injected unilaterally into the medullary dorsal horn causes ipsilateral facial scratching.[138,139] Modulation of the serotoninergic pathway and involvement of prostaglandins or histamine may also be important.[135] In addition, stimulation of opioid receptors in the skin by opioids cannot be excluded.[141]

Treatment of opioid-induced pruritus remains a challenge. Several treatment modalities have been tried, but none was fully satisfactory. Opioid antagonists may have a role in the prevention of opioid-induced pruritus; however, both naloxone and naltrexone decreased the analgesia, especially at higher doses.[141–145] Nalbuphine, as a 40-mg intravenous bolus, effectively prevents pruritus without increasing pain, but the treatment was associated with increased drowsiness.[141] However, nalbuphine was shown to be ineffective in the treatment of postoperative opioid-induced pruritus in pediatric patients.[146] The use of 5-HT$_3$ receptor antagonists (ondansetron, dolasetron) remains controversial. Some authors reported good efficacy,[134,143,147–149] while others denied it.[150–152] In addition, antihistaminics, droperidol, propofol, alizapride, tenoxicam, and diclofenac have been tried with varying success.[127,135,142,153] Another interesting option of pruritus prevention is the reduction of opioid dose by the combination of opioid with other drugs, e.g., sufentanil with bupivacaine.[154] Such combination offers satisfactory analgesia with a very low incidence of pruritus.[154]

## 31.5 Pruritus Induced by HES

HES is an artificial colloid commonly used for clinical fluid management.[155] The chemical synthesis of HES involves partial hydrolysis of amylopectin corn starch and hydroethylation of the constituents at the C2, C3, and C6 positions.[155] This drug can be produced with differing average molecular masses as well as with the different extent and pattern of substitution with hydroxyethyl groups resulting in numerous variants of HES.[155] The use of HES can be complicated with well-defined side effects including coagulopathy, clinical bleeding, anaphylactoid reactions, and pruritus.[155]

Because of the delayed onset of pruritus after HES administration, this symptom had not been recognized as a complication of HES for a long time. First case reports were published in the early 1980s,[156,157] but this side effect was not widely reported until the early 1990s.[155,158–161] The frequency of pruritus after HES administration varied depending on the studied population from 12.6 to 54%.[159,162–165] Pruritus may appear even after administration of small volumes of HES, but it seems that the use of higher doses is associated with higher frequency and more severe pruritus.[162,163,165] The symptom appears usually as pruritic crises lasting from 2 min to 1 h and is trigerred by friction, bathing in warm water, or physical stress.[155,165,166] Pruritus may be generalized or localized involving any part of the body, and there is no site predilection.[155,161,165] As mentioned above, the onset of pruritus is delayed, and it usually starts 1–6 weeks after HES infusion.[155,163] Pruritus is often very severe and may last for several weeks or months. In the study of Kimme et al.,[165] the median onset of pruritus after the administration of HES was 4 weeks and the median duration was 15 weeks. In another study, the symptoms resolved spontaneously after the median period of 10 months.[166] In individual patients pruritus was observed for as long as 18–24 months.[155,166]

The pathogenesis of pruritus induced by HES is still not fully clear. No degranulation of basophils, no release of histamine from mast cells, and no release of substance P from macrophages was observed.[160,161] However, it seems that pruritus may be elucidated by the storage of HES in tissues and direct activation of pruritogenic nerves. A deposition of HES in the skin, mainly in dermal macrophages, endothelial cells of blood, and lymph vessels, some perineuronal cells and endoneural macrophages of larger nerve fascicles, some keratinocytes and Langerhans cells has been reported by Jurecka et al.[160] Gall et al. found HES deposits mainly in macrophages and endothelial cells.[161] The storage of HES within the skin was also noted by Reimann et al.[167] All patients given HES had lysosomal deposits in the macrophages; some of them also had them in cutaneous epithelium and endothelium. The extent of lysosomal storage correlated with the amount of infused HES and the interval between biopsy and the last HES infusion.[167] Consecutive biopsies in some cases demonstrated a definite decrease over the years of HES deposits in the vacuoles.[167] In another study, a characteristic vacuolization of perivascular macrophages was noted in all skin biopsies as early as 1 day after a single infusion of 30 g HES, and immunoreactivity for HES was demonstrable within the vacuoles.[168] The size and number of vacuoles in the macrophages increased concomitantly with the cumulative dosage of HES and following administration of higher HES dosages. Vacuoles were demonstrable in endothelial cells of blood and lymphatic vessels, basal keratinocytes, epithelia of sweat glands, and small peripheral nerves, the last being associated with pruritus.[168] A subsequent reduction of the vacuoles in size and number could be demonstrated within 52 months.[168] In nerves, HES deposits persisted for no longer than 17 months paralleling the cessation of pruritus. Biopsies taken after 94 months exhibited no HES deposits in the skin.[168] HES deposits were also observed in other organs like liver, muscles, spleen, or intestine, and the HES storage was dose dependent, decreased in all organs with time, and was greater in patients suffering from pruritus.[169]

It seems that pruritus is caused by the deposition of HES in small peripheral nerves or in Schwann cells of cutaneous nerves.[155,166] It was noted that pruritus after high cumulative doses of HES was closely correlated with HES deposition in cutaneous nerves. It has been suggested that HES deposits may mechanically irritate nerve endings, thus provoking pruritus.[155,161,166] Metze et al.[166] found that deposition of HES in peripheral nerves was strictly confined to those patients who suffered from pruritus. A characteristic vacuolization was sporadically visible even at the light microscopic level in the perineural and endoneural cells.[166] Vacuoles partially filled with amorphous material could also be seen in Schwannian cells of small myelinated nerve fibers. In addition, Schwann cells surrounding unmyelinated axons also contained distinctly labeled vacuoles and vesicles.[166] Remarkably, no immunoreactivity was detected in the axonal elements.[166] Whether other HES-containing cells such as macrophages, endothelial cells, keratinocytes, or Langerhans cells also partake in provoking pruritic reaction or exert a more direct effect on sensory nerves fibers is unclear.[155]

Treatment of HES-induced pruritus still remains a challenge, as most currently available antipruritic strategies are not effective. Generally, no improvement was observed with antihistamic drugs, which are the most widely used antipruritic agents.[158–160,165] Glucocorticoids, neuroleptics, oil baths, or acetaminophen were shown to be ineffective, too.[155] One study documented good response to topical capsaicin, but this treatment regimen is frequently poorly tolerated due to burning sensations.[170] Some patients may respond to oral naltrexone,[171] and finally gradual relief has been reported over a period of several weeks with ultraviolet therapy in part of the studied population.[170] However, no controlled studies have been performed to date assessing these methods of treatment in HES-induced pruritus. Because of the severity of the symptoms and poor efficacy of the therapy, patients with HES-induced pruritus often present sleep disturbances and impaired quality of life.[155,162] Some patients may also need support for psychiatric conditions due to anxiety, and even suicides due to HES-induced pruritus have been reported.[155]

# References

1. Limauro DL, Chan-Tompkins NH, Carter RW, et al. Amoxicillin/clavulanate-associated hepatic failure with progression to Stevens-Johnson syndrome. *Ann Pharmacother*. 1999;33:560–564.
2. Orme S, da Costa D. Generalised pruritus associated with amlodipine. *Br Med J*. 1997;315:463.
3. Shirin H, Schapiro JM, Arber N, et al. Erythromycin base-induced rash and liver function disturbances. *Ann Pharmacother*. 1992;26:1522–1523.

4. Ständer S, Streit M, Darsow U, et al. Diagnostisches und therapeutisches Vorgehen bei chronischem Pruritus. *J Dtsch Dermatol Ges.* 2006;4:350–370.

5. Morton A, Muir J, Lim D. Rash and acute nephritic syndrome due to candesartan. *Br Med J.* 2004;328:25.

6. Adcock BB, Rodman DP. Ampicillin-specific rashes. *Arch Fam Med.* 1996;5:301–304.

7. Ball P. Ciprofloxacin: an overview of adverse experiences. *J Antimicrob Chemother.* 1986;18:(suppl D):187–193.

8. Gaut PL, Carron WC, Ching WT, et al. Intravenous/oral ciprofloxacin therapy versus intravenous ceftazidime therapy for selected bacterial infections. *Am J Med.* 1989;87:169S–175S.

9. Gonzalo-Garijo MA, de Argila D. Erythroderma due to aztreonam and clindamycin. *Investig Allergol Clin Immunol.* 2006;16:210–211.

10. Goulden V, Glass D, Cunliffe WJ. Safety of long-term high-dose minocycline in the treatment of acne. *Br J Dermatol.* 1996;134:693–695.

11. Hessen MT, Ingerman MJ, Kaufman DH, et al. Clinical efficacy of ciprofloxacin therapy for gram-negative bacillary osteomyelitis. *Am J Med.* 1987;82:262–265.

12. Kapoor K, Chandra M, Nag D, et al. Evaluation of metronidazole toxicity: a prospective study. *Int J Clin Pharmacol Res.* 1999;19:83–88.

13. Kaufmann D, Pichler W, Beer JH. Severe episode of high fever with rash, lymphadenopathy, neutropenia, and eosinophilia after minocycline therapy for acne. *Arch Intern Med.* 1994;154:1983–1984.

14. Lamb HM, Figgitt DP, Faulds D. Quinupristin/dalfopristin: a review of its use in the management of serious gram-positive infections. *Drugs.* 1999;58:1061–1097.

15. Report to the Research Committee of the British Tuberculosis Association by the Clinical Trials Subcommittee. Comparison of side-effects of tetracycline and tetracycline plus nystatin. *Br Med J.* 1968;4:11–15.

16. Ruskin J, LaRiviere M. Low-dose co-trimoxazole for prevention of *Pneumocystis carinii* pneumonia in human immunodeficiency virus disease. *Lancet.* 1991;337:468–471.

17. Wendel GD Jr, Stark BJ, Jamison RB, et al. Penicillin allergy and desensitization in serious infections during pregnancy. *N Engl J Med.* 1985;312:1229–1232.

18. Gonasun LM, Langrall H. Adverse reactions to pindolol administration. *Am Heart J.* 1982;104:482–486.

19. Jeck T, Edmonds D, Mengden T, et al. Betablocking drugs in essential hypertension: transdermal bupranolol compared with oral metoprolol. *Int J Clin Pharmacol Res.* 1992;12:139–148.

20. Ochoa PG, Arribas MT, Mena JM, et al. Cutaneous adverse reaction to furosemide treatment: new clinical findings. *Can Vet J.* 2006;47:576–578.

21. Ackerman BH, Townsend ME, Golden W, et al. Pruritic rash with actinic keratosis and impending exfoliation in a patient with hypertension managed with minoxidil. *Drug Intell Clin Pharm.* 1988;22:702–703.

22. Haider Z, Bano KA. Experience with anti-hypertensive drug therapy in a hypertension Clinic - 1972–1983. A retrospective analysis. *J Pak Med Assoc.* 1990;40:91–93.

23. Kashyap ML, McGovern ME, Berra K, et al. Long-term safety and efficacy of a once-daily niacin/lovastatin formulation for patients with dyslipidemia. *Am J Cardiol.* 2002;89:672–678.

24. Sharma M, Sharma DR, Singh V, et al. Evaluation of efficacy and safety of fixed dose lovastatin and niacin (ER) combination in Asian Indian dyslipidemic patients: a multicentric study. *Vasc Health Risk Manag.* 2006;2:87–93.

25. Stoebner PE, Michot C, Ligeron C, et al. Simvastatin-induced lichen planus pemphigoides. *Ann Dermatol Venereol.* 2003;130:187–190.

26. Fitzgerald DA, Heagerty AH, Stephens M, et al. Follicular toxic pustuloderma associated with allopurinol. *Clin Exp Dermatol.* 1994;19:243–245.

27. Grant JA, Weiler JM. A report of a rare immediate reaction after ingestion of acetaminophen. *Ann Allergy Asthma Immunol.* 2001;87:227–229.

28. Levy MB, Fink JN. Anaphylaxis to celecoxib. *Ann Allergy Asthma Immunol.* 2001;87:72–73.

29. Roll A, Wüthrich B, Schmid-Grendelmeier P, et al. Tolerance to celecoxib in patients with a history of adverse reactions to nonsteroidal anti-inflammatory drugs. *Swiss Med Wkly.* 2006;136:684–690.

30. Schwarz N, Ham Pong A. Acetaminophen anaphylaxis with aspirin and sodium salicylate sensitivity: a case report. *Ann Allergy Asthma Immunol.* 1996;77:473–474.

31. Thumb N, Kolarz G, Scherak O, et al. The efficacy and safety of fentiazac and diclofenac sodium in peri-arthritis of the shoulder: a multi-centre, double-blind comparison. *J Int Med Res.* 1987;15:327–334.

32. Torricelli R, Kurer SB, Kroner T, et al. Delayed allergic reaction to Chlorambucil (Leukeran). Case report and literature review. *Schweiz Med Wochenschr.* 1995;125:1870–1873.

33. MacLaughlin EJ, Fitzpatrick KT, Sbar E, et al. Anaphylactoid reaction to enoxaparin in a patient with deep venous thrombosis. *Pharmacotherapy.* 2002;22:1511–1515.

34. Shimokata K, Suetsugu S, Umeda H, et al. Evaluation of T-2588 in the treatment of respiratory tract infection. *Jpn J Antibiot.* 1986;39:2897–2913.

35. Sonoda T, Matsuda M, Nakano E, et al. Clinical evaluation of cefixime (CFIX) in the treatment of urinary tract infection. *Hinyokika Kiyo.* 1989;35:1267–1275.

36. Theopold M, Benner U, Bauernfeind A. Effectiveness and tolerance of cefixime in bacterial infections in the ENT area. *Infection.* 1990;18:(suppl 3):S122–S124.

37. Holloway WJ, Palmer D. Clinical applications of a new parenteral antibiotic in the treatment of severe bacterial infections. *Am J Med.* 1996;100:52S–59S.

38. Chapman TM, Perry CM. Cefepime: a review of its use in the management of hospitalized patients with pneumonia. *Am J Respir Med.* 2003;2:75–107.

39. Childs SJ, Kosola JW. Update of safety of cefotaxime. *Clin Ther.* 1982;5:(suppl A):97–111.

40. Cook JA, Silverman MH, Schelling DJ, et al. Multiple-dose pharmacokinetics and safety of oral amifloxacin in healthy volunteers. *Antimicrob Agents Chemother.* 1990;34:974–979.

41. Cox CE. A comparison of the safety and efficacy of lomefloxacin and ciprofloxacin in the treatment of complicated or recurrent urinary tract infections. *Am J Med.* 1992;92:82S–86S.

42. Cox CE, Gentry LO, Rodriguez-Gomez G. Multicenter open-label study of parenteral ofloxacin in treatment of pyelonephritis in adults. *Urology.* 1992;39:453–456.

43. Torum B, Block SL, Avila H, et al. Efficacy of ofloxacin otic solution once daily for 7 days in the treatment of otitis externa: a multicenter, open-label, phase III trial. *Clin Ther.* 2004;26:1046–1054.

44. Williams DJ, Hopkins S. Safety and tolerability of intravenous-to-oral treatment and single-dose intravenous or oral prophylaxis with trovafloxacin. *Am J Surg.* 1998;176:(suppl): 74S–79S.

45. Walker-Renard P. Pruritus associated with intravenous rifampin. *Ann Pharmacother.* 1995;29:267–268.

46. Siboulet A, Bohbot JM, Lhuillier N, et al. "One-minute treatment" with thiamphenicol in 50,000 cases of gonorrhea: a 22-year study. *Sex Transm Dis.* 1984;11:(suppl): 391–395.

47. Adebayo RA, Sofowora GG, Onayemi O, et al. Chloroquine-induced pruritus in malaria fever: contribution of malaria parasitaemia and the effects of prednisolone, niacin, and their combination, compared with antihistamine. *Br J Clin Pharmacol.* 1997;44:157–161.

48. Ajayi AA, Kolawole BA, Udoh SJ. Endogenous opioids, μ-opiate receptors and chloroquine-induced pruritus: a double-blind comparison of naltrexone and promethazine in patients with malaria fever who have an established history of generalized chloroquine-induced itching. *Int J Dermatol.* 2004;43:972–977.

49. Johnson BF, Eisner GM, McMahon FG, et al. A multicenter comparison of adverse reaction profiles of isradipine and enalapril at equipotent doses in patients with essential hypertension. *J Clin Pharmacol.* 1995;35:484–492.

50. Bernink PJ, de Weerd P, Ten CF, et al. An 8-week double-blind study of amlodipine and diltiazem in patients with stable exertional angina pectoris. *J Cardiovasc Pharmacol.* 1991;17:(suppl 1):S53–S56.

51. Gonzalo Garijo MA, Pérez Calderón R, de Argila Fernández-Durán D, et al. Cutaneous reactions due to diltiazem and cross reactivity with other calcium channel blockers. *Allergol Immunopathol (Madr).* 2005;33:238–240.

52. Kilo C, Dudley J, Kalb B. Evaluation of the efficacy and safety of Diamicron in non-insulin-dependent diabetic patients. *Diabetes Res Clin Pract.* 1991;14(suppl 2):S79–S82.

53. Cederberg J, Knight S, Svenson S, et al. Itch and skin rash from chocolate during fluoxetine and sertraline treatment: case report. *BMC Psychiatry.* 2004;4:36.

54. Richard MA, Fiszenson F, Jreissati M, et al. Cutaneous adverse effects during selective serotonin reuptake inhibitors therapy: 2 cases. *Ann Dermatol Venereol.* 2001;128:759–761.

55. Fischer JH, Patel TV, Fischer PA. Fosphenytoin: clinical pharmacokinetics and comparative advantages in the acute treatment of seizures. *Clin Pharmacokinet.* 2003;42:33–58.

56. Knapp LE, Kugler AR. Clinical experience with fosphenytoin in adults: pharmacokinetics, safety, and efficacy. *J Child Neurol.* 1998;13:(suppl 1):S15–S18.

57. Ochoa JG. Pruritus, a rare but troublesome adverse reaction of topiramate. *Seizure.* 2003;12:516–518.

58. Prosser TR, Lander RD. Phenytoin-induced hypersensitivity reactions. *Clin Pharm.* 1987;6:728–734.

59. Wellington K, Goa KL. Oxcarbazepine: an update of its efficacy in the management of epilepsy. *CNS Drugs.* 2001;15:137–163.

60. Freilich RJ, Seidman AD. Pruritis caused by 3-hour infusion of high-dose paclitaxel and improvement with tricyclic antidepressants. *J Natl Cancer Inst.* 1995;87:933–934.

61. Love RR, Nguyen BD, Nguyen CB, et al. Symptoms associated with oophorectomy and tamoxifen treatment for breast cancer in premenopausal Vietnamese women. *Breast Cancer Res Treat.* 1999;58:281–286.

62. Hejna M, Valencak J, Raderer M. Anal pruritus after cancer chemotherapy with gemcitabine. *N Engl J Med.* 1999;340: 655–656.

63. Hamm J, Schiller JH, Cuffie C, et al. Dose-ranging study of recombinant human granulocyte-macrophage colony-stimulating factor in small-cell lung carcinoma. *J Clin Oncol.* 1994;12:2667–2676.

64. Dias VC, Tendler B, Oparil S, et al. Clinical experience with transdermal clonidine in African-American and Hispanic-American patients with hypertension: evaluation from a 12-week prospective, open-label clinical trial in community-based clinics. *Am J Ther.* 1999;6:19–24.

65. Groth H, Vetter H, Knüsel J, et al. Transdermal clonidine application: long-term results in essential hypertension. *Klin Wochenschr.* 1984;62:925–930.

66. Miró N. Controlled multicenter study on chronic suppurative otitis media treated with topical applications of ciprofloxacin 0.2% solution in single-dose containers or combination of polymyxin B, neomycin, and hydrocortisone suspension. *Otolaryngol Head Neck Surg.* 2000;123: 617–623.

67. Szepietowski J, Reich A, Bialynicki-Birula R. Itching in atopic dermatitis: clinical manifestation, pathogenesis and the role of pimecrolimus in itch reduction. *Dermatol Klin.* 2004;6:173–176.

68. Lieberman DA, Keeffe EB, Stenzel P. Severe and prolonged oral contraceptive jaundice. 1. *J Clin Gastroenterol.* 1984;6: 145–148.

69. Medline A, Ptak T, Gryfe A, et al. Pruritus of pregnancy and jaundice induced by oral contraceptives. *Am J Gastroenterol.* 1976;65:156–159.

70. Steckelings UM, Artuc M, Wollschläger T, et al. Angiotensin-converting enzyme inhibitors as inducers of adverse cutaneous reactions. *Acta Derm Venereol.* 2001;81:321–325.

71. Velayudham LS, Farrell GC. Drug-induced cholestasis. *Expert Opin Drug Saf.* 2003;2:287–304.

72. Cundiff J, Joe S. Amoxicillin-clavulanic acid-induced hepatitis. *Am J Otolaryngol.* 2007;28:28–30.

73. de Haan F, Stricker BH. Liver damage associated with the combination drug amoxicillin-clavulanic acid (Augmentin). *Ned Tijdschr Geneeskd.* 1997;141:1298–1301.

74. Hunt CM, Washington K. Tetracycline-induced bile duct paucity and prolonged cholestasis. *Gastroenterology.* 1994;107: 1844–1847.

75. Katsinelos P, Vasiliadis T, Xiarchos P, et al. Ursodeoxycholic acid (UDCA) for the treatment of amoxycillin-clavulanate potassium (Augmentin)-induced intra-hepatic cholestasis: report of two cases. *Eur J Gastroenterol Hepatol.* 2000;12: 365–368.

76. Larrey D, Vial T, Micaleff A, et al. Hepatitis associated with amoxycillin-clavulanic acid combination report of 15 cases. *Gut.* 1992;33:368–371.

77. Quattropani C, Schneider M, Helbling A, Zimmermann A, Krähenbühl S. Cholangiopathy after short-term administration of piperacillin and imipenem/cilastatin. *Liver.* 2001;21: 213–216.

78. Soza A, Riquelme F, Alvarez M, et al. Hepatotoxicity by amoxicillin/clavulanic acid: case report. *Rev Med Chil.* 1999;127:1487–1491.

79. Kowdley KV, Keeffe EB, Fawaz KA. Prolonged cholestasis due to trimethoprim sulfamethoxazole. *Gastroenterology.* 1992;102:2148–2150.

80. Gavras H. A multicenter trial of enalapril in the treatment of essential hypertension. *Clin Ther.* 1986;9:24–38.

81. Mulinari R, Gavras I, Gavras H. Efficacy and tolerability of enalapril monotherapy in mild-to-moderate hypertension in older patients compared to younger patients. *Clin Ther.* 1987;9:678–689.

82. Nunes AC, Amaro P, Maçôas F, et al. Fosinopril-induced prolonged cholestatic jaundice and pruritus: first case report. *Eur J Gastroenterol Hepatol.* 2001;13:279–282.

83. Parker WA. Captopril-induced cholestatic jaundice. *Drug Intell Clin Pharm.* 1984;18:234–235.

84. Thestrup-Pedersen K. Adverse reactions in the skin from antihypertensive drugs. *Dan Med Bull.* 1987;34:(suppl 1):3–5.

85. Thind GS. Angiotensin converting enzyme inhibitors: comparative structure, pharmacokinetics, and pharmacodynamics. *Cardiovasc Drugs Ther.* 1990;4:199–206.

86. Hagmeyer KO, Stein J. Hepatotoxicity associated with carvedilol. *Ann Pharmacother.* 2001;35:1364–1366.

87. Chitturi S, Farrell GC. Drug-induced cholestasis. *Semin Gastrointest Dis.* 2001;12:113–124.

88. Burgunder JM, Abernethy DR, Lauterburg BH. Liver injury due to verapamil. *Hepatogastroenterology.* 1988;35:169–170.

89. Odeh M, Oliven A. Verapamil-associated liver injury. *Harefuah.* 1998;134:36–37.

90. Salti Z, Cloche P, Weber P, et al. A case of cholestatic hepatitis caused by amiodarone. *Ann Cardiol Angiol (Paris).* 1989;38:13–16.

91. Amaro P, Nunes A, Maçôas F, et al. Ticlopidine-induced prolonged cholestasis: a case report. *Eur J Gastroenterol Hepatol.* 1999;11:673–676.

92. Nammour FE, Fayad NF, Peikin SR. Metformin-induced cholestatic hepatitis. *Endocr Pract.* 2003;9:307–309.

93. Mikhail NE. Methimazole-induced cholestatic jaundice. *South Med J.* 2004;97:178–182.

94. Larrey D, Amouyal G, Pessayre D, et al. Amitriptyline-induced prolonged cholestasis. *Gastroenterology.* 1988;94:200–203.

95. Chlumská A, Curík R, Boudová L, et al. Chlorpromazine-induced cholestatic liver disease with ductopenia. *Cesk Patol.* 2001;37:118–122.

96. Moradpour D, Altorfer J, Flury R, et al. Chlorpromazine-induced vanishing bile duct syndrome leading to biliary cirrhosis. *Hepatology.* 1994;20:1437–1441.

97. Radzik J, Grotthus B, Leszek J. Disorder of liver functions in a schizophrenic patient after long-term risperidone treatment - case report. *Psychiatr Pol.* 2005;39:309–313.

98. Regal RE, Billi JE, Glazer HM. Phenothiazine-induced cholestatic jaundice. *Clin Pharm.* 1987;6:787–794.

99. Topal F, Ozaslan E, Akbulut S, et al. Methylprednisolone-induced toxic hepatitis. *Ann Pharmacother.* 2006;40:1868–1871.

100. Chamouard P, Walter P, Baumann R, et al. Prolonged cholestasis associated with short-term use of celecoxib. *Gastroenterol Clin Biol.* 2005;29:1286–1288.

101. Wilhelm MP. Vancomycin. *Mayo Clin Proc.* 1991;66:1165–1170.

102. Rocha JL, Kondo W, Baptista MI, et al. Uncommon vancomycin-induced side effects. *Braz J Infect Dis.* 2002;6:196–200.

103. Bertolissi M, Bassi F, Cecotti R, et al. Pruritus: a useful sign for predicting the haemodynamic changes that occur following administration of vancomycin. *Crit Care.* 2002;6:234–239.

104. Levy M, Koren G, Dupuis L, et al. Vancomycin-induced red man syndrome. *Pediatrics.* 1990;86:572–580.

105. Renz C, Lynch J, Thurn J, et al. Histamine release during rapid vancomycin administration. *Inflamm Res.* 1998;47:(suppl. 1):S69–S70.

106. Renz CL, Thurn JD, Finn HA, et al. Oral antihistamines reduce the side effects from rapid vancomycin infusion. *Anesth Analg.* 1998;87:681–685.

107. Valero R, Gomar C, Fita G, et al. Adverse reactions to vancomycin prophylaxis in cardiac surgery. *J Cardiothorac Vasc Anesth.* 1991;5:574–576.

108. Southorn PA, Plevak DJ, Wright AJ, et al. Adverse effects of vancomycin administered in the perioperative period. Mayo Clin Proc. 1986;**61**:721–724.

109. Rosemberg JM, Wahr JA, Smith KA. Effects of vancomycin infusion on cardiac function in patients scheduled for cardiac operations. J Thorac Cardiovasc Surg. 1995;**109**:561–564.

110. O'Sullivan TL, Ruffing MJ, Lamp KC, et al. Prospective evaluation of red man syndrome in patients receiving vancomycin. *J Infect Dis.* 1993;168:773–776.

111. Ajayi AA, Kolawole BA, Udoh SJ. Endogenous opioids, μ-opiate and chloroquine-induced pruritus: a double-blind comparison of naltrexone and promethazine in patients with malaria fever who have an established history of generalized chloroquine-induced itching. *Int J Dermatol.* 2004;43:972–977.

112. Ekpechi OL, Okoro AN. A pattern of pruritus due to chloroquine. *Arch Dermatol.* 1964;89:631–632.

113. Olayemi O, Fehintola FA, Osungbade A, et al. Pattern of chloroquine-induced pruritus in antenatal patients at the University College Hospital, Ibadan. *J Obstet Gynaecol.* 2003;23:490–495

114. Bussaratid V, Walsh DS, Wilairatana P, et al. Frequency of pruritus in *Plasmodium vivax* malaria patients treated with chloroquine in Thailand. *Trop Doct.* 2000;30:211–214.

115. Spencer HC, Poulter NR, Lury JD, et al. Chloroquine associated pruritus in a European. *Br Med J.* 1982;285:1703.

116. Kaseje DC, Sempebwa EK, Spencer HC. Malaria chemoprophylaxis to pregnant women provided by community health workers in Saradidi, Kenya. Reason for non-acceptance. *Ann Trop Med Parasitol.* 1987;81:77–82.

117. Adebayo RA, Sofowora GG, Onayemi O, et al. Chloroquine-induced pruritus in malaria fever: contribution of malaria parasitaemia and the effects of prednisolone, niacin, and their combination, compared with antihistamine. *Br J Clin Pharmacol.* 1997;44:157–161.

118. Osifo NG. The antipruritic effects of chlorpheniramine, cyproheptadine and sulphapyridine monitored with limb activity meters on chloroquine induced pruritus among patients with malaria. *Afr J Med Med Sci.* 1995;24:67–73.

119. Ademowo OG, Sodeine O, Walker O. The disposition of chloroquine and its main metabolite desethylchloroquine in volunteers with and without chloroquine-induced pruritus: evidence for decreased chloroquine metabolism in volunteers with pruritus. *Clin Pharmacol Ther*. 2000;67:237–241.

120. Onyeji CO, Ogunbona FA. Pharmacokinetic aspects of chloroquine-induced pruritus: influence of dose and evidence for varied extend of metabolism of the drug. *Eur J Pharm Sci*. 2001;13:195–201.

121. Onigbogi O, Ajayi AA, Ukponmwan OE. Mechanism of chloroquine-induced body scratching behavior in rats: evidence of involvement of endogenous opioid peptides. *Pharmacol Biochem Behav*. 2000;65:333–337.

122. Ajayi AA, Akinleye AO, Udoh SJ, et al. The effect of prednisolone and niacin on chloroquine-induced pruritus in malaria. *Eur J Clin Pharmacol*. 1991;41:383–385.

123. Ezeamuzie IC, Igbigbi PS, Ambakederemo AW, et al. Halofantrine-induced pruritus amongst subjects who itch to chloroquine. *J Trop Med Hyg*. 1991;94:184–188.

124. Holme SA, Holmes SC. Hydroxychloroquine-induced pruritus. *Acta Derm Venereol*. 1999;79:333.

125. Jiménez-Alonso J, Tercedor J, Jáimez L, et al. Antimalarial drug-induced aquagenic-type pruritus in patients with lupus. *Arthritis Rheum*. 1998;48:744–745.

126. Jiménez-Alonso J, Tercedor J, Reche I. Antimalarial drugs and pruritus in patients with lupus erythematosus. *Acta Derm Venereol*. 2000;80:458.

127. Swegle JM, Logemann C. Management of common opioid-induced adverse effects. *Am Pham Phys*. 2006;74:1347–1354.

128. Chamberlin KW, Cottle M, Neville R, et al. Oral oxymorphone for pain management. *Ann Pharmacother*. 2007;41: 1144–1152.

129. de Beer J de V, Winemaker MJ, Donnelly GA, et al. Efficacy and safety of controlled-release oxycodone and standard therapies for postoperative pain after knee or hip replacement. *Can J Surg*. 2005;48:277–283.

130. Hadi MA, Kamaruljan HS, Saedah A, et al. A comparative study of intravenous patient-controlled analgesia morphine and tramadol in patients undergoing major operation. *Med J Malaysia*. 2006;61:570–576.

131. Jacobson L, Chabal C, Brody MC, et al. Intrathecal methadone: a dose-response study and comparison with intrathecal morphine 0.5 mg. *Pain*. 1990;43:141–148.

132. Lane S, Evans P, Arfeen Z, et al. A comparison of intrathecal fentanyl and diamorphine as adjuncts in spinal anaesthesia for Caesarean section. *Anaesthesia*. 2005;60:453–457.

133. Möhrenschlager M, Glöckner A, Jessberger B, et al. Codeine caused pruritic scarlatiniform exanthemata: patch test negative but positive to oral provocation test. *Br J Dermatol*. 2000;143:663–664.

134. Kyriakides K, Hussain SK, Hobbs GJ. Management of opioid-induced pruritus: a role for 5-HT$_3$ antagonists? *Br J Anaesth*. 1999;82:439–441.

135. Szarvas S, Harmon D, Murphy D. Neuraxial opioid-induced pruritus pruritus: a review. *J Clin Anesth*. 2003;15: 234–239.

136. Herman NL, Choi KC, Affleck PJ, et al. Analgesia, pruritus, and ventilation exhibit a dose-response relationship in parturients receiving intrathecal fentsanyl during labor. *Analg Anesth*. 1999;89:378–383.

137. Ko MCH, Song MS, Edwards T, et al. The role of central μ opioid receptors in opioid-induced itch in primates. *J Pharmacol Exp Ther*. 2004;310:169–176.

138. Thomas DA, Hammond DL. Microinjection of morphine into the rat medullary dorsal horn produces a dose-dependent increase in facial scratching. *Brain Res*. 1995;695:267–270.

139. Thomas DA, Williams GM, Iwata K, et al. The medullary dorsal horn. A site of action of morphine in producing facial scratching in monkeys. *Anesthesiology*. 1993;79:548–554.

140. Tohda C, Yamaguchi T, Kuraishi Y. Intracisternal injection of opioids induces itch-associated response through μ-opioid receptor in mice. *Jpn J Pharmacol*. 1997;74:77–82.

141. Waxler B, Dadabhoy ZP, Stojiljkovic L, et al. Primer of postoperative pruritus for anaesthesiologists. *Anesthesiology*. 2005;103:168–178.

142. Charuluxananan S, Kyokong O, Somboonviboon W, et al. Nalbuphine versus propofol for treatment of intrathecal morphine-induced pruritus after cesarean delivery. *Anesth Analg*. 2001;93:162–165.

143. Charuluxananan S, Kyokong O, Somboonviboon W, et al. Nalbuphine versus ondansetron for prevention of intrathecal morphine-induced pruritus after cesarean delivery. *Anesth Analg*. 2003;96:1789–1793.

144. Kendrick WD, Woods AM, Daly MY, et al. Naloxone versus nalbuphine infusion for prophylaxis of epidural morphine-induced pruritus. *Anesth Analg*. 1996;82:641–647.

145. Okutomi T, Saito M, Mochizuki J, et al. Prophylactic epidural naloxone reduces the incidence and severity of nuraxial fentanyl-induced pruritus during labour analgesia in primiparous parturients. *Can J Anesth*. 2003;50:961–962.

146. Nakatsuka N, Minogue SC, Lim J, et al. Intravenous nalbuphine 50 microg × 1 kg(−1) is ineffective for opioid-induced pruritus in pediatrics. *Can J Anaesth*. 2006;53:1103–1110.

147. Han DW, Hong SW, Kwon JY, et al. Epidural ondansetron is more effective to prevent postoperative pruritus and nausea than intravenous ondansetron in elective cesarean delivery. *Acta Obstet Gynecol Scand*. 2007;86:683–687.

148. Iatrou CA, Dragoumanis CK, Vogiatzaki TD, et al. Prophylactic intravenous ondansetron and dolasetron in intrathecal morphine-induced pruritus: a randomized, double-blind, placebo-controlled study. *Anesth Analg*. 2005;101: 1516–1520.

149. Larijani GE, Goldberg ME, Rogers KH. Treatment of opioid-induced pruritus with ondansetron: report of four patients. *Pharmacotherapy*. 1996;16:958–960.

150. Korhonen AM, Valanne JV, Jokela RM, et al. Ondansetron does not prevent pruritus induced by low-dose intrathecal fentanyl. *Acta Anaesthesiol Scand*. 2003;47:1292–1297.

151. Waxler B, Mondragon SA, Patel S, et al. Prophylactic ondansetron does not reduce the incidence of itching induced by intrathecal sufentanil. *Can J Anesth*. 2004;51:685–689.

152. Wells J, Paech MJ, Evans SF. Intrathecal fentanyl-induced pruritus during labour: the effect of prophylactic ondansetron. *Int J Obstet Anesth*. 2004;13:35–39.

153. Horta ML, Morejon LCL, da Cruz AW, et al. Study of the prophylactic effect of droperidol, alizapride, propofol and promethazine on spinal morphine-induced pruritus. *Br J Anaesth*. 2006;96:796–800.

154. Demiraran Y, Ozdemir I, Kocaman B, et al. Intrathecal sufentanil (1.5 μg) added to hyperbaric bupivacaine (0.5%) for

elective cesarean section provides adequate analgesia without need for pruritus therapy. *J Anaesth*. 200;20:274–278.

155. Bork K. Pruritus precipitated by hydroxyethyl starch: a review. *Br J Dermatol*. 2005;152:3–12.

156. Bode U, Deisseroth AB. Donor toxicity in granulocyte collections: association of lichen planus with the use of hydroethyl starch leukapheresis. *Transfusion*. 1981;21:83–85.

157. Parker NE, Porter JB, Williams HJ, et al. Pruritus after administration of hetastarch. *Br Med J (Clin Res Ed)*. 1982;284:385–386.

158. Schneeberger R, Albegger K, Oberascher G, et al. Pruritus – a side effect of hydroxyethyl starch? First report. *HNO*. 1990;38:298–303.

159. Albegger K, Schneeberger R, Franke V, et al. Itching following therapy with hydroxyethyl starch (HES) in otoneurological diseases. *Wien Med Wochenschr*. 1992;142:1–7.

160. Jurecka W, Szépfalusi Z, Parth E, et al. Hydroxyethylstarch deposits in human skin – a model for pruritus? *Arch Dermatol Res*. 1993;285:13–19.

161. Gall H, Schultz KD, Boehncke WH, et al. Clinical and pathophysiological aspects of hydroxyethyl starch-induced pruritus: evaluation of 96 cases. *Dermatology*. 1996;192:222–226.

162. Sharland C, Hugett A, Nielson MS, et al. Persistent pruritus after after pentastarch infusions in intensive care patients. *Anaesthesia*. 1999;54:500–501.

163. Morgan PW, Berridge JC. Giving long-persistent starch as volume replacement can cause pruritus after cardiac surgery. *Br J Anaesth*. 2000;85:696–699.

164. Murphy M, Carmichael AJ, Lawler PG, et al. The incidence of hydroethyl starch-associated pruritus. *Br J Dermatol*. 2001;144:973–976.

165. Kimme P, Jannsen B, Ledin T, et al. High incidence of pruritus after large doses of hydroxyethyl starch (HES) infusions. *Acta Anaesthesiol Scand*. 2001;45:686–689.

166. Metze D, Reimann S, Szepfalusi Z, et al. Persistent pruritus after hydroxyethyl starch infusion therapy: a result of long-term storage in cutaneous nerves. *Br J Dermatol*. 1997;136:553–559.

167. Reimann S, Szépfalusi Z, Kraft D, et al. Hydroxyethyl starch accumulation in the skin with special reference to hydroxyethyl starch-associated pruritus. *Dtsch Med Wochenschr*. 2000;125:280–285.

168. Ständer S, Szápfalusi Z, Bohle B, et al. Differential storage of hydroxyethyl starch (HES) in the skin: an immunoelectronmicroscopical long-term study. *Cell Tissue Res*. 2001; 304:261–269.

169. Sirtl C, Laubenthal H, Zumtobel V, et al. Tissue deposits of hydroxyethyl starch (HES): dose-dependent and time-related. *Br J Anaesth*. 1999;82:510–515.

170. Szeimies RM, Stolz W, Wlotzke U, et al. Successful treatment of hydroxyethyl starch-induced pruritus with topical capsaicin. *Br J Dermatol*. 1994;131:380–382.

171. Metze D, Reimann S, Beissert S, et al. Efficacy and safety of neltrexone, an oral opiate receptor antagonist, in the treatment of pruritus in internal and dermatological diseases. *J Am Acad Dermatol*. 1999;41:533–539.

# Section 5
# Psychosomatics and Psychiatry

# Chapter 32
# Interaction Between Pruritus and Stress or Other Psychosomatic Factors

Laurent Misery

Itch is a suffering as well as pain. Its impact on the quality of life and psychism can be considerable. Vice versa, stress and psychological factors can influence it.

## 32.1 Impact on the Quality of Life

The impact of itch on the quality of life has been studied in numerous studies. Most of these studies are about chronic itch. Usually, itch is one of the factors of a specific disease (atopic dermatitis, psoriasis, urticaria) in these studies and there is no specific study about the impact of itch on the quality of life measured through a scale. Suffering from a chronic (or acute) itch can widely modify the life of patients with important effects on sleep, social life, sexual life and mental life. It represents a major stress, does strong damage to the quality of life and has impact on each moment of the day.

To give some examples, 60% of patients with psoriasis reported that pruritus affected their mood, 47% their concentration, 35% their sleep, 21% their sexual desire and 11% their appetite.[1] From another point of view, coping with itch has a cost and itchings and their treatment have a financial impact.[2] The strong association of chronic itch with psychosocial factors was confirmed in a logistic regression on a large population.[3] Itch intensity is significantly correlated with sleeplessness in children with atopic dermatitis and there is a negative impact on the quality of life of these children and their parents.[4] Sulfur mustard-exposed Iranian veterans suffered from severe itching, which induced a strong alteration of their quality of life.[5]

There is a need to conduct new studies about the specific role of itch in the deterioration of the quality of life in skin diseases and to get new instruments to measure it. The itch severity scale (ISS) is a new questionnaire with four questions about the clinical characteristics of itch and three questions about the effects of itch on mood, sleep and sexual life.[6] ISS scores correlate moderately with physical and mental health composite scores of the general scale RAND-36 but strongly with Dermatology Life Quality Index scores. ItchyQoL is a new quality of life instrument which is pruritus specific.[7] This 22-item questionnaire is reliable with high internal consistency and reproducibility, is responsive, and has been validated. Nonetheless, additional studies are warranted to use ItchyQoL with confidence in a general population.

## 32.2 Impact on Mental Functioning

The negative impact of itch on the quality of life has logical consequences on mental life. But the specific role of itch is rarely dissociated from the general role of skin diseases in the studies.[8] In a correlation study with pruritus patients and healthy controls, the average level of depression was significantly higher in patients than in controls.[9] In patients with skin diseases, itch-related coping has a strong influence on psychosocial morbidity.[10] In a study on psychiatric comorbidity, using a questionnaire on more than 4,000 dermatological out patients, pruritus was found to be a comorbidity of psychiatric disorders in 30%.[11] More than 70% of inpatients suffering from pruritus had 1–6 associated psychiatric disorders.[12] Psychiatric comorbidity is detailed in Chapter 33 of this section.

## 32.3 Effects of Stress on Pruritus

Stress and psychological factors are known to be able to induce itch. But they are, above all, able to modulate itch in all conditions. Recent insights into the neuroendocrinology and neuroimmunology of stress responses have improved our understanding of these phenomena.[13] Because stress induces the release of many mediators, these mediators (mainly opioid peptides) are responsible for itch intensification after stress.

Many patients with chronic skin diseases believe that there is a relationship between external stressors and their skin disease and it has been confirmed by numerous studies. While there have been no prospective studies on this subject, some experimental and cross-sectional studies indicate that stress factors can influence itch.[14] For example, perceived stress affects the capability of healthy subjects to discriminate among itch stimuli.[15] Major and minor life events have been shown to be associated with higher levels of itch in the general population and in patients with skin diseases.[16–18] High stress reactors (patients who indicate that their disease severity is strongly associated with stress) report more itch and stronger itch-scratch cycle than low reactors, which suggest that stressors may have different effects on the itch symptom in different subgroups of patients.[19, 20]

## 32.4 Effects of Psychological Factors

The total experienced itch, its distribution over time, peak itch experience, and its timing depends on personality variables.[8] A multivariate regression modelling demonstrated that around 70% of the total variance in these measures was predicted by personality variables (excluding neuroticism and trait anxiety) and depression measures. A state of anxiety or prior skin disease or reported severity of past experience of itch was predictive. The results imply that suggested psychological modulators of itch experience may be confounded by personality-based differences in reporting experiences with visual analogic scale (VAS), as shown by Psouni.

The search for a specific personality trait which could be responsible for more itching is a failure,[14] even in patients with diseases like prurigo nodularis[21] or psychogenic pruritus.[22] Nonetheless, anxiety and depression are consequences of itch as well as aggravating factors for an itch condition and scratching. In more than two-thirds of the patients with atopic dermatitis, psychosomatic factors play a major role in triggering and in the severity of episodes of itching.[12] Worrying and helplessness, as well as the behavioral response of scratching have been

indicated as possible worsening factors.[14] On the contrary, acceptance seems to be correlated with less itch intensity and lower psychological distress.[23]

Itching has to be addressed during psychiatric assessment. In a study among psychiatric patients (excluding patients with eczema, psoriasis or systemic disease), one-third of these patients with schizophrenia, affective disorders or other psychiatric disorders reported itch.[24]

## 32.5 Conclusions

Affective dimension, rather than sensory dimension, may be the most important predictor of pruritus-related psychological morbidity.[25] Interactions between pruritus and psychological factors are numerous and their relationship is complex and reciprocal. This suggests that a psychosocial support, and sometimes psychotherapy, is necessary for patients suffering from pruritus.

## References

1. Amatya B, Wennersten G, Nordlind K. Patients' perspective of pruritus in chronic plaque psoriasis: a questionnaire-based study. *J Eur Acad Dermatol Venereol*. 2008;22:822–826.
2. Van Os-Medendorp H, Eland-De Kok PC, Ros WJ, Bruijnzeel-Koomen CA, Grypdonck M. The nursing programme "Coping with itch": a promising intervention for patients with chronic pruritic skin diseases. *J Clin Nurs*. 2007;16:1238–1246.
3. Dalgard F, Lien L, Dalen I. Itch in the community: associations with psychosocial factors among adults. *J Eur Acad Dermatol*. 2007;21:1215–1219.
4. Weisshaar E, Dipegen TL, Bruckner T, et al. Itch intensity evaluated in the German Atopic Dermatitis Intervention Study (GADIS): correlations with quality of life, coping behaviour and SCORAD severity in 823 children. *Acta Derm Venereol*. 2008;88:234–239.
5. Panahi Y, Davoudi SM, Sadr SB, Naghizadeh MM, Mohammed-Mofrad M. Impact of pruritus on quality of life in sulphur mustard-exposed Iranian veterans. *Int J Dermatol*. 2008;47:557–561.
6. Majeski CJ, Davison SN, Lauzon GJ. Itch Severity Scale: a self-report instrument for the measurement of pruritus severity. *Br J Dermatol*. 2007;156:667–673.
7. Desai NS, Pointdexter GB, Miller Monthrope Y, Bendeck SE, Swerlick RA, Chen SC. A pilot study quality-of-life instrument for pruritus. *J Am Acad Dermatol*. 2008; 59:234–244.

8. Gieler U, Niemeier V, Brosig B, Kupfer J. Psychosomatic aspects of pruritus. *Dermatol Psychosom.* 2002;3:6–13.

9. Sheehan-Dare RA, Henderson MJ, Cotterill JA. Anxiety and depression in patients with chronic urticaria and generalized pruritus. *Br J Dermatol.* 1990;123:769–774.

10. Van Os-Medendorp, Eland-De Kok PCM, Grypdonck M, Bruinzeel-Koomen CAFM, Ros WJG. Prevalence and predictors of psychosocial morbidity in patients with chronic pruritic skin diseases. *J Eur Acad Dermatol Venereol.* 2006;20:810–817.

11. Picardi A, Abeni D, Melchi CE, Pasquini P. Psychiatric morbidity in dermatological outpatients. An issue to be recognized. *Br J Dermatol.* 2000;143:983–991.

12. Schneider G, Driesch G, Heuft G, Evers S, Luger TA, Stander S. Psychosomatic cofactors and psychiatric comorbidity in patients with chronic itch. *Clin Dermatol.* 2006;31:762–767.

13. Paus R, Schmelz M, Biro T, Steinhoff M. Frontiers in pruritus research: scratching the brain for more effective itch therapy. *J Clin Invest.* 2006;116:1174–1185.

14. Verhoeven EWM, De Klerk S, Kraaimaat FW, Van De Kerkhof PCM, De Jong EMGJ, Evers AWM. Biopsychosocial mechanisms of chronic itch in patients with skin diseases: a review. *Acta Derm Venereol.* 2008;88:211–218.

15. Edwards AE, Shellon WV, Wright ET, Dignam TF. Pruritic skin diseases, psychological stress and the itch sensation. A reliable method for the induction of experimental pruritus. *Arch Dermatol.* 1976;112:339–343.

16. Gupta MA, Gupta AK, Kirby S, Weiner HK, Mace TM, Schork NJ. Pruritus in psoriasis: A prospective study of some psychiatric and dermatologic correlates. *Arch Dermatol.* 1988;124:1052–1057.

17. Gupta MA, Gupta AK. Stressful major life events are associated with a higher frequency of cutaneous sensory symptoms: an empirical study of non-clinical subjects. *J Eur Acad Dermatol Venereol.* 2004;18:560–565.

18. Dalgard F, Svensson A, Sundby J, Dalgard OS. Self-reported skin morbidity and mental health. A population survey among adults in a Norwegian city. *Br J Dermatol.* 2005;153:145–149.

19. Niemeier V, Nippesen M, Kupfer J, Schill WB, Gieler U. Psychological factors associated with hand dermatoses: which subgroup needs additional psychological care? *Br J Dermatol.* 2002;146:1031–1037.

20. Zachariae R, Zachariae A, Blomqvist K, Davidsson S, Molin L, Mork C. Self-reported stress reactivity and psoriasis-related stress of Nordic psoriasis sufferers. *J Eur Acad Dermatol Venereol.* 2004;18:27–36.

21. Schneider G, Hockmann J, Stander S, Luger TA, Heuft G. Psychological factors in prurigo nodularis in comparison with psoriasis vulgaris: results of a case-control study. *Br J Dermatol.* 2006;154:61–66.

22. Misery L. Psychogenic pruritus or functional itch disorder. *Expert Rev Dermatol.* 2008;3:49–53.

23. Evers AW, Lu Y, Duller P, Van Der Valk PG, Kraaimaat FW, Van De Kerkhof PC. Common burden of chronic skin diseases? Contributors to psychological distress in adults with psoriasis and atopic dermatitis. *Br J Dermatol.* 2005;152:1275–1281.

24. Zachariae R, Zachariae COC, Lei U, Pedersen AF. Affective and sensory dimensions of pruritus severity: associations with psychological symptoms and quality of life in psoriasis patients. *Acta Derm Venereol.* 2008;88:121–127.

25. Mazeh D, Melamed Y, Cholostoy A, Aharonovitzch V, Weizman A, Yosipovitch G. Itching in the psychiatric ward. *Acta Derm Venereol.* 2008;88:128–131.

# Chapter 33
# Psychosomatic Aspects and Psychiatric Conditions

Gudrun Schneider

## 33.1 Psychosomatic Aspects

Both the skin and the central nervous system have their embryologic origin in the ectoderm; they are functionally closely connected. Colloquially, we therefore speak of "the skin as the mirror of the soul."

### 33.1.1 Developmental Psychological Aspects

*Skin* is a *communicative organ* and plays an important role in *personal development* and in *social contacts throughout life*. It is sensitive to tactile impulses and "replies" to emotional stimuli (i.e., blushing in the case of shame, turning pale in the case of fear, etc.)

Cutaneous stimuli during childhood seem to be an important factor for cell growth and maturation of the central nervous system; this has been demonstrated both in animal experiments as well as in premature children. A chronic itching dermatosis during infancy influences tactile stimulation: For example, an infant with neurodermatitis may experience environmental conditions that healthy children find agreeable, i.e., warmth, touching, hugging by primary care givers, to trigger or to increase itching; this might be experienced as unpleasant, eliciting crying thus making the principle care givers feel insecure in their reaction to the child. Itching may also lead to sleeping disorders, reduced concentration and a worsening of school performance, noticeable skin lesions may lead to teasing, stigmatization, and thus influencing self-confidence, choice of profession, and choice of partner. Chronic itching may thus have a strong influence on the development of body perception, communication, and relational experience.

### 33.1.2 State of Research

Psychosomatic aspects of skin diseases have a long tradition in the scientific literature. Since Sack established psychosomatic dermatology in 1933 with his article "Skin and Psyche," numerous papers that approached the subject clinically in presenting case reports have been published, and these were in part interpreted psychodynamically or psychoanalytically (the "anecdotic phase"). This was followed by a phase of systematic investigations on larger samples employing psychometric instruments and a control group design.

Maximum information about psychosomatic factors in chronic itching is available for *atopic eczema* (comprehensive review, cf.[1]). At present, one assumes a multifactorial pathogenesis, a hereditary disposition seems verified.

#### 33.1.2.1 Personality Aspects

Conspicuous personality profiles have been reported for patients with neurodermatitis: increase in neuroticism, anxiety and depression, increase in agitation, and inadequate coping with stress. These may also be found in other psychosomatically influenced diseases and are therefore not necessarily specific for neurodermatitis. Considering the stress involved with itching and conspicuous skin alterations as well as the early onset of the illness, it must be assumed that certain personality traits may rather be results than causes of the disease and interact with the course of the illness. On the whole, no specific personality type could be consistently demonstrated for all patients with neurodermatitis; however, psychologically conspicuous subgroups have been demonstrated.

L. Misery and S. Ständer (eds.), *Pruritus*,
DOI 10.1007/978-1-84882-322-8_33, © Springer-Verlag London Limited 2010

## 33.1.2.2 Life Events/Stress

During "life-event-research" in the 60s, the simple model was that the sum of "critical" life events irrespective of the context and person lead to illness; in the 1970s and 1980s subjective experience of the event, the role of personality aspects and social support in coping were emphasized. Psychosocial stressors in the form of burdening life events and psychic stress are regarded to be important triggers for the exacerbation of atopic dermatitis. The largest sample yet investigated were 1,457 patients with atopic dermatitis after the earthquake in Hanshin (January 17, 1995). Thirty-eight percent of the neurodermatitis subjects from the most severely affected area A, and 34% of the moderately affected area B reported a worsening of their skin disease compared to only 7% in the control group. Sixty-three percent of the A group, 48% of the B, and 19% of the undamaged area reported subjective stress due to the earthquake. In the multiple logistic regression analyses, subjective stress was the best predictor for the exacerbation of skin disease.[2] In an investigation of King and Wilson[3], an increase in psychic stress was closely associated with a distinct worsening of the skin condition after 24 h; however, 24 h after the exacerbation of the skin disease an increase in subjective psychic stress was also reported, indicating the vicious circle, in which psychosocial stress may be both the cause as well as the result of skin disease.

## 33.1.2.3 Psychophysiologic and Psychoneuroimmunologic Aspects

Research in the past 20 years has led to important findings on the psychophysiological and psychoneuroimmunological relations of many skin diseases including itching dermatoses (e.g.[4]). The relationship between stress and skin alterations is mediated by different neuroendocrine, immunologic, and vegetative regulation mechanisms. Some mechanisms are known, much is as yet unknown. In guinea pigs, histamine release could be achieved by means of classical conditioning; stress enhanced the conditioning effects.[5] The dermatological effects of histamine in humans are distinctly influenced by cognition: After a histamine prick test including dramatizing instructions (the histamine-induced itching is uncontrollable and unpredictable) 90% of the sample with atopic dermatitis reacted with increased itch and/or increase in hives; the anticipation of itching could already elicit scratching. Besides focussing on itch, the perception of options to cope with and control the itching was much more relevant in eliciting scratching behavior than the actual self-report on the severity of the itching.[6]

## 33.1.2.4 Social and Behavioral Aspects

Specific dermatologic stress factors are both the itching as well as the impairment of the outward appearance due to the conspicuous morphology of lesions.

Because of the easy accessibility, lesions may be easily reached. Therefore behavioral aspects (scratching, chafing, overdoing or neglecting the necessary skin care) may lead to new lesions and complicate the course of the disease. Reactive scratching is quite often experienced as automatic and uncontrollable. In the short term, scratching provides relief, in the long term, it leads to increased damage of the skin and therefore to an increased itching and a worsening of the skin condition. Many of those afflicted focus their attention on the itch; this leads to an increased perception, intensifies the suffering, and once more sets *the vicious circle of itching and scratching* in motion. The "itch-scratch-circle" is perceived as a loss of control and helplessness and is often associated with despondency and distinct feelings of guilt. In the sense of conditioning, scratching instantly improves itching and may perhaps reduce tension and is thus negatively reinforced. Perhaps the patient perceives relief of the tension by scratching in socially conflicting situations; these situations whether real or anticipated may become a conditioned stimulus to scratch. As the negative effect of scratching, the increase in skin lesions is a rather long-term effect, it is not effective in influencing the scratching behavior.

Both organic and psychic factors may have an influence in eliciting itching; the central nervous system and thus the psychic factors also play a decisive role in the subjective perception and especially in the coping with the itching sensation including the motoric response to this, i.e., scratching. These factors allow us to speak of *itching, similar as in the case of pain, as a psychosomatic-somatopsychic phenomenon.* In each individual case, the relevance of organic and psychogenic factors as well as their correlation in the development and persistence of chronic itching and scratching behavior must be evaluated.

## 33.2 Psychiatric Conditions

Table 33.1 presents an attempt at a systematization of the different psychic disorders in the context of chronic itching:

### 33.2.1 Chronic Itching as a Symptom of Psychic Disorders

There is an underlying psychic disorder that symptomatically manifests in itching (and perhaps other physical complaints) and/or the manipulation of the skin (A1-A3 in Table 33.1) without any organic disease eliciting the itch.

*Somatoform disorders* (Table 33.1, A1) are characterized by continuous physical symptoms, e.g., itching or burning skin in connection with an adamant demand for medical diagnostics despite continuous negative results and the doctors` continuous assurance that the symptoms are not physically explainable. At the same time, psychosocial burdens that induce and maintain the symptoms exist. The disorder may be monosymptomatic (only itching) or polysymptomatic (itching accompanied by other organically not explainable physical complaints).

*Schizophrenic and delusional disorders* (Table 33.1, A2) may manifest themselves in dermatology by tactile hallucinations of an itch or the delusional conviction to suffer from an infection due to parasites that elicit itching.

*Self-induced scratch artifacts with or without itching* (Table 33.1, A3): In factitious disorders, the main symptom is simulation, aggravation and/or production of physical and psychic symptoms often necessitating medical treatment. Genuine artefact disorders, in which damage to the skin occurs unconsciously, and as rule is not admitted, must be differentiated from "para-artefacts"; in the latter case, the patients are quite aware of damaging their skin, admit to the damage but are not able to stop it. Excessive scratching in this sense ("neurotic excoriation") may be classified according to the 10th version of the International Classification of Diseases (ICD-10) as loss of impulse control. Severe compulsive disorders, especially compulsive washing with consecutive desiccation and damage to the skin, resulting in eczema and super-infections may also lead to itching as a symptom.

### 33.2.2 Multifactorially Induced Itching, the Onset and Course of Which May Be Considerably Influenced by Psychic Factors

The diagnostic category "psychological and behavioral factors associated with disorders and diseases classified elsewhere" serves to record the psychic and behavioral influences that play an important role in the manifestation of physical diseases, which are classified in other chapters of the ICD-10 (e.g., in atopic eczema, chronic urticaria, prurigo simplex/nodularis, etc.). The psychic stress factors have often persisted for some time (e.g., worrying, emotional conflicts, expectational fear, stress, compliance problems) but are not so distinct as to justify another distinct psychic diagnosis. The influences of the psychological stress may in part be

**Table 33.1** Schematic of itch-associated psychic disorders

A. *Chronic itching as a result of psychic disorders*
  A1. Somatoform itching [ICD-10 (DSM-IV): F45.0 (300.81), F 45.1 (300.82), F 45.8 (300.81)]
  A2. Itching in coenaesthetic schizophrenia [ICD-10: F20.x; DSM-IV: 295.x]
  A3. Self-induced scratch artifacts with or without itching in habit and impulse disorder, unspecified [ICD-10: F63.9; DSM-IV: 312.30], factitious disorders [ICD-10: F68.1; DSM-IV: 300.xx), obsessive-compulsive disorders [F42.1; DSM-IV: 300.3]
B. *Multifactorially induced itching, the onset and course of which may be considerably influenced by psychic factors*, e.g., atopic eczema, chronic urticaria, prurigo simplex/nodularis [ICD-10: F54; DSM-IV: 316; psychological and behavioral factors associated with disorders and diseases classified elsewhere]
C. *Psychic disorders as a result of chronic itching*, e.g., reaction to severe stress and adjustment disorders [ICD-10: F 43; DSM-IV: 309.xx], depressive disorders [ICD-10: F 32.x, F33.x, F34.1; DSM-IV: 296.xx, 300.4, 311), anxiety disorders [ICD-10: F40.x, F41.x; DSM-IV: 300.2x, 300.01]
D. *From 1–3 independent co-morbidity with basically every psychic and psychosomatic disorder possible; these, for their part, complicate the handling of itching and thus influence the course of the disease* (e.g., compliance problems in the case of personality disorders, organic and schizophrenic psychoses, etc.)

explained by psychoneuroimmunological relationships (e.g., in the case of neurodermitis, psoriasis), and in part by behavioral aspects (cf. Section 33.1.2 above). They may be observed clinically, but the exact mechanisms are not fully understood yet.

### 33.2.3 Psychic Disorders as a Reaction to Chronic Itching

Chronic itching with or without skin alterations leads to considerable psychosocial burden, which is frequently under estimated as the condition is not usually life-threatening. Chronic itching as a psychosocial stressor demands coping mechanisms of the individual; and can be over-taxing the individual's abilities to cope. As a result clinically relevant problems such as problems in coping with the illness, depressive disorders, anxiety, sexual disorders etc. may develop. These must be diagnosed and treated where indicated.

### 33.2.4 Co-Morbidity with Psychic Disorders

Investigations in the general population demonstrated a prevalence of 20–25% of psychic disorders, i.e., in some of those afflicted by itching, a psychic disorder may co-exist, making coping with the itching difficult and thus influencing the course of the disease (e.g., compliance problems in the case of personality disorders, organic or schizophrenic psychoses, etc.). Co-morbid psychic disorders should be diagnosed and treated.

### 33.3 Frequency of Psychic Disorders in Patients With Itching

In an investigation we carried out, in over 70% of the sample of 109 dermatological in patients with the main symptom of itching, up to six psychiatric or psychosomatic diagnoses were given, demonstrating the high psychic co-morbidity in this population.[8] Other authors have also found, as a rule, a high prevalence of psychic

disorders more pronounced, in dermatological inpatients than in outpatients.[9,10]

In more than 60% of the patients investigated in our sample, psychotherapeutic or psychiatric treatment was indicated and more than 50% of all patients were advised to take up such a treatment, corresponding to the distinct psychic co-morbidity. In contrast to this, almost 90% of the patients had no previous psychotherapeutic experience and only nine of the 109 patients had had more than five psychotherapeutic sessions.

### 33.4 Therapeutic Approaches

Amazing results based solely on a single *psychiatric intervention* have been reported in one study, the aim of which was to investigate the connection between the onset of the skin disease and life-events. According to the treating dermatologists, in 40 of 64 patients, the skin improved within a few weeks. Ten of the 64 patients in this study suffered from not clearly defined "prurigo" and of these eight improved.[11]

Special *behavioral therapeutic programs* for dermatological patients include psycho-educative elements, stress training, training for social competence, and relaxation techniques. These programs aim at helping patients to cope better with the illness, help with the fears of losing control, and to breach the itch-scratch-circle. They are usually carried out as group programs either in an outpatient or inpatient setting. They have proven to be effective and practicable in controlled studies in patients with atopic eczema; their efficacy with regard to dermatologic findings and psychosocial parameters compared to solely dermatological treatment has been demonstrated. *Psychodynamic psychotherapy* in patients with dermatological problems has been described for a number of outpatients or has been carried out in an integrative inpatient setting. The pre-post-evaluation of integrative inpatient treatment of 40 neurdermatitis patients has shown satisfactory results (cf. overview[1]).

In view of the high psychic co-morbidity and psychic cofactors in eliciting itch and the course of chronic itching as well as in view of the proven psychotherapeutic treatment of patients with dermatological problems, an improvement of the psychosomatic and psychiatric consultation and in the liaison services in departments for dermatology must be strived for.

# References

1. Schneider G, Gieler U. Die Haut als Spiegel der Seele. Psychosomatische Dermatologie - aktueller Forschungsstand. *Z Psychosom Med Psychother.* 2001;47:307–331.

2. Kodama A, Horikawa T, Suzuki T, et al. Effect of stress on atopic dermatitis: Investigation in patients after the great Hanshin earthquake. *J Allergy Clin Immunol.* 1999;104:173–176.

3. King RM, Wilson GV. Use of a diary technique to investigate psychosomatic relations in atopic dermatitis. *J. Psychosom Res.* 1991;35:697–706.

4. Buske-Kirschbaum A, Geiben A, Hellhammer D. Psychobiological aspects of atopic dermatitis. *An overview. Psychother Psychosom.* 2001;70:6–16.

5. Dark K, Peeke HVS, Ellman G, Salfi M. Behaviorally conditioned histamine release. Prior stress and the conditionability and extinction of the response. *Ann N Y Acad Sci.* 1987;496:578–582.

6. Scholz OB, Hermanns N. Krankheitsverhalten und Kognitionen beeinflussen die Juckreiz-Wahrnehmung von Patienten mit atopischer Dermatitis. *Z Klin Psychol.* 1994; 23:127–135.

7. Niemeier V, Winckelsesser T, Gieler U. Hautkrankheit und Sexualität. Eine empirische Studie zum Sexualverhalten von Patienten mit Psoriasis vulgaris und Neurodermitis im Vergleich mit Hautgesunden. *Hautarzt.* 1997;48: 629–633.

8. Schneider G, Driesch G, Heuft G, Evers S, Luger TA, Ständer S. Psychosomatic cofactors and psychiatric comorbidity in patients with chronic itch. *Clin Exp Dermatol.* 2006;31:762–767.

9. Gupta MA, Gupta AK. Depression and suicidal ideation in dermatology patients with acne, alopecia areata, atopic dermatitis and psoriasis. *Br J Dermatol.* 1998;139: 846–850.

10. Picardi A, Abeni D, Melchi CF, Puddu P, Pasquini P. Psychiatric morbidity in dermatological outpatients: an issue to be recognized. *Br J Dermatol.* 2000;143:983–991.

11. Capoore HS, Rowland-Payne CME, Goldin D. Does psychological intervention help chronic skin conditions? *Postgrad Med J.* 1998;74:662–664.

# Chapter 34
# Psychosomatics and Psychiatry

## Psychological Approach

Sabine Dutray and Laurent Misery

*I really scratched myself, and I can say here that whoever has not known uninterrupted itching knows very little about hell...*

Lorette Nobécourt, La démangeaison [Itching], Editions J'ai lu, Paris, 1999

Defined as "an unpleasant sensation that provokes the desire to scratch oneself",[1] pruritus is one of the main functional signs in dermatology, specific to this speciality.[2] Lying on the skin and some mucosa, it disturbs the functions of these organs without creating a necessarily observable lesion on it. And in the end, it is always in the brain that the sensation is or is not perceived. As a conscious perception, it unites skin and brain - without "the brain, no itch."[3] Hence, there is a subjective side. The sign exists at the cerebral, physiological, psychological, and verbal levels. It is from this plurality that a link between soma and psyche can be formed. The use of the terms "displeasure" and "desire," and notions with a dual interpretation (physical and mental), to define pruritus express this complexity well. It is why the skin can be the starting point for a somatic and psychological expression of the subject, as well as the destination, a dead end where it becomes impossible to exist outside the itching. As a result it becomes a vicious circle, a suffering that can hold such a central position that it affects social, professional, emotional, and mental life. The subject becomes the pruritus: "...at the edge of one's self, on one's skin, the subject acts out not only his identity, his connections to others and his relationship to time, but his humanity as well."[4]

## 34.1 Link between Skin, Pruritus, and Psyche: an Aid in Diagnosis

The International Forum for the Study of Itch (IFSI) offers a specific classification for chronic pruritus (cf. Part II, Subchapter 4, Psychosomatic and Psychiatric Conditions) using the clinical study of the skin, noting the cutaneous variations according to the presence or absence of lesions, and distinguishing the primary injuries (i.e., caused by a dermatosis) from secondary injuries (created or maintained by the patient).[5] In this structure, the link between the itch and the psyche is explicitly present in two of three groups: with and without clinical manifestations of the pruritus. This does not mean that the psychological impact is excluded from the first group, which is reserved for pruritus on inflamed skin. Patients may be found to be overrun by the "unpleasant" nature of the itching and the irrepressible nature of the scratching, losing control of themselves.

We see how this close link between the body and the mind makes doctors' clinical work complex, with the need to integrate their clinical impressions and observations, as well as what the patients feel in order to best understand what is at stake.[6]

It is why the patient-practitioner relationship can rest on a special link between dermatological ailments and psychological (psychological or psychiatric) problems. In order to look into it more clearly, this continuum between soma and psyche was subjected to different classifications starting in 1929. Following Sylvie Consoli's classification,[6] Laurent Misery and Myriam Chastaing[7] took the history of the disease and its pathogenesis as classification criteria. As a result, four major groups could be drawn out:

1. Psychological problems resulting from pre-existing dermatological ailments: The character exhibited or the chronic development of the dermatological disease disturbs the patients' mental equilibrium, which may involve, for instance, depression or anxiety.

L. Misery and S. Ständer (eds.), *Pruritus*,
DOI 10.1007/978-1-84882-322-8_34, © Springer-Verlag London Limited 2010

In the context of a dermatological ailment, such as atopic dermatitis, pruritus can be an aggravating factor in the experience of the disease. It represents an additional element of discomfort and suffering, as well as a powerlessness that reminds patients at each attack or during the development of the disease of something against which it is difficult for them to fight, if not to give in to and satisfy it by scratching.

2. Psychological problems involving skin ailments: Patients suffer from psychological problems that bring about unpleasant skin sensations or that lead them to inflict skin injuries on themselves.

As a result in the case of exceptional skin perceptions, we find ourselves with a patient whose body becomes the place where a mental suffering is expressed. With respect to pruritus sine materia,[8] the pruritic functional disturbance, for example, remains just as disconcerting for the practitioners as for the patients (cf. Part II, Subchapter 4, Psychogenic Itch). The latter feel it even more acutely since they watch out for its appearance, pile up theories concerning its source, and despair when faced with the caution of their doctors who offer them different treatments for relief. Sometimes, a psychogenic pruritus can predominate with respect to an organogenic pruritus - such as aquagenic pruritus (cf. Part II, Subchapter 1, Aquadynia and Aquagenic pruritus):

For Marianne, 44 years old, each shower was subject to an immutable ritual involving long psychological and physical preparation for this confrontation with the water, and a meticulous organisation of her exit from the water in order to try to funnel the surge in itching through these obsessive reference points. This led her to remain alone after her shower in order to be able to scratch, sometimes for hours. This developed in her such an apprehension that the prospect of washing anticipated the physical and psychological suffering felt during the pruritus, creating a crippling phobic avoidance. During the psychotherapy she has started, she emphasized on the onset of itching in the periods where she has the impression of losing control over her environment, in particular when she is in conflict with her spouse. She feared both verbal and physical abuse from him; this expressed a massive anguish faced with what might happen and what she feared above all: to be "swallowed up," "destroyed." As a result, she sought to put a distance between herself and other people, no longer enduring closeness, while the pruritus provokes this space that is both necessary and unbearable.

In the elderly subject (cf. Part II, Subchapter 5, Geriatric Itch), "senile" pruritus, which may also have many somatic explanations, such as dryness of the skin, may be the expression of solitude, loss of a bond, and social isolation.[6] It is to be monitored immediately, as the slide towards a delusional parasitosis, Ekbom's syndrome, is possible, in particular among women of presenile age who do not suffer from any other organic or psychiatric disorder.[4,10–12] The context of ageing here finds an anchorage in a demand for attention and for connection in the doctor-patient relationship.[6] Practitioners then find themselves hearing as much about the mental suffering as about the somatic complaint.

In addition, genital pruritus (cf. Part II, Subchapter 5, Gynaecology) may be expressed in a context of fear of venereal disease or cancer, a fear frequently linked to a sexuality experienced with guilt or shame.[6] Particularly, anal pruritus that may start over a genuine somatic problem can develop in a subject whose mental functioning is of a fairly obsessive nature, expressing itself in a depressive way, and with anxious elements.[6,13]

Attribution to a psychological origin remains a difficult step for the subject to take, as for the dermatologist. Attacking one's own skin, attacking oneself, represents an aggression even less thinkable as it appears voluntary and conscious, as may be the case with excoriations:

Marjorie, 24 years old, scrapes her hands, her forearms, and her face. She cannot bear scabs and seeks to restore smooth skin. An insignificant scratch or reversal of the aggressiveness against herself, each scratch effect leaves a mark that is more visible each time. She willingly admits her inability to accept frustration, or to tolerate a change or an intrusion into her world. The attack she feels translates into these wounds, accompanied by an emotion of emptiness and sadness. She sets upon her skin during her days off, in the evenings, and in moments of boredom, when she cannot fill her mind, especially through work. Itches and irritation join into a single movement, the overflowing of a diffuse anguish that then engulfs her.

3. Dermatological ailments influenced by psychological difficulties: Patients suffer from a dermatological ailment, the pathophysiogenesis of which is complex, including psychological problems. Hormones and neurotransmitters (group three) play a central role in the origin of the disease and modulate the

characteristics of the immunity and the skin cells.[14] Those for whom the dermatological ailment is partly or wholly induced by their psychological problems (groups two and three) can also have mental problems connected with their skin lesions (group one).

Psychological disorders and dermatoses accompanied by pruritus can be tightly interlinked,[6] as in the case of psoriasis, atopic dermatitis, or chronic urticaria:[15]

Mona is 19 years old. She asks for an emergency dermatological consultation for an especially virulent attack of urticaria. She is suffering greatly and this has led her to seek out a doctor in the middle of the night. She straightaway links this attack to a recent family situation. In effect, she fears the impending release of her brother from prison, because he threatened her not only verbally but also physically. He criticizes her for not having supported him during his trial, even though Mona felt disappointed and betrayed by this brother she idolized so much. She expresses both her fear of violence from her brother and her wish not to knuckle under. She is in anguish awaiting what might happen.

4. Dermatological ailments and psychological problems without an obvious link between them.

This classification makes it possible to have a few clinical reference points for that which isn't immediately obvious during the consultation. And from this point of view, pruritus is a disorder that is even more difficult to grasp, as it remains subjective in its description, its intensity, and its impact on the subject's life.

This specificity questions the place of the skin in the mental functioning and structuring of the subject. How is it that by it, through it, on it, and for it, the patient and the dermatologist seek to unite, in a single therapeutic dialogue?

## 34.2   Skin, Pruritus, and Psyche: a History with Several Voices

Starting in embryogenesis, the skin and the brain are connected through their ectodermal origin. It is the first sign of an inevitable union in the development and functioning of the subject, as physiological as it is mental. Intended to protect and regulate, the cutaneous covering is an essential organ of relational life, both social and emotional, like the brain - defining oneself like taking one's bearings through exchange with others.

Psychoanalysis, the theory of the subject and its mental functioning founded on the idea of the unconscious, at the turn of the twentieth century proposed the first hypotheses on the parallel and possible link between the skin and the psyche. Sigmund Freud, an Austrian doctor specialising in neurology, elaborated a protection system, the "protective shield," intended to filter outside stimulations that could endanger the body by their intensity.[16] For him, this system took the shape of an envelope resting on the body: first the sensory organs, then the skin.

Additionally, the physical surface, sensations, and tactile experiences play a preponderant role in the psychological constitution of the individual, through the structuring of the Ego: "The ego is above all a physical ego, it is not only a surface being, but it is itself the projection of a surface."[17] And at the time of the English translation (1927) he added: "The ego is in the end derived of physical sensations, mainly from those that have their source in the surface of the body. It can therefore be considered a mental projection of the surface of the body, and furthermore, as we said above, it represents the surface of the mental apparatus."

In fact, the Ego is an authority intended to check psychological stimulations while standing up to prevent those that may be coming from the outside from breaking in. For this reason, it takes on a function as a boundary between outside perceptions and the interior psychological apparatus. It plays a role as an interface able to pinpoint and distinguish what belongs to the interior world from what is of the outside world, with the purpose of identifying aggressions that are internal (unpleasant emotions or feelings) as well as external in order to protect oneself from them, or to welcome the satisfying elements (perceptions, for example).[18] Consequently, ideas of surface, exchange, protection, and filter take on both physiological and mental meanings.

These take root through the first exchanges between the mother and the baby. As a result, the research of American ethologist and psychologist Harry F. Harlow using monkeys[19] showed the importance of a gentle, warm, skin-to-skin contact in the baby's attachment to his mother. This satisfying experience, a source of comfort, is the foundation for building self-confidence and a feeling of internal safety. And it is from this that the child can move towards others and exchange.[4]

In the course of the '50s, the English psychiatrist and psychoanalyst John Bowlby offered a theory of attachment in children that underlines the importance of the first contacts with the mother during the first years of life.[20] In effect, five elements seem to contribute to building a satisfying bond: the solidity of holding, the warmth of the embrace, the gentleness of the touch, the exchange of smiles, and during nursing, the interaction of sensory and motor signals. This lets an essential security take root in the child to meet his need for protection. Consequently, early on in the child's life, exchanges with the mother that are closest to skin-to-skin seem to play a vital role in the foundations of his psychological structuring.

Then, the paediatrician and psychoanalyst Donald W. Winnicott extended this thinking through the involvement of the mother in the baby's relationship to the outside world.[21] In effect, the baby, due to his physical and emotional immaturity, must rely on his mother who rightly plays the role of a "protective shield" (see above). As a result, she takes on the function of interface and filter, and protects the infant from external perceptions that are too intense, that could be received as aggressions, while favorably welcoming those that seem satisfying, until the child acquires the physiological maturity which allows him to accomplish this by himself. For this reason, when she appropriately ceases this function, the child can progressively invest his skin and sensory organs as effective boundaries to protect him from stimuli that are too strong. The "protective shield" system coming from the outside can then become internal. And it is from this process that the baby opens up to the world surrounding him, able to internalise satisfying experiences. It is in the back and forth between his own physical experiences of grasping and holding his mother - anchoring and protection points - and his moments of exploration, that he distinguishes himself from her and becomes autonomous.[22] As a result, she is the initial mediator between the child and the outside world, an "external skin" helping him, when she can play the role satisfactorily, to gradually recognise his own physical limits as efficient, and little by little construct his feeling of internal safety, to move confidently towards the outside.

Bringing the functions of the skin and its psychological representations together leads the French psychologist and psychoanalyst Didier Anzieu to elaborate and propose the concept of the "Skin Ego": "By Skin Ego, I refer to a representation which the Ego of the child makes use of during the early phases of its development to represent itself as an Ego containing psy-

chological content, from its experience of the body's surface."[23] The skin, a cutaneous covering, takes on a psychological meaning, therefore conceived as an envelope fulfilling different functions that echo those it exercises on the physiological level:

- The function of the "bag" or container, collecting the good and the solid that the baby will have felt during nursing, care, and the bath of words
- The function of the "interface," delimiting the inside from the outside, establishing a protective barrier against the aggressions produced by beings or things
- The function of the "place" and the "means of communication" with others to establish meaningful relationships, and a "surface for inscribing" the traces they leave

Through early tactile, harmonious exchanges and a reassuring attachment relationship, and from a "shared skin" with his mother, the baby gradually appropriates his skin as his own effective surface, which gives the child confidence and safety.

But when this process cannot completely take place, the distortion of certain functions of the skin and of the Skin Ego question the limits of the subject. And in this context, the onset of a pruritus can be perceived as both an external and internal aggression, likely to damage the cutaneous and psychological barrier, a source or an expression of anxiety for the subject. The few points of psychoanalytic understanding presented above can be linking supports between the "somatic skin" and the "psychological skin,"[18] in order to better grasp the role played by the itch in the subject's psychological economy, which comes to demand help and support from the doctor.

## References

1. Bernhard JD. *Itch. Mechanisms and Management of Pruritus.* New York: McGraw-Hill; 1994.
2. Misery L. *La peau neuronale - Les nerfs à fleur de peau.* Paris: Ellipses; 2000.
3. Misery L. Le prurit: nouveautés physiologiques. *Abstract Dermatologie.* 2007;521:16–17.
4. Consoli SG, Consoli SM. *Psychanalyse, Dermatologie, Prothèses - D'une Peau à l'autre.* Paris: PUF; 2006.
5. Ständer S, Weisshaar E, Mettang T, et al. Clinical classification of itch: a position paper of the international forum for the study of itch. *Acta Derm Venereol.* 2007;87:291–294.
6. Consoli SG. Psychiatrie et dermatologie. *Encycl Méd Chir, Dermatologie, 98–874-A-10.* Paris: Elsevier; 2001.
7. Misery L, Chastaing M. Joint consultation by a psychiatrist and a dermatologist. *Dermatol Psychosom.* 2003;4:160–164.

8. Cambazard F, Misery L. Thérapeutiques Germatologiques. Paris: Médecines-Sciences Flammarion; 2001.

9. Misery L, Alexandre S, Dutray S, et al. Functional itch disorder or psychogenic pruritus: Suggested diagnosis criteria from the French psychodermatology group. Acta Derm Venereol. 2007;87:341–344.

10. Dubreuil A, Hazif-Thomas C. Prurit et psychisme chez la personne âgée, interactions et intrications. Rev Gériatr. 2004; 29:319–327.

11. Bouree P, Benattar B, Perivier S. Une fausse ectoparasitose: le syndrome d'Ekbom. Rev Prat. 2007;57(6):585–589.

12. Consoli SG. La parasitophobie existe-t-elle encore aujourd'hui? Dermatol Prat. 2007;306:3–4.

13. Zuccati G, Lotti T, Mastrolorenzo A, Rapaccini A, Tiradritti L. Pruritus ani. Dermatol Ther. 2005;18:355–362.

14. Misery L. Are biochemical mediators the missing link between psychosomatics and dermatology? Dermatol Psychosom. 2001;2:178–183.

15. Gupta MA, Gupta AK. Depression modulates pruritus preception, a study of pruritus in psoriasis, atopic dermatitis and chronic idiopathic urticaria. Ann NY Acad Sci 1999;885: 394–395.

16. Freud S. "Au-delà du principe de plaisir" ["Beyond the Pleasure Principle"] (1920). Essais de psychanalyse. Paris: Payot; 1981:43–115.

17. Freud S, "Le Moi et le Ça" ["The Ego and the Id"] (1923). Essais de psychanalyse. Paris: Payot; 1981:230–239.

18. Consoli SG. Le moi-peau. Méd Sci. 2006;22:197–200.

19. Harlow HF. The nature of love. Am Psychol. 1958;13:673–685.

20. Bowlby J. "L'attachement" ["Attachment"]. Attachement et perte, Tome 1 [Attachment and Loss. Vol. I. Paris: PUF; 1978.

21. Winnicott DW. "La préoccupation maternelle primaire" [The primary maternal preoccupation] (1956). De la pédiatrie à la psychanalyse [Through Pediatrics to Psychoanalysis]. Paris: Payot; 1969:285–291.

22. Winnicott DW. "Le développement affectif primaire" ["Primary Emotional Development"] (1945). De la pédiatrie à la psychanalyse [Through Pediatrics to Psychoanalysis]. Paris: Payot; 1969:57–71.

23. Anzieu D. Le Moi-peau. Paris: Dunod; 1985.

# Chapter 35
# Psychogenic Pruritus

Laurent Misery

## 35.1 Definitions and Reality

Among extra-dermatological itchings, psychogenic pruritus is sometimes provided as a diagnosis. Unfortunately, it is too often mislabeled as idiopathic pruritus because the patient is anxious or the doctor has no other diagnosis to propose! Think about the movie of Nani Morretti: "*Caro diaro*"....

The existence of psychogenic pruritus is sometimes discussed by some dermatologists but most of them agree to recognize psychogenic pruritus as a specific disease, which is cited in most reviews about pruritus. Nonetheless, only 31 papers with this key word were referenced by PubMed in July 2007![1]

Regarding international classifications of psychiatric diseases, psychogenic pruritus is not cited in the (International Classification of Diseases-version 10) ICD-10 but pruritus is reported in the diagnosis termed "other somatoform disorders" (F45.8) along with dysmenorrhea, dysphagia, psychogenic stiff neck and bruxism. These disorders are classified among somatoform disorders, which are included in the broader category "neurotic disorders, stress-linked disorders and somatoform disorders."

Dermatologists are convinced of the reality of psychogenic pruritus because they know patients with this disease. One study reports that 6.5% of outpatients at a university department of dermatology, which is specialized in psychosomatic dermatology, suffered from "somatoform pruritus" according to a definition close to those of the (Diagnostic and Statistical Manual-version 4) DSM-IV.[2] However, this is a very rare condition for psychiatrists. The term "psychogenic pruritus" is not used in the DSM-IV, but we suggest that it can be recognized among the following four diagnoses in DSM-IV:

- Undifferentiated somatoform disorders (300.81): one or several somatic complaints without any medical or mental disease present to explain the presence or intensity of these symptoms, lasting for six months or more. This symptom is not intentionally self-induced or simulated.
- Pain disorder associated with psychological factors (307.80): psychological factors play a critical role in the triggering, intensity, aggravation or persistence of the pain.
- Unspecified somatoform disorder (300.82): all disorders with somatoform symptoms which do not fit the criteria of any specific somatoform disorder.
- "Conversion Disorder" (300.11): "unexplained symptoms or deficits affecting voluntary motor or sensory function that suggest a neurological or other general medical condition. Psychological factors are judged to be associated with the symptoms or deficits."

It is well known that psychogenic factors frequently enhance somatic sensations, such as pruritus or pain.[3] Fried[4] suggests that neither psychogenic nor organic pruritus exists in a pure form. The majority of patients with pruritus suffer from a somatic disease and their symptoms are modulated by psychosomatic factors, like depression. Yet, some have only a somatic disease and others have a specific psychogenic pruritus.

The French Psycho-Dermatology Group (FPDG) has proposed to define psychogenic pruritus as "an itch disorder where itch is at the centre of the symptomatology and where psychological factors play an evident role in the triggering, intensity, aggravation or persistence of the pruritus" and has suggested a preference for "functional itch disorder" (FID).[5] This definition has been completed by 10 diagnostic criteria. (Table 35.1). Three criteria are compulsory and seven are optional. To diagnose FID, all three compulsory criteria and at least three out of seven of the optional ones are necessary.

L. Misery and S. Ständer (eds.), *Pruritus*,
DOI 10.1007/978-1-84882-322-8_35, © Springer-Verlag London Limited 2010

**Table 35.1** Diagnostic criteria of FID (or psychogenic pruritus) from the French psychodermatology group (previously published in *Acta Derm Venereol.* 2007;87:341–344.)

Three compulsory criteria:
- Localized or generalized pruritus *sine material* (without primary skin lesion)
- Chronic pruritus (>6 weeks)
- No somatic cause

Three of seven optional criteria:
- A chronological relationship of the occurrence of pruritus with one or several life events that could have psychological repercussions
- Variations in intensity associated with stress
- Nycthemeral variations
- Predominance during rest or inaction
- Associated psychological disorder
- Pruritus that could be improved by psychotropic drugs
- Pruritus that could be improved by psychotherapies

It is very important to use a precise definition in order to avoid misdiagnoses. FID is not an idiopathic pruritus: it is necessary to associate both negative (no somatic cause) and positive criteria (clinical characteristics, association with psychological disorders or stressful life events). At the individual level, patients ask for an adequate diagnosis. At the collective level, a better understanding of FID is only possible through clinical and physiopathological studies using diagnostic criteria.

Concerning the terminology "psychogenic pruritus" the FPDG[5] had discussed other possibilities such as "non-organic pruritus" "psychosomatic pruritus" "somatoform pruritus" "itch disorder associated with psychological factors" and "FID." This last terminology appeared to be the best because it includes psychogenic pruritus among functional disorders and avoids the word "psychogenic" which may be too interpretative. "Somatoform pruritus" might be more acceptable outside dermatological societies with regard to the ICD-10 definition.

The FPDG preferred the terminology of "functional disorders" since the term "somatoform disorders" suggests a psychiatric definition because the consensual opinion was that there is neither a somatic nor a psychiatric underlying diagnosis for FID, although an internal psychological conflict is possible. Functional disorders, on the other hand, suggest a definition from the medical point of view, where no somatic cause can be found but an associated mental disorder or disease is possible. An associated psychological conflict preceding

the onset of the symptoms or a psychiatric disorder is not necessarily found when the diagnosis of FID is made but can be revealed later.

The International Forum for Studies on Itch (IFSI) uses the words "somatoform pruritus."[6] European guidelines for itch are in favor of the words "somatoform itch" which is convenient for easy international use and avoids the word "psychogenic."

This discussion is probably not very important. All these words are related to a pruritus with a psychological factor as the main cause.

## 35.2 Similar Disorders

Somatoform itch (FID) belongs to a family of disorders that we suggest naming "functional muco-cutaneous disorders" or "somatoform muco-cutaneous," like cutaneous psychogenic pain or paresthesia, vulvodynia, stomatodynia, glossodynia, some trichodynias and some reactive/sensitive/hyperreactive/irritable skin.[7] These disorders are similar to other disorders which are not in the muco-cutaneous field, like psychogenic pain, psychogenic cough and irritable bowel syndrome.[8] Fibromyalgia and multiple chemical sensitivities[9] could be added to this broad family of medically unexplained physical symptoms (MUPS).[10,11]

Psychodermatological classifications (associated skin and psychological disorders) have included pruritus *sine materia* among "psychological disorders responsible for skin sensations"[12] "functional cutaneous and mucous disorders"[13] or "conditions in which strong psychogenic factors are imputed."[14] There are some differential diagnoses of FID: psychogenic urticaria, psychogenic dermographism, and psychogenic excoriations without pruritus and dermatitis artifact.

## 35.3 Pathogenesis

Selective pathways for pruritus have been described.[15] In the brain, sensory, motor, and affective areas are activated at the same time when pruritus occurs.[16-19] Hence, a new definition of pruritus or itch could be "a sensation which is accompanied by the contralateral activation of the anterior cortex and the predominantly ipsilateral activation of the supplementary motor areas and the inferior parietal lobule; scratching may follow"[20] reflecting the fact that "it is the brain that itches, not the skin."[21] This very important role of the brain in the pathogeny of pruritus confirms that a psychological component could be present in every case of pruritus[22] and that a specific psychogenic pruritus is possible.[21] Itch can be mentally induced.[23] Opioids[24] and other neurotransmitters, such as acetylcholine,[25] are probably involved in this phenomenon.

Why do people with FID or other causes of itch scratch more, inducing nerve hyperplasia in the skin and more pruritus, i.e., do they not have another possibility? Scratch transiently inhibits itch sensation; then there are peripheral and central sensitizations.[21,26–28] The release of inflammatory mediators by scratching sensitize pruriceptors (peripheral sensitization), whereas this chronic skin inflammation facilitates spinal and cerebral itch processing, resulting in touch-evoked pruritus (central sensitization). The existence of central sensitization for itch improves our understanding of FID.

## 35.4 Psychopathology

The understanding of these MUPS, and especially FID, could be helped by neurophysiological or psychological data (see Chapter 33 of this section and Chapter 50 of Section 4 of Part III).

From the psychopathological point of view, concepts of Ego-skin (*Moi-peau*)[29] and somatoform dissociation[10] are very useful. The *Moi-peau* designates a fantasized reality that a child uses during its early development to represent itself as "me" based on its experience of the body surface, and is completed along his/her life. The child, enveloped in its mother's care, fantasizes of a skin shared with its mother: on one side the mother (the outer layer of the *Moi-peau*), and on the other side the child (the inner layer of the *Moi-peau*). These two layers must separate gradually if the child is to acquire its own ego-skin.[30] However, ego remains partly identified by the skin. This theory helps to understand why psychological conflicts may be translated in skin symptoms. Dissociation is defined as a disruption in the usually integrated functions of consciousness, memory, identity or perception of the environment in the DSM-IV. Symptoms of psychological and somatoform dissociation are correlated. Itching appears as a symptom of somatoform dissociation and, even milder degrees of dissociation may play a role in its genesis.[10]

## 35.5 Quality of Life

Somaticians who are not familiar with psychological concepts could believe that FID might be associated with pleasure. The underlying idea that pruritus might be something like a psychological masturbation has been propagated by some psychoanalysts. Like pain, pruritus represents suffering and never pleasure, even though scratching can sometimes provide a pleasant feeling. Itch, including FID, causes considerable physical and psychological distress, adversely affecting quality of life and inducing psychiatric co-morbidity.[31–33]

FID is obviously unpleasant. There is a vicious cycle itch/scratch/itch. The hedonic experience is not related to itch but to scratching, as confirmed by studies[26] showing that scratching actives hedonic cerebral areas, releasing opioids, which induce itch! A recent study[23] showed that itch and scratching could be induced purely by visual stimuli in a public lecture on itching. Hence, itch is contagious not only for patients but for those around them!

## 35.6 Announcement of the Diagnosis

To provide a diagnosis of FID to a patient supposes that this diagnosis has been made through diagnostic criteria (Table 35.1), in order to avoid misdiagnosis. In addition, some patients could unintentionally feel guilty about their itch if they are told that it is simply psychological. In order to prevent this, it is necessary to talk about this possible diagnosis at the first consultation for a pruritus without dermatological disease. After clinical, biological, and radiological exams and conversations with patients to know them better, this diagnosis will be naturally inferred or confirmed, like another diagnosis. It is important to explain to the patient that they are not responsible for the induction of the itch, to approach a patient suffering from psychogenic pruritus with the same objectively derived list of differential diagnoses and the same comprehensive treatment plan given to any other patient. Patients need to be told and to feel that their suffering is genuinely understood.

## 35.7 Treatments

Due to the recent definition of diagnostic criteria, there is no clinical trial concerning treatments for somatoform itch. An interesting three-level approach has been proposed by Fried:[4] lesional, emotional, and cognitive levels. In all patients, treatment of scratching lesions and prurigo will be made by occlusion, topical corticosteroids or calcineurin inhibitors, anti-pruritic emollients (containing capsaicin, doxepin, lidocaine, menthol, glycin, endocannabinoids, raffinose or others). PUVA or UVB are sometimes helpful.

The approach of the emotional level can be made through a doctor-patient alliance and emotional support; and then through personalized psychoanalysis, psychotherapies, hypnosis or behavioral therapies. The cognitive ability of the patient needs to be improved by making them understand their disease and relieving them of their sense of guilt, teaching them appropriate washing attitude and alternative behaviors for scratching.

Psychopharmacologic drugs can be very helpful, with an acceptable potentiality of adverse events: hydroxyzin, doxepin, and serotonin uptake antagonists (fluoxetine, sertraline, paroxetine, citalopram, fluvoxamine, escitalopram).[34] Psychopharmacological drugs appear as the most adequate and in the future these drugs ought to be further effective both for depression or anxiety and on pruritus (through antihistaminic rather than anticholinergic effects for better tolerance). Due to peripheral and central sensitization to itch, all drugs which could be used against itch might be interesting in FID.

## References

1. Misery L. Psychogenic pruritus or functional itch disorder. *Expert Rev Dermatol*. 2008;3:49–53.
2. Stangier U, Gieler U. Somatoforme Störungen in der Dermatologie. *Psychotherapie*. 1997;2:91–101.
3. Gieler U, Niemeier V, Brosig B, Kupfer J. Psychosomatic aspects of pruritus. *Dermatol Psychosom*. 2002;3:6–13.
4. Fried RG. Evaluation and treatment of "psychogenic" pruritus and self-excoriation. *J Am Acad Dermatol*. 1994;30:993–999.
5. Misery L, Alexandre S, Dutray S, et al. Functional itch disorder or psychogenic pruritus: suggested diagnosis criteria from the French psychodermatology group. *Acta Derm Venereol*. 2007;87:341–344.
6. Stander S, Weisshaar E, Mettang T, et al. Clinical classification of itch: a position paper of the international forum for the study of itch. *Acta Derm Venereol*. 2007;87:291–294.
7. Misery L, Myon E, Martin N, et al. Sensitive skin: psychological effects and seasonal changes. *J Eur Acad Dermatol Venereol*. 2007;21:620–628.
8. Misery L. Are pruritus and scratching the cough of the skin? *Dermatology*. 2008;216:3–5.
9. Barnig C, Kopferschmitt MC, de Blay F. Syndrome d'hypersensibilité chimique multiple: phsyiopathologie et clinique. *Rev Fr Allergol Immunol Clin*. 2007;47:250–252.
10. Gupta MA, Gupta AK. Medically unexplained cutaneous sensory symptoms may represent somatoform dissociation. *An Empirical study. J Psychosom Res*. 2006;60:131–136.
11. Richardson RD, Engel CC. Evaluation and management of medically unexplained physical symptoms. *Neurologist*. 2004;10:18–30.
12. Misery L, Chastaing M. Joint consultation by a psychiatrist and a dermatologist. *Dermatol Psychosom*. 2003;4:160–164.
13. Consoli SG. ed. *Psychiatrie et dermatologie*. Paris: Elsevier; 2001.
14. Koblenzer CS. Psychosomatic concepts in dermatology. *Arch Dermatol*. 1983;119:501–512.
15. Misery L. Voies spécifiques du prurit? *Ann Dermatol Venereol*. 2005;132:1007.
16. Darsow U, Drzezga A, Frisch M, et al. Processing of histamine-induced itch in the human cerebral cortex: a correlation analysis with dermal reactions. *J Invest Dermatol*. 2000;115: 1029–1033.
17. Drzezga A, Darsow U, Treede RD, et al. Central activation by histamine-induced itch: analogies to pain processing: a correlational analysis of O-15 $H_2O$ positron emission tomography studies. *Pain*. 2001;92:295–305.
18. Mochizuki H, Tashiro M, Kano M, Sakurada Y, Itoh M, Yanai K. Imaging of central itch modulation in the human brain using positron emission tomography. *Pain*. 2003;105: 339–346.
19. Walter B, Sadlo MN, Kupfer J, et al. Brain activation by histamine prick test-induced itch. *J Invest Dermatol*. 2005;125: 380–382.
20. Savin JA. How should we define itching? *J Am Acad Dermatol*. 1998;39:268–269.
21. Paus R, Schmelz M, Biro T, Steinhoff M. Frontiers in pruritus research: scratching the brain for more effective itch therapy. *J Clin Invest*. 2006;116:1174–1185.
22. van Os-Medendorp H, Eland- de Kok PCM, Grypdonck M, Bruijnzeel-Koomen CA, Ros WJG. Prevalence and predictors of psychosocial morbidity in patients with chronic pruritic skin. *J Eur Acad Dermatol Venereol*. 2006;20: 810–817.
23. Niemeier V, Kupfer J, Gieler U. Observations during an itch-inducing lecture. *Dermatol Psychosom*. 1999;1:15–19.
24. Krishnan A, Koo J. Psyche, opioids, and itch: therapeutic consequences. *Dermatol Ther*. 2005;314–322.
25. Arnold LM, Auchenbach MB, McElroy SL. Psychogenic excoriation. Clinical features, proposed diagnostic criteria, epidemiology and approaches to treatment. *CNS Drugs*. 2001;15:351–359.
26. Ikoma A, Steinhoff M, Stander S, Yosipovitch G, Schmelz M. The neurobiology of itch. *Nat Rev Neurosci*. 2006;7:535–547.
27. Stander S, Schmelz M. Chronic itch and pain – similarities and differences. *Eur J Pain*. 2006;10:473–478.
28. Yosipovitch G, Greaves MW, Schmelz M. Itch. *Lancet*. 2003;361:690–694.
29. Anzieu D. *Le moi-peau*. Paris: Bordas; 1985.

30. Consoli SG. The "Moi-peau". *Med Sci (Paris)*. 2006;22: 197–200.
31. van Os-Medendorp H, Eland-de Kok PC, Grypdonck M, Bruijnzeel-Koomen CA, Ros WJ. Prevalence and predictors of psychosocial morbidity in patients with chronic pruritic skin diseases. *J Eur Acad Dermatol Venereol*. 2006;20:810–817.
32. Schneider G, Driesch G, Heuft G, Evers S, Luger TA, Stander S. Psychosomatic cofactors and psychiatric comor-bidity in patients with chronic itch. *Clin Exp Dermatol*. 2006;31:762–767.
33. Misery L, Finlay AY, Martin N, et al. Atopic dermatitis: impact on the quality of life of patients and their partners. *Dermatology*. 2007;215:123–129.
34. Shaw RJ, Dayal S, Good J, Bruckner AL, Joshi SV. Psychiatric medications for the treatment of pruritus. *Psychosom Med*. 2007;69:970–978.

# Chapter 36
# Pruritus in Children

Matthieu Gréco and Laurent Misery

The aetiologies and treatment of pruritus in children tally, to a certain degree, with what is observed in adults. Moreover, the aetiological assessment to be made for an isolated case of pruritus in a child is identical to the one proposed for an adult. Nevertheless, the existence of more specifically pediatric pruritic dermatoses, as well as the location of the atopic dermatitis, justifies the dedication of a separate chapter for an examination of the causes of pruritus in children.

## 36.1 Genodermatoses Associated with Pruritus

### 36.1.1 Ichthyosis: Sjögren-Larsson Syndrome[1]

This hereditary ichthyosis is characterized by an intense and constant pruritus. Dermatosis is transmitted in the recessive autosomal form and is associated with the mutation of a gene found on chromosome 17, which is the coding for the alcohol dehydrogenase of long-chain fatty acids. At birth, the skin is thick and lichenified in appearance, which is often associated with a grey desquamation. Lesions are predominantly found in the large folds, in the cervical region, and around the umbilicus. The ichthyosic appearance develops gradually during infancy and remains most obvious in the large folds, sparing the middle section of the face. There is often major erythema.

Along with the cutaneous lesions, the clinical picture is marked by a spastic paresis of the lower limbs (and to a lesser degree of the upper limbs) as well, which becomes apparent around the age of 3, along with mental impairment and occasional convulsions.

Other abnormalities may be observed: growth retardation, microcephalus, multiple skeletal dysplasias, dental dysplasias, low implantation of ears, and retinal degeneration. Neurological impairment and mental deterioration are progressive and lead to death.

The anatomopathological examination shows hyperkeratosis with parakeratosis possible in some places. The epidermis is acanthotic and papillomatous, and the stratum granulosum may be slightly thickened. Horny plugs are present. There is a perivascular infiltrate of the dermis. Using electronic microscopy, lamellar inclusions were observed in the cytoplasm of the squamous and granulous cells and of the horny cells.

Treatment with Zileuton has proved quite effective for monitoring the pruritus in this syndrome.[2]

### 36.1.2 Netherton Syndrome

This genodermatosis, which is transmitted autosomally, recessively, is secondary to a mutation of the SPINK5 gene coding for the LEKT1 protein, which is a serine protease inhibitor acting on the inflammation channels.

The clinical picture combines severe atopic pseudodermatitis lesions with intense pruritus, and hair abnormalities (short and sparse): more often than not, there is *trichorrhexis invaginata* (Bamboo Hair), and more rarely, pili torti or trichorrexis nodosa. In newborn babies, the picture may be complicated by erythroderma with secondary hydro-electrolytic problems. In older children, the highly pruritic cutaneous legions adopt a more specific appearance, namely serpiginous, polycyclic, and erythematous migratory plaques with a double collarette edge (circumflex ichthyosis). The severity of the lesions may cause growth problems.

L. Misery and S. Ständer (eds.), *Pruritus*,
DOI 10.1007/978-1-84882-322-8_36, © Springer-Verlag London Limited 2010

At puberty, the lesions may improve with partial remission. Once the complications have been treated, life expectancy is normal.

The primary purpose of therapeutic treatment is to control the complications: hypernatraemia and growth retardation, associated with water and heat loss due to damage to the cutaneous barrier. Topical emollient treatments play an important role, but they must not contain keratolytic agents, as these may aggravate the skin condition. Topical calcineurine inhibitors are effective against pruritus, but they must be used sparingly due to the significant increase in systemic absorption.[3,4]

### 36.1.3 Cholestases of Genetic Origin

As in adults, hepatic cholestasis is an aetiology to be eliminated in an assessment of pruritus. However, there are specific causes of cholestasis in children. Most genetic cholestases develop in the neonatal period, and a diagnosis is often made before the pruritus appears, which is not before the age of 5 months.

*Alagille Syndrome* is often accompanied by severe pruritus secondary to cholestasis. This syndrome represents between 10% and 15% of the causes of neonatal cholestasis (one in every 100,000 births). It is characterized by the combination of five major criteria: a distinctive facies (bulging forehead, small angular chin and hypertelorism), a posterior embryotoxon, vertebral abnormalities of the "butterfly-wing" vertebrae type, a peripheral stenosis of the branches of the pulmonary artery, and a chronic cholestasis caused by a paucity of interlobular hepatic ducts. The diagnosis is made when at least three of these five criteria are combined. The paucity of hepatic ducts is defined by the absence of visible hepatic ducts in more than 50% of the Kiernan's spaces on a liver autopsy containing at least ten complete Kiernan's spaces. Progression to cirrhosis is not constant and may occur from adolescence onwards.[5]

*Progressive familial intrahepatic cholestases* (PFIC) are transmitted autosomally, recessively. There are three types. In the first two (PFIC1 and PFIC2), cholestasis often starts at the neonatal stage, with ferocious pruritus after a few months, despite always normal serum activity of the γ–glutamyl-transferase (GGT). Unlike the first two, PFIC3 often starts later in life and is often complicated by the occurrence of portal hypertension and hepatocellular insufficiency later on. Pruritus is inconstant and moderated, with an increased serum activity of the GGT and a ductular proliferation despite normal hepatic ducts. The reference treatment is a liver transplant, but certain children afflicted by PFIC can benefit from treatment using ursodesoxycholic acid or an external biliary derivation.[6]

Treatment using Rifampicin has proven to be effective at controlling cholestatic pruritus in children.[7]

### 36.1.4 Erythropoietic Protoporphyria[8]

Intense pruritus (or pain) occurs a few minutes after exposure to light. Erythropoietic protoporphyria is transmitted in a dominant autosomic mode but with variable expressivity. It is characterized by a decrease in heme synthetase activity. Protoporphyrin is increased in all cells which have a heme biosynthetic activity (erythrocites and hepatic cells).

Clinical signs are dominated by episodes of early photosensitivity, leaving variable dystrophic sequellae. The ailment starts before the age of 5 in 75% of cases. Attacks are triggered by sunlight or, more rarely, by artificial light. They may occur in winter, under a misty sky, even after exposure through glass. In the first few minutes after exposure, intense pruritus, burning sensations, or skin pain occur. Within about 10 h, a mauvish pseudo-urticaria erupts on the face and the back of the hands. Petechia, ecchymotic plaques occur occasionally. In 25% of cases, vesicles and bullae appear 1–3 days after the start. Small, crusty ulcerations follow in their wake.

The sequella vary in intensity. They may be discrete, or better still, nonexistent. In most cases, cupiliform scars are distributed around the forehead, nose, and cheeks, giving an "orange skin" appearance. The teguments are yellowish, sclerous, or pachydermatous. There may also be the appearance of dry eczema on the ridge of the nose, ears, fingers, and verruciform papules on the hands. Dysonychia are frequent: absence of lunula, bluish-grey coloring. The mucosae are unaffected. Development is usually favorable, and cutaneous signs improve spontaneously when the sufferers enter adulthood. The main complication is cholelithiasis, which may appear before 20 years and be accompanied by cirrhosis, the decomposition of which is occasionally sudden and very soon leads to death.

The diagnosis is confirmed by an orangey-red fluorescence between 10% and 30% of the erythrocytes circulating at 400 nm, and an increase in erythrocytic protoporphyrin (ten times the normal rate).

## 36.2 Acquired Pruritic Dermatoses in Children

### 36.2.1 Atopic Dermatitis[9]

Atopic eczema is a form of dermatosis characterized by pruritus in all patients. However, more often than not, pruritus is only evident between 4 and 6 months of age, when the baby is able to scratch.

Atopic dermatitis is the most common form of inflammatory dermatoses in children. Its pathogenesis is multifactorial, with polygenic transmission, and, in particular, combined with a mutation of the filaggrin gene. Environmental factors are combined with genetic factors. There is immunodysregulation with hyperproduction of E immunoglobulins but, above all, there is an abnormality in the Th1/Th2 balance influenced by multiple cytokines.

Skin lesions usually appear after the age of 3 months on the convexities of limbs and the face, sparing the mediofacial area. There is badly defined erythema, with squamous development which is occasionally vesicular and oozing. Dermatosis develops in successive growth stages, but the skin is rarely completely normal between two episodes. More often than not, skin xerosis persists. During the second year of life, the symptomatology changes, whereby the dermatosis tends to occur mainly in the flexion creases. The skin is dry, and if the dermatosis is very chronic, there is frequent secondary lichenification when scratching. After the age of 3–4 years, the skin symptomatology improves spontaneously. However, the child will often still experience skin xerosis. At this age too, respiratory signs occur (asthma and rhinitis, etc.). Occasionally, atopic dermatitis persists, with significant repercussions on social relationships.

Certain clinical presentations of atopic dermatitis are important to know, such as the nummular forms, in which the lesions are well defined and occasionally thick, resistant to treatment, and often confused with infectious dermatoses. Strophulus infantum is also often seen within the context of atopic dermatitis.

Pruritus remains the central symptom in the various clinical forms.

Regardless of the severity of the atopic dermatitis, topical treatment is essential. Few lesions will resist properly administered topical treatment. The most frequent reason for failure is a reluctance to use topical corticoids. First line treatment is based on the application of topical corticoids, combined with simple hygiene and dietary rules, as well as the regular application of emollients. Emollients actually reduce skin xerosis and play an important role in improving pruritus, which is often present away from the inflammatory lesions if not treated. If resistance to or dependence on topical corticoids occurs, topical calcineurin inhibitors can prove to be highly effective, particularly in controlling pruritus. Few studies about the clinical effectiveness of type 1 antihistamines (AH1) have been carried out on infants. The clinical results obtained with the orally administered nonsedative AH1s are comparable with the AH1 sedatives and not very different from the placebo. Therefore, oral antihistamines are not routinely prescribed at the acute stage. This may happen in severe pruritus and for short periods of time. Topical antihistamines have no place in the treatment of atopic dermatitis. For serious forms, the use of phototherapy or systemic immunosuppression treatment such as Ciclosporin may be required.

In rare cases, the atopic dermatitis is part of a more complex set of symptoms (Job-Buckley syndrome, Wiskott-Aldrich syndrome, etc.); there are associated clinical signs, particularly repeated bacterial infections, which rapidly lead to a specialist opinion. Netherton syndrome also needs to be considered (cf. supra).

### 36.2.2 Urticaria[10,11]

Urticaria lesions are characterized by moving pruritic and short-lived papules. In small children, the appearance is readily ecchymotic.

When the oedema reaches the deep section of the dermis or hypodermis, lesions adopt the appearance of firm and pale swellings, which are more painful than pruritic and may persist between 48 and 72 h. This is a deep urticaria, also called angio-oedema. Almost 50% of sufferers exhibit a combination of these two forms of urticaria. Pruritus is, therefore, the central symptom of common urticaria. In contrast, pruritus may be completely absent in the case of an isolated angio-oedema. A dietary cause of a facial angio-oedema in a child must be looked for. A hereditary angioneurotic oedema must also be ruled out by looking for an impairment in the quantity or quality of the C1 esterase inhibitor.

In a child, depending on the symptomatology, we need to know how to recognize a chronic infantile urticaria syndrome: chronic, infantile, neurological, cutaneous, and articular (CINCA) syndrome, hyper-IgD syndrome, Mückle–Wells syndrome and Still's disease. It should be noted that the urticarian rupture observed in CINCA syndrome is nonpruritic.

Chronic urticaria is defined as the persistence of lesions beyond 6 weeks. Chronic urticaria is exceptional in children and has few characteristics. The psychological, and particularly the academic repercussions, are often significant; this may affect the quality of life and cause anxiety both in the child and his/her parents. When faced with a case of childhood urticaria, the person questioning the child and his/her parents must systematically research the trigger or aggravating factors, placing emphasis on various points:

- Family and personal history (atopy, urticaria, and general illness)
- Chronology of outbreaks
- Any drugs taken (aspirin and nonsteroid anti-inflammatories such as ibuprofen, codeine and other histamine-releasing drugs)
- Dietary habits (overconsumption of histamine releasers)
- The concept of contact urticaria (latex is particularly found in balloons and swimming caps)
- Circumstances which trigger physical urticaria (effort, rubbing, pressure, heat, cold, water, exposure to the sun. and vibrations)
- The role of "stress" as an aggravating feature
- Accompanying signs indicating general illness. A fixed eruption which lasts longer than 24 h and is mildly pruritic, indicates urticarian vasculitis, particularly when combined with other elemental lesions, particularly purpuric lesions. It is also necessary to distinguish chronic urticaria from polymorphic erythema, mastocytosis and pemphigoid in the pre-bullous stage in children.

The assessment and treatment of a chronic urticaria in children are no different from what is recommended for adults, except for the fact that certain molecules do not have an MA (marketing authorisation) for children.

### 36.2.3 Hyperimmunoglobulinemia D Syndrome[12]

Hyperimmunoglobulinemia D Syndrome, which starts in childhood (in four out of five cases before the age of 1 year) and is familial in over a third of the cases (probably transmitted autosomally, recessively), involves attacks of urticaria which are pruritic to some extent lasting for between 3 and 7 days, persistent, with a highly variable frequency (between once a week and twice a year), including erythematous maculas followed by papules which are sometimes petechial, annular, hypodermic nodules without topical bile production or mucosa lesions (oral aphtose in two out of three cases). They are accompanied by a fever higher than 40°C preceded by chills, arthralgia or nondestructive symmetric arthritis affecting the large joints, adenopathies, occasional hepatosplenomegaly, abdominal pains (with diarrhoea, vomiting, occasional pseudosurgical).

### 36.2.4 Mückle–Wells Syndrome[13,14]

Mückle–Wells syndrome is defined as the combination of an urticaria, an essentially renal amyloidosis, and a neurosensorial hearing loss. It is transmitted through a dominant autosomic mode. In addition to the urticaria which defines the disease, clinical inflammatory attacks comprise a disorder in the joints involving arthralgia or arthritis and a conjunctivitis type of symptoms in the eye. Other symptoms, which suggest the clinical heterogeneity of this syndrome have been described.

### 36.2.5 Juvenile Idiopathic Arthritis[15]

Juvenile idiopathic arthritis (or juvenile chronic arthritis), formerly called Still's disease, combines systemic inflammatory systems, attacks of joint inflammation and cutaneous symptoms. Cutaneous symptoms are found in 90% of cases and must be looked into carefully because they help significantly with diagnosis. These are localized, short-lived, and often very discrete erythemas which are triggered by exposure to air, bathing and particularly at the time of the febrile peak. More rarely, there is a more intense urticarian outbreak. Pruritus is inconstant.

## 36.2.6 Childhood Psoriasis[16]

Pruritus, which is sometimes severe, is found in 30% of the cases. The disease, psoriasis starts before the age of 10 in approximately 15% of the cases. In the childhood psoriasis, girls are more often affected than boys and there is a family history in half of the cases. The childhood forms differ from the adult forms in terms of individual symptoms and topographical factors. There are delicate diagnosis problems for psoriasis in babies. Finally, we should point out the frequency of psoriasis in children treated with growth hormone (Turner syndrome).

All aspects of adult psoriasis can be encountered in children. However, some forms are more peculiar to children. This is the case for guttate psoriasis, which is the most common initial form. It frequently follows a rhinopharyngeal infection, or sometimes a vaccination. The eruption appears quickly, is monomorphic, and often febrile. After a rapid extension phase, the lesions stabilize and may recede after a few weeks or months. This receding, which is helped by antibiotic therapy, may even, in some cases, be definitive. These are the only cases of psoriasis that can be cured. Nummular psoriasis frequently follows the previous form and often takes an annular appearance on the trunk. Similarly, psoriasis spinulosa is more common in children: it causes plaques on the elbows and knees, rough keratosis pilaris, and causes delicate problems for diagnosis with the lichen or Pityriasis rubra pilaris. Pruritus can be observed in these various clinical presentations.

## 36.2.7 Mastocytoses[17]

Mastocytoses are defined as an abnormal accumulation of mast cells in one or more tissues. Pure cutaneous mast cells are distinguished from systemic mast cells. Predominantly observed in Caucasian populations, with a *sex ratio* of 1, mastocytoses particularly affect children in almost two-thirds of cases, more often than not in a purely cutaneous form. The condition recedes spontaneously at puberty in almost 50% of the sufferers.

Generalized pruritus readily accompanies *flushes* and congestive outbreaks of lesions; more rarely, it can be permanent. It is observed in 50% of the mastocytosis cases and improves with the age of the lesions. The intensity of the pruritus depends on the type of cutaneous mastocytosis. In pigmentary urticaria, it is often a central symptom observed in 33% to 46% of the patients. In diffuse cutaneous mastocytosis, the pruritus is often very intense. Diffuse cutaneous mastocytosis without a permanent lesion remains debatable, with six reported cases of pruritus related to a very significant increase in dermal mast cells.[18]

Besides the prevention of factors which may promote mast cell degranulation, the treatment of pruritus in relation to mastocytosis relies on anti-$H_1$ antihistamines, often combined with anti-H antihistamines$_2$. Antihistamines are the key first line treatments used for blocking the release of mediators, via mast cell receptors. Ketotifen seems to be effective against pruritus. Oral sodium cromoglycate (in an ampoule for drinking), a mast cell membrane stabilizer, acts on digestive manifestations at a dose of 400 mg/day for children. It also acts on pruritus. Finally, leukotriene inhibitors (montelukast) can also be offered for the treatment of pruritus.

## 36.2.8 Eruptive Diseases in Children[19]

Eruptive diseases in children are very frequently polymorphic. They are accompanied by pruritus which varies in intensity. The aetiologies are multiple, essentially viral but also bacterial and drug-related.

*Varicella* is characterized by a particularly pruritic vesicular eruption. Due to the herpes varicellae virus, this is a highly contagious ailment, which generally occurs between two and 10 years of age. The incubation is 14–16 days, followed by a very short invasion period (24 h) with general malaise and a febricula of 38°C. In fact, this stage is often inapparent. The eruption starts with pink macules, which become covered within 24 h with vesicles measuring between 1 and several millimeters in diameter, with regular contours and clear contents. The lesion will wither within 24–48 h. A brownish scab will replace the vesicle. Around day eight to ten, it will fall off without leaving a scar, except in the case of superinfection or inadvertent scratching. The eruption will appear on the face and thorax, before spreading to affect the scalp, palms and soles of the feet. It will be marked by a small temperature increase in two or three successive attacks. There may be a small buccal, conjunctival or laryngeal enanthema and discrete micropolyadenopathies, particular cervical ones. This is cured within 10–15 days. Treatment of the common form is purely symptomatic, by means of a combination of a sedative antihistamine to calm the pruritus and an antiseptic or drying topical to avoid superinfection. If superinfection does occur in spite of everything, it will require antibiotic therapy. In immunosuppressed children, immunosuppressant treatment must be stopped for a short time, if possible, and antiviral treatment must be started quickly using systemically administered acyclovir.

*Herpes zoster* corresponds to the recurrence of a *Herpes varicellae* virus infection, the primary infection of which is varicella. This is exceptional in babies and rare in children. It is more often observed in subjects suffering from an immune deficiency. The eruption occurs in the form of strictly unilateral erythematous plaques with a radicular topography, which are covered in vesicles before they join together to form bullae. The pain, which is not very intense in children as a rule, will disappear within a few days. Occasionally there will be no pain, but pruritus instead. There may be a febricula and painful satellite adenopathy. There are multiple topographic forms. The only problematic ones are those which attack the nervous trigeminus, particularly herpes zoster ophthalmicus. As the eruption is a characteristic, the diagnosis is primarily clinical. However, there may be a doubt at the pre-eruptive phase, if the eruption is discrete, or if pruritus is the only functional symptom without any associated pain. If in doubt, the virus can be shown in vesicles by using PCR. In nonimmunosuppressed children, treatment is limited to the disinfection of the lesions and possibly analgesics. In immunosuppressed children, the same antivirals are prescribed as for serious cases of varicella.

*Viral erythematous eruptions* are associated with inconstant pruritus, with varying degrees of intensity (measles, rubella, Epstein-Barr virus, cytomegalovirus, Human Herpes Virus 6, Enterovirus, etc.). Pruritus is also frequently observed during *scarlet fever*.

Pruritus may be the key factor in certain *drug-related exanthema*. These occur 7–24 days after the introduction of the molecule, but if the trigger drug is taken away the period is very short (1–3 days). All types of morbilliform, roseoliform and scarlatiniform erythema may occur, and pruritus can sometimes be the inaugural symptom. They may be caused by any type of drug. Nevertheless, they are most frequently caused by the following: penicillins (without any of their associated side effects, particularly if associated with childhood mononucleosis), sulfamides, anti-convulsants and nonsteroid anti-inflammatories. Symptoms subside quickly once the drug that caused the problem is no longer taken. The imputibility diagnosis is made using a probability method. Only the reintroduction of the test, which is occasionally dangerous, makes a formal confirmation possible, as a negative test does not eliminate the diagnosis.

### 36.2.9 Pityriasis Rubra Pilaris (PRP)[20,21]

PRP is a rare pathology in children, the origin of which is not explained. It combines three semiologic elements to various degrees: a follicular horny papule, an orangish palmoplantar keratoderma and erythematosquamous lesions. Pruritus can be found in approximately 20% of the patients. The Griffiths classification, which is based on the clinical presentation, distinguishes five types: types I and II affect adults, whereas types III to V affect children. Type VI, combined with HIV, is rarely encountered in children. Type III is the most common form in children. The clinical presentation is similar to the typical adult form, but the condition develops more quickly. The age when the condition occurs varies depending on the series; between five and 10 years for some, but a frequency peak between 16 and 19 years has also been observed. Type IV is the most common type and corresponds to a localized form. The most commonly affected areas are the elbows and the palmoplantar regions, followed by the knees, nails, hands, and the dorsal surfaces of the feet, the legs, and the arms. Type V is an atypical generalized form in children starting early in childhood with palmoplantar keratoderma, which is occasionally sclerodermiform. It corresponds to the majority of familial cases and is similar to ichthyosis type of keratinisation disorders.

## 36.2.10 Oxyuriasis[22]

Nocturnal anal pruritus is the most pathognomonic element of this intestinal parasitos in children, causing scratching lesions and being responsible for insomnia and nightmares. In young girls, vulvar pruritus is sometimes observed, accompanied by vulvo-vaginitis with leukorrhoea and cystitis.

Oxyuriasis is a cosmopolitan helminthiasis. Invasion occurs through the ingestion of eggs that are conveyed to the mouth by dirty hands, sucked objects or fingers, or with food. The oxyurises, which are 1 cm-long white nematodes, are found in the caecum. The females travel through the colon to lay their eggs at night in the anal seam, thereby causing anal pruritus.

Treatment is based on flubendazole administered orally, combined with hygiene measures: washing of hands, nails cut short, washing of underwear, concomitant treatment of the whole family.

## 36.2.11 Pityriasis Versicolor (PV)[23]

This very common dermatophytosis, caused by *Malassezia,* type lipophilic yeast is seldom pruritic. However, pruritus is readily present in the follicular forms. More common in adolescents and young adults, PV can also be found in children, particularly those originating from tropical areas. A clinical examination reveals clearly delimited, rounded maculas, between two and several dozen millimeters in diameter, with a uniform color, in which desquamation only occurs after scratching. The monochrome form is highly visible after tanning. The pigmented form is marked to some degree or another: the lesions are chamois colored to dark brown and occasionally erythematous. Guttate, confetti, nummular, plaque, plate, and mixed lesions can be observed. The top of the thorax, the shoulders, arms, and neck are most commonly affected. The large folds (inguinopubic, ulnar and popliteal) and the scalp are not particularly spared when examined under a Wood's light. The face is more commonly affected in children from tropical areas.

Topical treatments use imidazole and ciclopirox olamine for lesions which are in their early stages and limited. Following treatment, the achromic lesions only become repigmented after a variable period, after exposure to the sun.

## 36.2.12 Autoimmune Bullous Dermatoses in Children

### 35.2.12.1 Bullous Pemphigoid in Children[24,25]

Although bullous pemphigoid essentially affects older people, it can occur at any age, particularly in children. As in adults, the pruritus is, more often than not, very marked. Attacks of the oral mucosa, palms, soles of the feet and face are most commonly observed in pemphigoid in children.

### 36.2.12.2 Herpetiform Dermatitis[26]

This is a pruritic disease, characterized by a papulovesicular eruption, sitting symmetrically on the affected areas and developing over time. In its characteristic form, it begins with a pruritus or painful burning sensation on the skin. Then urticarian erythematopapular and vesicobullous lesions, which are small in size and quickly excoriated appear. Lesser signs are chronic urticarian plaques or papular elements and exzemaform aspects which are lichenified to varying degrees. The seat of the lesions is characterized by its symmetry, an important sign in deceptive forms. In a decreasing order of frequency, the following areas are affected: extensor aspects of the limbs, elbows and knees, buttocks, less commonly the scalp, nape of the neck, the sacral region, the shoulders, and more exceptionally the face. The initial attack may be localized on the palms. The mucosa attack is not rare, with an oral predominance causing vesicular stomatitis, which is more often than not purpuric and erosive. The clinical examination and questioning must look for digestive signs, which are rarely present. Malabsorption with diarrhoea is found in at least 5% of the cases. Herpetiform dermatitis is related to celiac disease. Shared mechanisms are described for these two diseases. The triggering role of an infection (adenovirus) is removed.

Herpetiform dermatitis is very closely linked to certain class I and II HLA antigens. The B8 HLA antigen is found in approximately 80% of cases, as is the DR3 antigen. There is a strong link to the DQ region. This link is found for celiac disease with class II HLA antigens.

The main form of treatment is dapsone (Disulone®) and a gluten-free diet.

### 36.2.12.3 Linear IgA Dermatosis in Children[27]

Its place next to linear IgA dermatosis in adults has not yet been properly stated: different illness or expression of a single pathology at different ages. The clinical aspect in children is far more stereotypical. The disease generally begins in the second stage of childhood and is equally common in both sexes. It typically affects the perioral and perineal areas. The rash is very pruritic and more often than not vesicular. The vesicles are arranged in herpetiform clumps or rosettes. The trunk and limbs are commonly affected; conversely, the mucosa attack is inconstant but may be severe if it does occur. The association with gluten enteropathy and haplotype HLA-B8-DR3 is less common than in herpetiform dermatitis. The immunopathological aspects identical to those of the adult form suggest an identity for the target antigen in adults and children.

With treatment, the disease evolves favorably, within 2 years on average. In some patients it has been reported that the disease takes longer to evolve (up to 10 years). Spontaneous remission is possible. The first line general treatment of the disease is based on Disulone®, initially at a posology of 100 mg/day, which is increased if this level proves ineffective.

### 36.2.12.4 Acquired Epidermolysis Bullosa in Children

Rare cases have been reported in young children. Therefore, the mucosa attack often dominates the clinical picture. Serious forms have been described with very extensive peeling. The dystrophic cicatricial evolution may cause therapeutic problems; however, it would seem that the long-term prognosis is better than in adults with recovery. Pruritus is particularly present in the acute inflammatory form, and more rarely in the chronic form.[28]

## 36.2.13 Polymorphous Light Eruptions in Children

### 36.2.13.1 Hydroa Vacciniforme[29]

The picture starts, after significant exposure, with pruritus or a burning sensation. Other prodromes are rarely noticed: general malaise, digestive problems, and febricula. Lesions occur after between 1 and 48 h. They are predominant on the cheekbones, the dorsum of the nose, the pinna of the ears and on the back of the hands and forearms. The mucosa attack is possible in the labial mucosa and ocular mucosa (photophobia, keratitis, conjunctivitis). Other locations are rarer: trunk, arms, and scalp. The elemental lesion defines the hydroa vacciniforme. Vesicles, which are occasionally confluent, appear on a slightly erythematous base. A central umblication covered with a brownish crust appears very quickly. When it falls off, a depressed varioliforme scar will be left. The number of lesions varies considerably.

The evolution of the hydroa vacciniforme is characteristic. It evolves in attacks lasting between 1 and 3 weeks, at a rate governed by exposure to sunlight. Long-term evolution is chronic. Lesions recur each year depending on exposure to sunlight. In some cases, the eruption can occur throughout the year. Typically, attacks become rarer and less serious after puberty, before finally clearing up more often than not between the ages of 20 and 30, leaving permanent scarring, which is occasionally severe.

On a recent lesion, an anatomopathological examination shows a focal necrosis of the epidermis and the adjacent dermis, causing the formation of a vesicle or bulla, as well as a lymphohistiocytic dermal inflammatory infiltrate. The direct immunofluorescence is negative.

The dosage of urinary, fecal and erythrocytic porphyrins must always be given so that it eliminates porphyria. A photobiological exploration authenticates the picture: positive test results are only obtained with high doses of UVA ($30–50$ J/cm$^2$) repeated after 48 h.

Photoprotection is often ineffective, as is betacarotene and synthetic antimalarials. The best results are obtained with phototherapy (UVB).

*Hydroa aestivale* is for some people a minor form of hydroa vacciniforme and for other people a clinical form of polymorphous light eruption, because it occurs more commonly in girls and only leaves infrequent and discrete scars.

### 36.2.13.2 Juvenile Spring Photodermatosis or Spring Eruption of the Ears[30]

Pruritus may also be replaced by a burning sensation in this clinical picture, affecting children between the ages of 5 and 12, much more commonly found in males, which can be explained by haircuts away from the ears. Juvenile spring photodermatosis seems to be triggered by both exposure to sunlight and the cold. The eruption is papulo-oedemato-vesicular, or initially vesicular. Exceptionally, it may be bullous. It is found electively on the free margin of the helix, on the tragus and the antihelix. The inconstant attack of the back of the hands and the extensor aspects of the wrists defines the bipolar form of juvenile spring photodermatosis. In this location, the lesions often adopt the appearance of polymorphous erythema. The evolution is benign. The lesions disappear spontaneously within a fortnight or so, without leaving any sequelae. The only possible complication is superinfection. Recurrences each spring are not rare. They gradually fade away after two or three attacks.

The anatomopathological examination reveals epidermic necrosis with major exoserosis. The photobiological exploration is negative in the very few cases where it is carried out. Hydroa vacciniforme, erythropoietic protoporphyria and polymorphous light eruption, which can remain for some time confined to the ears or adopt a bipolar topography, must be eliminated.

Besides prevention, the treatment continues through the wearing of ear protectors combined with a local corticotherapy, which reduces the duration of the attack.

## 36.2.14 Polymorphous Light Eruption in Children[31]

Pruritus precedes the eruption by a few hours. The concept of a burning sensation is found in 30–60% of cases. Occasionally pruritus will occur without an eruption. The conditions for the appearance and recurrence of this pruritus without eruption are a minor equivalent of polymorphous light eruption which is sometimes called "actinic pruritus."

The variety of semiological aspects explains the existence of several clinical forms: papulovesicular, plaques (pseudo-urticarian), tags ("polymorphic pseudo-erythema") and hemorragic. Scales, hyperkeratosis, lichenification or scars are not primary lesions but can appear as secondaries, linked with scratching. The eruption is mainly found on uncovered parts of the body, particularly the face, forehead, cheekbones and the retroauricular regions. This is characteristic of an attack. Normally the areas with little exposure, such as the orbital regions, the edge of the upper lip and the submental triangle, are respected. The neckline is commonly affected, as well as the extensor aspect of the upper limbs and the back of the hands. The attack may spread, depending on the clothing that is usually worn, to the front side of the legs and to the back of the feet. It may spread to covered areas, partly due to the sufferer wearing clothes which are partially transparent to UVA.

The ailment can begin at any age, but particularly between the ages of 10 and 30, with a peak in the prepuberty period. The circumstances surrounding the development of this ailment are an element of the diagnosis. The eruption appears in spring (March-April), as soon as the first rays of sunshine appear (70% of cases). More rarely, it occurs during the first months of summer. It occurs in current life conditions, in cloudy or clear weather. Sensitivity to long wavelengths explains the appearance of an eruption through glass. The duration of the triggering exposure varies from 10 min to several hours. Irradiation triggers the formation of photoproduct in affected subjects (endogenous photoallergen), stimulating a cellular mediated immune reaction which causes cutaneous lesions.

The long-term evolution of the disease is chronic and incapacitating. Although the pruritus disappears within a few days, the eruption persists for 2 or 3 weeks in the absence of exposure. Any further exposure causes a recurrence during the entire sunny period. In the long term, the ailment recurs every year for 10 years on an average. Spontaneous improvement is possible but the ailment often worsens, with the eruption spreading gradually to the covered areas and starting earlier and earlier for lower and lower levels of exposure.

The repetitive phototest makes it possible to reproduce lesions. Irradiation is produced in the total spectrum every 2 days, at a dose of two to three MED in order to avoid too intense a phototoxic reaction which conceals the reaction.

## 36.2.15 Actinic Prurigo (AP)

Two ailments with obvious semiological similarities have been described, firstly in Amerindians and secondly, but much more exceptionally, in Caucasians.

#### 36.1.2.15.1 Actinic Prurigo in Amerindians[32]

This is an idiopathic photodermatosis which is found in Indian populations in Canada, Chilean Indians from the high plateaus in Colombia and the Metis populations in Mexico. AP is usually familial, which has led to it also being called *hereditary polymorphic light eruption*. It is more common in girls (70%) and occurs particularly in socially deprived populations. There is a significant correlation with certain HLA groups.

It starts before the age of 10 and evolves chronically, before being perpetuated at an adult age. The eruption is made up of prurigo and eczematous lesions, predominantly on areas of the body that are exposed during the summer, but they can also occur on covered areas of the body, even persisting in winter. The combination with cheilitis of the upper lip is found in over 85% of cases. Conjunctivitis and eyebrow alopecia are often frequently observed.

#### 36.2.15.2 Caucasian Actinic Prurigo[33]

Previously called Hutchinson's *summer prurigo*, this differs clinically and epidemiologically. It is much rarer and does not appear to be familial or linked to socioeconomic conditions. It is combined with atopic dermatitis in 10–40% of cases and electively affects children (80% of cases occur before the age of 10 years), particularly girls.

Clinically, the eruption consists of lichenified plaques and prurigo lesions which leave very unsightly punctiform scars. The distal part of the nose and cheilitis are typically affected, but the eyebrow tail is not affected. The eruption mainly occurs on areas of the body that are exposed in summer, but it can also affect unexposed areas and last into winter, which, for a time, could make people question the actual role of light. Adolescence usually sees an improvement.

The polychromatic phototest makes it possible to reproduce the lesions and the UVA phototest. The histology at the acute stage of AP is completely comparable with that of polymorphous light eruption. Differential diagnosis arises with photosensitive atopic dermatitis.

#### 36.2.16  Acne and Excoriated Acne[34]

Acne may be pruritic. Treatment normally clears up the pruritus. However, facial excoriations (combined or not with other excoriations) may persist after the acne lesions have cleared up. This can enter the realms of psychopathological complexes

### 36.3  Treatment of Pruritus in Children

The basic treatment will depend on the etiological diagnosis, which more often than not is atopic dermatitis or varicella. In the forms for which the inflammatory attack and pruritus are intense, local corticotherapy may be effective and is often prescribed initially in order to try to relieve the child of the symptoms. However, sometimes only powerful topical corticoids (class II) are effective, but these expose the child to a not inconsiderable systemic uptake in newborn babies or on erythrodermic skin. The effectiveness of local corticotherapy varies according to the etiology. Erythroderma and pruritus, which are steroid-responsive during atopic dermatitis, are often steroid-dependent or steroid-resistant, as they are for the Netherton syndrome or immune deficiency diseases. Topical calcineurin inhibitors can prove to be more effective in controlling pruritus in certain cases of atopic dermatitis.

Neutral emollient creams often cause a not insignificant improvement in the pruritus, particularly in the case of xerosis. These creams must be reapplied several times a day if there is major desquamation or ichthyosis.

Sedative antihistamines (dexchlorpheniramine, hydroxyzine) may be useful for pruritus combined with insomnia. New-generation antihistamines (desloratadine syrup from the age of 1 year, levocetirizine tablet from the age of 6 years) should preferably be used for urticaria.

Scratching is possible from the age of four to six months onwards. This does not mean that the pruritus did not affect children who are less than 4–6 months of age; therefore, treatment for pruritus in children needs to be considered (see Part III).

### References

1. Lacour M. Update on Sjögren-Larsson syndrome. *Dermatology*. 1996;193:77–82.
2. Willemsen MA, Lutt MA, Rotteveel, et al. Clinical and biochemical effects of zileuton in patients with the Sjgren-Larsson syndrome. *Eur J Pediatr*. 2001;160:711–717.

3. Saif GB, Al-Khenaizan S. Netherton syndrome: successful use of topical tacrolimus and pimecrolimus in four siblings. *Int J Dermatol.* 2007;46:290–294.

4. Shah KN, Yan AC. Low but detectable serum levels of tacrolimus seen with the use of very dilute, extemporaneously compounded formulations of tacrolimus ointment in the treatment of patients with Netherton syndrome. *Arch Dermatol.* 2006;142:1362–1363.

5. Lykavieris P, Hadchouel M, Chardot C, et al. Outcome of liver disease in children with Alagille syndrome: a study of 163 patients. *Gut.* 2001;49:431–435.

6. Van Mil SW, Houwen RH, Klomp LW. Genetics of familial intrahepatic cholestasis syndromes. *J Med Genet.* 2005;42:449–463.

7. Cynamon HA, Andres JM, Iafrate RP. Rifampin relieves pruritus in children with cholestatic liver disease. *Gastroenterology.* 1990;98:1013–1016.

8. Lecha M. Erythropoietic protoporphyria. *Photodermatol Photoimmunol Photomed.* 2003;19:142–146.

9. Proceedings of the consensus conference on the management of atopic dermatitis in children. *Ann Dermatol Venereol.* 2005;132–290.

10. Poonawalla T, Kell, B. Urticaria: a review *Am J clin Dermatil.* 2009,10:9–21

11. Zuberbier T. EAACI/GA2LEN/EDF guideline: management of urticaria. *Allergy.* 2006;61:321–327. European Academy of Allergology and Clinical Immunology.

12. Bader-Meunier B, Venencie PY, Vieillefond A, et al. Hyperimmunoglobulinemia D and familial urticaria in children *Ann Dermatol Vénéréol.* 1996;123:398–400.

13. Muckle TJ, Wells M. Urticaria, deafness, and amyloidosis: a new heredo-familial syndrome *Q J Med.* 1962;31:235–248.

14. Feldmann J, Prieur AM, Quartier P, et al. Chronic infantile neurological cutaneous and articular syndrome is caused by mutations in CIAS1, a gene highly expressed in polymorphonuclear cells and chondrocytes. *Am J Hum Genet.* 2002;71:198–203.

15. Petty RE, Southwood TR, Baum J, et al. Revision of the proposed classification criteria for juvenile idiopathic arthritis. *J Rheumatol.* 1998;25:1991–1994.

16. Léauté-Labrèze C. Treatment of psoriasis in children. *Ann Dermatol Venereol.* 2001;128:286–290.

17. Valent P, Horny HP, Escribano L, et al. Diagnostic criteria and classification of mastocytosis: a consensus proposal. *Leuk Res.* 2001;25:603–625.

18. Legrain V, Taieb A, Bioulac-Sage P, et al. Diffuse cutaneous mastocytosis without permanent lesions. *Ann Dermatol Venereol.* 1994;121:561–564.

19. Mansouri S, Aractingi S. Erythema: diagnostic orientation. *Rev Prat.* 1997;47:891–895.

20. Griffiths WA, Ozluer S. Pityriasis rubra pilaris. *Ann Dermatol Venereol.* 2001;128:931–934.

21. Misery L, Véron I, Saint-Marc T, et al. Pityriasis rubra pilaris in an AIDS patient. *Ann Med Interne.* 1994;145:199–200.

22. Bouree P. Oxyurose. In: Nozais JP, Datry A, Danis M, eds. *Medical Parasitology Compendium.* Paris: Pradel; 1987.

23. Gupta AK, Batra R, Bluhm R, et al. Skin diseases associated with Malassezia species. *J Am Acad Dermatol.* 2004;51:785–798.

24. Misery L, Jay P, Claudy A, et al. Pemphigoid in children. *Ann Dermatol Venereol.* 1994;12:623–625.

25. Nemeth AJ, Klein AD, Gould EW, et al. Childhood bullous pemphigoid. *Arch Dermatol.* 1991;127:378–386.

26. Hall RP. Dermatitis herpetiformis. *J Invest Dermatol.* 1992;99:873–881.

27. Zone JJ. Clinical spectrum, pathogenesis and treatment of linear IgA bullous dermatosis. *J Dermatol.* 2001;28:651–653.

28. Wojnarowska F, Mardsen RA, Bhogal, et al. Chronic bullous disease of childhood, childhood cicatricial pemphigoid and linear IgA disease of adults: a comparative study demonstrating clinical and immunopathologic overlap. *J Am Acad Dermatol.* 1988;19:792–805.

29. Gupta G, Man I, Kemmett D. Hydroa vacciniforme: a clinical and follow-up study of 17 cases. *J Am Acad Dermatol.* 2000;42:208–213.

30. Requena L, Alegre V, Hasson A. Spring eruption of the ears. *Int J Dermatol.* 1990;29:284–286.

31. Draelos ZK, Hansen RC. Polymorphic light eruption in childhood. *Clin Pediatr.* 1985;24:692–695.

32. Fusaro RM, Johnson JA. Hereditary polymorphic light eruption of American Indians: occurrence in non-Indians with polymorphic light eruption. *J Am Acad Dermatol.* 1996;34:612–617.

33. Lane PR, Hogan DJ, Martel MJ, et al. Actinic prurigo: clinical features and prognosis. *J Am Acad Dermatol.* 1992;26:683–692.

34. Reich A, Trybucka K, Szepietowski JC. Acne itch: do acne patients suffer from itching? *Acta Derm Venereol.* 2008;88:38–42.

# Chapter 37
# Pruritus Vulvae

Micheline Moyal-Barracco

Pruritus is a common motive of consultation both in gynaecological and vulvar clinics although the prevalence of this symptom in any given population is not known. As opposed to vulvar pain, pruritus vulva is almost always associated with visible lesions. An etiological diagnosis is mandatory if we are to correctly inform the patient and to treat her as efficiently as possible. The age of the patient, the chronology of pruritus (acute, chronic, recurrent), the response to previous treatments (antifungal, corticosteroid), the location and the aspect of the lesions will all help assessing, or at least orienting, the etiological diagnosis. Diagnostic tests are frequently indicated. This chapter focuses on the diagnostic approach and treatment. Only the most common causes of pruritus vulvae will be considered.

## 37.1 Definition

Pruritus vulva (or vulvar itch) is an unpleasant vulvar sensation that provokes the urge to scratch to obtain relief. The severity of pruritus is eminently variable. Whatever its cause, the symptom is often more prominent in the evening or at night, or when the area is touched during toilet or intercourse. Scratching may induce vulvar excoriations which are a source of burning pain. In this situation, the patient is aware that pain is a consequence of scratching and not the primary symptom. Indeed, pruritus must be differentiated from pain, an unpleasant sensation which does not provoke the urge to scratch. The differentiation between these two vulvar symptoms is essential because their etiological approach is different. Indeed, pruritus is almost always associated with abnormal visible findings, whereas vulvar pain in the absence of abnormal visible findings (vulvodynia) is a common vulvar condition.

## 37.2 Diagnostic Approach

Pruritus vulva is not a condition. It is the symptom of various - most often benign, sometimes malignant – disorders.[1] The diagnostic approach is aimed to search for an etiology in order to offer the most specific treatment.

### 37.2.1 Age

The cause of pruritus vulvae varies across the ages.[1] The available literature does not enable one to state the prevalence of the symptoms of pruritus vulvae according to the age of the afflicted patients. From the author's experience, in young patients, infections are the most common causes. In post menopausal patients, lichen sclerosus or lichen planus and intraepithelial neoplasia are more frequent than infections (Table 37.1).

### 37.2.2 Past History

Both past gynaecological *human papilloma virus* and yeast infections as well as familial or personal past history of an inflammatory dermatosis (psoriasis, atopic dermatitis, and lichen planus) should be searched for, as all these conditions may cause pruritus.

### 37.2.3 Symptoms' Analysis

#### 37.2.3.1 Evolution

Pruritus vulvae may be acute, chronic or recurrent (Table 37.2). Acute pruritus vulvae most frequently

L. Misery and S. Ständer (eds.), *Pruritus*,
DOI 10.1007/978-1-84882-322-8_37, © Springer-Verlag London Limited 2010

**Table 37.1** Main causes of pruritus vulvae according to age

| Girls | Irritant contact dermatitis |
|---|---|
| | Pinworms |
| | Atopic dermatitis |
| | Lichen sclerosus |
| Adults < 50 | Candidosis |
| | Lichen simplex |
| | Lichen sclerosus |
| | Psoriasis |
| | Lichen planus |
| | Classic VIN |
| Adults > 50 | Lichen sclerosus |
| | Lichen planus |
| | Classic VIN |
| | Paget's disease |
| | Differentiated VIN |

**Table 37.2** Main causes of pruritus vulvae according to its chronology

Acute (i.e., rapid onset and short course)
Yeast infection
Contact dermatitis
Chronic (i.e., persistent and lasting)
Lichen sclerosus
Lichen planus
Lichen simplex
Psoriasis
Intraepithelial neoplasia: classic, differentiated, Paget
Recurrent (i.e., alternately ceasing and beginning again)
Yeast infection
Contact dermatitis (if repeated contacts)
Herpes
Inflammatory dermatosis
Fixed drug reactions

reveal an infection, more rarely a contact dermatitis. Chronic pruritus vulvae are mainly related to inflammatory dermatosis. Intraepithelial neoplasia is a rarer cause. The causes of recurrent pruritus are more frequently infections (yeasts at first) than inflammatory or neoplastic.[2]

### 37.2.3.2 Consequences

Pruritus vulvae may have local, general, and psychosexual consequences. Scratching may provoke multiple painful, linear excoriations or a thickening of the skin. Conversely, thickening of the skin may be a cause of pruritus (itch-scratch-itch circle). Pruritus vulvae may be more intense in the evening or at night. It could wake up the patient during the night and be a source of

insomnia and fatigue. Conversely, insomnia and fatigue may both make the pruritus more intense and persistent. Pruritus vulvae, particularly when recurrent or chronic, are a distressing symptom: indeed, vulva is a secret sexually implicated area and any symptom in this area may induce feelings of dirtiness, infectiousness, or loss of feminity. In addition, pruritus vulvae, which urge to touch to obtain relief often produces a feeling of shame and guiltiness. Anxiety, depression, and sexual dysfunction (desire, arousal, and orgasm) are often associated with chronic or recurrent pruritus vulvae, particularly when the cause of the pruritus has not yet been identified.

### 37.2.3.3 Effect of Previous Treatments

The effect of previous treatments (mainly antifungal and topical corticosteroids) may help orienting the etiological investigation. The physician should be aware of some pitfalls in the interpretation of the data which are brought forward by the patient:

- When a patient says that a treatment is "not effective," she may mean that her disease has not been definitively cured by the treatment. Therefore, she should be invited to specify if the pruritus was controlled while she was following the treatment or immediately after she stopped it.
- Improvement after antifungal treatment is not synonymous with yeast infection.
- Improvement after topical corticosteroid treatment does not exclude a yeast infection.
- Absence of improvement immediately after appropriate antifungal treatment is usually an argument against the diagnosis of a yeast infection.

### 37.2.3.4 Hygiene Habits

Contrary to popular belief, hygiene habits are not a common cause of pruritus vulvae in adults. According to the author's experience, the marketed washing products or sanitary pads are a possible but rare source of well documented contact dermatitis. By contrast, in girls, nonspecific irritant dermatitis related to inadequate hygiene habits and to the fragile hypoestrogenized vulvar tegument is common.[3]

## 37.2.4 *Physical Findings*

Vulvar examination is an important part of the diagnosis process. The only condition which could possibly be diagnosed on a "phone call" is an episode of candidosis (acute pruritus associated with discharge). Ideally, the patient should be examined in a comfortable gynaecological position and have her vulva perfectly lighted during the examination. A lighted magnifying glass is helpful.

### 37.2.4.1 Location

The location of the pruritic lesions may orient the diagnosis. Mucosal lesions most frequently result from vaginal infection, whereas cutaneous lesions are usually related to inflammatory dermatosis. Vulvar intra-epithelial neoplasia (VIN) may involve either the mucosa or the skin of the vulva.

When the lesions are subtle, it is helpful to ask the patient to point out the pruritic area. In case of unilateral lesion comparative examination of both sides of the vulva may help better visualising the lesions.

### 37.2.4.2 Specific Features of the Lesions

Pruritic lesions of the vulva are mainly red or white. The color of the lesions may help orienting the diagnosis (Table 37.3).

**Table 37.3** Etiology of pruritus vulvae according to the colour of the lesions

|  | Frequent conditions | Rarer conditions |
|---|---|---|
| Red lesions | Candidosis | VIN |
|  | Lichen simplex | Paget's disease |
|  | Psoriasis | Herpes (preulcerative phase) |
|  | Lichen planus | Trichomonasis |
|  |  | Contact dermatitis |
|  |  | Tinea cruris |
| White lesions | Lichen sclerosus | VIN |
|  | Lichen simplex | Paget's disease |
| Dark lesions | Pubic lice | VIN |
|  |  | Fixed drug eruption |

### 37.2.4.3 Muco-Cutaneous Associated Extra-Vulvar Lesions

Examination of extra vulvar areas could detect contributory abnormalities. For example, in case of suspicion of a vulvar lichen planus, examination of mouth and skin may reveal lesions which are typical of this dermatosis. Suspicion of vulvar psoriasis may be reinforced by the presence of typical skin, scalp, or nail lesions.

## 37.3 Laboratory Tests

Diagnostic assessment frequently requires laboratory tests.

### 37.3.1 *Search for Infection*

The different tests are presented in 36.4.

### 37.3.2 *Cytology*

Cytology is rarely indicated in case of vulvar lesions. However, Tzanck test can rapidly confirm a herpes lesion (see below).

### 37.3.3 *Biopsy*

Biopsy is helpful to confirm a dermatosis or a VIN. The site of the biopsy and the aspect of the lesions as well as the diagnostic hypothesis will be specified to the pathologist. Vulvar biopsy is always performed under local anesthesia. A cream containing lidocaine and prilocaine (EMLA cream®) provides a satisfactory anesthesia within 10 min when applied on the mucosal aspect of the vulva.[4]

On the skin side, either a longer application of this cream (2 h under occlusion) or an injection of lidocaine is required. The specimen is easily taken with punch biopsy of 3–4 mm in diameter. Hemostasis is obtained either by pressure or electrocauterization or application of a topical hemostatic such as silver nitrate, ferric sulfate (Monsel's solution), or aluminum chloride. The pathological conclusion will always be confronted with the clinical features.

Patch tests can be performed in case of suspicion of contact dermatitis. The relevance of a positive test must always be discussed. Negative tests do not exclude a contact dermatitis for two reasons: 1. the dermatitis may result from irritation and not from allergy; 2. the patch tests are performed on the back or the upper limb, two areas which do not reproduce the specific humid and frictional environment of the vulva.[5]

## 37.4 Main Etiologies of Pruritus Vulvae

### 37.4.1 *Infections*

#### 37.4.1.1 Mycosis

- The most common vulvar mycosis is candidiasis, an opportunistic infection mainly related to *Candida albican*.[6]

Pruritus is typically associated with burning and a white creamy discharge. During the bouts of candidosis, the patient may suffer from a post coïtal balanoposthitis. The lesions mainly consist in a diffuse vestibular erythema, which may be associated to some degree of edema. The perineal area is sometimes involved by a symmetrical eczematous-like eruption.

The diagnosis of candidosis mainly relies on clinical examination. However in case of atypical features, resistance to treatment or suspicion of a recurrent candidosis (which will require a long term imidazole treatment), the diagnosis should be confirmed by microscopic examination and cultures. The specimens should be taken when the symptoms are present, and in the absence of a current or recent antifungal treatment. The results are obtained within a few days. When a vulvo-perineal rash is observed, specimens should be taken not only from the vagina but also from the cutaneous vulvo perineal area. The presence of pseudohyphae with budding yeast on a wet mount or potassium hydroxide preparation is considered as a feature of pathogenicity. *Candida albicans* is the most frequently isolated yeast. The presence of *Candida albicans* even

in small quantity on the skin should be considered as abnormal, whereas the isolation of a small number of colonies of Candida in the vagina in the absence of pseudohyphae on a wet mount specimen may not have a pathological significance. *Candida albicans* azole resistance is rare in vaginal isolates, and susceptibility testing is not warranted and even not totally reliable.

Short duration topical or oral azole effectively treats an episode of vulvovaginal candidosis. The treatment may either consist of insertions of a vaginal cream or suppository or a single 150 mg dose of fluconazole. No statistically significant differences are observed in clinical cure rates of anti-fungals administered by the oral and intra-vaginal routes for the treatment of uncomplicated vaginal candidiasis.[7]

In case of recurrent vulvovaginal candidiasis defined as four or more symptomatic episodes per year, two options can be offered: either treating each individual episode for a longer time (e.g., 7–14 days of topical therapy or a 100, 150, or 200 mg oral dose of fluconazole every third day for a total of three doses (day 1, 4, and 7) or prescribing a suppressive maintenance antifungal therapy weekly for 6 months, i.e., oral fluconazole (100, 150, or 200 mg dose) or vaginal imidazole suppository or cream. Suppressive maintenance antifungal therapies are effective in reducing recurrent vulvo-vaginal candidosis (RVVC). However, 30–50% of women will have recurrent disease after the maintenance therapy is discontinued. Treatment of sex partners does not seem to influence the rate of recurrences; it will be offered in case of postcoital balanoposthitis.

- Vulvar tinea is rare. This dermatophytosis is mainly caused by *Trichophyton rubrum, Epidermophyton floccosum,* and *Trichophyton mentagrophytes*. The disease should be diagnosed before an erythematous vulvar skin rash associated with a groin involvement. The erythematous patches typically have a characteristic central clearing and a scaly, sharply demarcated periphery. Deep tissue involvement may be responsible for nodular or papulo-pustular atypical lesions; these so-called Majocchi's granulomas may be elicited by iterative applications of topical corticosteroids or by systemic immunodepression. The diagnosis of tinea will be confirmed by direct examination and cultures performed on specimen taken both from the vulva and from the other susceptible sites such as groin, feet, and toenails, if lesions are present there. The specimens should be taken in the absence of a current or recent fungal treatment by scraping the periphery of the lesion. The results are obtained within 1–6 weeks. The treatment may be either topical (imidazole derivatives) or systemic (terbinafine).

## 37.4.1.2  Parasitic Infections

* *Phthirus pubis* infects the hairy part of the vulva (mons Venus and labia majora). The infection is usually transmitted by sexual contacts,[8] although contact with towels, blankets, sheets or clothes could be a source of contamination. The parasites appear as tiny (1 mm) rusty spots located at the base of the hair shaft. The ovale gray louse eggs (nits) are laterally attached to the hair. Associated sexually transmitted infections should be searched for. Treatment consists in the application of shampoos or creams containing permethrin or pyrethrins with piperonyl butoxide infection (Sexually Transmitted Diseases treatment guidelines). Decontamination of bedding and clothing with hot-water, machine washing or dry cleaning is essential to avoid re-infection.[10]

* Pinworm infection is caused by a small, white intestinal worm called *Enterobius vermicularis*. It is the most common worm infection in the United States. School age children, have the highest rates of infection. This infection is mainly responsible for pruritus ani. However, pinworm is a classical cause of pruritus vulvae in prepubertal girls. Pinworms live in the rectum of humans. Female pinworms leave the intestines through the anus and deposit eggs on the anal margin and the surrounding area. Pinworms are visible either in the stools or on the anal margin or on the vulva where they appear as small (1/2 in. size) white thread like worms. In the absence of visible live worms, a scotch tape test will look for eggs of *Enterobius vermicularis*. Treatment consists in the oral administration of one dose of mebendazole or pyrantel pamoate followed by a second dose 2 weeks later. All the members of the family will be simultaneously treated.[11]

* Scabies is a transmissible skin infection induced by an ectoparasite: *Sarcoptes scabiei*.[12] Scabies may provoke vulvar pruritic nodules on the labia majora. Pruritus is usually not restricted to this area. Usually, it also involves other sites of the body, particularly finger web spaces and ventral wrists where typical burrows (linear papules or vesicules) are observed. A deep scraping of burrows or nodules may yield the microscopic identification of a mite ova or scybala (feces). The treatment of choice of scabies is the topical use of permethrin (5%). Topical crotamiton and oral ivermectin are alternative drugs. If a topical preparation is used, a second treatment with the same product may be necessary 7–10 days later. All clothes, bedding, and towels used by the infested person during 2 days before the treatment should be washed in hot water, and dried in a hot dryer.

* Trichomoniasis is a common sexually transmitted disease caused by the protozoan parasite, *Trichomonas vaginalis*.[13] The vagina is the most common site of infection in women. When present, symptoms appear within 5–28 days after exposure. Pruritus vulva is associated with a frothy, smelly, yellow-green vaginal discharge, dyspareunia and vulvar burning during micturion. The vulvovaginal mucosa is uniformly red, with, sometimes a typical "strawberry" appearance. Trichomonasis is easily diagnosed on a wet mount of the vaginal secretions. *Trichomonas vaginalis* appear as small, rapidly moving, teardrop-shaped, flagellate organisms. There are a large number of neutrophils, vaginal pH is high and lactobacilli are absent. In women in whom trichomoniasis is suspected but not confirmed by microscopy, vaginal secretions should be cultured for. *Trichomonas vaginalis* sp. Recommended regimens include Metronidazole (2 g orally in a single dose or 1 g per day for 7 days) or Tinidazole 2 g orally in a single dose. Patients should be advised to avoid consuming alcohol during the treatment and for 24 h after completion of metronidazole or 72 h after completion of tinidazole. The sex partners should be simultaneously treated. In pregnant women, metronidazole will be preferred to tinidazole.

## 37.4.1.3  Herpes[14]

Although genital herpes is mainly responsible for painful ulcers, pruritus vulvae may be a symptom, either as a prodrome or associated with the preulcerative papulovesicular phase of the infection. Therefore, herpes will be suspected in case of recurrent episodes of localized pruritus rapidly replaced by a burning sensation.

The duration of each episode varies from 2 to 10 days. Different tests could be used to confirm the presence of *Herpes simplex virus (HSV)* mainly Type II on the lesions either indirectly (cytology) or directly (virus, antigens, DNA). Whatever the test used, the specimens should be taken appropriately by scraping or energically swabbing a fresh, vesicular or ulcerative lesion. Tzanck preparation consists in fixing with alcohol, staining with Giemsa, and then examining the collected cells under a microscope. Herpes causes formation of giant basophilic cells with multiple nuclei. This costless and rapid test is not considered as sensitive enough. Cultures are considered as the gold standard technique. The virus can be grown and identified within 3–7 days from the time the specimen has been collected. The viral antigens can also be detected by rapid methods, such as immunofluorescence testing (IF) and enzyme linked immunosorbent assays (ELISA), which will give the results on the same day. These tests utilize monoclonal antibodies directed against HSV-1 and HSV-2 respectively. Recently, sensitive laboratory techniques have been developed. Polymerase chain reaction (PCR) is a more recent, sensitive technique based on the molecular detection of viral DNA. Whatever the technique used, a negative result does not exclude the diagnosis of herpes. In case of consistent clinical suspicion, the test should be repeated. Antibody detection is useful to confirm a primary HSV infection. Oral antiviral treatment by acyclovir, valaciclovir, or famciclovir is the mainstay of management. These drugs have a beneficial clinical impact but neither eradicate latent virus nor affect the risk, frequency, or severity of recurrences after they are discontinued. Topical therapy with antiviral drugs offers minimal clinical benefit. Systemic antiviral drugs are mainly used to treat first clinical episodes (7–10 days regimen) and recurrent infection defined as 6 episodes or more per year. Indeed, suppressive therapy reduces the frequency of genital herpes recurrences by 70–80%.[15]

### 37.4.1.4  Rare Infectious Causes of Pruritus

*Streptococcus A* infection,[16] molluscum contagiosum (when inflamed, usually soon before spontaneous regression)[17] and Schistosomiasis during the invasion phase could be responsible for pruritus.

## 37.4.2  *Inflammatory Dermatosis*

### 37.4.2.1  Lichen Simplex

Lichen simplex is probably the most common itchy vulvar condition and represents a reaction to chronic scratching associated with atopic dermatitis or psoriasis rather than an authentic dermatosis.[18] The lesions are mainly located on the cutaneous aspect of the vulva. Anal lichen simplex is frequently associated. The skin is thickened, pink, white or pigmented. The hair may be cut by the chronic itch and excoriatons may be seen. Pruritus tends to thicken the skin and the thickened skin is a source of pruritus (itch-scratch cycle). Mucosa is less frequently involved; in that case the thickened area is usually pale. Lichen simplex of the vulva may be either "primary" (i.e., no associated dermatosis) or "secondary" representing a feature of atopic dermatitis[19] or psoriasis. In these cases, past history or the presence of specific extravulvar lesions will contribute to assess the diagnosis. Biopsy will exclude lichen sclerosus and VIN (classic VIN, differentiated VIN, and Paget's disease). Topical corticosteroids are the mainstay of the treatment (Table 37.4). Recurrences are common.

### 37.4.2.2  Psoriasis

As opposed to extra genital psoriasis, vulvar psoriasis is frequently itchy. The lesions mainly involve the hairy portion of the vulva and the vulvar folds (i.e., inter labial fold, anterior commissure close to the mons pubis). The lesions are typically, red, thickened, sharply demarcated plaques, more or less scaly according to the level of the occlusion of the involved area. Past history and associated lesions may substantiate the diagnosis. Topical corticosteroids (Table 2.4) and moisturizing creams are the first line treatment of vulvar psoriasis. The role of calcineurin inhibitors in the treatment of vulvar psoriasis needs to be specified.[20] Recurrences are common.

### 37.4.2.3  Lichen Sclerosus

Lichen sclerosus (LS), an inflammatory auto-immune disorder, is one of most frequent motive for consultation in vulvar clinics. The mean age of the patients is about 50.

**Table 37.4** Topical corticosteroid treatment of inflammatory itchy vulvar dermatosis (based on experts' experience, not on controlled trials)

| Dermatose | First line treatment | Maintenance therapy | Recurrence |
|---|---|---|---|
| Lichen simplex | Class 4<br>Once a day × 3 weeks | Class 3<br>Once a day × 3 weeks, then twice a week × 2 months | Class 4 or 3<br>Episodic: once a day × 15 days or restart the whole treatment (first line + maintenance) |
| Psoriasis | Class 4<br>One a day × 3 weeks | Class 3<br>Once a day × 3 weeks, then twice a week × 2 months | Class 4 or 3:<br>Episodic: once a day × 15 days or restart the whole treatment (first line + maintenance) |
| Lichen sclerosus | Class 4 or 3<br>Once a day × 3 months | Class 3 twice a week × 9 months | Restart the whole protocol (First line + maintenance) |
| Lichen planus | Class 4 or 3<br>Once a day × 3 months | Class 3 twice a week × 9 months | Restart the whole protocol (First line + maintenance) |

Topical corticosteroid potency: Class 1: mil; Class 2: moderate; Class 3: potent; Class 4: very potent. (Refer to classification in another chapter, I suppose.)

Pruritus vulva is the most common symptom although LS can be asymptomatic or be responsible for burning or dyspareunia. Vulvar lichen sclerosus mainly involves the mucosal aspect of the vulva (labia minora, vestibule, interlabial folds), but vulvar skin and anal margin may also be involved. The main features of vulvar LS are palor, atrophy, and architectural modification. These abnormalities are diversely associated in each patient. The palor, either focal or diffuse is typically shiny. Atrophy is responsible for a thin, sometimes wrinkled aspect of the skin and mucosa. Architectural modifications are the results of mucosal synechiae (i.e., adhesions of contiguous involved mucosa). They include burying of the clitoris, resorption of the labia minora contours and posterior synechiae of the labia minora. Many clinical variants are observed: bullous, pigmented, ecchymotic, and leucoplastic. Approximately 60% of squamous carcinoma are associated with lichen sclerosus. However the risk of progression of vulvar lichen sclerosus (VLS) to cancer is low (less than 5%). Precursors of squamous cell carcinoma associated with VLS are differentiated VIN, epithelilial hyperplasia, and classical VIN.[21] Medical treatment consists in the application of corticosteroids (Table 2.4).[22] The role of calcineurin inhibitors in the treatment of vulvar lichen sclerosus needs to be determined.[23] Surgery is needed in case of leucoplakia or focal resistance to corticosteroids or in case of symptomatic interlabial or clitoral synechiae.

### 37.4.2.4 Lichen Planus

Like lichen sclerosus, lichen planus (LP) is an inflammatory auto-immune mucocutaneous disorder which frequently involves the genital mucosa.[24] Vulvar lichen planus (VLP) exhibits widely variable morphology. Nonerosive VLP is easy to recognize; violaceous small flat topped papules, annular display, fern like patter are all classical features. Pruritus, when present, is easily controlled by topical corticosteroids. By contrast, erosive vulvar lichen planus (EVLP) may be clinically misleading; the eruption consists in erosive well demarcated plaques predominantly located on the posterior vestibule; they are usually surrounded by a halo of pale mucosa. Architectural modifications are frequently associated; they result from synechiae which lead to a resorption of the vulvar contours. Burning is the major symptom. Pruritus is generally not on the first line. Histology is not always specific. However, it will help excluding VIN. Erosive lichen planus may not only involve the vulva but also the vagina and other mucosal sites such as mouth, oesophagus, eye, and external ear. Typical cutaneous lesions may be associated; their presence will help substantiating the diagnosis. Response of EVLP to topical corticosteroids is usually satisfactory.[25] However, the therapeutical response of vaginal lesions may be poor; synechia and atrophy may comprise the coital function despite surgical intervention. Long term follow up of EVLP is mandatory both to help the patient to alleviate the vulvar pain and to detect, as early as possible, complications such as VIN or squamous cell carcinoma both of which are a rare complications of EVLP.

Contact dermatitis is a classical cause of pruritus vulvae. This dermatitis may result either from irritation or allergic.[26] Urines or hygiene products (poorly rinsed or too frequently applied antiseptic soap for example) may induce an irritant dermatitis characterized by a dry, wrinkled, sometimes erosive erythema involving not only the vulva but also the adjacent regions (perineum, inner thighs). Pruritus is associated with burning. Allergic vulvar dermatitis is mainly related to topical treatments or hygiene products. Like in irritant vulvitis, the lesions involve not only the vulvar skin but also the adjacent regions. The eruption consists in red eczematous plaques with a vesicular or oozing surface and ill defined borders. Patch tests may identify the allergizing product which has to be definitively withdrawn. A positive patch test to a product does not necessarily mean that the application of this product is the cause of the pruritus vulvae. The relevance of the test has to be demonstrated (rash produced by the application of the incriminated product and improvement after withdrawal). Conversely, a negative test does not exclude an allergic dermatitis: indeed, the patch tests performed on the back or the upper limb do not reproduce the specific humid and frictional environment of the vulva. Adapted patch testing has been proposed.[27] Topical corticosteroid may help in reducing pruritus, burning, and the duration of the rash.

### 37.4.2.5 Rare Dermatological Causes of Pruritus Vulvae

- Fox Fordyce disease is a rare disorder of unknown etiology characterized by a keratin plug in the follicular infundibulum and the adjacent apocrine acrosyringium.[28] It consists of a chronic pruritic papular eruption localized to apocrine glands-bearing areas. It mainly affects adolescents or young women. Pruritus is the main symptom, often more prominent in the premenstrual period. The lesions are located not only in the hairy parts of the vulva but also in the axillae and on the areolas. Therapeutic options include topical corticosteroids, topical or oral retinoids, topical antibiotics (clindamycine, erythromycin), and immunosuppressants (pimecrolimus, tacrolimus)
- Vulvar syringomas are benign tumors of the sweat glands resulting from malformation of the sweat ducts.[29] They consist in multiple small papules (a few millimetres to 1 cm in diameter) mainly located on the labia majora. Although usually asymptomatic, they may provoke itching.
- Hailey-Hailey disease, also called familial benign pemphigus, is a chronic autosomal dominant disorder with incomplete penetrance. An overall defect in keratinocyte adhesion appears to be secondary to

a primary defect in a calcium pump protein, ATP2C.[30] Commonly, patients may not have symptoms until the age of 30–49. Vesicles, fissures, and erythematous plaques with overlying crusts typically occur on the vulva, as well as the chest, neck, and axillary areas. Burning and itching accompany the eruption, and a malodorous oozing may occur as a result of a secondary infection. A history of multiple relapses and remissions is characteristic. Heat, friction, and infection are all exacerbating factors. Microscopic examination reveals intraepidermal and suprabasilar acantholysis. The treatment mainly consists of topical corticosteroids and topical or systemic antibiotics. Dermabrasion, carbon dioxide laser ablation, and pulsed dye laser therapy have been tried with variable success. Patient should be advised to wear cool and comfortable clothing that reduces heat, friction, and sweating.

### 37.4.3 Vulvar Intraepithelial Neoplasia

Squamous VIN are divided into two categories.[31,32]

- Classic VIN is related to high risk Human papillomavirus (HPV) mainly type 16 or 18. Cytological and architectural atypia are present on the whole thickness of the epithelium. Lesions are polymorphous in terms of clinical features of prognosis. They may consist of raised or macular, red, white or pigmented patches; their surface may be smooth or verrucous. The risk of progression to squamous cell carcinoma is globally low (less than 5%). This risk is higher in immunocompromised patients with extensive lesions and, probably, in patients with erythroplastic lesions. Several therapeutical options exist: surgical excision, electrocautery, cryotherapy, laser vaporisation, photodynamic therapy, imiquimod;[33,34] The rate of recurrence is about 30%. The follow up will focus not only on the vulva but also on the cervix, the vagina, and the anus as VIN is often part of a multicentric infection.
- Differentiated VIN is histologically characterized by the presence of atypia confined to the basal and suprabasal layers of the epithelium. This type of VIN is not related to HPV infection but to an inflammatory dermatosis, i.e., active or quiescent lichen

sclerosus or lichen planus. Differentiated VIN appears as a leucoplastic or erythematous lesion which does not regress after topical treatment with corticosteroids. The risk of progression to squamous cell carcinoma is higher than for classic VIN.[35] Therefore, surgical excision is the most appropriate treatment as it allows a pathological examination.

### 37.4.4 Vulvar Paget's disease[36]

Paget's disease is an intraepithelial adenocarcinoma, affecting women over 65. Most of the time, this condition is restricted to the epithelium and does not compromise the prognosis. In rare cases however, vulvar Paget's disease is invasive (abnormal Paget's cell present in the dermis) or is associated with a contiguous adenocarcinoma (skin, rectum, colon, urethra). The lesions are usually responsible for chronic pruritus and burning. They consist in red sometimes erosive plaques typically punctuated by white thickened areas. In case of periurethral involvement, search for a bladder or urethral carcinoma will be performed. In case of perianal involvement, a rectocoloscopy is indicated to rule out an associated adenocarcinoma. Treatment will be as conservative as possible. Therapeutic options include, surgery which yield a risk of recurrence of 30–40%,[37] imiquimod, or careful follow-up without treatment if the symptoms are not too bothering for the patient.

### 37.4.5 Idiopathic Vulvar Pruritus

Pruritus without any skin findings or underlying disease (old term: pruritus sine materia or idiopathic pruritus) is rare. Most of the time, pruritus vulva is related to an identifiable vulvar condition. If no lesion is visible while the patient is symptomatic (first see how to perform an appropriate clinical vulvar inspection) the diagnosis of pruritus on unchanged skin (or idiopathic pruritus) can be made. The management of this condition includes symptomatic measures as well as a psychological approach.

Squamous cell carcinoma is not per se a source of pruritus vulvae. The lesions are usually ulcerated and mainly produce pain. However, the precursors of this tumor (VIN either differentiated or classic, lichens) may be pruritic.

## References

1. Bohl TG. Overview of vulvar pruritus through the life cycle. *Clin Obstet Gynecol.* 2005;48:786–807.
2. Boardman LA, Botte J, Kennedy CM. Recurrent vulvar itching. *Obstet Gynecol.* 2005;105:1451–1455.
3. Paek SC, Merritt DF, Mallory SB. Pruritus vulvae in prepubertal children. *J Am Acad Dermatol.* 2001;44:795–802.
4. Yrne MA, Taylor-Robinson D, Harris JR. Topical anaesthesia with lidocaine-prilocaine cream for vulval biopsy. *Br J Obstet Gynaecol.* 1989;96(4):497–499.
5. Akashin K. Sanitary napkin contact dermatitis of the vulva: location-dependent differences in skin surface conditions may play a role in negative patch test results. *J Dermatol.* 2007;34:834–837.
6. Sobel JD. Vulvovaginal candidosis. *Lancet.* 2007; 369(9577):1961–1971.
7. Nurbhai M, Grimshaw J, Watson M, et al. Oral versus intravaginal imidazole and triazole anti-fungal treatment of uncomplicated vulvovaginal candidiasis (thrush). *Cochrane Database Syst Rev.* 2007;(4):CD002845.
8. Varela JA, Otero L, Espinosa E, et al. Phthirus pubis in a sexually transmitted diseases unit: a study of 14 years. *Sex Transm Dis.* 2003;30:292–296.
9. Pierzchalski JL, Bretl DA, Matson SC. Phthirus pubis as a predictor for chlamydia infections in adolescents. *Sex Transm Dis.* 2002;29:331–334.
10. CDC's Sexually Transmitted Disease Treatment Guidelines, 2006. MMWW 2006;55:1–94.
11. St Georgiev V. Chemotherapy of enterobiasis (oxyuriasis). *Expert Opin Pharmacother.* 2001;2:267–275.
12. Johnstone P, Strong M. Scabies. *Clin Evid.* 2006;15: 2284–2290.
13. Wendel KA, Workowski KA. Trichomoniasis: challenges to appropriate management. *Clin Infect Dis.* 2007;44(suppl 3):S123–S129.
14. Gupta R, Warren T, Wald A. Genital herpes. *Lancet.* 2007; 370:2127–2137.
15. Patel R, Stanberry L, Whitley RJ. Review of recent HSV recurrent-infection treatment studies. *Herpes.* 2007;14: 23–64.
16. Echeverría Fernández M, López-Menchero Oliva JC, Marañón Pardillo R, et al. Isolation of group A beta-hemolytic Streptococcus in children with perianal dermatitis]. *Pediatr (Barc).* 2006;64:153–157.
17. Hanna D, Hatami A, Powell J, et al. A prospective randomized trial comparing the efficacy and adverse effects of four recognized treatments of molluscum contagiosum in children. *Pediatr Dermatol.* 2006;23:574–579.
18. O'Keefe RJ, Scurry JP, Dennerstein G, et al. Audit of 114 non-neoplastic vulvar biopsies. *Br J Obstet Gynaecol.* 1995;102:780–786.
19. Lynch PJ. Lichen simplex chronicus (atopic/neurodermatitis) of the anogenital region. *Dermatol Ther.* 2004;17:8–19.
20. Martín Ezquerra G, Sánchez Regaña M, Herrera Acosta E, et al. Topical tacrolimus for the treatment of psoriasis on the face, genitalia, intertriginous areas and corporal plaques. *J Drugs Dermatol.* 2006;5:334–336.
21. Jones RW, Sadler L, Grant S, et al. Clinically identifying women with vulvar lichen sclerosus at increased risk of

squamous cell carcinoma: a case-control study. *J Reprod Med.* 2004;49:808–811.

22. Neill SM, Tatnall FM, Cox NH; British association of dermatologists. Guidelines for the management of lichen sclerosus. *Br J Dermatol.* 2002;147:640–649.

23. Strittmatter HJ, Hengge UR, Blecken SR. Calcineurin antagonists in vulvar lichen sclerosus. *Arch Gynecol Obstet.* 2006;274:266–270.

24. Moyal-Barracco M, Edwards L. Diagnosis and therapy of anogenital lichen planus. *Dermatol Ther.* 2004;17:38–46.

25. Ooper SM, Wojnarowska F. Influence of treatment of erosive lichen planus of the vulva on its prognosis. *Arch Dermatol.* 2006;142:289–294.

26. Arage MA. Vulvar susceptibility to contact irritans and allergens: a review. *Arch Gynecol Obstet.* 2005;272:167–172.

27. Farage MA, Maibach H. Cumulative skin irritation test of sanitary pads in sensitive skin and normal skin population. *Cutan Ocul Toxicol.* 2007;26:37–43.

28. Zcan A, Senol M, Aydin NE, et al. Fox-fordyce disease. *J Eur Acad Dermatol Venereol.* 2003;17:244–245.

29. Dereli T, Turk BG, Kazandi AC. Syringomas of the vulva. *Int J Gynaecol Obstet.* 2007;99:65–66.

30. Oggia L, Hovnanian A. Calcium pump disorders of the skin. *Med Genet C Semin Med Genet.* 2004;131C:20–31.

31. Scurry J, Campion M, Scurry B, et al. Pathologic audit of 164 consecutive cases of vulvar intraepithelial neoplasia. *Int J Gynecol Pathol.* 2006;25:176–181.

32. Ideri M, Jones RW, Wilkinson EJ, et al. Squamous vulvar intraepithelial neoplasia: 2004 modified terminology, ISSVD Vulvar Oncology Subcommittee. *J Reprod Med.* 2005;50:807–810.

33. van Seters M, van Beurden M, Heijmans-Antonissen C et al. Treatment of vulvar intraepithelial neoplasia with topical imiquimod. *N Engl J Med.* 2008;358:1465–1473.

34. Hillemanns P, Wang X, Staehle S, et al. Evaluation of different treatment modalities for vulvar intraepithelial neoplasia (VIN): $CO_2$ laser vaporization, photodynamic therapy, excision and vulvectomy. *Gynecol Oncol.* 2006;100:271–275.

35. Roma AA, Hart WR. Progression of simplex (differentiated) vulvar intraepithelial neoplasia to invasive squamous cell carcinoma: a prospective case study confirming its precursor role in the pathogenesis of vulvar cancer. *Int J Gynecol Pathol.* 2007;26:248–253.

36. Parker LP, Parker JR, Bodurka-Bevers D, et al. Paget's disease of the vulva: pathology, pattern of involvement, and prognosis. *Gynecol Oncol.* 2000;77(1):183–189.

37. Black D, Tornos C, Soslow RA, et al. The outcomes of patients with positive margins after excision for intraepithelial Paget's disease of the vulva. *Gynecol Oncol.* 2007;104:547–550.

**Part III**
**Treatment**

# Chapter 38
# General Principles and Guidelines[*]

Elke Weisshaar

General standardized recommendations for pruritus therapy do not exist and should not be given, considering the diversity of the underlying causes of pruritus. According to recent neurophysiologic findings, antipruritic therapies aim to influence both, cutaneous and central mechanisms of pruritus. Topical and systemic antipruritic therapies have to be worked out individually in recognition of age, preexisting diseases, medications, allergies, severity of pruritus, and impact on quality of life. The first step is to identify any underlying disease and its causative therapy. Depending on the underlying cause this may range from a specific treatment of an underlying dermatosis, avoidance of a contact allergen, discontinuation of a medication, specific internal, neurological, and psychiatric therapies up to a surgical therapy of an underlying tumor.[1,2] The early start of the therapy aims to prevent the sensitization of the nerve system and thereby chronification of pruritus. The second step is to advise the patient about the general, pruritus-relieving measures (Table 38.1) followed by a step by step, symptomatic, antipruritic treatment (Table 38.2). Pruritus often stops quickly when the underlying disease improves, e.g., removal of an underlying tumor. It should be considered that especially chronic pruritus is frequently caused by several factors and may be supported by cofactors suggesting a multifactorial origin.[3,4] Especially in the elderly, several factors causing pruritus may be identified.[3]

Some general principles should be followed[1,2] (Table 38.1). It is important to evaluate the condition of the individual patient in the light of his/her age, preexisting diseases and medications, and the quality and intensity of pruritus. On the basis of this an individual therapy regimen should be set up.[2] As the care for a patient especially with chronic pruritus often extends over a longer period of time with a long period of uncertainty about the aetiology of the pruritus, frustration because of the failure of past therapies and general psychological stress frequently occur. The extent of the planned diagnostic procedures and therapy should be discussed with the patient in order to achieve best possible compliance. It has to be considered that some topical and systemic therapies may be performed as "off-label use" and require informed consent. When treating pruritus with a systemic medication patients have to be informed carefully about possible side effects. In opioid receptor antagonists and gabapentin they need to be instructed that a drivers' vigilance may be reduced while driving. If such off-labels therapies cannot be initiated in the physician's office, co-operation with a specialized center for pruritus is helpful and beneficial for the patient.[2]

As a next step, the patient should be informed about general, pruritus-relieving measures[2] (Table 38.1). Creams/lotions, e.g., with menthol, camphor, urea, polidocanol, or tannin can temporarily reduce pruritus. They can be applied by the patients themselves in case of day or night time pruritus. Prior to any further symptomatic therapy, a careful diagnostic evaluation and therapeutic treatment of any underlying diseases is of high priority (see Part II, Section 1, Chapter 13). If pruritus still persists, a combined or consecutive, step by step, symptomatic treatment is necessary (see the following subchapters). The use of antihistamines, e.g., hydroxycine 25 mg up to 100 mg daily may be helpful in serving as an additional therapy for a certain time period before other causal or aetiology-orientated therapies work. Short-term treatment with topical

[*]No funding Sources supported these book chapters. The author has no conflict of interest.

L. Misery and S. Ständer (eds.), *Pruritus*,
DOI 10.1007/978-1-84882-322-8_38, © Springer-Verlag London Limited 2010

**Table 38.1** General therapeutic measure to relieve pruritus[1,2]

- Avoidance of factors that increase skin dryness, such as dry climate, heat (e.g., sauna), alcoholic compresses, ice pack, frequent washing and bathing.
- Avoidance of contact with irritating substances (e.g., compresses with, e.g., rivanol, camomile, tea tree oil).
- Avoidance of hot and very spicy foods, large amounts of hot drinks, and alcohol.
- Avoidance of excitement and stress.
- Use of mild, nonalkaline soaps, moisturizing syndets or shower and bath oils (oil with low amount of tensid). Use of lukewarm water, maximum bathing time of 20 min. After showering/bathing immediate application of a topical in consideration of the individual skin condition.
- In case of preexisting dermatoses: drying the body skin without vigorous rubbing because this can cause further damage and peeling of the already predamaged skin.
- Regular moisturizing of the skin with hydrating skincare products adjusted to the individual skin condition.
- Wearing of adequate, soft, loose-fitting clothes, e.g., made of cotton (no wool, no synthetic materials).
- In case of atopic individuals: avoidance of house dust or house dust mites which can aggravate pruritus.
- Short-term pruritus relief / in case of nocturnal pruritus: application of creams/lotions containing urea, camphor, menthol, polidocanol, tannic acid, moist or cooling compresses, cool showers, black tea compresses.
- Education of the patient to deal with pruritus by using adequate methods of interrupting the itch–scratch-cycle, e.g., by application of a cold wash cloth, application of light pressure. Asking the patient not to scratch does not help. Distraction and attention of a caregiver works better especially in children.
- Relaxation exercises (autogenous training), relaxation therapy, stress avoidance, informing and influencing the psychosocial environment.

**Table 38.2** Therapeutic approach in chronic pruritus by step[2]

|  | Therapy |
| --- | --- |
| Step 1 | • General therapeutic measures (Table 38.1)<br>• Diagnoses of any underlying disease and causal therapy<br>• Initial symptomatic therapy: oral antihistamines (solely or in combination), cooling lotions, polidocanol, menthol, urea, tannin, topical glucocorticosteroids |
| Step 2 | • Symptomatic and causal therapy |
| Step 3 | • Symptomatic topical and/or systemic therapy, e.g., capsaicin, calcineurin inhibitors, cannabinoid agonists, montelukast, naltrexone, gabapentin, UV-therapy<br>• In most severe cases: systemic glucocorticosteroids, immunosuppressants (cyclosporine A) |
| Accompanying therapy during each step | • In case of sleep disorders: sedating antihistamines, tranquilizer, tricyclic antidepressants or neuroleptics<br>• Psychosomatic care, behavioral therapy<br>• In case of erosive scratch artefacts: disinfecting substances (e.g., fusidic acid), topical glucocorticosteroids |

Steps 1 through 3 can be performed additively or consecutively.

glucocorticosteroids may serve as a first aid treatment in uncontrolled local pruritus but is only helpful for pruritus in inflammatory skin diseases.

There is a significant lack of controlled therapy studies (RCT). This can be explained by the diversity and complexity of this symptom, the multifactorial aetiologies of pruritus and the lack of defining an outcome of assessment (e.g., defining successful treatment, varying scales for measuring itch and scratch). The differing characteristics of the patients and especially the high number of different forms of pruritus (e.g., uremic pruritus, haematologic pruritus) complicate identifying any evidence. Randomized controlled therapy studies exist for simple types of pruritus but with conflicting results (e.g., naltrexone in renal pruritus). Still, there is no study focusing on the major types of pruritus and the new therapies. Nevertheless, new systematic therapeutic concepts for improved medical care have been established. Guidelines incorporate a grading system that describes the quality of evidence used to make recommendations and their strength. An interdisciplinary group of physicians has recently published the first version of a guideline for diagnosis and treatment of chronic pruritus for the German speaking countries.[2] A group of European physicians is currently working out a guideline for chronic pruritus.

# References

1. Weisshaar E, Kucenic MJ, Fleischer AB. Pruritus: a review. *Acta Derm Venereol.* 2003;213(suppl):5–32.
2. Ständer S, Streit M, Darsow U, et al. Diagnostic and therapeutic measures in chronic pruritus. *J Dtsch Dermatol Ges.* 2006;4:350–370.
3. Sommer F, Hensen P, Böckenholt B, et al. Underlying diseases and co-factors in patients with severe chronic pruritus: a 3-year retrospective study. *Acta Derm Venereol.* 2007;87:510–516.
4. Weisshaar E, Apfelbacher CJ, Jäger G, et al. Pruritus as a cardinal symptom - clinical characteristics and quality of life in German and Ugandan patients. *Br J Dermatol.* 2006; 155:957–964.

# Chapter 39
# Menthol

Laurent Misery and Sonja Ständer

Menthol is a naturally occurring cyclic terpene alcohol $(C_{10}H_{20}O)$[10]. Its use in dermatology is very old and very ubiquitous: cooling, antipruritic, analgesic, antiseptic, etc. For decades, it has not been known as to how this chemical product can initiate a cold sensation. In fact, its mechanism of action has been recently described.

## 39.1 Mechanisms of Action

Transient receptor channels (TRP) are a family of sensory receptors that can be activated by both chemical and physical factors[3]. It is not clear if these channels directly transduce the stimuli or are part of a downstream signaling pathway[5]. TRPM8 (TRP-melastatin-8) is activated by chemical agents like menthol or when in ambient temperature drop below $26°C$[1,6,9]. Its activation leads to a cold sensation, through primary afferent sensory neurons. The absence of TRPM8 clearly demonstrates that it is the principal detector of environmental cold[1]. TRPM8 is expressed almost exclusively in the subpopulation of C-fibres[8].

Some cold-responsive neurons respond to temperatures below $20°C$, probably through TRPA1 (TRP ankyrin 1). TRPA1 is robustly activated by substances like mustard oil or garlic but it has been recently demonstrated that menthol could also activate TRPA1 with a bimodal action[7]. Ubmicromolar to mow-micromolar concentrations cause channel activation whereas higher concentrations lead to a reversible channel block. Hence, TRPA1 appears as a highly-sensitive menthol receptor, as well as TRPM8. Recent arguments are in favor of the role of TRP in the pathogenesis of itch and its treatment[2]. Temperature-sensitive TRP channels establish a basic syntax and molecular substrate of pruriception. Among them are TRPM8 and TRPA1. Itch is known to be aggravated by warmth and attenuated by cold. Hence, menthol and also eucalyptol or icilin appear as good candidates for the treatment of itch.

## 39.2 Clinical Data

Menthol induces a feeling of cold and can thereby reduce the sensation of pruritus[6]. The antipruritic effect of menthol has been proved in an experimentally induced pruritus[4]. Creams and lotions containing 1–5% menthol are used since decades for the quick relief of pruritus. Menthol had a subjective cooling effect lasting up to 70 min[11]. Thereby, it does not affect the cold and heat threshold. Usually, creams containing menthol are applied for short term reduction of pruritus. No clinical study data are available concerning the efficacy of menthol in pruritic dermatoses or chronic pruritus of various origins.

## References

1. Bautista DM, Siemens J, Glazer JM, et al. The menthol receptor TRPM8 is the principal detector of environmental cold. *Nature*. 2007;448:204–208.
2. Biro T, Toth BI, Marincsak R, Dobrosi N, Geczy T, Paus R. TRP channels as novel players in the pathogenesis and therapy of itch. *Biochem Biophys Acta*. 2007;1772:1004–1021.
3. Boulais N, Misery L. The epidermis: a sensory tissue. *Eur J Dermatol*. 2008;18:119–127.
4. Bromm B, Scharein E, Darsow U, Ring J. Effects of menthol and cold on histamine-induced itch and skin reactions in man. *Neurosci Lett*. 1995;187:157–160.

L. Misery and S. Ständer (eds.), *Pruritus*,
DOI 10.1007/978-1-84882-322-8_39, © Springer-Verlag London Limited 2010

5. Christensen AP, Corey DP. TRP channels in mechansosensation: direct or indirect activation? *Nat Rev Neurosci.* 2007;8:510–521.
6. Green BG, Schoen KL. Thermal and nociceptive sensations from menthol and their suppression by dynamic contact. *Behav Brain Res.* 2007;176(2):284–291.
7. Karashima Y, Damann N, Prenen J, et al. Bimodal action of menthol on the transient recptor potential channel TRPA1. *J Neurosci.* 2007;27:9874–9884.
8. Lumpkin EA, Caterina MJ. Mechanisms of sensory transduction in the skin. *Nature.* 2007;445:858–865.
9. Macpherson LJ, Hwang SW, Miyamoto T, Dubin AE, Patapoutian A, Story GM. More than cool: promiscuous relationships of menthol and other sensory compounds. *Mol Cell Neurosci.* 2006;32(4):335–343.
10. Patel T, Ishiuji Y, Yosipovitch G. Menthol: a refreshing look at this ancient compound. *J Am Acad Dermatol.* 2007;57:873–878.
11. Yosipovitch G, Szolar C, Hui XY, Maibach H. Effect of topically applied menthol on thermal, pain and itch sensations and biophysical properties of the skin. *Arch Dermatol Res.* 1996;288(5–6):245–248.

# Chapter 40
# Capsaicin

Laurent Misery

Capsaicin is a naturally occurring trans-8-methyl-N-vanillyl-6-noneamide, extracted from the hot pepper plant and other peppers from the genus *Capsicum* (no relation with black pepper).[1] It is found in the 'placenta', the white fibrous material that holds the seeds.[2] In dermatology it is used to treat abnormal sensations: pain (post-zoster, neuralgias, vulvodynia, HIV neuropathy, etc.), paresthesias (diabetes), and pruritus. Capsaicin is traded in some countries (Zostrix® or Axsain®) but it is prepared in lot of countries (*Capsicum* tincture 12.5 g with a cosmetic base 37.5 g).

## 40.1 Mechanisms of Action

Transient receptor channels (TRP) are a family of sensory receptors that can be activated by both chemical and physical factors.[3] It is not clear if these channels directly transduce the stimuli or are part of a downstream signaling pathway.[4] Growing arguments are in favor of a role for TRP in the pathogenesis of itch and its treatment.[5] Temperature-sensitive TRP channels establish a basic syntax and molecular substrate of pruriception. TRPV1 is one among them.

TRPV1 is a transient receptor, a potential vanilloid 1. The capsaicin receptor was previously named vanilloid receptor 1 or VR1 but it has been demonstrated that it belongs to the TRP family[6] and is now named TRPV1. TRPV1 is activated by physical (temperature > 42°C, osmotic pression) or chemical (capsaicin, protons, endocannabinoids, diphenyl compounds) factors.[7] TRPV1 is broadly expressed in the skin: on nerve fibers, mast cells, epithelial cells, Langerhans cells, sebocytes, endothelial cells, and smooth muscle cells but not melanocytes.[8,9] Its expression is upregulated by capsaicin and protons, allowing the induction of its expression on fibroblasts.[10]

Itch is aggravated by heat and acidosis through TRPV1. TRPV1 can be indirectly activated by many substances known as pruritogens through their specific receptors. TRPV1 is probably expressed on pruriceptors. Hence, TRPV1 can function as a 'central integrator' molecule in the itch pathway.[5]

The local application of capsaicin excites C nerve fibers and causes the release of substance P (responsible for side effects), then prolonged repeat applications deplete the sensory nerve endings in substance P and other neurotransmitters.[11] Chronic or high-dose use induces nerve ending degeneration that can eventually be permanent.

## 40.2 Clinical Data

### 40.2.1 Effects on Pruritus

Capsaicin is widely used as an antiprutitic agent in various diseases. Because of the central role of TRPV1, capsaicin can be used against pruritus of different mechanisms. Capsaicin prevents histamine-induced itch[12] and can be effective when itch is not induced by histamine.

Capsaicin can effectively interrupt the vicious itch circle in 70% of the patients with nostalgia paresthetica,[13] 12/15 patients with brachioradial pruritus,[14] aquagenic pruritus,[15] psoriasis,[16] pruritus ani,[17] prurigo nodularis[18] or hydroxyethyl-starch-induced pruritus.[19] Its effects are

L. Misery and S. Ständer (eds.), *Pruritus*,
DOI 10.1007/978-1-84882-322-8_40, © Springer-Verlag London Limited 2010

disappointing in uremic pruritus,[20] aquadynia,[21] and atopic dermatitis.[22]

### 40.2.2 Side Effects

The nerve desensitization is preceded by some adverse events which are secondary to the neurogenic inflammation induced by neuropeptide release: pain, burning, heat hyperalgesia, and erythema. Many patients discontinue treatment because of these side effects, which are present only for 1 week. These effects can be prevented by pre-treatment with topical anesthesic EMLA 1 h before application of capsaicin.[23]

### 40.2.3 Practical Use

Consequently, it is necessary to inform patients on the side effects and to advise them to use EMLA or to be confident about the spontaneous disappearance of these side effects. The usual concentrations of capsaicin are 0.025% and 0.075%. The number of applications varies from 2 to 5. The treatment has to be performed for 4 weeks or more. Pharmaceutic preparations need to be preserved at 4°C.

### 40.3 Other Vanilloids

Considering that capsaicin can be badly tolerated, a therapeutic challenge is to find a TRPV1 agonist which cause only minor receptor excitation but still possess a significant desensitization power.[5] Nowadays, the most promising product might be resiniferatoxin (RTX), a vanilloid extracted from the cactus-lie plant, Euphorbia resinifera.[24] At present, RTX is undergoing clinical trials. RTX is, however, expensive to isolate from natural sources, difficult to synthesize and cannot be given orally. Therefore, the synthesis of simplified and orally active vanilloids is an ongoing objective. Unsaturated 1,4-dialdehydes and triprenyl phenols might provide new clues for vanilloid drug development. But we lack clinical trials. Only one vanilloid has shown some antipruritic effects in mice.[25]

### References

1. Paul C, Chosidow O, Francès C. La capsaïcine en dermatologie. *Ann Dermatol Venereol*. 1993;120:563–570.
2. Norton SA. Useful plants of dermatology. V. Capsicum and capsaicin. *J Am Acad Dermatol*. 1998;39:626–628.
3. Boulais N, Misery L. The epidermis: a sensory tissue. *Eur J Dermatol*. 2008;18:119–127.
4. Christensen AP, Corey DP. TRP channels in mechansosensation: direct or indirect activation? *Nat Rev Neurosci*. 2007;8: 510–521.
5. Biro T, Toth BI, Marincsak R, Dobrosi N, Geczy T, Paus R. TRP channels as novel players in the pathogenesis and therapy of itch. *Biochem Biophys Acta*. 2007;1772: 1004–1021.
6. Caterina MJ, Schumacher MA, Tominaga M, Rosen TA, Levine JD, Julius D. The capsaicin receptor: a heat-activated ion channel in the pain pathway. *Nature*. 1997;389: 816–824.
7. Lumpkin EA, Caterina MJ. Mechanisms of sensory transduction in the skin. *Nature*. 2007;445:858–865.
8. Stander S, Moorman C, Schumacher M, et al. Expression of vanilloid receptor subtype 1 in cutaneous sensory nerve fibers, mast cells and epithelial cells of appendage structures. *Exp Dermatol*. 2004;13:129–139.
9. Bodo E, Kovacs I, Telek A, et al. Vanilloid receptor-1 (VR1) is widely expressed on various epithelial and mesnchymal cell types of human skin. *J Invest Dermatol*. 2004;123:4 10–413.
10. Kim SJ, Lee SA, Yun SJ, et al. Expression of vanilloid receptor 1 in cultured fibroblast. *Exp Dermatol*. 2006;15: 362–367.
11. Markovits E, Gilhar A. Capsaicin – an effective topical treatment in pain. *Int J Dermatol*. 1997;36:401–404.
12. Weisshaar E, Heyer G, Forster C, Handwerker HO. Effect of topical capsaicin on the cutaneous reactions and itching to histamine in atopic eczema compared to healthy skin. *Arch Dermatol Res*. 1998;290:306–311.
13. Wallengren J, Klinker M. Successful treatment of nostalgia paresthetica with topical capsaicin: vehicle-controlled, double-bind, crossover study. *J Am Acad Dermatol*. 1995;32: 287–289.
14. Texeira F, Miranda-Vega A, Hijyo-Tomoka T, Dominguez-Soto L. Solar-brachioradial pruritus – response to capsaicin cream. *J Am Acad Dermatol*. 1995;32:594–595.
15. Lotti T, Teofoli P, Tsampau D. Treatment of aquagenic pruritus with topical capsaicin cream. *J Am Acad Dermatol*. 1994;30: 232–235.
16. Kurkcuoglu N, Alaybeyi F. Topical capsaicin for psoriasis. *Br j Dermatol*. 1990;123:549–550.
17. Lysy J, Sistiery-Ittah M, Israelit Y, et al. Topical capsaicin - a novel and effective treatment for idiopathic intractable pruritus ani: a randomised, placebo controlled, crossover study. *Gut*. 2003;52:1323–1326.
18. Ständer S, Luger T, Metze D. Treatment of prurigo nodularis with topical capsaicin. *J Am Acad Dermatol*. 2001;44: 471–478.
19. Szeimies RM, Stolz W, Wlotzke U, Korting HC, Landthaler M. Successful treatment of hydroxyethyl-starch-induced

pruritus with topical capsaicin. *Br J Dermatol.* 1994;131: 380–382.

20. Breneman DL, Cardone S, Blusack RF, Lather RM, Searle EA, Pollack VE. Topical capsaicin for treatment of hemodialysis-related pruritus. *J Am Acad Dermatol.* 1992; 26:91–94.

21. Misery L, Meyronet D, Pichon M, Brutin JL, Pestre P, Cambazard F. Aquadynie: rôle du VIP? *Ann Dermatol Venereol.* 2003;130:195–198.

22. Marsella R, Nicklin CF, Melloy C. The effects of capsaicin topical therapy in dogs with atopic dermatitis: a randomized, double-blinded, placebo-controlled, cross-over clinical trial. *Vet Dermatol.* 2002;13:131–139.

23. Yosipovitch G, Maibach HI, Rowbotham MC. Effect of EMLA pre-treatment on capsaicin-induced burning and hyperalgesia. *Acta Derm Venereol.* 1999;79:118–121.

24. Sterner O, Szallasi A. Novel natural vanilloid receptor agonists: new therapeutic targets for drug development. *Trends Pharmacol Sci.* 1999;20:459–465.

25. Kim DH, Ahn BO, Kim SH, Kim WB. Antipruritic effect of DA-5018, a capsaicin derivative, in mice. *Arch Pharm Res.* 1999;22:549–553.

# Chapter 41
# Topical Immunomodulators

Laurent Misery

Topical immunomodulators (steroids or calcineurin inhibitors) are known for their efficacy on numerous inflammatory skin diseases. This effect is due to their immunosuppressive and anti-inflammatory properties, allowing amelioration of numerous skin diseases. A specific effect of calcineurin inhibitors (ciclosporin, tacrolimus, and pimecrolimus) on pruritus also exists.

## 41.1 Anti-Pruritic Effect of Calcineurin Inhibitors

Among calcineurin inhibitors, only tacrolimus and pimecrolimus are available in topical forms. They allow a more rapid improvement in the treatment of pruritus than steroids[2,3] and they can treat the pruritus of noninflammatory pruritic diseases.[1] Unfortunately, there are very few reports about nonatopic dermatoses. An extensive study was made of 20 patients with prurigo nodularis, gentioanal pruritus, or generalized pruritus of unknown origin.[1] Anecdoctic dramatic improvements of pruritus were also reported in psoriasis, rosacea,[4] chronic irritative hand dermatitis,[5] graft-versus-host disease,[6] lichen sclerosus,[7] lichen planus,[8] epidemolysis bullosa,[8] uremic pruritus, primary biliary cirrhosis,[9] etc. In uremic pruritus, results are controversial; one prospective study being in favor of an interesting effect[10] and the other not so.[11]

## 41.2 Other Neural Effects of Calcineurin Inhibitors

Tacrolimus and pimecrolimus are safe treatments of atopic dermatitis[12] and probably many pruritic disorders. Nonetheless, there are obviously adverse events. Among them, burning sensations and pruritus in the first days of application are common.[12] These sensations are transient, lasting 15–20 min. They are often associated with a feeling of warmth. They occur in 15–60% of the patients and usually disappear after one week. They are more frequent in patients with severe atopic dermatitis.

Other side effects, which are rarer (6–7%), are associated with alcohol drinking: erythema at application sites[13] or facial flushing.[14]

## 41.3 Understanding: a Capsaicin-Like Mechanism

Burning sensations, or alcohol-associated erythema, followed by a dramatic improvement of pruritus evokes an initial release of neuropeptides (mainly substance P followed by an inhibition of this release). Such effects are very well known with capsaicin.[15,16]

This has been confirmed by some recent studies. Tacrolimus activates capsaicin- and bradykinin-sensitive dorsal root ganglia (DRG) neurons and cutaneous C-fibers.[17] Morphological and then biochemical studies have shown a neuropeptide (substance P and calcitonin-gene related peptide (CGRP)) release and mast cell degranulation in the skin of mice after application of tacrolimus or pimecrolimus.[18] It may be speculated that calcineurin inhibitors bind to transient receptor protein-vanilloid (TRPV1) or other receptors or stimulate intracellular signaling pathway, such as macrophilins. A study in a coculture of neurons and keratinocytes has shown that tacrolimus was able to initially induce substance P release, which is followed by a Ca-dependant TRPV1 desensitization after repeated applications.[19]

L. Misery and S. Ständer (eds.), *Pruritus*,
DOI 10.1007/978-1-84882-322-8_41, © Springer-Verlag London Limited 2010

# References

1. Stander S, Schürmeyer-Horst F, Luger TA, Weisshaar E. Treatment of pruritic diseases with topical calcineurin inhibitors. *Ther Clin Risk Manag*. 2006;2:213–218.
2. Meurer M, Fölster-Horst R, Wozel G, et al. Pimecrolimus cream in the long-term management of atopic dermatitis in adults: a six-month study. *Dermatology*. 2002;205: 271–277.
3. Reitamo S, Van Leent EJ, Ho V, et al. Efficacy and safety of tacrolimus ointment compared with that of hydrocortisone acetate ointment in children with atopic dermatitis. *J Allergy Clin Immunol*. 2002;109:539–546.
4. Goldman D. Tacrolimus ointment for the treatment of steroid-induced rosacea: a preliminary report. *J Am Acad Dermatol*. 2001;44:995–998.
5. Cherill R, Tofte S, MacNaul R, et al. SDZ ASM 981 1% cream is effective in the treatment of chronic irritant hand dermatitis. *J Eur Acad Dermatol Venereol*. 2000;14 (suppl 1):128.
6. Choi CJ, Nghiem P. Tacrolimus ointment in the treatment of chronic cutaneous graft-versus-host disease: a case series of 18 patients. *Arch Dematol*. 2001;137:1202–1206.
7. Böhm M, Friedling U, Luger TA, et al. Successful treatment of anogenital lichen sclerosus with topical tacrolimus. *Arch Dermatol*. 2003;139:922–924.
8. Banky JP, Sheridan AT. Storer EL, et al. Successful treatment of epidermolysis bullosa pruriginosa with topical tacrolimus. *Arch Dermatol*. 2004;140:794–796.
9. Aguilar-Bernier M, Bassas-Vila J, Sanz-Munoz S, et al. Successful treatment of pruritus with topical tacrolimus in a patient with primary biliray cirrhosis. *Br J Dermatol*. 2005;152:808–809.
10. Kuypers DR, Claes K, Evenpoel P, et al. A prospective proof of concept study of the efficacy of tacrolimus ointment on uraemic pruritus (UP) in patients on chronic dialysis therapy. *Nephrol Dial Transplant*. 2004;19:1895–1901.
11. Duque MI, Yosipovitch G, Fleischer AB, et al. Lack of efficacy of tacrolimus ointment 0.1% for treatment of hemodialysis-related pruritus: a randomized double-blinded, vehicle-controlled study. *J Am Acad Dermatol*. 2005;52: 519–521.
12. Rustin MHA. The safety of tacrolimus ointment for the treatment of atopic dermatitis: a review. *Br J Dermatol*. 2007;157: 861–873.
13. Calza AM, Lübbe J. Tacrolimus ointment-associated alcohol intolerance in infants receiving ethanol-containing medication. *Br J Dermatol*. 2005;152:569.
14. Milingou M, Antille C, Sorg O, Saurat JH, Lübbe J. Alcohol intolerance and facial flushing in patients treated with topical tacrolimus. *Arch Dermatol*. 2004;140:1542–1544.
15. Trevisani M, Smart D, Gunthorpe MJ, et al. Ethanol elicits and potentiates nociceptor response via the vanilloid-receptor 1. *Nat Neurosci*. 2002;5:546–551.
16. Stander S, Luger TA. Antipruritic effects of pimecrolimus and tacrolimus. *Hautartzt*. 2003;54:413–417.
17. Senba E, Katanosaka K, Yajima H, et al. The immunosuppressant FK506 activates capsaicin- and bradykinin-sensitive DRG neurons and cutaneous C-fibers. *Neurosci Res*. 2004; 50:257–262.
18. Stander S, Stander H, Seelinger S, Luger TA, Steinhoff M. Topical tacrolimus and pimecrolimus transiently induce neuropeptide release and mast cell degranulation in murine skin. *Br J Dermatol*. 2007;156:1020–1026.
19. Pereira U, Boulais N, Dorange G, Misery L. Impact of tacrolimus on cutaneous neurogenic inflammation (CNI). *J Invest Dermatol*. 2480;2007:127.

# Chapter 42
# Cannabinoid-Receptor Agonists

Sonja Ständer

## 42.1 Cannabinoid-Receptor Agonists

Endogenous and synthetic cannabinoids are known for their psychotic and analgesic potency upon systemic administration. Topical cannabinoid agonists are a new modality in chronic pruritus since a couple of years. Both cannabinoid receptors CB1 and CB2 were found to be expressed on cutaneous sensory nerve fibres, mast cells, and keratinocytes. The physiological role of cutaneous cannabinoids and their receptors is still under investigation, however, recent data suggest that they are involved in inflammation of especially allergic contact dermatitis, keratinocyte proliferation and are neurosensory as well (see Chapter 2 of Part I). It was demonstrated that during inflammation, CB1 expression in primary afferent neurons and transport to peripheral axons is increased and contributes thereby to enhanced antihyperalgesic efficacy of locally administered CB1 agonist.[1] In addition, injections of the CB2 agonist N-Palmitoylethanolamin (PEA) may inhibit experimental NGF-induced thermal hyperalgesia.[2] Experimentally induced pain, itch, and erythema could be reduced by application of a topical cannabinoid agonist.[3,4]

In Europe and USA, the cannabinoid agonist N-PEA is available as a cream and lotion. In clinical trials and case series, this preparation proved to have antipruritic effects in atopic dermatitis, renal pruritus, prurigo, and pruritus of unknown origin.[5–7] In a multinational clinical prospective cohort-study, 2,456 patients with subacute and chronic atopic deramtitis including 923 children up to age of 12 received the cream twice daily. A reduction of erythema, scaling, and scratch lesions was observed. Pruritus showed reduction of 60% (mean reduction of pruritus intensity of VAS 4.89 points to 1.97 points.)[7] Thirty eight percent patients with renal pruritus reported a relief of pruritus within three weeks of therapy with this CB2 agonist.[5] Another study demonstrated relief of pruritus in 64% of patients with prurigo, lichen simplex, and pruritus of unknown origin.[6] Mean pruritus reduction was 86.4%. In addition, unpublished observations exist for application of this cream in aquagenic and brachioradial pruritus as well as burning pain in postzosteric neuralgias. These preliminary data show that topically applied cannabinoid agonists may be an interesting option of antipruritic therapy in the future.

## References

1. Amaya F, Shimosato G, Kawasaki Y, et al. Induction of CB1 cannabinoid receptor by inflammation in primary afferent neurons facilitates antihyperalgesic effect of peripheral CB1 agonist. *Pain*. 2006;124:175–183.
2. Farquhar-Smith WP, Rice AS. A novel neuroimmune mechanism in cannabinoid-mediated attenuation of nerve growth factor-induced hyperalgesia. *Anesthesiology*. 2003;99:1391–1401.
3. Rukwied R, Watkinson A, McGlone F, Dvorak M. Cannabinoid agonists attenuate capsaicin-induced responses in human skin. *Pain*. 2003;102:283–288.
4. Dvorak M, Watkinson A, McGlone F, Rukwied R. Histamine induced responses are attenuated by a cannabinoid receptor agonist in human skin. *Inflamm Res* 2003;52:238–245.
5. Szepietowski JC, Szepietowski T. Reich A. Efficacy and tolerance of the cream containing structured physiological lipids with endocannabinoids in the treatment of uremic pruritus: a preliminary study. *Acta Dermatovenerol Croat*. 2005; 13:97–103.
6. Ständer S, Reinhardt HW, Luger TA. Topische Cannabinoid-Agonisten: Eine effektive, neue Möglichkeit zur Behandlung von chronischem Pruritus. *Hautarzt* 2006;57:801–807.
7. Eberlein B, Eicke C, Reinhardt HW, Ring J. Adjuvant treatment of atopic eczema: assessment of an emollient containing N-palmitoylethanolamine (ATOPA study). *JEADV*. 2008; 22:73–82.

L. Misery and S. Ständer (eds.), *Pruritus*,
DOI 10.1007/978-1-84882-322-8_42, © Springer-Verlag London Limited 2010

# Chapter 43
# Other Topical Treatments

Laurent Misery

Numerous topical treatments have been proposed in the treatment of pruritus. The preceding chapters were dedicated to main topical treatments. Etiological treatments are often effective against pruritus. In this chapter, we would like to name some of the specific topical treatments of itch (alphabetic order).

## 43.1 Anesthetics

Local anesthetics are sometimes used against itch: eutectic mixture of local anesthetics (EMLA). EMLA has been successfully used against postburn pruritus in children[4] and experimental pruritus induced by papain or cowhage[9] but not histamine-induced pruritus.[13] Polidocanol has been successfully used against itch in uremic pruritus, atopic dermatitis, and psoriasis.[12]

## 43.2 Antihistamines

Topical antihistamines are widely used but their efficacy is low and many cases of allergy were registered.

## 43.3 Calamine

Calamine is a very old treatment for pruritus. This natural product is zinc carbonate with small quantity of iron oxide. A randomized double-blind study in 69 patients is in favor of the efficacy of a cream containing calamine and zinc oxide for the treatment of pruritus ani.[7]

## 43.4 Camphor

Camphor might be useful in the treatment of pruritus because this naturally occurring product is an agonist of TRPV3 and other transient receptor protein (TRP) channels.[8] Unfortunately, its allergic and irritant properties limit its use.

## 43.5 Doxepin

A cream containing 5% of doxepin (Zonalon®, Doxederm®), an antagonist of histamine and acetylcholine, is effective in reducing pruritus in patients with atopic dermatitis.[3] Some cases of contact eczema were reported.

## 43.6 Icilin

Like menthol, icilin is an agonist of TRPM8 and TRPA1 receptors (see Chapter 39). It induces a cold sensation and might be used against itch.

## 43.7 Methylene Blue

Intradermal injections of methylene blue have been successfully used for the treatment of pruritus ani in 24/30 patients[5] and in some other studies. A neurotoxic effect is suggested.

L. Misery and S. Ständer (eds.), *Pruritus*,
DOI 10.1007/978-1-84882-322-8_43, © Springer-Verlag London Limited 2010

## 43.8 Phenol

Phenol is used in numerous creams against pruritus but it is usually associated with other compounds.

## 43.9 Prostaglandin D2 Agonists

TS-022 is a prostanoid DP(1) receptor agonist. Clinical trials on mice showed suppression of scratching and improvement of the skin inflammation in the NC/Nga (NC) mouse, a model of atopic dermatitis. The potent anti-pruritic activity of TS-022 might be attributable to the decrease of endogenous prostaglandin D(2) production and increase of prostanoid DP(1) receptor expression in atopic dermatitis.[10]

## 43.10 Raffinose

Raffinose is an oligosaccharide with effects on cell degranulation. Interesting results were observed in pruritus following burns[1,6] and atopic dermatitis.

## 43.11 Salicylic Acid and Aspirin

A randomized double-blind study showed a significant reduction of pruritus in patients with neurodermatitis after applications of aspirin solution.[14] It does not seem to be related to nonsteroidal anti-inflammatory properties.

Salicylic acid may be effective against scalp pruritus[2] and in pruritus in patients with psoriasis.

Salicylic compounds diethylamine salicylate and salicylamide were effective on serotonin-induced scratching in rats, through the slow release of acetylsalicylic acid.[11]

## 43.12 Strontium Nitrate

Strontium nitrate could reduce sensory irritation and inflammation when applied topically. A 20% strontium nitrate decreased the magnitude of histamine-induced itch in a pilot study.[15]

## References

1. Campech M, Gavroy JP, Ster F, et al. Etude de l'effet antiprurigineux du raffinose sur le tégument récemment épidermisé du grand brulé. *Brûlures.* 2002;11:219–222.
2. Draelos Z. An evaluation of topical 3% salicylic acid and 1% hydrocortisone in the maintenance of scalp pruritus. *J Cosmet Dermatol.* 2005;4:193–197.
3. Drake LA, Fallon JD, Sober A. Relief of pruritus in patients with atopic dermatitis after treatment with topical doxepin cream. *J Am Acad Dermatol.* 1994;31:613–616.
4. Kopecky E, Jacobson S, Bch M, et al. Safety and pharmacokinetics of EMLA in the treatment of postburn pruritus in pediatric patients: a pilot study. *J Burn Care Rehabil.* 2001; 22:235–242.
5. Mentes B, Akin M, Leventoglu S, Gultekin F, Oguz M. Intradermal methylene blue injection for the treatment of intractable idiopathic pruritus ani: results of 30 cases. *Tech Coloproctol.* 2004;8:11–14.
6. Misery L, Liège P, Cambazard F. Evaluation de l'efficacité et de la tolérance d'une crème contenant du raffinose au cours de la dermatite atopique. *Nouv Dermatol.* 2005;24: 339–341.
7. Misery L, Mazharian R, Teurquety L, et al. Efficacité du Gel de Calamine dans le prurit anal. *Nouv Dermatol.* 2004;23:7–9.
8. Moqrich A, Hwang SW, Earley TJ, et al. Impaired thermosensation in mice lacking TRPV3, a heat and camphor sensor in the skin. *Science (New York, NY).* 2005;307:1468–1472.
9. Shuttleworth D, Hill S, Marks R, Connelly D. Relief of experimentally induced pruritus with a novel eutectic mixture of local anaesthetic agents. *Br J Dermatol.* 1988;119: 535–540.
10. Sugimoto M, Arai I, Futaki N, et al. The anti-pruritic efficacy of TS-022, a prostanoid DP1 receptor agonist, is dependent on the endogenous prostaglandin D2 level in the skin of NC/Nga mice. *Eur J Pharmacol.* 2007;564:196–203.
11. Thomsen JS, Simonsen L, Benfeldt E, Jensen SB, Serup J. The effect of topically applied salicylic compounds on serotonin-induced scratching behavior in hairless rats. *Exp Dermatol.* 2002;11:370–375.
12. Twycross R, Greaves MW, Handwerker H, et al. Itch: scratching more than the surface. *Q J Med.* 2003;96:7–26.
13. Weisshaar E, Forster C, Dotzer M, Heyer G. Experimentally induced pruritus and cutaneous reactions with topical antihistamine and local analgesics in atopic eczema. *Skin Pharmacol.* 1997;10:183–190.
14. Yosipovitch G, Sugeng MW, Chan H, Goon A, Ngim S, Goh CL. The effect of topically applied aspirin on localized circumscribed neurodermatitis. *J Am Acad Dermatol.* 2001;45: 910–913.
15. Zhai H, Hannon W, Hahn GS, Harper RA, Pelosi A, Maibach H. Strontium nitrate decreased histamine-induced itch magnitude and duration in man. *Dermatology (Basel, Switzerland).* 2000;200:244–246.

# Section 3
# Systemical

# Chapter 44
# Antihistamines

Caroline Gaudy-Marqueste

## 44.1 Introduction

Histamine, first characterized nearly a century ago, is a key mediator of numerous biologic reactions including "allergic" ones, some of which are involved in usual dermatosis pathophysiology. There are conceptually three ways to counteract the biological effects of histamine: (1) to decrease its synthesis, (2) to inhibit its release and (3) to prevent its fixation at the surface of the receptors. Antihistamines act via his third way and two main families of drugs actually exist: H1-antihistamines counteracting effects mediated through H1-receptors and H2-antihistamine counteracting effects mediated through H2 histamine receptors.

Antihistamines, and especially the H1 ones, are widely used in dermatological practice mainly for itching dermatosis even if histamine is not always involved in their pathophysiology.

In this chapter, we will briefly review the physiological and pharmacological properties of antihistamines and data supporting their interest in itchy dermatosis treatment.

## 44.2 Physiopathological and Pharmacologic Properties of Histamine and Its Receptors

### 44.2.1 Histamine

Histamine is a biogenic amine formed by decarboxylation of L-Histidine. It is synthesized and stored within cytoplasmic secretory granules of human mast cells, basophils, gastric enterochromaffin cells, and histaminergic neurons and released by degranulation following various stimuli that may or may not involve the IgE. IgE mediated degranulation can be triggered by the cross-linking of two surface IgE molecules bound to high affinity receptors (FCεRIαβγ) even by specific allergens (type I hypersensibility) or autoantibodies. Non IgE mediated stimuli include cytokines, physical factors (nettle contact), amphipathic molecules including opioids such as codeine and morphine, anaphylotoxins, neuropeptides (P substance), antibiotics (vancomycin or quinolones), and viral or bacterial antigens. Histamine release is followed by its binding to specific receptors located at the surface of the target cells. Four types of receptors (H1, H2, H3, and H4) are individualized to date. Most of the effects of Histamine in allergic diseases are mediated by the H1 receptors. H1 and H2 vascular receptors are both involved in the occurrence of hypotension, tachycardia, flushing, and headache.[1] Stimulation of H1 and H3 receptors may result in cutaneous itch and nasal congestion.[2,3] Most recently H4 receptor antagonism was shown to reduce pruritus in mice through potential action on peripheral neurons.[4] Besides its role in early allergic response to antigen, Histamine also stimulates cytokines production and the expression of cell-adhesion molecules and class II antigens, thus contributing to the late allergic response.[5] Through its four types of receptors, Histamine also modulates immune responses.

### 44.2.2 Histamine Receptors

All the four types of Histamine Receptors belong to the G-protein-coupled receptors family and display a constitutive activity (spontaneous activity in the absence

L. Misery and S. Ständer (eds.), *Pruritus*,
DOI 10.1007/978-1-84882-322-8_44, © Springer-Verlag London Limited 2010

of histamine).[6] They differ in their cellular expression, signal transduction effectors, and function.

### 44.2.2.1 H1-Receptors

H1-receptors, widely expressed in the human body, mediate most of the effects of Histamine. Activation of the H1-receptor-coupled Gq/11 stimulates the inositol phospholipide signaling pathways resulting in the formation of inositol-1,4,5-triphosphate (InsP3) and diacylglycerol (DAG) leading to C protein kinase activation and increase in intracellular calcium.[7] H1-receptor can also activate other signaling pathways including phospholipase, D and A2,[7] NOS[8] and the transcription factor NF-kB.[9] H1-receptor stimulation leads to vasodilatation, increase in vascular permeability, smooth contraction of muscle, mucus secretion and viscosity, activation of the sensory nerve endings contributing to pruritus, decreased conduction time of the atrio-ventricular node, and coronary vasospasm. H1-receptors also support histamine participation in allergic inflammation and immune modulation via macrophages and eosinophils activation, increased expression of adhesion molecules such as intercellular adhesion molecule-1 (ICAM-1), vascular cell adhesion molecule-1 (VCAM-1) and P-selectin, increased antigen-presenting cell capacity, costimulatory activity on B-cells, decrease of humoral immunity and IgE production, induction of cellular immunity (Th1), increased IFNγ autoimmunity, and polarization of human dendritic cells into Th2 cell-promoting effectors dendritic cells.[10–13]

### 44.2.2.2 H2-Receptors

H2-receptors are, like H1-receptors, widely expressed, mainly at the surface of lymphocytes and basophiles, coronary and pulmonary vessels, cardiac tissue and gastric parietal cells. They are coupled to Gs proteins and mediate an intracellular response most characterized by elevations in intracellular levels of cyclic-AMP following adenylate cyclase activation, protein kinase A activation and $Ca^{2+}$ flux modulation.[14] Together with H1-Receptors, H2-receptors stimulation lead to vasodilation and increase in vascular permeability. They also mediate effects on the cardiovascular system (positive cardiotropic and inotropic effect), gastrointestinal tractus (increase in gastric

acid and pepsin secretion) and respiratory system (airway relaxation, activation of mucus secretion). Histamine, via an action on H2-receptors can also inhibit some lymphocytes functions such as proliferative response to mitogens, antibody synthesis by antibody-secreting B cells, cell mediated cytolysis and lymphokines production[14] and recruitment of T CD4 helpers lymphocytes.[15] Stimulation of H2-receptors inhibits TNF alpha production, stimulates IL10 production,[16] and promotes the polarization of dendritic cells into Th2 cell-promoting effector dendritic cells.[13] Finally, H2-receptor stimulation can inhibit the chemotactic responsiveness of basophils and the histamine release from mast cells and basophils[14] leading to a decrease of histamine release.

### 44.2.2.3 H3-Receptor

H3-receptor was identified in the central and peripheral nervous systems as a presynaptic receptor controlling the release of histamine and other neurotransmitters. It is a $G_{i/o}$ protein coupled receptor whose stimulation inhibits adenylate cyclase leading to reduced production of cAMP and inhibition of $Ca^{2+}$ influx. Stimulation of the H3-receptor also leads to a decrease in acetylcholine, neurokinines, and catecholamines liberation, modulating the stimulating effect of the H1 receptors.[17] Finally, H3-receptors regulate histaminergic neurotransmission: their stimulation induces a decrease in histaminergic transmission leading to impairment of vigilance, cognitive and cochleo-vestibular functions.[18] It has been shown that like all the others Histamine receptors,[6] H3 receptors display high constitutive activity.[19]

### 44.2.2.4 H4-Receptors

H4-receptors were the latest to be identified. They are highly expressed on bone marrow and peripheral hematopoietic cells, neutrophils, eosinophils, and T cells and moderately expressed in spleen, thymus, lung, small intestine, colon, heart, and brain.[20, 21] Like H3-receptors, they are functionally coupled to protein $G_{i/o}$, and their activation inhibits forskolin-induced cAMP formation.[20] Histamine H4-receptor activation promotes the accumulation of inflammatory cells (mainly eosinophils and mast cells) at the sites of allergic inflammation.[10] It is also suggested that H4 receptors are involved together with the H2 receptors in the control of IL16 release from human lymphocytes. Most of the effects of their stimulation on target cells and tissues remain to be defined.

## 44.3 H1-Antihistamines

H1-antihistamines, discovered by Bovet and Staub in 1937, were initially developed to counteract physiological effects following fixation of histamine on H1-receptors. They have been considered for a long time as H1- blockers or H1-receptor antagonists until recent works showed that they were rather inverse agonists of these receptors. Indeed, it is now proven that, under basal conditions, the H1-receptor is present both at an active and an inactive state coexisting in a reversible equilibrium and that fixation of the H1-antihistamines stabilizes the inactive conformation of the receptor by shifting the equilibrium toward the inactive state leading not only to a blockage of Histamine fixation on the receptor but also to a decrease of the constitutive receptor activity.[22]

H1-antihistamines are nitrogenous bases containing an aliphatic side chain sharing the common core structure of a substituted ethylamine with histamine [23] allowing fixation of the molecule on the receptor. Two classes of H1-antihistamines are individualized: first generation H1 antihistamines and second generation ones. Differences between these groups mainly result from specificity or selectivity of histamine receptors and penetration into the central nervous system while no differences have been established regarding antiH1 activity. (Table 44.1)

### 44.3.1 First Generation H1 Antihistamines

First generation H1 antihistamines were the first developed and include six chemical groups: ethylenediamines, ethanolamines, alkylamines, phenotiazines, piperazines and piperidines. Their fixation on the H1-receptor is defined as competitive as they inhibit the binding of histamine on the receptor in a reversible and concentration-dependent way. Their fixation can thus be reversed by their dissociation from the receptor

or in the presence of high levels of histamine.[24] Most of these molecules also exhibit other pharmacological effects due to their lack of specificity for the histamine receptor and structural analogy with other amines. First generation H1-antihistamines bind also to serotoninergic, muscarinic and $\alpha$-adrenergic receptors explaining some of their usual side effects: weight gain relative to antiserotoninergic activity, atropinic side effects such as urine retention, intra ocular hypertension, eye dryness, and antinaupathic effect due to the anticholinergic properties. Due to the penetration into the central nervous system, H1 first class antihistamines induce side effects in the central nervous system and often drowsiness with potential impact on daily life activities including work and driving abilities. All first class H1-antihistamines undergo liver metabolism (P450 cytochrome) with the ultimate clearance of the active drug or metabolites via feces or urine. Drugs interactions with others medications known to interfere with P450 cytochrome may thus result in diminished efficacy or side effects. Short half-life of some of these molecules may require multiple daily dosages. Agonist effect can occur at the beginning of the treatment, with transitory aggravation of the symptoms.

### 44.3.2 Second Generation H1-Antihistamines

Second generation H1-antihistamines were designed at the beginning of the 1980s. The main differences between first and second generation H1-antihistamines depend on receptor binding-dissociation kinetic and central system penetration. Fixation of the drug on the H1-Receptor is defined as "noncompetitive,"[24] as the biding site is not the same as the histamine one. Binding on the receptor is thus more stable, slowly reversible, and cannot be easily suppressed by a new histamine afflux. Second generation H1-antihistamines are further more specific and selective for the peripheral H1-receptors, allowing for reduction of side effects mainly muscarinic ones. Lipophobicity of these molecules and involvement of P-glycoprotein efflux transporters for which they constituted substrates[25] reduces the blood-brain barrier penetration decreasing side effects, but second generation H1-antihistamines are not totally free of side effects in the central nervous

C. Gaudy-Marqueste

**Table 44.1** H-1 Antihistamines available on the European market

| Molecule | Formulation | Use in pregnancy | Lactation | Use in children | Population requiring precaution | Interactions |
|---|---|---|---|---|---|---|
| *First generation* | | | | | | |
| Hydroxyzine | tb/syrup/injection | Allowed 2 and 3 Trr | Inadvisable | tb > 6 years/syrup > 30 months | Elderly | Alcohol |
| Brompheniramine | tb/syrup | Allowed 2 and 3 Tr | Inadvisable | tb > 12 years/syrup > 2 months | Hepatic or renal dysfunction elderly | Alcohol |
| Cyproheptadine | tb | ci | Inadvisable | > 6 years | Hepatic or renal dysfunction sun (photosensitivity) | Alcohol |
| Promethazine | tb/syrup/injection | Allowed 2 and 3 Tr | Inadvisable | tb/ injection ci syrup > 1 year | Hepatic or renal dysfunction sun (photosensitivity), cardiac disease | Alcohol sultopride |
| Dexchlorpheniramine | tb/syrup/injection | allowed 1 and 2 Tr | inadvisable | tb > 6 years/syrup > 2 months injection > 30 months | Hepatic or renal dysfunction elderly | Alcohol |
| Mequitazine | tb/syrup | allowed 2 and 3 Tr | allowed | tb > 6 years/syrup: newborn | Hepatic or renal dysfunction elderly, epilepsia | Alcohol |
| Alimemazine | tb/syrup solution/ injection | Allowed 2 and 3 Tr | Inadvisable | tb > 6 years syrop/solution > 1 year injection ci | Hepatic or renal dysfunction sun (photosensitivity) | Alcohol sultopride |
| *Second generation* | | | | | | |
| Cetirizine | tb/syrup/injection | Allowed 2 and 3 Tr | Inadvisable | tb > 6 years/sol > 2 years | Hepatic or renal dysfunction | Alcohol |
| Ebastine | tb | ci | Inadvisable | >12 years | Hepatic or renal dysfunction | Alcohol |
| Mizolastine | tb | Allowed 2 and 3 Tr | Inadvisable | >12 years | Hepatic dysfunction | Imidazole antifungals macrolide antibiotics |
| Loraradine | tb/syrup | ci | Inadvisable | tb > 12 years/syrup > 2 years | Hepatic dysfunction | Imidazole antifungals macrolides antibiotics |
| Fexofenadine | tb/syrup | ci | inadvisable | tb > 6 years/syrup > 6 months | Renal dysfunction | |
| Desloratadine | tb/syrup | ci | Inadvisable | tb > 12 years/syrup > 2 years | Renal dysfunction | Erythromycine/ketoconazole anti-ulcer drugs |
| Levocetirizine | tb/syrup | ci | Inadvisable | tb/syrup > 6 years | Renal dysfunction | |

tb, tablets; sol, solution; ci, contra indicated; Tr, trimester.

system as occupancy of the central nervous system H1-receptors varies from 0% to 30%.[22]

The latest molecules developed mainly derive from older ones. For example, desloratadine and fexofenadine are metabolites of loratadine and terfenadine, and levocetirizine is an enantiomer of cetirizine. Some of the second generation H1-antihistamines (azelastine, ebastine, loratadine, mizolastine) undergo extensive metabolism involving the P450 cytochrome while other molecules (acrivastine, fexofenadine, cetirizine, levocetirizine, and desloratadine) are not metabolized as extensively through the P450 cytochrome system.[26] Fexofenadine and levocetirizine are not metabolized and are cleared unchanged in the urine and feces respectively. Long half life of many of the molecules allows for once-daily dosing. Hepatic impairment (cetirizine, ebastine, loratadine) and renal dysfunction (cetirizine, fexofenadine, loratadine, and acrivastine) may require dose adjustment.[27,28]

### 44.3.3 Antiallergic and Anti-Inflammatory Activities of Antihistamines

Many H1-antihistamines have been shown to display antiallergic activities including inhibition of the mediators' release (cetirizine, loratadine), reduction of eosinophils chemotaxis (cetirizine, levocetirizine, desloratadine, and loratadine), inhibition of cell adhesion molecules expression (cetirizine, loratadine, desloratadine, and fexofenadine[29] and down regulation of the H1-receptor activated nuclear factor-κB (cetirizine, azelastine).[9]

H1-antihistamines must be used carefully in young children, old people, pregnant women, and patients suffering from renal or hepatic impairment.[22] Concomitant medication with macrolides, imidazoles, and cytochrome P450 inductors, and alcohol consumption should be avoided when using molecules with liver metabolism involving P450 cytochrome. Grapefruit juice may also lead to increased concentrations of loratadine and terfenadine.[30] Congenital malformation risk following exposure to H1-antihistamines has been evaluated in several studies showing no increase in the teratogenic risk[31] even if some cases of oral clefs were reported with the first generation brompheniramine and diphenhydramine.[31] No malformative effects have

been reported with chlorpheniramine and dexchlorpheniramine in animals and never in humans. Thus these two drugs should be used preferentially during pregnancy. A few human data are available regarding second generation H1-antihistamines and most of them have to be prescribed carefully during the first trimester of the pregnancy. Hypospadias have been reported after fetal exposure to loratadine or desloratadine in one but not subsequent studies.[32] H1-antihistamine medication of lactating women has never been reported to cause serious adverse events in the nursing infant but a few cases of irritability and drowsiness have been reported with first generation molecules. Withdrawal manifestations have been reported in the newborn babies of women receiving supratherapeutic dosage of diphenhydramine (150 mg/j) and hydroxyzine.[31]

### 44.3.4 Adverse Effects of H1-Antihistamines

#### 44.3.4.1 Central Effects

First generation H1-antihistamine, known to cross the blood–brain barrier, can impair physical and intellectual capacities. Clinical symptoms may include drowsiness, dizziness, sedation, decrease in coordination, cognitive function, memory and psychomotor performance, and occasionally paradoxal stimulation with dystonia, dyskinesia, and agitation. This sedative effect can be of interest as it can allow for limiting the objective perception of the symptoms, mainly pruritus, and first generation H1-antihistamines are sometimes prescribed at sleeping time. Several studies have, however, shown that the sedative effect of the drug was maintained during the entire day following an evening dosage.[33] Data supporting the occurrence of a tolerance to adverse effects of first generation H1 antihistamines, in the CNS after a few days are conflicting.[33] Second generation H1-antihistamines are considered as nonsedative molecules at clinically recommended dosage but some of them such as loratadine, cetirizine, ebastine, and mizolastine can be sedative when given at a higher dosage.[33] No central side effect have been reported to date with fexofenadine, even at a supra therapeutic dosage.[34] All H1-antihistamines except rupatadine,[35] fexofenadine, desloratadine[36] and levocetirizine,[37] may impair driving performance. Use of diphenhydramine have been shown to impair driving ability as much as alcohol even if users do not feel drowsy[38] and first generation H1-antihistamines have been implicated in the loss of productivity by workers, injuries, and deaths in aviation and traffic accidents.[39] Coadministration of alcohol or benzodiazepines with first generation H1-antihistamines (clemastine, chlorpheniramine, cyproheptadine, diphenydramine) can increase side effects of the CNS. Such effects were not reported to date with the second generation molecules.[33] In children, first generation H1-antihistamines are known to impair cognitive functions and to reduce school performance.[40] Such effects are not observed with second generation molecules and school performance amelioration was even reported in children suffering from allergic rhinitis and treated with loratadine.[41] The lack of impact on psychomotor development and cognitive function after 18 months of daily dose of cetirizine and levocetirizine was confirmed in atopic children aged 12–24 months.[41,42]

### 44.3.4.2 Cardiac Effects

Cardiac side effects can occur with both first and second generation H1-antihistamines. They are mainly explained by increased plasma levels of H1-antihistamines following abnormal metabolism (liver metabolism impairment following concomitant medication with cytochrome P450 inhibitors such as ketoconazole, itraconazole and macrolides antibiotics, impaired liver function due to cirrhosis or ethanol abuse). Pre-existing cardiac dysfunctions and electrolyte imbalance may also enhance cardiac arrhythmias as well as coadministration of other drugs known to prolong the interval between the onset of the Q wave and the end of the T wave in the electrocardiogram (QT-interval) such as tricyclic antidepressant and antipsychotic drugs. Cardiac arrhythmias with torsades de pointe, ventricular tachycardia, atrio-ventricular blockage, and even cardiac arrest have been reported with 2 second-generation H1-antihistamines: terfenadine and astemizole, which were later withdrawn from the market. Cardiac side effects of antihistamines are not relative to the antihistaminic activity but to the blockage of the delayed potassium rectifier current in the myocardium leading to the prolongation of the QT interval.[43] Other second generation molecules (loratadine, desloratadine, ebastine, and mizolastine) can also inhibit potassic channels

in vitro but not in vivo. Cetirizine, levocetirizine and fexofenadine have no effect on potassic channels. No QT prolongation was reported with loratadine, mizolastine, cetirizine, fexofenadine, and azelastine even at a supratherapeutic dosage.[43] However prolongation of the QT interval can occur with ebastine or mizolastine at high dosage or following association with ketoconazole.[43] Association with ketoconazole or macrolides of loratadine or fexofenadine did not prolong the QT interval.[43] Second generation H1-antihistamines such as cetirizine, desloratadine, fexofenadine, and loratadine appear to be relatively free of cardiac toxic effects.

### 44.3.4.3 Digestive Side Effects

Digestive side effects have only been reported with first generations drugs (pyrilamine, antazoline, tripelennamine) that induced nausea, diarrhea, anorexia, and epigastralgia. No gastrointestinal disturbance has been reported to date with second generation molecules.

### 44.3.4.4 Anticholinergic Effects

Anticholinergic effects including mouth, eye and nose dryness, blurred vision, and urinary retention can be provoked by first generation H1-antihistamine. Thus, use of first generation molecules is contraindicated in patients suffering from glaucoma or prostatic hypertrophy.

### 44.3.4.5 Cutaneous Eruptions

Cutaneous eruptions have been reported with both first and second generation H1-anti-histamines. This includes eczematiform eruption following diphenhydramine,[44] urticaria following cetirizine and hydroxyzine[45] and fixed drug eruption following hydroxyzine, loratadine, diphenhydramine, and cetirizine.[46–48]

## 44.4 Antihistamines for Pruritus Treatment

Prescription of H1-antihistamines is common in dermatological practice. If urticaria remains the first indication for H1-antihistamines prescription, these drugs are also widely prescribed for other pruriginous dermatosis, even when they are not histamine mediated, sometimes for their soporific properties. If the use of H1-antihistamines in urticaria is supported by numerous publications, a few studies are available in the literature when looking at other indications.

## 44.4.1 Urticaria

Due to the usual, highly itchy character of urticaria and the known implication of histamine on its pathophysiology, H1-antihistamines are widely used in the treatment of both its acute and chronic forms. Several studies have demonstrated their efficiency in decreasing pruritus and reducing the number, size, and duration of urticarian lesions. Antihistamines have been proven as efficient in the treatment of acute urticaria together with the eviction of the causative agent. Superiority of some of the second generation H1-antihistamines (loratadine, cetirizine) against chlorpheniramine have been reported,[49,50] while no difference was evidenced against first generation molecules (hydroxyzine, diphenhydramine).[51,52] Two studies assessing histamine-induced wheal-and-flare inhibition show a superiority of levocetirizine against desloratadine,[53] fexofenadine, loratadine, and mizolastine[54] but the clinical correlation remains unknown. H2-antihistamines are not efficient by themselves but can be combined with H1-antihistamines to improve early regression of the lesions.[55–58]

H1-antihistamines are the treatment of choice for chronic urticaria as several studies have demonstrated their efficacy on pruritus, œdema, and wheals decrease. Superiority against placebo has been proven for hydroxyzine,[59] loratadine,[59] mizolastine,[60] cetirizine,[61] ketotifen,[62] ebastine,[63] fexofenadine,[64] desloratadine,[65] levocetirizine,[66] and rupatadine.[67] Second generation molecules were found globally equivalent to first generation ones; however, hydroxyzine was considered more efficient than diphenhydramine,[68] loratadine than cetirizine[69] and cetirizine than fexofenadine[70] regarding efficacy and rapidity of action. Coadministration of the H1-antihistamines hydroxyzine and chlorpheniramine with the H2-antihistamine cimetidine have been found a little bit more efficient than H1-antihistamines alone[71,72] in the decrease of pruritus and wheals, but there is no sufficient data to date to support such an association in the usual practice. Treatment of physical urticarias remains a challenge and few H1-antihistamines are

efficient. Among the few studies available, cetirizine and acrivastine have been found more efficient than a placebo[73,74] and hydroxyzine more efficient than chlorpheniramine in the treatment of dermographism.[75] Coadministration of H1 and H2-antihistamines especially hydroxyzine and cimetidine was also efficient[76] as well as the association of chlorpheniramine and cimetidine was found to be more efficient than chlorpheniramine administrated alone.[77] Cetirizine has been reported as most effective as a placebo for delayed pressure urticaria,[78] solar urticaria,[79] and cholinergic urticaria.[80] Hydroxyzine has been proposed for aquagenic urticaria[81] and cholinergic urticaria.[82] Ebastine for acquired cold urticaria[83] Efficacy of the association H1-antihistamine/antileucotrien was reported in delayed pressure urticaria[84,85] and cold urticaria[86] as well as those of the association of H1 and H2-antihistamines in cold[87] and local heat urticaria.[88]

Health related quality of life (HRQoL) assessment has become a current issue when evaluating the efficacy of treatment on dermatological diseases. Chronic urticaria is known to severely impact the quality of life of patients due to usual chronicity and unpredictability of the disease. Validity of the usual dermatologic specific questionnaires (DLQI and VQ-Derm)[89] and chronic urticaria specific questionnaire (CU-QoL)[90] have been established in such population. Only a few studies have, however, considered this issue to date and HRQoL amelioration following H1-antihistamine therapy was reported for desloratadine[91] fexofenadine,[92] levocetirizine[66] and rupatadine.[93]

## 44.4.2 Atopic Dermatitis (AD)

Histamine implication in the pathophysiology of pruritus occurring during AD has been advocated[94] and H1-antihistamines are frequently employed as antipruritic agents in AD treatment. No robust study with a high level of evidence exists to support this practice even if efficacy of cyproheptadine,[95,96] hydroxyzine,[95,96] cetirizine,[97,98] loratadine[99] and fexofenadine[100] was punctually reported. Some data support the interest of a long course H1-antihistamine therapy in children as in one study with a high level of evidence showing a topical glucocorticoids-sparing effect in children who underwent a 18 months course of treatment with cetirizine[101] and even a delay in asthma development in those who were sensitized to grass pollen and dust mite.[102] Combination of the second generation H1-antihistamine, fexofenadine, with topical glucocorticoids (60 mg × 2/j) was found more efficient than a placebo.[103] One of the explanations may result in the modification of immune parameters (IgE amount, lymphocytes proliferative index and decrease in CD4: CD8 index.[104)

### 44.4.3 Mastocytosis

H1-antihistamines are widely employed when treating mastocytosis despite a few available studies. Efficacy of azelastine, chlorpheniramine,[105] cyproheptadine,[106] ketotifene,[107] and hydroxyzine[108] has been punctually reported but none of these molecules were compared to a placebo. No studies are available with the second generation molecules.

### 44.4.4 Insect Bites Reactions

Loratadine,[109] ebastine,[110] and cetirizine[111] were found more efficient than a placebo to prevent whealing and delayed papules from mosquito bites in children and adults. However when compared to loratadine and a placebo, cetirizine and ebastine were more efficient in decreasing œdema and pruritus.[112] Most recently, levocetirizine was found effective to decrease the size of wheals and the pruritus following mosquito bites in adults.[113]

### 44.4.5 Drug Eruption

Treatment of drug eruption is constituted by causative drug identification and arrest, but, due to the usual itchy character of such eruptions, H1-antihistamines are often prescribed. No study can support such a medication outside the subgroup of urticarian drug eruptions.

### 43.4.6 Other Pruritic Dermatosis

A few studies and case reports report the efficacy of H1-antihistamines in the treatment of various itchy

dermatosis. Thus, coadministration of cetirizine and cimetidine was found efficient in reducing the itching score in patients suffering from burns.[114] Systemic administration of oxatomide was reported efficient for the treatment of senile pruritus[115] and topical administration of oxatomide efficient to improve vulvar pruritus among women suffering from vulvar lichen sclerosus[116] or idiopathic vulvar pruritus.[117]Administration of dimethindene maleate efficiently controlled pruritus caused by varicella zoster virus in children.[118]

## 44.5 Conclusion

H1-antihistamines are an efficient treatment for urticaria where their efficacy is widely evidenced. They should not be prescribed for all pruritic dermatosis but logically reserved for diseases involving histamine. Second generation molecules should be the first to be prescribed due to low side effects and the best pharmacokinetic profile. All second generation molecules are equivalent in terms of efficacy and most of them are free of sedative and cardiac side effects.

## References

1. Spittle MM, Hammer A, Malli R, et al. Functional analysis of histamine receptor subtypes involved in endothelium-mediated relaxation of the human uterine artery. *Clin Exp Pharmacol Physiol.* 2002;29:711–716.
2. Sugimoto Y, Iba Y, Nakamura Y, et al. Pruritus-associated response mediated by cutaneous histamine H3 receptors. *Clin Exp Allergy.* 2004;34:456–459.
3. McLeod RL, Mingo GG, Herczku C, et al. Combined histamine H1 and H3 receptor blockade produces nasal decongestion in an experimental model of nasal congestion. *Am J Rhinol.* 1999;13:391–399.
4. Dunford PJ, Williams KN, Desai PJ, et al. Histamine H4 receptor antagonists are superior to traditional antihistamines in the attenuation of experimental pruritus. *J Allergy Clin Immunol.* 2007;119:176–183.
5. MacGlashan D Jr. Histamine: a mediator of inflammation. *J Allergy Clin Immunol.* 2003;112:S53–S59.
6. Leurs R, Church MK, Taglialatela M. H1-antihistamines: inverse agonism, anti-inflammatory actions and cardiac effects. *Clin Exp Allergy.* 2002;32:489–498.
7. Hill SJ, Ganellin CR, Timmerman H, et al. Classification of histamine receptors. *Pharmacol Rev.* 1997;49:253–278.
8. García-Cardeña G, Fan R, Shah V, et al. Dynamic activation of endothelial nitric oxide synthase by Hsp90. *Nature.* 1998;392:821–824.

9. Bakker RA, Schoonus SB, Smit MJ, et al. Histamine H(1)-receptor activation of nuclear factor-kappa B: roles for G beta gamma- and G alpha(q/11)-subunits in constitutive and agonist-mediated signaling. *Mol Pharmacol.* 2001;60:1133–1142.

10. Akdis CA, Simons FE. Histamine receptors are hot in immunopharmacology. *Eur J Pharmacol.* 2006;533(1–3):69–76.

11. Pincus SH, DiNapoli AM, Schooley WR. Superoxide production by eosinophils: activation by histamine. *J Invest Dermatol.* 1982;79:53–57.

12. Triggiani M, Gentile M, Secondo A, et al. Histamine induces exocytosis and IL-6 production from human lung macrophages through interaction with H1 receptors. *J Immunol.* 2001;166:4083–4091.

13. Caron G, Delneste Y, Roelandts E, et al. Histamine polarizes human dendritic cells into Th2 cell-promoting effector dendritic cells. *J Immunol.* 2001;167:3682–3686.

14. Hill SJ. Distribution, properties, and functional characteristics of three classes of histamine receptor. *Pharmacol Rev.* 1990;42:45–83.

15. Gantner F, Sakai K, Tusche MW, et al. Histamine h(4) and h(2) receptors control histamine-induced interleukin-16 release from human CD8(+) T cells. *J Pharmacol Exp Ther.* 2002;303:300–307.

16. Sirois J, Menard G, Moses AS, et al. Importance of histamine in the cytokine network in the lung through H2 and H3 receptors: stimulation of IL-10 production. *J Immunol.* 2000;164:2964–2970.

17. Varty LM, Hey JA. Histamine H3 receptor activation inhibits neurogenic sympathetic vasoconstriction in porcine nasal mucosa. *Eur J Pharmacol.* 2002;452:339–345.

18. Arrang JM. Le récepteur H3 de l'histamine: une cible pour de nouveaux médicaments. *Ann Pharm Fr.* 2003;61:173–184.

19. Schwartz JC, Morisset S, Rouleau A, et al. Therapeutic implications of constitutive activity of receptors: the example of the histamine H3 receptor. *J Neural Transm Suppl.* 2003;64:1–16.

20. Nakamura T, Itadani H, Hidaka Y, et al. Molecular cloning and characterization of a new human histamine receptor. *HH4R. Biochem Biophys Res Commun.* 2000;279(2):615–620.

21. Cogé F, Guénin SP, Rique H, et al. Structure and expression of the human histamine H4-receptor gene. *Biochem Biophys Res Commun.* 2001;284:301–309.

22. Bakker RA, Wieland K, Timmerman H, et al. Constitutive activity of the histamine H(1) receptor reveals inverse agonism of histamine H(1) receptor antagonists. *Eur J Pharmacol.* 2000;387:R5–R7.

23. Trzeciakowski J, Levi R. Antihistamines. In: Middleton E Jr, Reed CE, Ellis EF, eds. *Allergy, Principles and Practice.* 2nd ed. Mosby: St Louis, MO; 1983:575–592.

24. Passalacqua G, Canonica GW. Structure and classification of H1-antihistamines and overview of their activities. In: Simons FER, ed. *Histamine and H1-Antihistamines in Allergic Disease.* New York: Marcel Dekker; 2002:65–100.

25. Chen C, Hanson E, Watson JW, et al. P-glycoprotein limits the brain penetration of nonsedating but not sedating H1-antagonists. *Drug Metab Dispos.* 2003;31:312–318.

26. Renwick AG. The metabolism of antihistamines and drug interactions: the role of cytochrome P450 enzymes. *Clin Exp Allergy.* 1999;29:116–124.

27. Robbins DK, Horton MW, Swan SK, et al. Pharmacokinetics of fexofenadine in patients with varying degrees of renal impairment. *Pharm Res.* 1996;13:S431. Abstract.

28. Matzke GR, Yeh J, Awni WM, et al. Pharmacokinetics of cetirizine in the elderly and patients with renal insufficiency. *Ann Allergy.* 1987;59:25–30.

29. Walsh GM. The anti-inflammatory effects of the second generation antihistamines. *Dermatol Ther.* 2000;13:349–360.

30. Holgate ST, Canonica GW, Simons FE, et al. Consensus group on new-generation antihistamines (CONGA): present status and recommendations. *Clin Exp Allergy.* 2003;33:1305–1324.

31. Schatz M. H1-antihistamines in pregnancy and lactation. In: Simons FER, ed. *Histamine and H1-Antihistamines in Allergic Disease.* New York: Marcel Dekker; 2002:421–436.

32. Kallen B. Effect of perinatal (prenatal?) Loratadine exposure on male rat reproductive organ development. *Reprod Toxicol.* 2004;18:453.

33. Welch MJ, Meltzer EO, Simons ER. H1-antihistamines and the central nervous system. In: Simons FER, ed. *Histamine and H1-Antihistamines in Allergic Disease.* New York: Marcel Dekker; 2002:337–388.

34. Hindmarch I, Shamsi Z, Kimber S. An evaluation of the effects of high-dose fexofenadine on the central nervous system: a double-blind, placebo-controlled study in healthy volunteers. *Clin Exp Allergy.* 2002;32:133–139.

35. Vuurman E, Theunissen E, van Oers A, et al. Lack of effects between rupatadine 10 mg and placebo on actual driving performance of healthy volunteers. *Hum Psychopharmacol.* 2007;22:289–297.

36. Vuurman EF, Rikken GH, Muntjewerff ND, et al. Effects of desloratadine, diphenhydramine, and placebo on driving performance and psychomotor performance measurements. *Eur J Clin Pharmacol.* 2004;60:307–313.

37. Verster JC, Volkerts ER. Antihistamines and driving ability: evidence from on-the-road driving studies during normal traffic. *Ann Allergy Asthma Immunol.* 2004;92:297–303.

38. Angello JT, Druce HM. Drug effects on driving performance. *Ann Intern Med.* 2000;132(5):354–363.

39. Simons FE, Fraser TG, Reggin JD, et al. Adverse central nervous system effects of older antihistamines in children. *Pediatr Allergy Immunol.* 1996;7:22–27.

40. Vuurman EF, van Veggel LM, Uiterwijk MM, et al. Seasonal allergic rhinitis and antihistamine effects on children's learning. *Ann Allergy.* 1993;71:121–126.

41. Stevenson J, Cornah D, Evrard P, et al. Long-term evaluation of the impact of the h1-receptor antagonist cetirizine on the behavioral, cognitive, and psychomotor development of very young children with atopic dermatitis. *Pediatr Res.* 2002;52:251–257.

42. Simons FE. Early prevention of asthma in atopic children (EPAAC) study group. Safety of levocetirizine treatment in young atopic children: an 18-month study. *Pediatr Allergy Immunol.* 2007;18(6):535–542. Epub 2007 Jun 11.

43. Yap YG, Camm AJ. Potential cardiotoxicity of H1-antihistamines. In: Simons FER, ed. *Histamine and H1-Antihistamines in Allergic Disease.* New York: Marcel Dekker; 2002;389–420.

44. Lawrence CM, Byrne JP. Eczematous eruption from oral diphenhydramine. *Contact Dermatitis.* 1981;7:276–277.

45. Tella R, Gaig P, Bartra J, et al. Urticaria to cetirizine. *J Investig Allergol Clin Immunol.* 2002;12:136–137.

46. Assouere MN, Mazereeuw-Hautier J, Bonafe JL. Toxidermie à deux antihistaminiques ayant une parenté

chimique: la cétirizine et l'hydroxyzine. *Ann Dermatol Venereol.* 2002;129:1295–1298.

47. Dwyer CM, Dick D. Fixed drug eruption caused by diphenhydramine. *J Am Acad Dermatol.* 1993;29:496–497.

48. Pionetti CH, Kien MC, Alonso A. Fixed drug eruption due to loratadine. *Allergol Immunopathol (Madr.).* 2003;31: 291–293.

49. Roman IJ, Kassem N, Gural RP, et al. Suppression of histamine-induced wheal response by loratadine (SCH 29851) over 28 days in man. *Ann Allergy.* 1986;57:253–256.

50. Snyman JR, Sommers DK, Gregorowski MD, et al. Effect of cetirizine, ketotifen and chlorpheniramine on the dynamics of the cutaneous hypersensitivity reaction: a comparative study. *Eur J Clin Pharmacol.* 1992;42:359–362.

51. Gengo FM, Dabronzo J, Yurchak A, et al. The relative antihistaminic and psychomotor effects of hydroxyzine and cetirizine. *Clin Pharmacol Ther.* 1987;42:265–272.

52. Simons FE, Fraser TG, Reggin JD, et al. Comparison of the central nervous system effects produced by six H1-receptor antagonists. *Clin Exp Allergy.* 1996;26:1092–1097.

53. Denham KJ, Boutsiouki P, Clough GF, et al. Comparison of the effects of desloratadine and levocetirizine on histamine-induced wheal, flare and itch in human skin. *Inflamm Res.* 2003;52:424–427.

54. Grant JA, Riethuisen JM, Moulaert B, et al. A double-blind, randomized, single-dose, crossover comparison of levocetirizine with ebastine, fexofenadine, loratadine, mizolastine, and placebo: suppression of histamine-induced wheal-and-flare response during 24 hours in healthy male subjects. *Ann Allergy Asthma Immunol.* 2002;88:190–197.

55. Pontasch MJ, White LJ, Bradford JC. Oral agents in the management of urticaria: patient perception of effectiveness and level of satisfaction with treatment. *Ann Pharmacother.* 1993;27:730–731.

56. Watson NT, Weiss EL, Harter PM. Famotidine in the treatment of acute urticaria. *Clin Exp Dermatol.* 2000;25:186–189.

57. Moscati RM, Moore GP. Comparison of cimetidine and diphenhydramine in the treatment of acute urticaria. *Ann Emerg Med.* 1990;19:12–15.

58. Lin RY, Curry A, Pesola GR, et al. Improved outcomes in patients with acute allergic syndromes who are treated with combined H1 and H2 antagonists. *Ann Emerg Med.* 2000;36:462–468.

59. Monroe EW, Bernstein DI, Fox RW, et al. Relative efficacy and safety of loratadine, hydroxyzine, and placebo in chronic idiopathic urticaria. *Arzneimittelforschung.* 1992;42:119–1121.

60. Brostoff J, Fitzharris P, Dunmore C, et al. Efficacy of mizolastine, a new antihistamine, compared with placebo in the treatment of chronic idiopathic urticaria. *Allergy.* 1996;51:320–325.

61. Breneman DL. Cetirizine versus hydroxyzine and placebo in chronic idiopathic urticaria. *Ann Pharmacother.* 1996;30: 1075–1079.

62. Kamide R, Niimura M, Ueda H, et al. Clinical evaluation of ketotifen for chronic urticaria: multicenter double blind comparative study with clemastine. *Ann Allergy.* 1989;62: 322–325.

63. Kalis B. Double blind multicenter comparative study of ebastine, terfenadine and placebo in the treatment of chronic idiopathic urticaria in adults. *Drugs.* 1996;52:30634.

64. Kulthanan K, Gritiyarangsan P, Sitakalin C, et al. Multicenter study of the efficacy and safety of fexofenadine 60 mg.

Twice daily in 108 Thai patients with chronic idiopathic urticaria. *J Med Assoc Thai.* 2001;84:153–159.

65. Monroe E, Finn A, Patel P, et al. Efficacy and safety of desloratadine 5 mg once daily in the treatment of chronic idiopathic urticaria: a double-blind, randomized, placebo-controlled trial. *J Am Acad Dermatol.* 2003;48:535–541.

66. Kapp A, Pichler WJ. Levocetirizine is an effective treatment in patients suffering from chronic idiopathic urticaria: a randomized, double blind, placebo controlled, parallel, multi-center study. *Int J Dermatol.* 2006;45:469–474.

67. Gimenez-Arnau A, Pujol RM, Ianosi S, et al. Rupatadine in the treatment of chronic idiopathic urticaria: a double blind, randomized, placebo controlled multicenter study. *Allergy.* 2007;62:539–546.

68. Sussman G, Jancelewicz Z. Controlled trial of H1 antagonists in the treatment of chronic idiopathic urticaria. *Ann Allergy.* 1991;67:433–439.

69. Guerra L, Vincenzi C, Marchesi E, et al. Loratadine and cetirizine in the treatment of chronic urticaria. *J E Acad Dermatol Venereol.* 1994;3:148–152.

70. Handa S, Dogra S, Kumar B. Comparative efficacy of cetirizine and fexofenadine in the treatment of chronic idiopathic urticaria. *J Dermatolog Treat.* 2004;15:55–57.

71. Simons FE, Sussman GL, Simons KJ. Effect of the H2-antagonist cimetidine on the pharmacokinetics and pharmacodynamics of the H1-antagonists hydroxyzine and cetirizine in patients with chronic urticaria. *J Allergy Clin Immunol.* 1995;95:685–693.

72. Bleehen SS, Thomas SE, Greaves MW, et al. Cimetidine and chlorpheniramine in the treatment of chronic idiopathic urticaria: a multi-centre randomized double-blind study. *Br J Dermatol.* 1987;117:81–88.

73. Sharpe GR, Shuster S. The effect of cetirizine on symptoms and wealing in dermographic urticaria. *Br J Dermatol.* 1993;129:580–583.

74. Boyle J, Marks P, Gibson JR. Acrivastine versus terfenadine in the treatment of symptomatic dermographism - a double blind, placebo-controlled study. *J Int Med Res.* 1989;17: 9B–13B.

75. Matthews CN, Kirby JD, James J, et al. Dermographism: reduction in weal size by chlorpheniramine and hydroxyzine. *Br J Dermatol.* 1973;88:279–282.

76. Breathnach SM, Allen R, Ward AM, et al. Symptomatic dermographism: natural history, clinical features laboratory investigations and response to therapy. *Clin Exp Dermatol.* 1983;8:463–476.

77. Kaur S, Greaves M, Eftekhari N. Factitious urticaria (dermographism): treatment by cimetidine and chlorpheniramine in a randomized double-blind study. *Br J Dermatol.* 1981;104:185–190.

78. Kontou-Fili K, Maniatakou G, Demaka P, et al. Therapeutic effects of cetirizine in delayed pressure urticaria: clinicopathologic findings. *J Am Acad Dermatol.* 1991;24:1090–1093.

79. Monfrecola G, Masturzo E, Riccardo AM, et al. Cetirizine for solar urticaria in the visible spectrum. *Dermatology.* 2000;200:334–335.

80. Zuberbier T, Munzberger C, Haustein U, et al. Double-blind crossover study of high-dose cetirizine in cholinergic urticaria. *Dermatology.* 1996;193:324–327.

81. Medeiros M, Jr. Aquagenic urticaria. *J Investig Allergol Clin Immunol.* 1996;6:63–64.

82. Kobza Black A, Aboobaker J, Gibson JR, et al. Acrivastine versus hydroxyzine in the treatment of cholinergic urticaria. A placebo-controlled study. *Acta Derm Venereol*. 1988;68:541–544.

83. Magerl M, Schmolke J, Siebenhaar F, et al. Acquired cold urticaria symptoms can be safely prevented by ebastine. *Allergy*. 2007;62:1465–1468.

84. Nettis E, Pannofino A, Cavallo E, et al. Efficacy of montelukast, in combination with loratadine, in the treatment of delayed pressure urticaria. *J Allergy Clin Immunol*. 2003;112:212–213.

85. Nettis E, Colanardi MC, Soccio AL, et al. Desloratadine in combination with montelukast suppresses the dermographometer challenge test papule, and is effective in the treatment of delayed pressure urticaria: a randomized, double blind, placebo-controlled study. *Br J Dermatol*. 2006;155:1279–1282.

86. Bonadonna P, Lombardi C, Senna G, et al. Treatment of acquired cold urticaria with cetirizine and zafirlukast in combination. *J Am Acad Dermatol*. 2003;49:714–716.

87. Duc J, Pecoud A. Successful treatment of idiopathic cold urticaria with the association of H1 and H2 antagonists: a case report. *Ann Allergy*. 1986;56:355–357.

88. Irwin RB, Lieberman P, Friedman MM, et al. Mediator release in local heat urticaria: protection with combined H1 and H2 antagonists. *J Allergy Clin Immunol*. 1985;76:35–39.

89. Lennox RD, Leahy MJ. Validation of the dermatology life quality index as an outcome measure for urticaria-related quality of life. *Ann Allergy Asthma Immunol*. 2004;93: 142–146.

90. Baiardini I, Pasquali M, Braido F, et al. A new tool to evaluate the impact of chronic urticaria on quality of life: chronic urticaria quality of life questionnaire (CU-qol). *Allergy*. 2005;60:1073–1078.

91. Grob JJ, Stalder JF, Ortonne JP, et al. Etude multicentrique randomisée en double insu, contre placebo, comparant les effets d'un traitement quotidien par desloratadine 5 mg ou placebo pendant six semaines sur la qualité de vie d'adultes atteints d'urticaire chronique idiopathique. *Rev Fr Allergo Immunol Clin*. 2004;44:127.

92. Thompson AK, Finn AF, Schoenwetter WF. Effect of 60 mg twice-daily fexofenadine hcl on quality of life, work and classroom productivity, and regular activity in patients with chronic idiopathic urticaria. *J Am Acad.Dermatol*. 2000;43:24–30.

93. Mullol L, Bousquet J, Bachert C, et al. Rupatadine in allergic rhinitis and chronic urticaria. *Allergy*. 2008;63:5–28.

94. Reitamo S, Ansel JC, Luger TA. Itch in atopic dermatitis. *J Am Acad Dermatol*. 2001;45:S55–S56.

95. Baraf CS. Treatment of pruritus in allergic dermatoses: an evaluation of the relative efficacy of cyproheptadine and hydroxyzine. *Curr Ther Res Clin Exp*. 1976;19:32–38.

96. Klein GL, Galant SP. A comparison of the antipruritic efficacy of hydroxyzine and cyproheptadine in children with atopic dermatitis. *Ann Allergy*. 1980;44:142–145.

97. Hannuksela M, Kalimo K, Lammintausta K, et al. Dose ranging study: cetirizine in the treatment of atopic dermatitis in adults. *Ann Allergy*. 1993;70:127–133.

98. La Rosa M, Ranno C, Musarra I, et al. Double-blind study of cetirizine in atopic eczema in children. *Ann Allergy*. 1994;73:117–122.

99. Monroe EW. Relative efficacy and safety of loratadine, hydroxyzine, and placebo in chronic idiopathic urticaria and atopic dermatitis. *Clin Ther*. 1992;14:17–21.

100. Kawakami T, Kaminishi K, Soma Y, et al. Oral antihistamine therapy influences plasma tryptase levels in adult atopic dermatitis. *J Dermatol Sci*. Aug;2006;43(2):127–134. Epub 2006 Jul. 14.

101. Diepgen TL. Long-term treatment with cetirizine of infants with atopic dermatitis: a multi-country, double-blind, randomized, placebo-controlled trial (the ETAC trial) over 18 months. *Pediatr Allergy Immunol*. 2002;13:278–286.

102. Warner JO. ETAC study group, early treatment of the atopic child. A double-blind, randomized, placebo-controlled trial of cetirizine in preventing the onset of asthma in children with atopic dermatitis: 18 months treatment and 18 months post treatment follow-up. *J Allergy Clin Immunol*. 2001;108:929–937.

103. Kawashima M, Tango T, Noguchi T, et al. Addition of fexofenadine to a topical corticosteroid reduces the pruritus associated with atopic dermatitis in a 1-week randomized, multicentre, double-blind, placebo-controlled, parallel-group study. *Br J Dermatol*. 2003;148:1212–1221.

104. Guzik TJ, Adamek-Guzik T, Bzowska M, Miedzobrodzki J, Czerniawska-Mysik G, Pryjma J. Influence of treating atopic dermatitis with oral antihistamine and topical steroids on selected parameters of cell and humoral immunity. *Folia Med Cracov*. 2002;43:79–93.

105. Friedman BS, Santiago ML, Berkebile C, Metcalfe DD. Comparison of azelastine and chlorpheniramine in the treatment of mastocytosis. *J Allergy Clin Immunol*. 1993;92:520–526.

106. Gasior-Chrzan B, Falk ES. Systemic mastocytosis treated with histamine H1 and H2 receptor antagonists. *Dermatology*. 1992;184:149–152.

107. Czarnetzki BM. A double-blind cross-over study of the effect of ketotifen in urticaria pigmentosa. *Dermatologica*. 1983;166:44–47.

108. Povoa P, Ducla-Soares J, Fernandes A, et al. A case of systemic mastocytosis; therapeutic efficacy of ketotifen. *J Intern Med*. 1991;229:475–477.

109. Karppinen A, Kautiainen H, Reunala T, Petman L, Reunala T, Brummer-Korvenkontio H. Loratadine in the treatment of mosquito-bite-sensitive children. *Allergy*. 2000;55: 668–671.

110. Karppinen A, Petman L, Jekunen A, et al. Treatment of mosquito bites with ebastine: a field trial. *Acta Derm Venereol*. 2000;80:114–116.

111. Reunala T, Lappalainen P, Brummer-Korvenkontio H, et al. Cutaneous reactivity to mosquito bites: effect of cetirizine and development of anti-mosquito antibodies. *Clin Exp Allergy*. 1991;21:617–622.

112. Karppinen A, Kautiainen H, Petman L, et al. Comparison of cetirizine, ebastine and loratadine in the treatment of immediate mosquito-bite allergy. *Allergy*. 2002;57:534–537.

113. Karppinen A, Brummer-Korvenkontio H, Petman L, et al. Levocetirizine for treatment of immediate and delayed mosquito bite reactions. *Acta Derm Venereol*. 2006;86(4): 329–331.

114. Baker RA, Zeller RA, Klein RL, et al. Burn wound itch control using H1 and H2 antagonists. *J Burn Care Rehabil*. 2001;22:263–268.

115. Dupont C, de Maubeuge J, Kotlar W, et al. Oxatomide in the treatment of pruritus senilis. A double-blind placebo-controlled trial. *Dermatologica*. 1984;169:348–353.

116. Origoni M, Ferrari D, Rossi M, et al. Topical oxatomide: an alternative approach for the treatment of vulvar lichen sclerosus. *Int J Gynaecol Obstet*. 1996;55:259–264.

117. Origoni M, Garsia S, Sideri M, et al. Efficacy of topical oxatomide in women with pruritus vulvae. *Drugs Exp Clin Res*. 1990;16:591–596.

118. Englisch W, Bauer CP. Dimethindene maleate in the treatment of pruritus caused by varizella zoster virus infection in children. *Arzneimittelforschung*. 1997;47:1233–1235.

# Chapter 45
# Anticonvulsants for the Treatment of Pruritus

Nora V. Bergasa and Deewan Deewan

Pruritus or itch is the most common symptom of skin diseases. Liver and kidney diseases and various forms of cancer can also be complicated by pruritus. The origin of pruritus can be peripheral, as with conditions of the skin, or central, as associated with conditions of the central nervous system including multiple sclerosis and brain infarcts. There is still a vacuum in the understanding of the pathophysiology of pruritus, but it is accepted that pruritus leads to scratching behavior, a well conserved reflex, which is believed to have been passed on as a protective reaction to an unpleasant or harmful stimulus. The lack of understanding of the pathophysiology of pruritus has led to the use of many interventions, sometimes without a clear rationale, for the treatment of this complication, which can be maddening. In this chapter, the use of anticonvulsants to treat pruritus will be reviewed and in Table 45.1, a select number of published experiences with the use of anticonvulsants in the treatment of pruritus is provided.

## 45.1 Neurophysiology of Pruritus

Stimulation of polymodal (i.e., that respond to more than one type of stimuli) nociceptors (i.e., sensory fibers that respond to nociceptive stimuli) has been reported to result in pruritus. Neurons that respond to histamine alone have been defined as itch transmitting.[1]

Functional magnetic resonance imaging (fMRI)s[2–5] and positron emission tomography (PET)[6–9] studies have been conducted to explore areas of activation after stimulation with allergens and the pruritogen histamine. The studies have revealed that the administration of histamine to the skin of volunteers was associated with activation of certain brain areas that included the

anterior cingular cortex, areas of the insula, and the posterior cingular cortex, which concern emotional processing, and of the basal ganglia, and supplemental pre motor areas, which concern the planning of movement. These data provide a visual depiction of what has been interpreted as the sensory input and the behavioral expression of pruritus; however, the areas of the brain that are involved in the spontaneous sensation of pruritus, such as that experienced by patients with internal medicinal causes of pruritus are still unknown.

## 45.2 Insight from Behavioral Studies in Pruritus

One of the major obstacles in the study of pruritus has been the lack of inclusion of behavioral methodology in clinical studies. Pruritus is a sensation, and, as it is a sensation it cannot be directly quantitated; in contrast, the behavior that results in pruritus, scratching, can be measured by available instruments that allow for the recording of scratching activity independently from gross body movements. The prototype of these instruments is the scratching activity monitoring system (SAMS).[10] The SAMS consists of a scratch transducer made of piezoelectric film, attached to a fingernail or to a prosthetic device on the fingernail. The signals derived from the vibrations generated by the fingernail in the act of scratching, independent from gross body movements, are amplified, transmitted, and processed by the supporting electronics. The piezo film functions as a contact microphone on the fingernail of the subject from whom scratching behavior is being recorded. The data can be extracted as hourly scratching activity (HSA). The SAMS has been applied in clinical trials of therapeutic interventions on the pruritus of cholestasis

L. Misery and S. Ständer (eds.), *Pruritus*,
DOI 10.1007/978-1-84882-322-8_45, © Springer-Verlag London Limited 2010

**Table 45.1** Selected published experiences of anticonvulsants for the treatment of pruritus

| Drug | Rationale to use drug | Study duration | Cause of pruritus | N | Design of study | Method to assess pruritus | Results | Reference |
|---|---|---|---|---|---|---|---|---|
| Gabapentin | Relief of neuropathic pain | 4 months | Brachioradial pruritus | 1 | Case report | Oral report | Improvement of pruritus at high doses* | 24 |
| Gabapentin | Relief of itch in patients with diabetic neuropathy to treat diabetic | 4 weeks | Uremic pruritus in patient in hemodialysis | 25 | Double blind randomized placebo controlled cross over study. | Visual analogue scale | Improvement in the mean VAS for pruritus from 8.4 to 1.2 (p = 0.0001); on placebo half of the patients decreased the VAS by more than 50% | 26 |
| Gabapentin | Reports on its ameliorating effect on pruritus. | 9 months | Pruritus of Unknown origin | 2 | Case series | Oral report | Improvement in pruritus | 59 |
| Gabapentin | Reported to increase threshold to nociception | 4 weeks | Pruritus of cholestasis | 16 | Double blind, randomized, placebo controlled | VAS and HSA | Increased pruritus and HAS in contrast to placebo | 16 |
| Lamotrigine | Reported to relief neuropathic pain. | 18 months | Brachioradial Pruritus | 1 | Case report | Oral report | Improvement in complain of pruritus | 57 |
| Phenobarbital | Improvement of liver panel in animal studies | 7–12 months | Cholestasis | 15 | Open label | Oral reports | Relief of pruritus | 22 |
| Pregabalin | Similar to gabapentin, which was reported to relief neuropathic pain. | 17 days | Cetuximab induced itch. | 1 | Case report | NRS | Improvement in pruritus on high doses from 9 to 3 on NRS scale. | 60 |
| Pregabalin | Decreases neuronal hyperexcitability | 6 months | Chronic pruritus of unknown origin. | 3 | Case report | VAS | Improvement in pruritus on high doses** from 8 to 3 on NRS scale | 56 |

VAS, visual analogue score; NRS, numerical rate scale; HAS, hourly scratching activity.

*600–1,800 mg daily.

**150 mg by mouth twice daily.

and allows for the incorporation of a well-defined endpoint i.e. changes in scratching activity.[11-16] Portable SAMSs that also use piezoelectric technology and can be used by individuals in their living environment have been developed.[17-19] This type of methodology allows for a systematic collection of behavioral data, which can be compared among different population of patients, and which has recently provided enlightening information on the placebo effect, which has direct impact on how the data are interpreted, especially when trying to assess the antipruritic effect of an intervention.

## 45.3 Rationale for the Use of Anticonvulsants to Treat Pruritus

Itch originating in the skin seems to result from the stimulation of the free nerve ending of specialized C-fibers by peripheral pruritogens.[1] The pruritogenic stimuli are processed in the central nervous system followed by scratching behavior, although the detailed neurotransmission of the itch and scratch cycle is still unknown. Pruritus is considered a second order of nociception, the first one being pain. It is this relationship that seems to have provided a rationale for the use of anticonvulsants, which have been used to treat neuropathic pain, in the treatment of pruritus.

## 45.4 Phenobarbital

Phenobarbital induces hepatic and microsomal enzymes.[20] It has been used to treat pruritus in cholestasis,[20-22] which is defined as impaired secretion of bile.[23] Studies have reported that the liver profile improved with the administration of phenobarbital to patients with cholestatic disorders. Phenobarbital reduces serum bilirubin and serum bile acid levels, the concetration of which, increases in cholestasis, and it enhances the excretion of organic anions that are cleared from the plasma by the liver and excreted into the bile;[22] thus, a choleretic effect of phenobarbital may contribute to its reported antipruritic effect. Phenobarbital acts in the central nervous system via its binding site in the GABA complex; thus, some of the reported antipruritic effects of phenobarbital may result from sedation.

## 45.5 Gabapentin

Gabapentin has been used to treat brachioradial pruritus[24, 25] pruritus secondary to uremia,[26-28] pruritus of cholestasis,[16] and pruritus associated with wound healing in burns.[29] Gabapentin is a drug used as an adjunct to treat partial and generalized tonic clonic seizures and for the treatment of post herpetic neuralgia.[30] The mechanism of action of gabapentin has not been completely elucidated. Gabapentin is not a gamma aminobutyric acid (GABA) mimetic.[30] It binds presynaptically to an exofacial epitope of the alpha-2 delta-1 and alpha-2 delta-2 auxiliary subunits of voltage gated calcium channels, which results in decreased depolarization induced by calcium influx at nerve terminals, decreasing the release of excitatory neurotransmitters.[30] A recent publication reported that gabapentin inhibits voltage gated calcium channels trafficking and their expression on plasma membranes, and that it exerts its inhibitory effect on synaptic neurotransmission by acting on intracellular alpha2 delta subunits mostly, rather than inhibiting calcium currents.[31] Altered expression and distribution of neuropetides and their receptors within the various layers of the skin of the patients with psoriasis and pruritus, including substance P, calcitonin-related peptide (CGRP), and somatostatin have been reported.[32] In one study the plasma concentration of CGRP was significantly increased in patients with pruritic psoriasis as compared to that of healthy subjects.[33] These data have been interpreted to suggest that these peptides are involved in itch. In the context of gabapentin, this drug inhibits the release of calcitonin gene-related peptide, a neuropetide, described as an itch mediator.[34] In an animal model of nociception, naloxone was reported to reverse the antinocipetive effects of gabapentin.[35] These results suggested that gabapentin might mediate some of its actions by opioid receptors.

Gabapentin was reported to increase the hyperpolarization activated current (Ih) in CA1 hippocampal neurons, which decreases the generation of action potentials and reduces neuronal excitability.[36] Ih has a significant impact on the resting properties of hippocampal neurons by considerably decreasing the input resistance.[37] As a result an increased Ih leads to a decreased input resistance, which makes the cell less sensitive to synaptic input; thus, it has been suggested that the gabapentin induced increase in Ih protects the CA 1 pyramidal cells against excessive synaptic or intrinsic activity.[36]

Gabapentin also increases the threshold to experience nociception,[38, 39] which formed part of the rationale used to study this drug in a double-blind, randomized, placebo controlled trial of 4 weeks duration in patients with pruritus secondary to cholestasis that included sixteen women. HSA was continuously recorded for up to 48 hour-periods at baseline and on treatment for at least 4 weeks in an in patient setting. Interviews and a visual analogue scale were used to assess the perception of pruritus. The placebo intervention was associated with a decrease in HAS, in contrast to gabapentin, which was associated with an increase. The mean visual analogue score (VAS) decreased significantly on placebo and in some patients on gabapentin.[16]

The results of this study, shown in figures and stunning and appreciable on inspection. It is clear that the patients on placebo (Fig. 45.2b) scratched less than those on gabapentin (Fig. 45.2a). The consistent decrease in

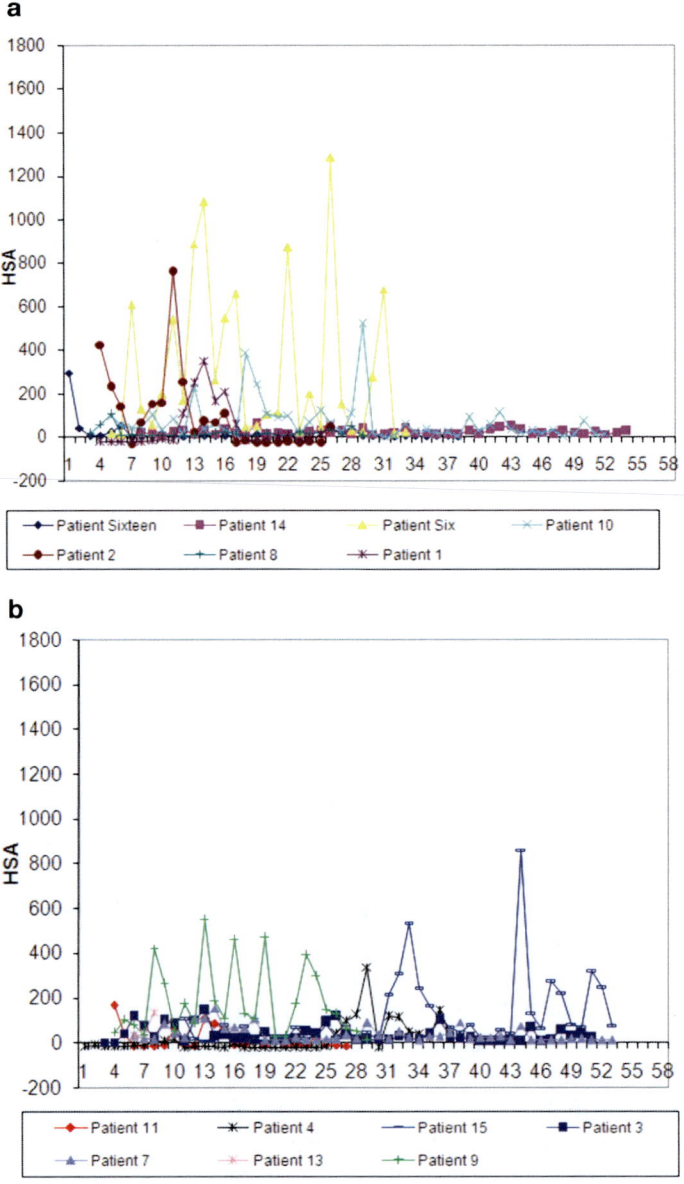

**Fig. 45.1** Baseline mean hourly scratching activity (HSA) from patients with cholestasis and pruritus who were subsequently randomized to gabapentin (a) and to placebo (b)[16]

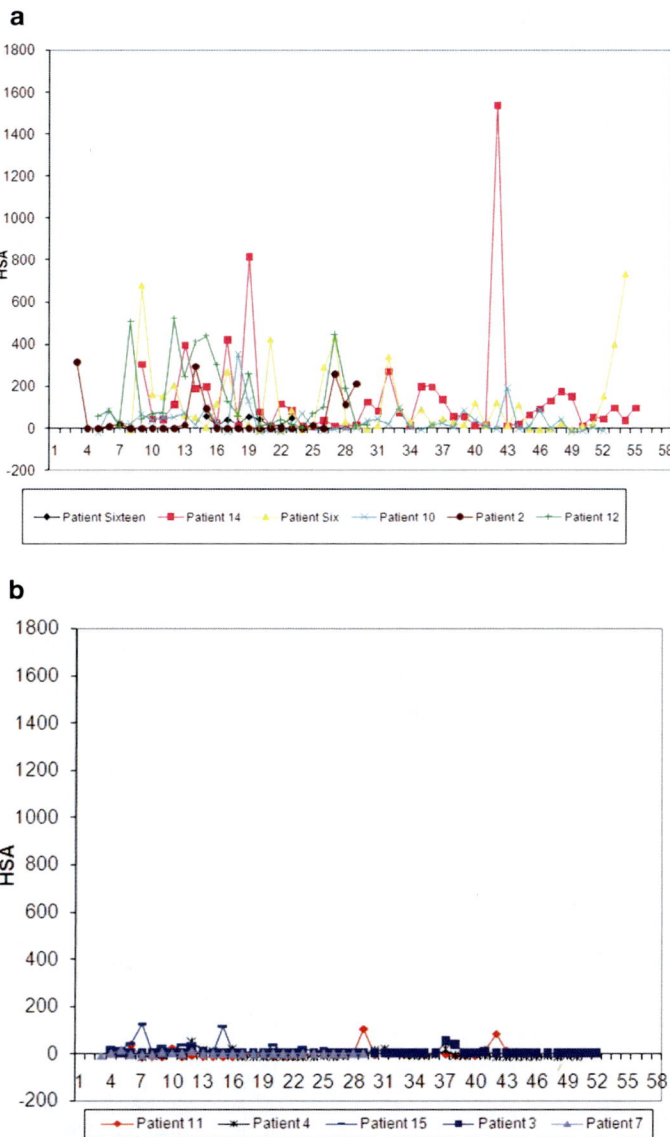

**Fig. 45.2**  Mean hourly scratching activity (HSA) from the patients randomized to gabapentin (a) and to placebo (b) after at least 4 weeks of treatment. The placebo intervention was associated with a decreased in HAS, in contrast to the gabapentin[16]

scratching behavior in patients on placebo indicates that the placebo effect resulted not only in a subjective improvement, but also in a change in behavior. On gabapentin, in contrast, some of the patients reported no relief of pruritus, and scratched more and had a higher mean VAS, some significantly, more than at baseline. In light of recent studies in patients with Parkinson's disease who responded to a placebo intervention with clinical improvement in association with dopamine release, as studied with PET,[40] the results of

the gabapentin trial suggested that the amelioration of pruritus in patients with cholestasis in association with the placebo intervention might have been also secondary to dopamine release. In this context, there is evidence to suggest that pruritus in patients with cholestasis is mediated, at least in part, by increased central opioidergic tone, which forms the basis for the treatment of this type of pruritus with opiate antagonists.[11–14, 41–47] In this regard, the pruritus that results from the central administration of morphine (i.e., pruritus secondary to increased opioidergic tone), which would be analogous to the pruritus of cholestasis, can be relieved effectively by droperidol,[48, 49] a short acting neuroleptic agent with affinity for the D2 dopamine receptor.[50] The acute effect of neuroleptic administration, which would be analogous to droperidol administration, is associated with the activation of dopamine neurons and dopamine release.[50] Thus, if droperidol decreases central, morphine-induced pruritus, endogenous dopamine release may decrease central, opioid-mediated pruritus (i.e., as it is hypothesized to occur in cholestasis). Accordingly, the activation of the nigrostriatal system (i.e., dopamine release) by the placebo intervention might have mediated the decrease in pruritus experienced by the patients in that study by signals transmitted via the neural networks between the basal ganglia and the cerebral cortex,[51, 52] where itch stimuli and the urge to scratch are represented.[6–8] It has been proposed that the active drug in this study, gabapentin, prevented the placebo effect that the intake of a study drug could have triggered, by blocking the release of dopamine, as gabapentin it has been reported to do in vitro[53] and in behavioral studies.[54] The results of this study have opened new areas of investigation in the field of the pruritus of cholestasis. In addition, these results underscore the importance of the placebo effect in the studies of pruritus and emphasize that the use of behavioral methodology should be included in clinical trials of medications for the treatment of pruritus.

## 45.6 Pregabalin

Pregabalin is a relatively new anticonvulsant medication that is approved for the treatment of neuropathic pain. The experience with gabapentin in the treatment of pruritus seems to have encouraged the use of pregabalin as a new therapeutic alternative for this symptom. Pregabalin is a GABA analog of gabapentin. It selectively binds to neuronal voltage-gated calcium channels, modulates presynaptic neurotransmitter release, and thereby neuronal activity.[55] As a result, neuronal hyperexcitability is reduced. It was hypothesized that the beneficial effect of pregabalin in chronic pruritus may result from counteracting the effects on the central sensitization processes involved in the generation of chronic itch.[56]

## 45.7 Lamotrigine

Lamotrigine was reported to decrease brachioradial pruritus in one case report.[57] Lamotrigine exerts its antiepileptic effect primarily by the blockade of sodium channels and calcium channels. It is reported that the efficacy of lamotrigine in relieving neuropathic pain seems related to the blockade of the sodium channels;[58] this process of suppression of pain threshold may be relevant to pruritus.

In summary, there are insufficient data to conclude that anticonvulsants are an effective therapeutic alternative to treat pruritus; however, encouraging results with some of the recently marketed drugs of this type should be confirmed in clinical studies that apply objective methodology. In this context, the study of gabapentin for the treatment of the pruritus of cholestasis has confirmed the large placebo effect that has been considered inherent to all studies of pruritus; therefore, clinical studies that use subjective methodology only should be traded in favor of those that include behavioral methodology.

## References

1. Schmelz M, Schmidt R, Bickel A, Handwerker HO, Torebjork HE. Specific C-receptors for itch in human skin. *J Neurosci*. 1997;17:8003–8008.
2. Walter B, Sadlo MN, Kupfer J, et al. Brain activation by histamine prick test-induced itch. *J Invest Dermatol*. 2005;125: 380–382.
3. Leknes SG, Bantick S, Willis CM, Wilkinson JD, Wise RG, Tracey I. Itch and motivation to scratch: an investigation of the central and peripheral correlates of allergen- and histamine-induced itch in humans. *J Neurophysiol*. 2007; 97:415–422.
4. Mochizuki H, Sadato N, Saito DN, Toyoda H, Tashiro M, Okamura N, Yanai K. Neural correlates of perceptual difference between itching and pain: a human fMRI study. *Neuroimage*. 2007;36:706–717.
5. Valet M, Pfab F, Sprenger T, Wöller A, Zimmer C, Behrendt H, Ring J, Darsow U, Tölle TR. Cerebral processing of histamine-induced itch using short-term alternating temperature modulation – an fMRI study. *J Invest Dermatol*. 2008;128(2):426–433.
6. Hsieh JC, Hagermark O, Stahle-Backdahl M, et al. Urge to scratch represented in the human cerebral cortex during itch. *J Neurophysiol*. 1994;72:3004–3008.
7. Mochizuki H, Tashiro M, Kano M, Sakurada Y, Itoh M, Yanai K. Imaging of central itch modulation in the human brain using positron emission tomography. *Pain*. 2003;105:339–346.
8. Drzezga A, Darsow U, Treede RD, et al. Central activation by histamine-induced itch: analogies to pain processing: a

correlational analysis of O-15 $H_2O$ positron emission tomography studies. *Pain.* 2001;92:295–305.

9. Darsow U, Drzezga A, Frisch M, et al. Processing of histamine-induced itch in the human cerebral cortex: a correlation analysis with dermal reactions. *J Invest Dermatol.* 2000;115:1029–1033.

10. Talbot TL, Schmitt JM, Bergasa NV, Jones EA, Walker EC. Application of piezo film technology for the quantitative assessment of pruritus. *Biomed Instrument Technol.* 1991;25:400–403.

11. Bergasa NV, Talbot TL, Alling DW, et al. A controlled trial of naloxone infusions for the pruritus of chronic cholestasis. *Gastroenterology.* 1992;102:544–549.

12. Bergasa NV, Alling DW, Talbot TL, Wells MC, Jones EA. Oral nalmefene therapy reduces scratching activity due to the pruritus of cholestasis: a controlled study. *J Am Acad Dermatol.* 1999;41:431–434.

13. Bergasa NV, Schmitt JM, Talbot TL, et al. Open-label trial of oral nalmefene therapy for the pruritus of cholestasis. *Hepatology.* 1998;27:679–684.

14. Bergasa NV, Alling DW, Talbot TL, et al. Effects of naloxone infusions in patients with the pruritus of cholestasis. A double-blind, randomized, controlled trial. *Ann Intern Med.* 1995;123:161–167.

15. Bergasa NV, Link MJ, Keogh M, Yaroslavsky G, Rosenthal RN, McGee M. Pilot study of bright-light therapy reflected toward the eyes for the pruritus of chronic liver disease. *Am J Gastroenterol.* 2001;96:1563–1570.

16. Bergasa NV, McGee M, Ginsburg IH, Engler D. Gabapentin in patients with the pruritus of cholestasis: a double-blind, randomized, placebo-controlled trial. *Hepatology.* 2006;44: 1317–1323.

17. Molenaar HA, Oosting J, Jones EA. Improved device for measuring scratching activity in patients with pruritus. *Med Biol Eng Comput.* 1998;36:220–224.

18. Stein H, Bijak M, Heerd E, et al. Pruritometer 1: portable measuring system for quantifying scratching as an objective measure of cholestatic pruritus. *Biomed Tech (Berl).* 1996;41:248–252.

19. Bijak M, Mayr W, Rafolt D, Tanew A, Unger E. Pruritometer 2: portable recording system for the quantification of scratching as objective criterion for the pruritus. *Biomed Tech (Berl).* 2001;46:137–141.

20. Cies JJ, Giamalis JN. Treatment of cholestatic pruritus in children. *Am J Health Syst Pharm.* 2007;64:1157–1162.

21. Ghent CN, Bloomer JR, Hsia YE. Efficacy and safety of long-term phenobarbital therapy of familial cholestasis. *J Pediat.* 1978;93:127–132.

22. Bloomer JR, Boyer JL. Phenobarbital effects in cholestatic liver diseases. *Ann Internal Med.* 1975;82:310–317.

23. Reichen J, Simon F: Cholestasis. In: Arias IM, Jakoby WB, Popper H, Schachter D, Schafritz DA, eds. *The Liver: Biology and Pathobiology.* 2nd ed. New York: Raven Press; 1988;1105–1124.

24. Bueller HA, Bernhard JD, Dubroff LM. Gabapentin treatment for brachioradial pruritus. *J Eur Acad Dermatol Venereol.* 1999;13:227–228.

25. Winhoven SM, Coulson IH, Bottomley WW. Brachioradial pruritus: response to treatment with gabapentin. *Br J Dermatol.* 2004;150:786–787.

26. Gunal AI, Ozalp G, Yoldas TK, Gunal SY, Kirciman E, Celiker H. Gabapentin therapy for pruritus in haemodialysis patients: a randomized, placebo-controlled, double-blind trial. *Nephrol Dial Transplant.* 2004;19:3137–3139.

27. Manenti L, Vaglio A, Costantino E, et al. Gabapentin in the treatment of uremic itch: an index case and a pilot evaluation. *J Nephrol.* 2005;18:86–91.

28. Naini AE, Harandi AA, Khanbabapour S, Shahidi S, Seirafiyan S, Mohseni M. Gabapentin: a promising drug for the treatment of uremic pruritus. *Saudi J Kidney Dis Transpl.* 2007;18:378–381.

29. Mendham JE. Gabapentin for the treatment of itching produced by burns and wound healing in children: a pilot study. *Burns.* 2004;30:851–853.

30. Taylor CP. The biology and pharmacology of calcium channel alpha2-delta proteins Pfizer satellite symposium to the 2003 society for neuroscience meeting. Sheraton New Orleans Hotel, New Orleans, LA November 10, 2003. *CNS Drug Rev.* 2004;10:183–188.

31. Hendrich J, Van Minh AT, Heblich F, et al. Pharmacological disruption of calcium channel trafficking by the alpha2delta ligand gabapentin. *Proc Natl Acad Sci USA.* 2008;105: 3628–3633.

32. Chang SE, Han SS, Jung HJ, Choi JH. Neuropeptides and their receptors in psoriatic skin in relation to pruritus. *Br J Dermatol.* 2007;156:1272–1277.

33. Reich A, Orda A, Wisnicka B, Szepietowski JC. Plasma concentration of selected neuropeptides in patients suffering from psoriasis. *Exp Dermatol.* 2007;16:421–428.

34. Fehrenbacher JC, Taylor CP, Vasko MR. Pregabalin and gabapentin reduce release of substance P and CGRP from rat spinal tissues only after inflammation or activation of protein kinase C. *Pain.* 2003;105:133–141.

35. Yoon MH, Choi JI, Jeong SW. Spinal gabapentin and antinociception: mechanisms of action. *J Korean Med Sci.* 2003;18:255–261.

36. Surges R, Freiman TM, Feuerstein TJ. Gabapentin increases the hyperpolarization-activated cation current Ih in rat CA1 pyramidal cells. *Epilepsia.* 2003;44:150–156.

37. Maccaferri G, Mangoni M, Lazzari A, DiFrancesco D. Properties of the hyperpolarization-activated current in rat hippocampal CA1 pyramidal cells. *J Neurophysiol.* 1993;69:2129–2136.

38. Gustafsson H, Flood K, Berge OG, Brodin E, Olgart L, Stiller CO. Gabapentin reverses mechanical allodynia induced by sciatic nerve ischemia and formalin-induced nociception in mice. *Exp Neurol.* 2003;182:427–434.

39. Rodrigues-Filho R, Campos MM, Ferreira J, Santos AR, Bertelli JA, Calixto JB. Pharmacological characterisation of the rat brachial plexus avulsion model of neuropathic pain. *Brain Res.* 2004;1018:159–170.

40. de la Fuente-Fernandez R, Ruth TJ, Sossi V, Schulzer M, Calne DB, Stoessl AJ. Expectation and dopamine release: mechanism of the placebo effect in Parkinson's disease. *Science.* 2001;293:1164–1166.

41. Bernstein JE, Swift R. Relief of intractable pruritus with naloxone. *Arch Dermatol.* 1979;115:1366–1367.

42. Thornton JR, Losowsky MS. Opioid peptides and primary biliary cirrhosis. *Br Med J.* 1988;297:1501–1504.

43. Carson KL, Tran TT, Cotton P, Sharara AI, Hunt CM. Pilot study of the use of naltrexone to treat the severe pruritus of cholestatic liver disease. *Am J Gastroenterol.* 1996;91: 1022–1023.

44. Wolfhagen FHJ, Sternieri E, Hop WCJ, Vitale G, Bertolotti M, van Buuren HR. Oral naltrexone treatment for cholestatic pruritus: a double-blind, placebo-controlled study. *Gastroenterology*. 1997;113:1264–1269.

45. Neuberger J, Jones EA. Liver transplantation for intractable pruritus is contraindicated before an adequate trial of opiate antagonist therapy. *Eur J Gastroenterol Hepatol*. 2001;13:1393–1394.

46. Terg R, Coronel E, Sorda J, Munoz AE, Findor J. Efficacy and safety of oral naltrexone treatment for pruritus of cholestasis, a crossover, double blind, placebo-controlled study. *J Hepatol*. 2002;37:717–722.

47. Mansour-Ghanaei F, Taheri A, Froutan H, et al. Effect of oral naltrexone on pruritus in cholestatic patients. *World J Gastroenterol*. 2006;12:1125–1128.

48. Horta ML, Ramos L, Goncalves ZR. The inhibition of epidural morphine-induced pruritus by epidural droperidol. *Anesth Analg*. 2000;90:638–641.

49. Horta ML, Ramos L, Goncalves Zda R, de Oliveira MA, Tonellotto D, Teixeira JP, de Melo PR. Inhibition of epidural morphine-induced pruritus by intravenous droperidol. The effect of increasing the doses of morphine and of droperidol. *Reg Anesth*. 1996;21:312–317.

50. Baldessarini RJ. Drugs and the treatment of psychiatric disorders. In: Molinoff PB, Ruddon RW, eds. *The Pharmacological Basis of Therapeutics*. New York: McGraw-Hill; 1996: 399–430.

51. Coté L, Crutcher M: The basal ganglia. In: Kandel ER, Scwartz JH, Jessell TM, eds. *Principles of Neural Science*. Norwalk: Appleton and Lange; 1991:647–659.

52. McFarland NR, Haber SN. Thalamic relay nuclei of the basal ganglia form both reciprocal and nonreciprocal cortical connections, linking multiple frontal cortical areas. *J Neurosci*. 2002;22:8117–8132.

53. Reimann W. Inhibition by GABA, baclofen and gabapentin of dopamine release from rabbit caudate nucleus: are there common or different sites of action? *Eur J Pharmacol*. 1983;94:341–344.

54. Andrews N, Loomis S, Blake R, Ferrigan L, Singh L, McKnight AT. Effect of gabapentin-like compounds on development and maintenance of morphine-induced conditioned place preference. *Psychopharmacology (Berl)*. 2001;157:381–387.

55. Shneker BF, McAuley JW. Pregabalin: a new neuromodulator with broad therapeutic indications. *Ann Pharmacother*. 2005;39:2029–2037.

56. Ehrchen J, Stander S. Pregabalin in the treatment of chronic pruritus. *J Am Acad Dermatol*. 2008;58:S36–S37.

57. Crevits L. Brachioradial pruritus – a peculiar neuropathic disorder. *Clin Neurol Neurosurg*. 2006;108:803–805.

58. Lindia JA, Kohler MG, Martin WJ, Abbadie C. Relationship between sodium channel NaV1.3 expression and neuropathic pain behavior in rats. *Pain*. 2005;117:145–153.

59. Jesudian P, Wilson NJ. Efficacy of gabapentin in the management of pruritus of unknown origin. *Arch Dermatol*. 2005;141:1507–1509.

60. Porzio G, Aielli F, Verna L, Porto C, Tudini M, Cannita K, Ficorella C. Efficacy of pregabalin in the management of cetuximab-related itch. *J Pain Symptom Manage*. 2006;32: 397–398.

# Chapter 46
# Opioid Receptor Antagonists or Agonists

Laurent Misery

The use of agonists or antagonists against itch is surprising. Indeed, itch is known to be induced by opioids, and the use of both agonists and antagonists of a peptide is very rare in pharmacology. Understanding the mechanism needs physiopathological data.

## 46.1 The Opioid System and Pruritus

Opioids have three receptors in primates: μ (MOR), κ(KOR), and δ (DOR). Opioid drugs (heroin, morphine, codeine, analgesics) can induce itch. Systemic administration of μ agonists produces scratching but κ agonists or δ agonists evoke scratching.[1] This phenomenon is not mediated by histamine. On the contrary, κ agonists are able to inhibit opioid-induced itch by preventing or reversing it,[2] as well as μ antagonists.[3] These agonists were developed for the treatment of heroin or alcohol dependence and for symptom reversal of postanesthetic depression, narcotic overdose, and opioid intoxication.

Physiological opioids (enkephalins, endorphins, dynorphins) are involved in itch pathophysiogeny, especially in atopic dermatitis (AD) and probably uremic or hepatic pruritus. The main peptides are β endorphin (MOR agonist) and dynorphin A (KOR agonist). They act at central, spinal, and peripheral levels. Histamine-independent opiate-dependent itch seems to be elicited in the epidermal unmyelinated C fibers.[4] Behavior experiments reveal that MOR and KOR knockout mice scratch less after induction of dry skin dermatitis than wild-type mice. These results indicate that MOR and KOR are important in skin homeostasis, epidermal nerve fiber regulation, and pathophysiology of itching.[5] Only the κ-opioid system, not the μ-opioid system, is downregulated in the epidermis of patients with AD.

The downregulation of the μ-opioid system and the restoration of the κ-opioid system by psoralen and ultraviolet A (PUVA) therapy were observed in patients with AD, concomitant with a decrease of itch visual analog scale (VAS) scores. These results suggest that epidermal opioid systems are strongly associated with the modulation of pruritus in AD.[6] This new finding may help us to understand the control mechanism of peripheral itch.

## 46.2 μ-Receptor Antagonists

The pharmacological control of opioid-induced itch was studied in many clinical trials. In a meta-analysis,[7] most MOR antagonists were efficacious: intravenous naloxone 0.25–2.4 μg/kg/h, relative risk 2.31 (95% confidence interval, 1.5–3.54), number needed to treat to prevent pruritus compared with control 3.5; oral naltrexone 9 mg, relative risk 2.80 (1.35–5.80), number needed to treat 1.7; naltrexone 6 mg was less effective and 3 mg did not work; different intravenous and epidural nalbuphine regimens, relative risk 1.71 (1.12–2.62), number needed to treat 4.2. Intravenous nalmefene 0.5 or 1 mg was not antipruritic.

Fifty patients with pruritus caused by internal diseases, hydroxyethyl starch, contact with water, cutaneous lymphoma, AD, xerosis cutis, macular amyloidosis, psoriasis, and other skin disorders as well as with pruritus of unknown origin were randomly selected to receive naltrexone 50 mg daily.[8] A significant therapeutic response was achieved in 35 of the 50 patients within 1 week (confidence limits of 0.55 and 0.82 at a confidence level of 0.95). Naltrexone had high antipruritic effect in 9 of 17 cases of prurigo nodularis and contributed to healing of the skin lesions. Tachyphylaxis was infrequent

L. Misery and S. Ständer (eds.), *Pruritus*,
DOI 10.1007/978-1-84882-322-8_46, © Springer-Verlag London Limited 2010

(6/50), occurred late, and could be counterbalanced by raising the dosage in two patients. Adverse drug effects were restricted to the first 2 weeks of treatment and included nausea (11/50), fatigue (3/50), dizziness, and heartburn and diarrhea (1/50 each).

Sixteen patients with pruritus of chronic cholestasis were randomized to receive naltrexone (4-week course of 50 mg naltrexone daily) or placebo.[9] Mean changes with respect to baseline were significantly different, in favor of the naltrexone group, for daytime itching (–54% vs. 8%) and nighttime itching (–44% vs. 7%). In four patients treated with naltrexone, side effects (transient in three cases) consistent with an opiate withdrawal syndrome were noted. Naltrexone and 6β-naltrexol levels did not differ between patients and controls, and there was no significant association with treatment response.

In uremic pruritus, one clinical trial proved efficacious,[10] another gave contradictory results,[11] and a third suggested that naltrexone is effective only in some patients.[12]

Eleven atopic patients participated in our double-blind study. Either 25 mg of naltrexone (Nemexin) or a placebo was given to the participants 60 min prior to the intracutaneous injection of acetylcholine.[13] A placebo stimulus with buffered saline served as control on the opposite forearm. Oral naltrexone reduced the perifocal itch significantly. In four of our observations, the area of alloknesis completely disappeared. Itch duration was reduced by 20 s and the intensity of itch was diminished, but not significantly. Naltrexone had no significant effects on cholinergic vasoreactions measured by the laser Doppler.

Naltrexone exerted an antipruritic effect on chloroquine-induced itch, but this effect was not clearly superior to that of promethazine.[14]

## 46.3 κ-Receptor Agonists

The inhibitory effects of KOR agonists TRK-820 on systemic skin scratching induced by the intravenous administration of morphine, a micro-opioid receptor agonist, were investigated in rhesus monkeys. Intravenous pretreatment with KOR agonists, either TRK-820 at 0.25 and 0.5 μg/kg or U-50488H at 64 and 128 μg/kg, inhibited systemic skin scratching induced by morphine at 1 mg/kg, i.v., in a dose-dependent manner.

By the intragastric route, apparent inhibitory effects on morphine-induced systemic skin scratching were evident following pretreatment with TRK-820 at 4 μg/kg but not with U-50488H from 512 to 2048 μg/kg. These results suggest that TRK-820 produces antipruritic effects on i.v. morphine-induced systemic skin scratching and is more readily absorbed intragastrically than U-50488H, resulting in high bioavailability in the intragastric route.[15] Similar results were observed in mice,[16] and KOR agonists are found to be effective in both antihistamine-sensitive and antihistamine-resistant pruritus.[16]

Two multicenter, randomized, double-blind, placebo-controlled studies enrolled 144 patients with uremic pruritus to postdialysis intravenous treatment with either nalfurafine or placebo for 2–4 weeks. A meta-analysis approach was used to assess the efficacy of nalfurafine. Statistically significant reductions in worst itching and itching intensity and sleep disturbances were noted in the nalfurafine group as compared with that of the placebo. Improvements in itching and excoriations were noted for the patients treated with nalfurafine. Nalfurafine showed similar types and incidences of drug-related adverse events as did placebo. In conclusion, nalfurafine was shown to be an effective and safe compound for use in this severely ill patient population.[17]

Intranasal butarphenol may be used in the treatment of itch but studies on this product are lacking, which is also an MOR antagonist.[18]

## 46.4 δ-Receptor Antagonists

Specific DOR antagonists are poorly studied. Nonetheless, intravenous or epidural droperidol 2.5 mg is efficacious on opioid-induced itch.[7,19]

## 46.5 Topical Treatments

Two separate studies to evaluate the efficacy of topically applied naltrexone were conducted with different objectives.[20] In the open study, more than 70% of the patients using the 1% naltrexone cream experienced a significant reduction of pruritus. The placebo-controlled, crossover trial demonstrated clearly that the cream containing naltrexone had an overall 29.4%

better effect compared with placebo. The formulation containing naltrexone required a median of 46 min to reduce the itch symptoms to 50%; for placebo it took 74 min. A liposomal butarphenol preparation could be useful in the treatment of itch,[21] but no clinical trial has been performed at the time of writing.

# References

1. Ko MC, Song MS, Edwards T, Lee H, Naughton NN. The role of central mu opioid receptors in opioid-induced itch in primates. *J Pharmacol Exp Ther.* 2004;310:169–176.

2. Ko MC, Lee H, Song MS, et al. Activation of kappa-opioid receptors inhibits pruritus evoked by subcutaneous or intrathecal administration of morphine in monkeys. *J Pharmacol Exp Ther.* 2003;305:173–179.

3. Ständer S, Weisshaar E, Luger T. Neurophysiological and neurochemical basis of modern pruritus treatment. *Exper Dermatol.* 2008;17:161–169.

4. Bigliardi-Qi M, Lipp B, Sumanovski LT, Buechner SA, Bigliardi PL. Changes of epidermal mu-opiate receptor expression and nerve endings in chronic atopic dermatitis. *Dermatology (Basel, Switzerland).* 2005;210:91–99.

5. Bigliardi-Qi M, Gaveriaux-Ruff C, Pfaltz K, et al. Deletion of mu- and kappa-opioid receptors in mice changes epidermal hypertrophy, density of peripheral nerve endings, and itch behavior. *J Invest Dermatol.* 2007;127:1479–1488.

6. Tominaga M, Ogawa H, Takamori K. Possible roles of epidermal opioid systems in pruritus of atopic dermatitis. *J Invest Dermatol.* 2007;127:2228–2235.

7. Kjellberg F, Tramer MR. Pharmacological control of opioid-induced pruritus: a quantitative systematic review of randomized trials. *Eur J Anaesthesiol.* 2001;18:346–357.

8. Metze D, Reimann S, Beissert S, Luger T. Efficacy and safety of naltrexone, an oral opiate receptor antagonist, in the treatment of pruritus in internal and dermatological diseases. *J Am Acad Dermatol.* 1999;41:533–539.

9. Wolfhagen FH, Sternieri E, Hop WC, Vitale G, Bertolotti M, Van Buuren HR. Oral naltrexone treatment for cholestatic pruritus:

10. Peer G, Kivity S, Agami O. Randomized cross-over trial of naltrexone in uremic pruritus. *Lancet.* 1996;348:1552–1554.

11. Pauli-Magnus C, Mikus G, Alscher D, et al. Naltrexone does not relieve uremic pruritus: Results of a randomized, double-blind, placebo-controlled crossover study. *J Am Soc Nephrol.* 2000;11:514–519.

12. Legroux-Crespel E, Cledes J, Misery L. A comparative study on the effects of naltrexone and loratadine on uremic pruritus. *Dermatology (Basel, Switzerland).* 2004;208:326–330.

13. Heyer G, Groene D, Martus P. Efficacy of naltrexone on acetylcholine-induced alloknesis in atopic eczema. *Exper Dermatol.* 2002;11:448–455.

14. Ajayi A, Kolawole B, Udoh S. Endogenous opioids, mu-opiate receptors and chloroquine-induced pruritus: a double-blind comparison of naletrexone and promethazine in patients with malaria fever who have an established history of generalized chloroquine-induced pruritus. *Int J Dermatol.* 2004;43:972–977.

15. Wakasa Y, Fujiwara A, Umeuchi H, et al. Inhibitory effects of TRK-820 on systemic skin scratching induced by morphine in rhesus monkeys. *Life Sci.* 2004;75:2947–2957.

16. Togashi Y, Umeuchi H, Okano K, et al. Antipruritic activity of the kappa-opioid receptor agonist, TRK-820. *Eur J Pharmacol.* 2002;35:259–264.

17. Wikstrom B, Gellert R, Ladefoged SD, et al. Kappa-opioid system in uremic pruritus: multicenter, randomized, double-blind, placebo-controlled clinical studies. *J Am Soc Nephrol.* 2005;16:3742–3747.

18. Dawn AG, Yosipovitch G. Butorphanol for treatment of intractable pruritus. *J Am Acad Dermatol.* 2006;54:527–531.

19. Lee IH, Lee IO. The antipruritic and antiemetic effects of epidural droperidol: a study of three methods of administration. *Anesth Analg.* 2007;105:251–255.

20. Bigliardi PL, Stammer H, Jost G, Rufli T, Buchner S, Bigliardi-Qi M. Treatment of pruritus with topically applied opiate receptor antagonist. *J Am Acad Dermatol.* 2007;56:979–988.

21. Lim GJ, Ishiuji Y, Dawn A, et al. In vitro and in vivo characterization of a novel liposomal butorphanol formulation for treatment of pruritus. *Acta dermato-venereologica.* 2008;88:327–330.

a double-blind, placebo-controlled study. *Gastroenterology.* 1997;113:1264–1269.

# Chapter 47
# Serotonin Reuptake Inhibitors and Other Antidepressants in the Treatment of Chronic Pruritus

Zbigniew Zylicz and Małgorzata Krajnik

## 47.1 Introduction

The idea that antidepressants may be useful in the treatment of chronic pruritus appeared sometime in the 1990s. Although Zylicz et al. published a report in 1998 involving a series of patients suffering from various types of pruritus who responded to paroxetine,[1] Browning et al.[2] reported in 2003 on a group of 32 patients with primary biliary cirrhosis, also suffering from pruritus and having been observed for a mean of 7.5 years. In six out of seven patients who had been given sertaline initially for the treatment of depressive symptoms pruritus unexpectedly improved considerably, and in three of those subjects it completely disappeared.

The first patient seen by Zylicz et al.[1] was a man with lung cancer suffering from intractable severe pruritus accompanying bullous pemphigoid. As this patient attempted suicide on the ward, he was diagnosed with major depression and started on paroxetine. To the surprise of the attending doctor, his pruritus ceased within 3 days and the skin, heavily damaged by bullae and scratching, healed within a week. Subsequently, the same authors treated four other patients with different types of pruritus with the same dose of paroxetine and observed a similar positive effect.[1]

Based on this first serendipitous anecdotal report, Diehn and Tefferi treated 10 patients suffering pruritus in the course of polycythemia vera with paroxetine 20 mg and one patient with fluoxetine.[3, 4] All the patients had a favorable response, which included complete or near-complete resolution of pruritus in 8 out of 10 patients. Patients rated paroxetine and hydroxyzine as the most effective antipruritic drugs. It was not until 2003 that the first controlled trials were published. The first was by Zylicz et al., who were looking at the effect of paroxetine on a population of patients mainly with paraneoplastic pruritus.[5] This was followed by a trial with sertraline, performed by Mayo et al.[6] on 21 patients with primary biliary cirrhosis. More recently, Ständer et al. published a large series of 72 patients randomized to either receive paroxetine or fluvoxamine for pruritus due to a variety of mainly dermatological conditions (Ständer et al., 2009)[7]. All three studies showed considerable efficacy in the treatment of severe pruritus. In addition, a single case of psychogenic pruritus was reported to respond to paroxetine.[8]

It is possible that mirtazapine may also have an antipruritic effect similar to selective serotonin reuptake inhibitors (SSRIs), without producing as many adverse effects. Indeed, an antipruritic effect has been reported[9–12] but controlled studies are still missing.

Interestingly, SSRIs, in a manner similar to other antipruritic agents, had occasionally been reported as drugs that caused pruritus.[13] Discontinuation of paroxetine may also trigger severe pruritus.[14] Pruritus had also been reported after eating chocolate while being treated with fluoxetine and paroxetine.[15]

## 47.2 The Strengths and Weaknesses of the Available Evidence

A trial by Zylicz et al.[5] with paroxetine was performed in two hospices, with a heterogeneous patient population representing this kind of environment: 17/26 patients had solid tumors; 4/26 had haematological malignancies; and 5/26 had various nonmalignant or idiopathic conditions. Because of the advanced nature of their diseases, the trial needed to be short and the crossover took place after one week. A later trial by a Ständer et al.[7] showed that although some patients

L. Misery and S. Ständer (eds.), *Pruritus*,
DOI 10.1007/978-1-84882-322-8_47, © Springer-Verlag London Limited 2010

respond rapidly within the first week of treatment, evaluation of the treatment could only be carried out several weeks later. Because of the lack of a wash-out period in the trial by Zylicz et al.,[1] the differentiation between the effects of the drug and those of the placebo might have been underestimated in their article, in that there was no carry-over effect. However, one patient who was treated with paroxetine in the first week without showing any significant response exhibited response in the second week while on placebo. In this trial there was no opportunity to titrate the dose to the effect, and many patients still experienced severe adverse effects, mainly nausea and vomiting. Two patients needed to discontinue treatment (they had both been on paroxetine) because of severe adverse effects. The secondary end point of treatment, which was a 50% reduction in itch intensity, was robust and probably compensated for other shortcomings in the trial. In general, this trial showed a mean difference between the placebo and paroxetine of 0.78 (95%CI 0.37–1.19). Nine out of 24 patients (37.5%) fulfilled the criteria of response.

The trial with sertraline performed by Mayo et al.[6] comprised a much more homogenous population of patients with primary biliary cirrhosis and tormented by itch. The drug was in the first open-label part of the study, carefully titrated to effect, and the patients were randomized to be either treated for 6 weeks with sertraline or placebo. After a robust 4-week wash-out period, the patients were crossed over to the other treatment, again for 6 weeks. Only 12/21 patients completed such a long and strenuous study. The dynamics of biliary cirrhosis could not be compared with those of advanced cancer, as in the trial by Zylicz et al.[5] However, it is still possible that the liver function and intensity of the itch might have changed over the course of 4 months and the first period might not be fully comparable with the second. Patients randomized to either sertraline or the placebo were not sertraline naïve, and the drug given in the open-label titration phase could have had a profound and durable effect on itch in the placebo group. In this trial, the optimum sertraline dose (75–100 mg/day) was well tolerated. Pruritus in patients treated with sertraline improved by 1.86 net raw points, while pruritus in patients treated with the placebo worsened by 0.38 points (net beneficial effect 2.24 points p = 0.009). As expected, the response rate in the open-label part of the study was much higher than in the double-blind

section. Blinding was not ideal, as the patients could recognize the active drug.

The third trial by Ständer et al.[7] comprised a much larger number of patients (72) but, again, the population was more heterogeneous. This time, the patients were recruited for the trial within the dermatology clinic and there were many patients with itch and dermatoses, something that was lacking in the previous two trials. Interestingly, this trial included numerous patients with itchy atopic dermatitis and other conditions traditionally seen as treatable with antihistamines. This trial, however, was not placebo-controlled and the patients were randomized either into the paroxetine or fluvoxamine arms. The observations carried out within this design gave valuable information about the time to response and time to relapse. Forty nine of the 72 patients (68.0%) experienced a weak ($n=9$), good ($n=16$) or very good ($n=24$) antipruritic effect. Statistical analysis proved that the efficacy of paroxetine and fluvoxamine was without significant difference suggesting class effect of the drugs.

## 47.3 What Kind of Pruritus Can Be Treated with SSRIs?

In general, the three trials discussed here, supported by noncontrolled observations,[3,4] suggest that SSRIs act on a wide range of pruritus types, from primary dermatoses complicated by itch to systemic diseases such as cholestasis and cancer. The result is not robust enough to state that SSRIs would reduce the intensity of all kinds of itch, and several types of itch were not fully represented in all three trials. We do not have any suggestion that paroxetine or fluvoxamine would be helpful in the case of itch in the course of Hodgkin lymphoma or in the case of neuropathic itch. Also, in the trial by Ständer et al.[7], none of the patients with cutaneous lymphoma responded to either paroxetine or fluvoxamine, which is consistent with unpublished observations by the authors of this chapter. There are enough data to suggest that SSRIs would be effective as the first-line treatment of itch in cholestasis and paraneoplastic itch. However, the authors of this chapter tried paroxetine several times when the opioid antagonists failed in the treatment of pruritus in cholestasis but found the treatment ineffective.[28,29]

The available data suggest that SSRIs act centrally upon the regulation of the conveyance of the itch and less so at the periphery.

## 47.4  Is the Effect of SSRIs a Class Effect or Can It Be Assigned to Specific Drugs?

This question is difficult to answer because only a few drugs in this class have been studied. The three drugs studied were paroxetine, sertraline, and fluvoxamine. These drugs do not differ widely in their ability to inhibit radioligand binding in vitro to rat brains.[30] Neither, clinically, are there any suggestions that one of these drugs is better than the other. The trial by Ständer et al.[7] compared paroxetine directly with fluvoxamine and found paroxetine insignificantly better and fluvoxamine insignificantly less toxic. The fact that some patients may also respond to mirtazapine[10] suggests that a wide range of drugs affecting serotonin reuptake may share similar properties. For the time being, clinicians should consider one of the three SSRIs tested and not 'just' an SSRI.

## 47.5  What Kinds of Side Effects Are Encountered During Treatment with SSRIs and What Are the Strategies to Overcome Them?

The most cumbersome adverse effects sometimes prompting the early discontinuation of therapy are nausea and vomiting. These adverse effects, however, are preventable by slow titration,[6] which may take weeks. When nausea and vomiting are present, cisapride may be effective,[5] although this drug has now been withdrawn from the market. In current clinical practice, ondansetron, which specifically inhibits $5HT_3$ receptors, is used most often. Ondansetron may also help to suppress pruritus.[31] Another problem signalled by some patients is sleeplessness and agitation. This adverse effect was studied in detail by Mayo et al.[6] However, sleeplessness due to pruritus was replaced by the insomnia induced by sertraline. These patients slept as well on sertraline as with the placebo. So, after

all, the patients did not experience it as being especially annoying. Some patients on long-term SSRIs suffer from sexual dysfunction and, when this is worse than the itch, the patient may be tried on mirtazapine, although the evidence for this move is lacking. Two patients in the trial by Mayo et al.[6] reported unusual visual hallucinations, not usually seen in depressed patients treated with SSRIs. Many patients reported an improvement in their mood, even though they were not previously thought to be depressed (see below).

## 47.6  What Is the Presumptive Mechanism of Action of SSRIs in Pruritus?

Based on the evidence obtained until now, one cannot say anything about the mechanism of action for SSRIs in pruritus. It is not even certain whether the quality one is looking for is dependent on the serotonin reuptake inhibition. If this is the case, SSRIs may act as a modulation on the conveyance of the ascending itch signals. By this effect, SSRIs may counterbalance the effects of opioids. There are multiple suggestions that SSRIs interact with the opioidergic system.[32–34] However, in the present context this remains speculative. SSRIs deplete the platelets from serotonin[35] and this mechanism may be important at least in the pruritus which is a complication of polycythemia vera.[36] However, all SSRIs, especially paroxetine, sertraline, and fluvoxamine are potent inhibitors of CYP2D6 oxidases.[37] This inhibition may interfere with the metabolism of one or more pruritogens, although evidence for this is equally lacking.

## 47.7  How Rapid Are the Antipruritic Effects of SSRIs and How Long Do Patients Need to Be Treated Before SSRIs Can Be Discontinued?

From the evidence published, one may infer that the effect of SSRIs on pruritus is usually rapid, although the full effectiveness of the therapy can be assessed only after several weeks. In the trial by Ständer et al.[7], the antipruritic effect was experienced within the first week in 12/49 patients (24.5% of responding patients), in the second week in 12/49 patients (24.5%), up to the fourth week in 11/49 patients (22.5%) or up to the eighth week in 8/49 patients (16.3%), while 6/49 patients responded after 8 weeks (12.2%). Accordingly, the duration for achieving the maximal antipruritic effect ranged from 3 days to 34 weeks. The trial by Mayo et al.[6] was not designed to assess the time to response because of its slow titration and randomization after titration. The trial by Zylicz et al.,[5] by its short observation time delivered from several single cases reported initially,[1] probably underestimated the efficacy by a factor of 3–4.

## 47.8 Is the Antipruritic Effect of SSRIs Sustained and Stable?

None of the trials was really designed to answer this important question. Ständer et al.[7] concluded that both the paroxetine and fluvoxamine effect on pruritus was prolonged and sustained. However, in several patients the authors needed to increase the dose of the drugs. During treatment of patients outside the trial, it was frequently noted by the authors of this chapter that the effect of paroxetine may sometimes subside after several weeks. They did not increase the dose to levels as high as those described by Ständer et al., probably because of their patients' poorer general condition. Tefferi, who reported on the longitudinal treatment of pruritus in polycythemia vera,[3, 4] informed the authors personally that none of his patients showed this kind of effect but, as he told us, one should never stop other cytoreductive measures and rely on antipruritic drugs alone. As in palliative care, when cytoreductive or disease-oriented options have been exhausted and the patients cannot tolerate high doses of SSRIs, it is probable that tachyphylaxis and loss of efficacy will be seen more often.

## 47.9 Does the Itch Come Back After Discontinuation of the SSRIs?

The itch suppressed by the SSRIs may reappear after discontinuation of the treatment. However, it was noted that the intensity that appeared after discontinuation of

treatment might last for much less time than before (unpublished observations). Two patients withdrawn from the study by Zylicz et al.[5] because of adverse effects reported that even after one and two doses of paroxetine, respectively, their itch was suppressed for a period of several weeks. One should not forget that pruritus may emerge after the discontinuation of paroxetine, even if the symptom did not exist prior to therapy.[14]

## 47.10 Do Patients Need to Be Depressed to Have an Antipruritic Response to SSRIs?

This problem was addressed both by Mayo et al.[6] and Ständer et al.[7] In both studies, patients were assessed for their depression, and in both studies it was found that depressed patients responded equally well to SSRIs as the nondepressed. The onset of an antipruritic effect can be very rapid (within days 5) but on average it is 4.9 weeks (Ständer et al.,[7]). This fact does not preclude that the antipruritic effect has nothing to do with the antidepressive effect of the drugs.

## 47.11 The Antipruritic Effect of Tricyclic Antidepressants

Also, other antidepressants, mainly tricyclic ones, have an antipruritic effect. For example, a favorable effect of doxepin, a tricyclic antidepressant, was reported in the treatment of pruritus. Doxepin was used topically as a 5% cream and was found to be effective in the prevention of pruritus induced by histamine[16] and acetylocholine[17] in volunteers. In the first study,[16] topical amitriptyline and diphenhydramine showed similar effects. The antipruritic effect of tricyclic antidepressants was attributed to the antihistaminic effect of these drugs. This concept was proven in patients with atopic dermatitis complicated by itch, who were treated with 5% doxepin in a one-week-long trial.[18] The results were favorable, although some patients (39/270) reported an unpleasant stinging sensation after application of the cream. Low-dose oral doxepin apparently also had a significant antipruritic effect.[19] In two controlled trials more recently, doxepin was found to be equally effective as hydroxizine in the treatment of pruritus induced by sulfur mustard.[20,21] Based on these scarce clinical data, doxepin, both oral and topical, is mentioned in numerous guidelines as the drug of choice.[22-27] Amitriptyline has never been reported to be clinically active as an antipruritic agent. Due to the presumptive antihistaminic effect of doxepin and the fact that many forms of chronic pruritus, especially those without dermatosis, are relatively insensitive to antihistamines, the authors decided to concentrate on the antipruritic effects of SSRIs in this chapter.

## 47.12 Conclusion

Evidence analyzed in this chapter suggests that SSRIs, here narrowed down to paroxetine, sertraline, and fluvoxamine, may be used as the first line of treatment for pruritus accompanying different conditions. Indications may include pruritus of cholestasis and paraneoplastic pruritus. However, other conditions may also be treated. If possible, the treatment should be accompanied by cytoreductive or disease-oriented treatment. In addition, patients should continue using moisturisers and other measures that help to control pruritus. In most cases, antihistamines can be discontinued with the exception of dermatological diseases usually sensitive to these drugs. The adverse effects are common but most appear in the first week(s) of treatment and can be avoided by careful titration or the use of specific drugs such as antiemetics. The antipruritic effect can have a rapid onset, but on average it takes several weeks to reach maximal effect. The effect is usually sustained but several patients may need dose escalation. The mechanism by which the antipruritic effect of SSRIs occurs is still unknown. It may be similar to the antidepressive effect.

## References

1. Zylicz Z, Smits C, Krajnik M. Paroxetine for pruritus in advanced cancer. *J Pain Symptom Manage*. 1998;16: 121–124.
2. Browning J, Combes B, Mayo MJ. Long-term efficacy of sertraline as a treatment for cholestatic pruritus in patients with primary biliary cirrhosis. *Am J Gastroenterol*. 2003;98: 2736–2741.
3. Diehn F, Tefferi A. Pruritus in polycythaemia vera: prevalence, laboratory correlates and management. *Br J Haematol*. 2001;115:619–621.
4. Tefferi A, Fonseca R. Selective serotonin reuptake inhibitors are effective in the treatment of polycythemia vera-associated pruritus. *Blood*. 2002;99:2627.
5. Zylicz Z, Krajnik M, Sorge AA, Costantini M. Paroxetine in the treatment of severe non-dermatological pruritus: a randomized, controlled trial. *J Pain Symptom Manage*. 2003;26: 1105–1112.
6. Mayo MJ, Handem I, Saldana S, Jacobe H, Getachew Y, Rush AJ. Sertraline as a first-line treatment for cholestatic pruritus. *Hepatology*. 2007;45:666–674.
7. Stander S, Bockenholt B, Schurmeyer-Horst F, Weishaupt C, Heuft G, Luger TA, Schneider G. Treatment of chronic pruritus with the selective serotonin re-uptake inhibitors paroxetine and fluvoxamine: results of an open-labelled, two-arm proof-of-concept study. *Acta Derm Venereol* 2009;89: 45–51.
8. Biondi M, Arcangeli T, Petrucci RM. Paroxetine in a case of psychogenic pruritus and neurotic excoriations. *Psychother Psychosom*. 2000;69:165–166.
9. Hundley JL, Yosipovitch G. Mirtazapine for reducing nocturnal itch in patients with chronic pruritus: a pilot study. *J Am Acad Dermatol*. 2004;50:889–891.
10. Davis MP, Frandsen JL, Walsh D, Andresen S, Taylor S. Mirtazapine for pruritus. *J Pain Symptom Manage*. 2003;25: 288–291.
11. Demierre MF, Taverna J. Mirtazapine and gabapentin for reducing pruritus in cutaneous T-cell lymphoma. *J Am Acad Dermatol*. 2006;55:543–544.
12. Dawn A, Yosipovitch G. Treating itch in psoriasis. *Dermatol Nurs*. 2006;18:227–233.
13. Spigset O. Adverse reactions of selective serotonin reuptake inhibitors: reports from a spontaneous reporting system. *Drug Saf*. 1999;20:277–287.
14. Mazzatenta C, Peonia G, Martini P. Pruritus induced by interruption of paroxetine therapy. *Br J Dermatol*. 2004; 150:787.
15. Cederberg J, Knight S, Svenson S, Melhus H. Itch and skin rash from chocolate during fluoxetine and sertraline treatment: case report. *BMC Psychiatry*. 2004;4:36.
16. Bernstein JE, Whitney DH, Soltani K. Inhibition of histamine-induced pruritus by topical tricyclic antidepressants. *J Am Acad Dermatol*. 1981;5:582–585.
17. Groene D, Martus P, Heyer G. Doxepin affects acetylcholine induced cutaneous reactions in atopic eczema. *Exp Dermatol*. 2001;10:110–117.
18. Drake LA, Fallon JD, Sober A. Relief of pruritus in patients with atopic dermatitis after treatment with topical doxepin cream. The Doxepin Study Group. *J Am Acad Dermatol*. 1994;31:613–616.
19. Smith PF, Corelli RL. Doxepin in the management of pruritus associated with allergic cutaneous reactions. *Ann Pharmacother*. 1997;31:633–635.
20. Shohrati M, Tajik A, Harandi AA, Davoodi SM, Akmasi M. Comparison of hydroxyzine and doxepin in treatment of pruritus due to sulfur mustard. *Skinmed*. 2007;6:70–72.
21. Shohrati M, Davoudi SM, Keshavarz S, Sadr B, Tajik A. Cetirizine, doxepin, and hydroxyzine in the treatment of pruritus due to sulfur mustard: a randomized clinical trial. *Cutan Ocul Toxicol*. 2007;26:249–255.
22. Greaves MW. Itch in systemic disease: therapeutic options. *Dermatol Ther*. 2005;18:323–327.

23. Arnold LM, Auchenbach MB, McElroy SL. Psychogenic excoriation. Clinical features, proposed diagnostic criteria, epidemiology and approaches to treatment. *CNS Drugs*. 2001;15:351–359.

24. Nowak MA, Tsoukas MM, Delmus FA, Falanga V, Brodell RT. Generalized pruritus without primary lesions. Differential diagnosis and approach to treatment. *Postgrad Med*. 2000;107:41–42, 5–6.

25. Greiding L, Moreno P. Doxepin incorporated into a dermatologic cream: an assessment of both doxepin antipruritic action and doxepin action as an inhibitor of papules, in allergen and histamine-caused pruritus. *Allergol Immunopathol (Madr)*. 1999;27:265–270.

26. Millikan LE. Treating pruritus. What's new in safe relief of symptoms? *Postgrad Med*. 1996;99:173–176, 9–84.

27. Anonymous. Doxepin cream for pruritus. *Med Lett Drugs Ther*. 1994;36:99–100.

28. Zylicz Z, Stork N, Krajnik M. Severe pruritus of cholestasis in disseminated cancer: developing a rational treatment strategy. A case report. *J Pain Symptom Manage*. 2005;29: 100–103.

29. Jones EA, Zylicz Z. Treatment of pruritus caused by cholestasis with opioid antagonists. *J Palliat Med*. 2005;8:1290–1294.

30. Johnson AM. The comparative pharmacological properties of selective serotonine re-uptake inhibitors in animals. In: Feighner JP, Boyer, W.F,, eds. *Selective Serotonin Re-uptake Inhibitors*. Chichester, Willey; 1991:37–70.

31. O'Donohue JW, Pereira SP, Ashdown AC, Haigh CG, Wilkinson JR, Williams R. A controlled trial of ondansetron in the pruritus of cholestasis. *Aliment Pharmacol Ther*. 2005;21:1041–1045.

32. Narita N, Hashimoto K, Tomitaka S, Minabe Y. Interactions of selective serotonin reuptake inhibitors with subtypes of sigma receptors in rat brain. *Eur J Pharmacol*. 1996;307: 117–119.

33. Gray AM. The effect of fluvoxamine and sertraline on the opioid withdrawal syndrome: a combined in vivo cerebral microdialysis and behavioural study. *Eur Neuropsychopharmacol*. 2002;12:245–254.

34. Gray AM, Spencer PS, Sewell RD. The involvement of the opioidergic system in the antinociceptive mechanism of action of antidepressant compounds. *Br J Pharmacol*. 1998;124: 669–674.

35. Hergovich N, Aigner M, Eichler HG, Entlicher J, Drucker C, Jilma B. Paroxetine decreases platelet serotonin storage and platelet function in human beings. *Clin Pharmacol Ther*. 2000;68:435–442.

36. Fjellner B, Hagermark O. Pruritus in polycythemia vera: treatment with aspirin and possibility of platelet involvement. *Acta Derm Venereol*. 1979;59:505–512.

37. Alfaro CL, Lam YW, Simpson J, Ereshefsky L. CYP2D6 inhibition by fluoxetine, paroxetine, sertraline, and venlafaxine in a crossover study: intraindividual variability and plasma concentration correlations. *J Clin Pharmacol*. 2000;40:58–66.

# Chapter 48
# Systemic Immunosuppressants in the Treatment of Pruritus

Silvia Moretti, Francesca Prignano, and Torello Lotti

## 48.1 Background

Pruritus is a sensation that, if sufficiently strong, will provoke scratching or the desire to scratch.[1] It is perhaps the most common dermatological symptom associated not only with numerous skin diseases but also with extracutaneous disorders in the absence of any kind of objective illness. Itch is propagated by complex mechanisms located both peripherally and within the central nervous system. The concern for the patient and physician alike is the cure of chronic itch. Traditional systemic treatments have limited efficacy and new options are emerging slowly. New insights have recently been obtained in the understanding of itch transmission and physiology, and such progress can contribute to further the development of more effective therapies. In fact, the therapeutic strategies rely mainly on a deep understanding of pruritus pathophysiology. Definitions of different types of itch have been described and, although no perfect classification system of pruritus exists, one of the most accepted is the clinical one proposed by Bernhard.[2] He classifies itch into six categories: (1) dermatologic (arising from skin disorders such as psoriasis, eczema, winter itch, scabies, and urticaria; (2) systemic (arising from internal diseases such as primary cholestatic liver disease, renal failure, Hodgkin's disease, polycythemia vera, and some multifactorial [e.g., metabolic] situations); (3) neurogenic/neuropathic (arising from disorders of the central or the peripheral nervous system, such as brain tumors, multiple sclerosis, neuropathy, and nerve compression or irritation [e.g., notalgia paresthetica and brachioradial pruritus]); (4) psychogenic; (5) mixed; and (6) others.

Another classification, mainly based on an underlying pathophysiology, divides pruritus into pruritoceptive (originating from skin diseases, as in scabies or urticaria), neurogenic (originating centrally but without evidence of neural pathology, as a consequence of neurochemical activity, such as the action of opioid peptides in cholestasis), neurophatic (resulting from a primary neurological disorder, such as a brain tumor), and psychogenic (associated with psychological abnormalities, as in the delusional state of parasitophobia).[3]

Identification of distinct pathways for each type of itch can allow new therapeutic targets to be detected; therefore medical strategy is to treat the pruritus according to the diverse pathogeneses. The pruritogens cover a wide spectrum of substances that can induce pruritus: apart from histamine, which is surely the earliest one, many substances do induce – directly or indirectly – itch: proteases, amines, neuropeptides, opioids, eicosanoids, endovanilloids, endocannabinoids, growth factors, and cytokines.[4] Some of these chemicals can act by causing histamine release from local mast cells and/or by sensitizing the relevant specialized C-fibers originating superficially in the skin, which mediate itch.[4]

However, among systemic treatments, the most classic therapy is represented by the H1 and H2 antihistamines, which are very effective when itching is histamine-induced; opiate receptor antagonists can efficiently inhibit itch transmission in the case of opioid-induced pruritus; various antidepressive agents are capable of reducing itch intensity in the central nervous system; and anti-epileptics are reported to have some success in neuropathic itch.[5,6] Recently, systemic immunosuppressants have been added to medications used against itching.

L. Misery and S. Ständer (eds.), *Pruritus*,
DOI 10.1007/978-1-84882-322-8_48, © Springer-Verlag London Limited 2010

## 48.2 Systemic Immunosuppressants and Itch

Systemic immunosuppressants are mainly used to treat dermatological or pruriceptive pruritus, according to the above-mentioned classifications,[2,3] originating in the skin, especially during inflammatory processes or conditions releasing cytokines and growth factors. In fact, the dominant role of intracutaneous inflammation in itch pathogenesis and the vicious cycles of neurogenic inflammation upregulating and perpetuating chronic itch must be taken into account.[7]

Among these medications, different classes of drugs are included: thalidomide, cyclosporine, mycophenolate mofetil, and some biological agents approved for the treatment of moderate to severe psoriasis.

Thalidomide can be included in the treatment of neuropathic and pruritoceptive itch. This drug has been used for years as an immunomodulatory agent, whose immunologic effects may be substantially related to the suppression of excessive tumor necrosis factor alpha (TNF-$\alpha$) production.[6] TNF-$\alpha$ does not exert any direct pruritogenic effect, but, being a proinflammatory cytokine, it is elevated in many pruritic dermatoses. Thus the antipruritic action of this drug could be secondary to inhibition of TNF-$\alpha$.[6,8] Another possibility is that thalidomide can act as both a peripheral and a central nerve depressant.[9] Thalidomide was reported to be effective in prurigo nodularis[10] and in recalcitrant prurigo nodularis in patients who are HIV positive and unresponsive to antihistamines, topical/intralesional corticosteroids, and phototherapy.[11] The dosage of thalidomide is about 100–200 or more mg/day and it is effective within 2–3 weeks, although the treatment is to be continued for months. Of course, the severe adverse side effects of this drug must be taken into account, particularly neuropathy and teratogenicity.[8,10] Peripheral neuropathy is characterized by an acute distal, symmetric axonal involvement, with painful paresthesias of hands and feet and sensory loss in lower extremities. Rigorous examination of sensory symptoms and dose adjustment can prevent motor involvement.[12] Teratogenicity (especially deformities of the upper and lower limbs) is the most devastating adverse effect, and women of reproductive age must be monitored strictly in order to avoid pregnancy by means of appropriate tests and birth control measures.[8,12] Less severe side effects are weight increase, sedation, constipation, and mood changes.[13]

Cyclosporine has also been known to decrease pruritus intensity, e.g., in atopic eczema.[14] It exhibits a potent inhibitory effect on T lymphocytes, suppressing the response to antigen by inhibiting cytokine secretion and proliferation. This action is produced through the inhibition of calcineurin, which is a cytoplasmic enzyme capable of promoting nuclear transcription of several cytokines, such as IL-2, $\gamma$-IFN, granulocyte-macrophage colony stimulating factor, IL-3, IL-4, TNF-$\alpha$, and others.[15] Cytokines, such as IL-2, which recruit and activate T cells, are known to be involved in inducing itch,[16] and this is the basis for the use of immunomodulators such as cyclosporine. The effectiveness of systemic cyclosporine in patients with severe atopic eczema has been recently assessed by a systematic review and meta-analysis of trials.[17] It appears that after 2 weeks of treatment, a dose-related response with a decrease in disease severity, including pruritus, is found. Reduction of symptoms severity is 22% under a low dose ($\leq 3$ mg/kg) and 40% at a dosage $\geq 4$ mg/kg.[16] Relapse after discontinuation of cyclosporine therapy is also reported, with 73% of patients relapsing within 24 weeks[18] and 86% within 9 months.[19] Adverse effects included an increase in creatinine by more than 30% compared to a baseline in 10.9% patients after months of active treatment with cyclosporine, newly diagnosed hypertension in up to 5.8%, infections in up to 12.4%, and gastrointestinal symptoms in up to 40.3%.[17] Adverse events and consequent withdrawals were observed more frequently in adults than in children and were more likely with higher dosages.[17,19]

Cyclosporine is also used in the treatment of severe chronic urticaria, and its activity seems due to, besides the potent inhibition of T lymphocytes,[15] the inhibition of basophil and mast cell degranulation.[20,21] The drug appears to be effective after at least 8 weeks of treatment.[21,22]

A new entrant into the field of immunosuppressive agents is mycophenolate mofetil, used in organ transplantation. Mycophenolate is the 2-morpho-linoethyl ester of mycophenolic acid and is rapidly adsorbed after oral administration. Mycophenolate is then hydrolyzed to its active metabolite mycophenolic acid, which potently, selectively, and reversibly inhibits inosine monophosphate dehydrogenase and thereby suppresses the de novo pathway of purine synthesis in T and B cells.[23] Lymphocytes require this pathway for purine biosynthesis, while other inflammatory cells also use a salvage pathway, making mycophenolate mofetil useful for selectively suppressing lymphocyte function and capable of minimizing unwanted effects on other cell types.[23] Mycophenolic acid also exerts its immuno-modulatory effects by inhibiting the leukocyte recruitment and glycosylation of lymphocyte glycoproteins involved in their adhesion to endothelial cells.[24] Recently, this molecule was demonstrated to have an inhibitory effect on endothelial prostaglandin E2 production, which might lower the benefits of the prostaglandin E2-triggered immune response after organ transplantation.[24] Mycophenolate appears to be a highly effective drug for treating moderate to severe atopic eczema at the dosage of 1 g twice daily for 4 weeks, followed by a dosage reduction to 500 mg twice daily during week 5 to week 8[24] or 1 g daily for the first week and 2 g daily for an additional 11 weeks,[25] with no serious adverse effects occurring in any patients. Given the favorable side-effect profile, this drug is also suggested for the treatment of severe childhood atopic dermatitis, where it has demonstrated safety and efficacy.[26] Mycophenolate mofetil may also be a valuable and safe treatment for patients with severe chronic urticaria who do not respond to antihistamines and/or corticosteroids, and who require aggressive therapy to control symptoms (pruritus!).[27] However, larger controlled trials are needed to confirm its efficacy.

As cytokines are involved in inducing itch,[4,7] the new cytokine- and T-cell-inhibiting biologics employed for psoriasis may have some role in pruritoceptive itch treatment, although all these biologics include itching as a side effect.[6] Efalizumab* is a humanized monoclonal antibody that blocks T-cell-dependent functions mediated by leukocyte function antigen-1 (LFA-1), specifically binding to the LFA-1 subunit CD11a and preventing the migration of T cells out of peripheral blood vessels into the skin and preventing T-cell stimulation.[28] Efalizumab has been shown to decrease pruritus significantly compared to a placebo during psoriasis treatment[29] and to induce significant clinical improvements in severe atopic dermatitis,[30] although controlled studies are required to test its efficacy and safety in atopic eczema. Infliximab, which is a human–mouse monoclonal antibody that binds and neutralizes soluble and receptor-bound TNF-α, has been reported to be effective in a case of long-standing severe atopic dermatis associated with contact allergy.[31] Etanercept, which is a fully human, soluble, TNF receptor-IgG1

fusion protein, was described to be a successful treatment for reducing symptoms in recalcitrant, erythroderma-associated pruritus.[32]

As new information becomes available about the links between cytokines and itching, new therapeutic options concerning immunosuppressants may be provided for patients suffering from chronic itch.

## References

1. Savin JA. How should we define itching *J Am Acad Dermatol.* 1998;38:268–269.
2. Bernhard JD. Itch and pruritus: what are they, and how should itches be classified? *Dermatol Ther.* 2005;18:288–291.
3. Yosipovitch G, Greaves MW, Schmelz M. Itch. *Lancet.* 2003;361:690–694.
4. Twycross R, Greaves MW, Handwerker H, Jones EA, Libretto SE, Szepietowski JC, Zylicz Z. Itch: scratching more than surface. *Q J Med.* 2003;96:7–26.
5. Teofoli P, Procacci P, Maresca M, Lotti T. Itch and pain. *Int J Dermatol.* 1996;35:159–166.
6. Summey BT, Yosipovitch G. Pharmacologic advances in the systemic treatment of itch. Dermatol Ther, 2005;18:328–332.
7. Paus R, Schmelz M, Birò T, Steinhoff M. Frontiers in pruritus research: scratching the brain for more effective itch therapy. *J Clin Invest.* 2006;116:1174–1185.
8. Wu JJ, Huang DB, Pang KR, Hsu S, Tyring SK. Thalidomide: dermatological indications, mechanisms of action and side-effects. *Br I Dermatol.* 2005;153:254–273.
9. Daly BM, Shuster S. Antipruritic action of thalidomide. *Acta Derm Venereol.* 2000;80:24–25.
10. Alfadley A, Al-Hawsasawi K, Therstrup-Pedersen K, Al-Aboud K. Treatment of prurigo nodularis with thalidomide: a case report and review of the literature. *Int J Dermatol.* 2003;42:372–375.
11. Maurer T, Ponceler A, Berger T. Thalidomide treatment for prurigo nodularis in human immunodeficiency virus-infected subjects. *Arch Dermatol.* 2004;140:845–849.
12. Mellin GW, Katzenstein M. The saga of thalidomide: neuropathy to embryopathy, with case reports of congenital anomalies. *N Engl J Med.* 1962;267:1184–1192.
13. Grosshans E, Illy G. Thalidomide therapy for inflammatory dermatoses. *Int J Dermatol.* 1984;23:598–602.
14. Munro CS, Levell NJ, Shuster S, Friedmann PS. Maintenance treatment with cyclosporine in atopic eczema. *Br J Dermatol.* 1994;130:376–380.
15. Berth-Jones J. The use of cyclosporine in psoriasis. *J Dermatol Treat.* 2005;16:258–277.
16. Yosipovitch G. The pruritus receptor unit: a target for novel therapies. *J Invest Dermatol.* 2007;127:1857–1859.
17. Schmitt J, Schmitt N, Meurer M. Cyclosporin in the treatment of patients with atopic eczema - a systematic review and meta-analysis. *J Eur Acad Dermatol Venereol* 2007;21:606–619.

---

* This drug is no more available at present in the market

18. Atakan N, Erden C. The efficacy, tolerability and safety of a new oral formulation of Sandimmun – Sandimmun Neoral in severe refractory atopic dermatitis. *J Eur Acad Dermatol Venereol.* 1998;11:240–246.

19. Harper JL, Ahmend I, Barclay G, et al. Cyclosporin for severe childhood atopic dermatitis: short course versus continuous therapy. *Br J Dermatol.* 2000;142:52–58.

20. Teofoli P, De Pità O, Frezzolini A, Lotti T. Antipruritic effect of oral cyclosporine A in essential senile pruritus. *Actd Derm Venereol.* 1998;78:232.

21. Kaplan AP. Chronic urticaria: pathogenesis and treatment. *J Allergy Clin Immunnol.* 2004;114:465–474.

22. Vena GA, Cassano N, Colombo D, Peruzzi E, Pigatto P. NEO-I-30 Study Group. Cyclosporine in chronic idiopathic urticaria: a double-bind, randomised, placebo controlled trial. *J Am Acad Dermatol.* 2006;55:705–709.

23. Murray ML, Cohen JB. Mycophenolate mofetil therapy for moderate to severe atopic dermatitis. *Clin Exp Dermatol.* 2006;32:23–27.

24. Grundmann-Kollmann M, Podda M, Ochsendorf F, Boehncke WH, Kaufmann R, Zollner TM. Myciphenolate mofetil is effective in the treatment of atopic dermatitis. *Arch Dermatol.* 2001;137:870–873.

25. Neuber K, Schwatz I, Itschert G, Dieck AT. Treatment of atopic eczema with oral mycophenolate mofetil. *Br J Dermatol.* 2000;143:385–391.

26. Heller M, Shin HT, Orlow SJ, Schaffer JV. Mycophenolate mofetil for severe childhood atopic dermatitis: experience in 14 patients. *Br J Dermatol.* 2007;157:127–132.

27. Shahar E, Bergman R, Guttman-Yassky E, Pollack S. Treatment of severe chronic idiopathic urticaria with oral myciphenolate mofetil in patients not responding to antihistamines and/or corticosteroids. *Int J Dermatol.* 2006;45:1224–1227.

28. Krueger J, Gottlieb AB, Miller B, Dedrick R, Garovoy M, Walicke P. Anti-CD11a treatment for psoriasis concurrently increases circulating T cells and decreases plaque T cells, consistent with inhibition of cutaneous T cell trafficking. *J Invest Dermatol.* 2000;115:333–339.

29. Menter A, Kosinski M, Bresnahan BW, Papp KA, Ware JE Jr. Impact of efalizumab on psoriasis-specific patient-reported outcomes. Results from three randomised, placebo-controlled clinical trials of moderate to severe plaque psoriasis. *J Drugs Dermatol.* 2004;3:27–38.

30. Takiguchi R, Tofte S, Simpson B, Harper E, Blauvelt A, Hanifin J, Simpson E. Efalizumab for severe atopic dermatitis: a pilot study in adults. *J Am Acad Dermatol.* 2007;56:222–227.

31. Cassano N, Loconsole F, Coviello C, Vena GA. Infliximab in recalcitrant severe atopic eczema associated with contact allergy. *Int J Immunopathol Pharmacol.* 2006;19:237–240.

32. Querfeld C, Guitart J, Kuzel TM, Rosen S. Successful treatment of recalcitrant, erythroderma-associated pruritus with etanercept. *Arch Dermatol.* 2004;140:1539–1540.

# Chapter 49
# Other Systemic Treatments

Sonja Ständer

Most of the systemic therapies have been discussed in previous chapters. There are only some therapies left to be mentioned. However, controlled studies are mostly missing and these therapies are less commonly used than others.

## 49.1 Leukotriene Receptor Antagonists

Several studies suggest a role of leukotrienes in the induction of pruritus. For example, intradermally injected leukotriene B4 is able to provoke scratching in mice.[1] Nociceptin acts on opioid receptor-like 1 (ORL1) receptor on the keratinocytes to produce leukotriene B4, which induces itch-associated responses in mice. Consequently, the leukotriene B4 receptor antagonist ONO-4057 reduces nociception-induced pruritus.[2] In addition, a correlation of nocturnal itch and high urinary leukotriene B4 levels was found in patients with atopic dermatitis (AD),[3] suggesting that leukotrienes may contribute to severe pruritus at night in AD. Leukotriene receptor-antagonists such as zafirlukast, zileuton, and montelukast block cysteinyl leukotriene receptors. Most commonly, montelukast, a leukotriene D4 receptor antagonist, is approved for asthma therapy. Montelukast has also proved its clinical efficacy in urticaria and urticaria factitia.[4, 5] According to our own experiences, patients suffering from aquagenic pruritus experienced improvement when treated with montelukast. Zafirlukast and zileuton have been demonstrated to suppress pruritus in AD patients.[6–8] However, controlled studies for the application of leukotriene receptor antagonists in chronic pruritus are missing.

## 49.2 Interferon Alpha

Interferon alpha (IFN-$\alpha$) inhibits the growth of the abnormal clone in patients with myeloproliferative disorders, leading to a reduction of the clinical and laboratory signs of the pathologic myeloproliferation. In addition, IFN-$\alpha$ also effectively inhibits the pruritus in polycythemia vera[9,10] and nonHodgkin-lymphoma.[11]

## 49.3 Cimetidine

Cimetidine effectively inhibited urticaria, angioedema, and urticaria factitia in case reports.[12, 13] Others have reported that high-dosage application of cimetidine (800–1,000 mg) relieves pruritus effectively in solid tumors and myeloproliferative diseases such as polycythemia vera and Hodgkin lymphoma.[14–17]

## 49.4 Aceytlsalicylic Acid

Few reports describe the effect of systemic acetylsalicylic acid (ASS) on pruritus. In an analysis of the Cochrane Pregnancy and Childbirth Group trials register, ASS was found to be more effective than chlorpheniramine in relieving itching during pregnancy when no rash is present (odds ratio 2. 39; 95%confidence interval 1.25–4.57). If there is a rash, chlorpheniramine was found to be more effective.[18] In several reviews and case reports, the effect of ASS on aquagenic pruritus[19–21] and polycythemia vera[22] (ASS 300 mg) is mentioned.

L. Misery and S. Ständer (eds.), *Pruritus*,
DOI 10.1007/978-1-84882-322-8_49, © Springer-Verlag London Limited 2010

However, ASS at 900 mg doses does not seem to influence chronic pruritus on inflamed skin (dermatoses other than urticaria).[23]

## 49.5 Nitrazepam

The effect of benzodiazepine was examined in a double-blind placebo-controlled crossover study in patients with AD.[24] Ten milligram nitrazepam was not effective in reducing the total duration of nocturnal scratching in patients with AD, although it decreased the frequency with which the bouts of nocturnal scratching occurred. There are no other studies investigating the antipruritic efficacy of nitrazepam.

## 49.6 Serotonin Receptor Antagonists

Serotonin receptor antagonists (5-HT3 antagonists) such as ondansetron (8 mg 1–3 times daily), tropisetron (5 mg/d), and granisetron (1 mg/d) were described to exhibit antipruritic efficacy in cholestatic pruritus,[25–28] renal pruritus,[29, 30] and intrathecal or epidural opioid-induced pruritus.[31–34] In addition, several cases and small case series have been reported regarding the response to 5-HT3 antagonists.[35–37] However, contradictory results have also been published concerning therapy with ondansetron of cholestatic pruritus[38, 39] and opiate-induced pruritus.[40–42] To date, controlled studies with large patient population evaluating the antipruritic potency of serotonin receptor antagonists are missing.

## 49.7 Thalidomide

Thalidomide (200–400 mg/d) has been described in the treatment of several diseases to have antipruritic effects. For example, actinic prurigo,[43, 44] prurigo nodularis,[45–48] psoriasis,[48] pruritus of HIV/AIDS,[49] renal pruritus,[50] and primary biliary cirrhosis[48, 51] responded to thalidomide. Though this seems to be an interesting treatment option, the risk of side effects has led to application of thalidomoide only under very strict conditions: over 50% of treated patients may develop permanent peripheral neuropathy.

## 49.8 Pentoxifylline

Pentoxyfilline[52, 53] and oxpentifylline[54] showed efficacious relief of pruritus in patients with renal pruritus,[52] keloids[54] and actinic prurigo[55] as well as HIV-infected patients with pruritic papular eruption.[53] In an open-label, uncontrolled study with 12 patients with HIV infection receiving pentoxifylline for 8 weeks, the average degree of pruritus was significantly reduced ($p = 0.0009$) from 6.5 at baseline examination to 3.6 at the end of the study.[53] Ten of 11 patients experienced a reduction in their pruritus ranging from 22.6% to 87.3%. Pentoyxifylline was also useful in the treatment of patients with actinic prurigo.[55] Ten patients with severe actinic prurigo received pentoxifylline in a 6-month open-label uncontrolled study. Clinical improvement of lesions was evident in all patients. Relief in pruritus was evident after 1 month of treatment and was maintained while receiving pentoxifylline.[55] However, in primary sclerosing cholangitis, pentoxifylline did not significantly alter pruritus or other parameters such as serum liver tests, serum tumor necrosis factor alpha (TNF-$\alpha$) or TNF receptor levels.[56]

## 49.9 Etanercept

TNF-$\alpha$ is a proinflammatory cytokine that may induce pruritus. Therefore, etanercept, a recombinant TNF-$\alpha$ receptor fusion protein, was applied in several pruritic conditions. For example, etanercept improved pruritus in 5/12 patients in keloids,[57] severe pruritus in erythroderma,[58] and pruritus in primary sclerosing cholangitis.[59]

## 49.10 Dronabinol

In an AD mouse model (NC mice), systemic administration of the selective cannabinoid CB2 receptor antagonist/inverse agonist JTE-907 suppressed spontaneous itch-associated responses.[60] In one clinical report, antipruritic effect of systemic applied dronabinol was shown in three patients with cholestatic pruritus.[61] Controlled studies in a large number of patients fail to judge the antipruritic potency of systemic cannabinoids.

# References

1. Andoh T, Kuraishi Y. Intradermal leukotriene B4, but not prostaglandin E2, induces itch-associated responses in mice. *Eur J Pharmacol.* 1998;353: 93–96.
2. Andoh T, Yageta Y, Takeshima H, Kuraishi Y. Intradermal nociceptin elicits itch-associated responses through leukotriene B(4) in mice. *J Invest Dermatol.* 2004;123:196–201.
3. Miyoshi M, Sakurai T, Kodama S. Clinical evaluation of urinary leukotriene E4 levels in children with atopic dermatitis. *Arerugi.* 1999;48:1148–1152.
4. Di Lorenzo G, Pacor ML, Mansueto P, et al. Is there a role for antileukotrienes in urticaria? *Clin Exp Dermatol.* 2006; 31:327–334.
5. Bernardini N, Roza C, Sauer SK, Gomeza J, Wess J, Reeh PW. Muscarinic M2 receptors on peripheral nerve endings: a molecular target of antinociception. *J Neurosci.* 2002;22:RC229.
6. Carucci JA, Washenik K, Weinstein A, Shupack J, Cohen DE. The leukotriene antagonist zafirlukast as a therapeutic agent for atopic dermatitis. *Arch Dermatol.* 1998;134:785–786.
7. Woodmansee DP, Simon RA. A pilot study examining the role of zileuton in atopic dermatitis. *Ann Allergy Asthma Immunol.* 1999;83:548–552.
8. Zabawski EJ Jr, Kahn MA, Gregg LJ. Treatment of atopic dermatitis with zafirlukast. *Dermatol Online J.* 1999;5:10.
9. Finelli C, Gugliotta L, Gamberi B, Vianelli N, Visani G, Tura S. Relief of intractable pruritus in polycythemia vera with recombinant interferon alfa. *Am J Hematol.* 1993;43: 316–318.
10. Muller EW, de Wolf JT, Egger R, Wijermans PW, Huijgens PC, Halie MR, Vellenga E. Long-term treatment with interferon-alpha 2b for severe pruritus in patients with polycythaemia vera. *Br J Haematol.* 1995;89:313–318.
11. Radossi P, Tison T, Vianello F, Dazzi F. Intractable pruritus in non-Hodgkin lymphoma/CLL: rapid response to IFN alpha. *Br J Haematol.* 1996;94:579.
12. Deutsch PH. Dermatographism treated with hydroxyzine and cimetidine and ranitidine. *Ann Intern Med.* 1984;101:569.
13. Farnam J, Grant JA, Guernsey BG, Jorizzo JL, Petrusa ER. Successful treatment of chronic idiopathic urticaria and angioedema with cimetidine alone. *J Allergy Clin Immunol.* 1984;73:842–845.
14. Berild D, Hasselbalch H. Itching of the skin in myeloproliferative disease treated with cimetidine. *Ugeskr Laeger.* 1985;147:1403–1404.
15. Easton P, Galbraith PR Cimetidine treatment of pruritus in polycythemia vera. *N Engl J Med.* 1978;299:1134.
16. Aymard JP, Lederlin P, Witz F, Colomb JN, Herbeuval R, Weber B. Cimetidine for pruritus in Hodgkin's disease. *Br Med J.* 1980;280:151–152.
17. Twycross R, Greaves MW, Handwerker H, Jones AE, Libretto SE, Szepietowski JC, Zylicz Z. Itch: scratching more than the surface. *QJM.* 2003;96: 7–26.
18. Young GL, Jewell D. Antihistamines versus aspirin for itching in late pregnancy. *Cochrane Database Syst Rev.* 2000;2:CD000027.
19. Bircher AJ. Water-induced itching. *Dermatologica.* 1990; 181(2):83–87.
20. Durand-Malgouyres C, Bazex J, Marguery MC. Aquagenic pruritus (A.P.). *Allerg Immunol (Paris).* 1990; 22:271–273.
21. Fjellner B, Hägermark O. Pruritus in polycythemia vera: treatment with aspirin and possibility of platelet involvement. *Acta Derm Venereol.* 1979;59:505–512.
22. Jackson N, Burt D, Crocker J, Boughton B. Skin mast cells in polycythaemia vera: relationship to the pathogenesis and treatment of pruritus. *Br J Dermatol.* 1987;116:21–29.
23. Daly BM, Shuster S. Effect of aspirin on pruritus. *Br Med J (Clin Res Ed).* 1986;293:907.
24. Ebata T, Izumi H, Aizawa H, Kamide R, Niimura M. Effects of nitrazepam on nocturnal scratching in adults with atopic dermatitis: a double-blind placebo-controlled crossover study. *Br J Dermatol.* 1998;138(4):631–634.
25. Schwörer H, Ramadori G. Improvement of cholestatic pruritus by ondansetron. *Lancet.* 1993;341:1277.
26. Schwörer H, Ramadori G. Treatment of pruritus: a new indication for serotonin type 3 receptor antagonists. *Clin Investig.* 1993;71:659–662.
27. Schwörer H, Hartmann H, Ramadori G: Relief of cholestatic pruritus by a novel class of drugs: 5-hydroxytryptamine type 3 (5-HT3) receptor antagonists: effectiveness of ondansetron. *Pain.* 1995;61:33–37.
28. Raderer M, Müller C, Scheithauer W. Ondansetron for pruritus due to cholestasis. *N Engl J Med.* 1994;330:1540.
29. Andrews PA, Quan V, Ogg CS. Ondansetron for symptomatic relief in terminal uraemia. *Nephrol Dial Transplant.* 1995;10:140.
30. Albares MP, Betlloch I, Guijarro J, Vergara G, Pascual JC, Botella R. Severe pruritus in a haemodialysed patient: dramatic improvement with granisetron. *Br J Dermatol.* 2003;148:376–377.
31. Han DW, Hong SW, Kwon JY, Lee JW, Kim KJ. Epidural ondansetron is more effective to prevent postoperative pruritus and nausea than intravenous ondansetron in elective cesarean delivery. *Acta Obstet Gynecol Scand.* 2007;86: 683–687.
32. Gulhas N, Erdil FA, Sagir O, Gedik E, Togal T, Begec Z, Ersoy MO Lornoxicam and ondansetron for the prevention of intrathecal fentanyl-induced pruritus. *J Anesth.* 2007;21:159–163.
33. Iatrou CA, Dragoumanis CK, Vogiatzaki TD, Vretzakis GI, Simopoulos CE, Dimitriou VK. Prophylactic intravenous ondansetron and dolasetron in intrathecal morphine-induced pruritus: a randomized, double-blinded, placebo-controlled study. *Anesth Analg.* 2005;101:1516–1520.
34. Pirat A, Tuncay SF, Torgay A, Candan S, Arslan G Ondansetron, orally disintegrating tablets versus intravenous injection for prevention of intrathecal morphine-induced nausea, vomiting, and pruritus in young males. *Anesth Analg.* 2005;101:1330–1336.
35. Frigon C, Desparmet J. Ondansetron treatment in a child presenting with chronic intractable pruritus. *Pain Res Manag.* 2006;11(4):245–247.
36. Ruiz Villaverde R, Sánchez Cano D, Villaverde Gutiérrez C. Ondansetron. A satisfactory treatment for refractory palmo-plantar pruritus. *Actas Dermosifiliogr.* 2006; 97(10): 681–682.
37. Zenker S, Schuh T, Degitz K. Therapy of pruritus associated with skin diseases with the serotonin receptor antagonist ondansetron. *J Dtsch Dermatol Ges.* 2003;1(9):705–710.
38. Müller C, Pongratz S, Pidlich J, et al. Treatment of pruritus in chronic liver disease with the 5-hydroxytryptamine receptor

type 3 antagonist ondansetron: a randomized, placebo-controlled, double-blind cross-over trial. *Eur J Gastroenterol Hepatol*. 1998;10:865–870.

39. O'Donohue JW, Haigh C, Williams R. Ondansetron in the treatment of cholestasis: a randomised controlled trial. *Gastroenterology*. 1997;112: A1349.

40. Larijani GE, Goldberg ME, Rogers KH. Treatment of opioid-induced pruritus with ondansetron: report of four patients. *Pharmacotherapy*. 1996;16:958–960.

41. Borgeat A, Stirnemann HR. Ondansetron is effective to treat spinal or epidural morphine-induced pruritus. *Anesthesiology*. 1999;90:432–436.

42 Kjellberg F, Tramer MR. Pharmacological control of opioid-induced pruritus: a quantitative systematic review of randomized trials. *Eur J Anaesthesiol*. 2001;18:346–357.

43. Londono F. Thalidomide in the treatment of actinic prurigo. *Int J Dermatol*. 1973;12:326–328.

44. Calnan CD, Meara RH. Actinic prurigo (Hutchinson's summer prurigo). *Clin Exp Dermatol*. 1977;2:365–372.

45 van den Broek H. Treatment of prurigo nodularis with thalidomide. *Arch Dermatol*. 1980;116:571–572.

46. Sheskin J. Zur Therapie der Prurigo nodularis Hyde mit Thalidomid. *Hautarzt*. 1975;26:215–217.

47. Winkelmann RK, Connolly SM, Doyle JA, Padilha-Goncalves A. Thalidomide treatment of prurigo nodularis. *Acta Derm Venereol*. 1984;64:412–417.

48. Daly BM, Shuster S. Antipruritic action of thalidomide. *Acta Derm Venereol*. 2000;80(1):24–25.

49 Maurer T, Poncelet A, Berger T. Thalidomide treatment for prurigo nodularis in human immunodeficiency virus-infected subjects: efficacy and risk of neuropathy. *Arch Dermatol*. 2004;140:845–849.

50. Silva SR, Viana PC, Lugon NV, Hoette M, Ruzany F, Lugon JR: Thalidomide for the treatment of uremic pruritus: a crossover randomized double-blind trial. *Nephron*. 1994;67:270–273.

51. McCormick PA, Scott F, Epstein O, Burroughs AK, Scheuer PJ, McIntyre N. Thalidomide as therapy for primary biliary cirrhosis: a double-blind placebo controlled pilot study. *J Hepatol*. 1994;21:496–499.

52. Mettang T, Krumme B, Bohler J, Roeckel A. Pentoxifylline as treatment for uraemic pruritus – an addition to the weak armentarium for a common clinical symptom? *Nephrol Dial Transplant*. 2007;22:2727–2728.

53. Berman B, Flores F, Burke G 3rd efficacy of pentoxifylline in the treatment of pruritic papular eruption of HIV-infected persons. *J Am Acad Dermatol*. 1998;38:955–959.

54. Wong TW, Lee JY, Sheu HM, Chao SC. Relief of pain and itch associated with keloids on treatment with oxpentifylline. *Br J Dermatol*. 1999;140(4):771–772.

55. Torres-Alvarez B, Castanedo-Cazares JP, Moncada pentoxifylline in the treatment of actinic prurigo. A preliminary report of 10 patients. *Dermatology*. 2004; 208(3):198–201.

56. Bharucha AE, Jorgensen R, Lichtman SN, LaRusso NF, Lindor KD. A pilot study of pentoxifylline for the treatment of primary sclerosing cholangitis. *Am J Gastroenterol*. 2000;95(9):2338–2342.

57. Berman B, Patel JK, Perez OA, et al. Evaluating the tolerability and efficacy of etanercept compared to triamcinolone acetonide for the intralesional treatment of keloids. *J Drugs Dermatol*. 2008;7(8):757–761.

58. Querfeld C, Guitart J, Kuzel TM, Rosen S. Successful treatment of recalcitrant, erythroderma-associated pruritus with etanercept. *Arch Dermatol*. 2004;140(12):1539–1540.

59. Epstein MP, Kaplan MM. A pilot study of etanercept in the treatment of primary sclerosing cholangitis. *Dig Dis Sci*. 2004;49(1):1–4.

60. Maekawa T, Nojima H, Kuraishi Y, et al. The cannabinoid CB2 receptor inverse agonist JTE-907 suppresses spontaneous itch-associated responses of NC mice, a model of atopic dermatitis. *Eur J Pharmacol*. 2006;542 (1–3):179–183.

61. Neff GW, O'Brien CB, Reddy KR, et al. Preliminary observation with dronabinol in patients with intractable pruritus secondary to cholestatic liver disease. *Am J Gastroenterol*. 2002;97 (8):2117–2119.

# Chapter 50
# Psychological Intervention

Sabine Dutray and Laurent Misery

Covered head to toe, I slipped on thick cotton pyjamas and decided to go back to bed for the day. Overwhelmed by such a sudden burst of this unexpected crisis, I felt an implacable need to sleep. And, knowing the treachery of my sickness, I bandaged my hands to make them two stumps useless for satisfying it…. The telephone rang around noon. Work was worried…. I hung up without a word, already knowing that I would not go back before having reached the end of my pitiful difference.

Lorette Nobécourt, La démangeaison [Itching], Editions J'ai lu, Paris, 1999

Does the appearance of pruritus always necessitate psychological treatment? The answer to this question remains subordinate to the dermatologist's clinical examination, including the psychological component (cf. Part II, Subchapter 4, Psychological Approach). The dermatologist's entire observational and clinical sense is mobilized. 'What is the patient telling me about his pruritus?' 'Is he psychically and physically overwhelmed by the itching?' 'Did this lead to changes in his daily life?' 'Is he only talking to me about his skin, or also about what it is to him as an individual?' Taking into account the psychological functioning of the subject under medical treatment permits a global approach to the patient.

The pruritus inevitably has a psychological dimension (as origin or impact) on account of the very subjectivity of this disorder. As a result, sometimes it is through the keen expression of the psychological dimension that a diagnosis, at first oriented towards a psychosomatic origin, is established on a genuine dermatosis.[1] And it is justly because a practitioner pays attention to the psychological suffering expressed by the patient and a dialogue can ensue between them.

However, it is important to take into account the patient's first demand: to treat his skin.[2] The subject has come to consult an organ doctor, a dermatologist. The initial subject of the consultation was the skin. And it is primarily to this that he/she must respond.

Moreover, in many situations appropriate dermatological supportive care that is attentive and containing is enough to soften the impact of the dermatosis on the patient's life. If this treatment necessitates additional therapy because the practitioner identifies a problem or a particular suffering, it must conform to what the patient feels himself capable of investing, and be appropriate to the symptoms, which often initially center on the quality of life and the psychological repercussions on the subject's mood. To introduce supportive care to the psychological aspect, the treatment may first focus on cutaneous therapy.

## 50.1 A Primary Necessity: Improvement of the Skin Condition

In effect, *therapeutic education* as applied to dermatology is intended to aid patients in better understanding their disease and certain signs in particular, such as pruritus.[2] The subject thereby develops skills in the area of care so that his/her compliance is appropriate and allows an appreciable and lasting cutaneous improvement, and he/she regains more comfort in daily life. The patient then becomes an active participant in his/her care. This therapy is therefore aimed at the patient, and also at his/her loved ones, those with whom he lives, so that they become provide support in the treatment of his cutaneous disease.

Accordingly, in the context of atopic dermatitis in children, education can target both the child and the parents. A study performed by the Therapy Education group of the French Dermatology Society has made it possible to establish a system of reference in the use of professionals to evaluate and develop three areas of

L. Misery and S. Ständer (eds.), *Pruritus*,
DOI 10.1007/978-1-84882-322-8_50, © Springer-Verlag London Limited 2010

competence:[3] knowledge about dermatosis, treatments, and triggering factors; expertise on care performed by patients and parents; and life skills in the ability to explain the disease and its care to others, knowing when and whom to contact. Therefore, in the event of the manifestation of the pruritus, the patient learns to implement alternatives to scratching, and to notify someone in case of acute pruritus. These are reference points that reassure patients and their loved ones, providing them with a certain degree of control over the situation.

A multicenter, randomized study performed jointly across seven German hospitals further shows that the major support that therapeutic education programmes constitute is structured and adapted to the age of the child or adolescent, in order to improve management of a dermatosis (such as atopic dermatitis), with pruritus among other aspects.[4] To do so, groups of parents with children who have atopic dermatitis (from 3 months to 7 years of age, and from 8 to12 years of age), and adolescents (13–18 years of age) suffering from atopic dermatitis, were formed. They attended weekly 2-h group sessions for 6 weeks, or they did not have any particular therapy. The therapy involved medical, nutritional, and psychological interventions performed by a multidisciplinary team. So, specifically for pruritus, the improvement is significant over the 'catastrophization' scales and 'coping' strategies (vide infra) on the 8–12 age group, while the improvement among the adolescents (13–18 years old) was only meaningful over the first scale.

When conjoined with therapeutic education, health psychology can provide some additional tools. The learning of 'coping' strategies can be combined with it in different forms: a behavioral form, such as confronting a problem (for example an avoidance behavior), or seeking out social support. This learning allows better management in terms of stress, pruritus crises or various events in daily life that intrude, overwhelm the subject, and produce significant stress.[2] Hence, the feasibility and effects of a pilot care programme 'Coping with Itch' were studied over the frequency and intensity of the pruritus and scratching, the associated strategies of adaptation, psychosocial morbidity, and quality of life.[5] This programme aimed to reduce pruritus and to aid the patient in managing crises. To accomplish this, patients suffering from chronic pruritus had one to four sessions, of 45 min each, over a period of 4 months. They included educational and cognitive–behavioral interventions, mental training, changes in habits, and relaxation exercises. The results showed that this programme was suited to

the objectives established, and that it seemed effective in reducing the frequency of the pruritus and scratching, an improvement in the adaptation to the pruritus, and a decrease in psychosocial comorbidity. These results appeared a short time after the sessions were set up and stabilized over 9 months. In addition, the multidisciplinary nature allowed better efficacy, since the alliance between therapeutic education and cognitive and behavioral intervention gave better results than each of the therapies performed individually.

In other respects, 'coping' strategies also find their expression in social support, such as that generated by the parents of patients (cf. above), groups of patients, and patient associations.[2] The function of this type of support is to provide emotional security, the sentiment of feeling understood by people who have similar daily experiences, of relying on a group identity, and of receiving information allowing concrete and tangible help for everyday life and for difficult situations.

## 50.2 Alternative Care, from the Body to the Mind

Also centered on the body, but taking a step back from standard dermatological care, *massage therapy* may allow a subject reinforce support for his body. As a result, in 20 burn patients whose moderate wounds were in the recovery stage and who were complaining of severe itch, the effects of therapeutic massage were examined in a randomized study of the reduction of this postburn pain and pruritus. Similarly, the effects of this technique were evaluated for reducing anxiety and depression across half of the subjects, while the other half (the control group) received standard medical care.[6] The latter consisted in clinical exams, treatment with drugs, and therapy centered on physical or occupational activity, while the first group's care included 30 min of massage twice per week for 5 weeks. The wound and its surrounding areas were specifically massaged. The results for the group receiving therapeutic massage showed a reduction in pruritus, anxiety, and depression as well as pain. Furthermore, this therapy allowed improvement across all the signs over the long term.

This approach based on physical sensations helps the patient to recover a calmer and more enhanced body image: and for massages intended for the entire body, to obtain a physical unity where the pruritus was singling out some surfaces more than others.[2] The skin can take back its surface and envelope functions both from a somatic and a psychological perspective, along with the idea of the boundary that the pruritus questions when it arouses one to scratch and attack one's own skin (cf. Part II, Subchapter 4, Psychological Approach). Further, it acts as a mediator to establish patient–therapist communication around the language of the body.[7]

Linking the body to the mind, different *relaxation techniques* can be proposed according to the patient's possibilities of cathexis.[2] Schultz autogenic training is an induction method based on active participation of the subject, to obtain a state of muscle relaxation and overall relaxation of the body, as opposed to the physiological manifestations of anxiety. The patient puts his environment and his own thoughts at a distance, focusing on sensations such as weight, warmth, the beating of the heart or breathing, for example.

Jacobson's progressive relaxation is above all a physiological method.[8] It methodically examines each functional muscle group to maximally reduce tonus, thereby inducing the largest possible decrease in excitability and emotional reactivity. For the patient, this means becoming aware of proprioceptive sensations of muscle contraction and relaxation. This technique can be used during the day when a situation invades, and difficulties in facing up to it are encountered.

*Analytical psychotherapy by relaxation* is a novel method, since it depends on two seemingly antinomic entities: the body as therapeutic mediator and psychoanalytic theory based on the idea of the unconscious. Their linking allows the emergence of a genuine therapeutic relationship and encourages the subject to express what he feels about his body and the effect this produces on his psyche.

These relaxation techniques are quite significant in the context of pruritus, as they allow the patient, while remaining centered on his body and his sensations, to work out the psychological impact of the pruritus, especially in terms of anguish, or the emergence of this anguish with itching as a possible consequence.

## 50.3  Thinking or Psyche: Therapies According to the Patient's Cathexis

Moving away from an anchorage on the body, *medical hypnosis* is a method of suggestion that can be used in dermatology, either to reduce pain or make it disappear, or to modify a mental or physical habit.[8] It can take two forms: '*neutral hypnosis*' through images of relaxation intended to reinforce the '*ego*', for issues concerning anxiety disorders (for example), or '*problem-centred*' hypnosis through direct or metaphorical suggestions, such as the reduction of compulsive acts. Hence, a review of the literature made over the period 1966–1998 cited studies revealing the possible effects of hypnosis on immediate immune reactions, as well as on allergic manifestations encountered in atopic dermatitis or urticaria.[2,9] Further, hypnosis seems to have also been used to improve good health behaviors, reduce or control harmful behaviors for the patient, such as scratching, or allow the expression of an immediate and lasting analgesia. With regard to the phenomenon of scratching, it is replaced under suggestion with another physical activity, such as exerting pressure on the area or the scratches, or with having an activity to discharge stress, such as physical exercise. The intensity of the pruritus itself seems to be modifiable or improvable through hypnosis; it may be a significant complement when allied with other therapies.

A study was moreover performed among three patients with HIV who were suffering from a persistent pruritus inducing significant scratching that was resulting in lesions.[10] They had six hypnosis sessions over a period of more than 6 weeks. These sessions were composed of muscle relaxation, a technique of intensification in order to improve relaxation, visualization of a pleasant scene and the use of images and suggestions to control the pruritus. At the end of the treatment, the three patients reported a significant reduction in the severity of the pruritus, including effects on the quality of their sleep. One patient also felt a significant decrease in suffering connected with the pruritus, and for another there was a significant reduction in the time devoted to the pruritus. For two people with whom it was possible to continue the study, the hypnosis treatment produced continuous, and increasing, effects.

However, one of the difficulties presented by medical hypnosis is the receptivity and sensitivity of patients to this type of method. This is why it must be integrated into a therapeutic plan appropriate for the subject.

*Behavioral and cognitive therapies* can be an appreciable recourse for various dermatoses, such as urticaria, atopic dermatitis, psoriasis or pruritus.[2,11] Behavioral therapy can intervene through simulation and gradual exposure of the subject to the situations that cause anxiety. Cognitive therapy, a complement to the former, can act on the subject's thoughts that present cognitive distortion, i.e., a dysfunction of mental schemas, leading the subject to false beliefs, as for example regarding contagion. These therapies are active methods, involving the patient and the therapist. They take place over four main phases: a pretreatment evaluation of the behaviors at work with respect to their factors of appearance, a choice of objective in the form of a contract with an agreement, the application of the appropriate programme, and an evaluation of results during and after the treatment.[7]

As a result, in light of what was practised in the treatment of 'bad manias' and tics, a change of habit was experimented within the context of atopic dermatitis - since the itch from it can be ferocious and the injuries caused by scratching significant. Forty six adults with atopic dermatitis were included in a randomized study[12] of four groups: the first two had to use a cortisone cream over 4 weeks, the other two a powerful steroid over 2 weeks, then the cortisone cream during the following two. One group of each also benefited from a habit-reversing technique, consisting in using an alternative to scratching (such as clenching one's fists and counting till 30, or tightly gripping an object), and in finding an alternative response to the pruritus, such as pinching one's skin on the area concerned. All the subjects had previously kept a journal for 1 week where they inventoried each moment of the pruritus, the scratching, the areas involved, and the durations. The two specific groups obtained significant results with respect to the pruritus and the scratching. However, their cutaneous recovery was not complete at the end of 4 weeks of treatment. In fact, it is necessary to distinguish the possibility of reducing scratching by 90% in 3 days thanks to behavioral and cognitive therapy and the improvement of the eczema. Therefore, the experiment was continued, stressing the patients' awareness of their mode of functioning in case of pruritus, so that they could best adhere to a new behavior, offered by the therapist or by themselves, which could be applied at any time on a daily basis.

These therapies can also undoubtedly take their place as part of a therapeutic education program. For children's atopic dermatitis, a cognitive–behavioral approach centered on pruritus and scratching behaviors was proposed as an accompaniment to appropriate treatment with medication, the acquisition of reference points in daily care, and the acquisition of tools for evaluating the programme.[13] The therapy took place in five stages. The first consisted in designing a methodical

approach to the care by assessing the existing situation. The second was specific to the presentation and appropriation of the program by the parents and children: returning medical information, sensitizing them to the situations which can induce pruritus and scratching, and so on. The third was reserved for introducing the change of habit itself with opposite behaviors, such as clenching one's fists, or pressing or tapping the skin, to be used individually or together according to the family's choice, parallel to the cutaneous treatment. The fourth stage endeavored to set up this program over time through close support. And finally, an evaluation of the method was performed during the fifth stage.

The patients could thereby possess concrete responses in order to emerge from the vicious circle of itch-scratch-itch, with a global and targeted treatment.

Patients may wish for a different approach when they wonder about their psychological functioning and wish to elaborate in depth about their suffering, in order to feel more in harmony with themselves.[2] *Psychoanalysis and analysis-inspired psychotherapies* can offer this possibility of working over the long term. Analysis[7] aims to reactualise the infantile conflicts, in order to encourage awareness of it and thereby permit the subject to reinvest his newly available pulsional energy differently and to enlarge the influence of the Ego over his entire psychological life (cf. Part II, Subchapter 4, Psychological Approach). In doing so, the therapeutic context has great importance: the subject's reclining position, outside the analyst's view, frequent sessions, steady pace, and similar duration of the sessions. On the patient's side, the fundamental rule is free association favored by the visual absence of the therapist, with the interplay of transference in which the subject reactualizes past relationships with the analyst. On the analyst's side, his/her neutrality favors the expression of archaic elements from the subject, and the analysis of the countertransference allows work on what is happening unconsciously in the course of treatment. With regard to analysis-inspired psychotherapies,[7] the objective (similar to the previous) is to uphold the awareness of the conflicts that underpin the expression of symptoms. They differ insofar as this involves working out the functioning of the Ego rather than making a change. The context for this type of work is also more flexible, since the subject faces the therapist, the sessions are shorter and less frequent during the week and the overall duration of the therapy is shorter. While the fundamental rule remains the same, the visual presence of the therapist cannot allow as straightforward a relaxation of conscious control, which produces a limit on the work, since the subject then takes the therapist's reactions into account. Choosing between the techniques depends on the psychological possibilities of the subject in having access to and expressing his unconscious fantasies and desires. Therefore, the second technique allows reinforcement and often more appropriate containment when soma and psyche overlap.[14] If the subject can broach the work with the 'disappearance' of the somatic symptom as his intention, the development can gradually make it possible to move away from this narrow demand, which imprisons one into a results-oriented process, in order to examine one's emotional and relational psychological life. He/she will then be able to size up what is comfortable to him/her overall and not only on the level of the skin. Moreover, the therapist must also take into account the patient's personality. In dermatology, the term 'alexithymia' is often mentioned, defined by Sifneos to mean mental functioning characterized by the inability to identify and express emotions verbally, the limitation of imaginary life, the tendency to resort to action to manage conflicts and the detailed description of facts and physical symptoms. From the psychoanalytic point of view, the term used instead is 'operational thinking,' according to P. Marty, merging similar components: *'thinking that is current, factual, motor, and blank without affect'*.[15] This type of functioning requires the context to be laid out, but it must not overshadow each patient's resources, even if these resources do not initially announce themselves. In this, the subject can find a certain support in the analyst when the latter takes into account the cutaneous signs, believes that the subject's psychological capacities can emerge and informs him of it, so he can then advance more confidently in this exploration that he perceives as so uncertain.[15]

When the limits are questioned, as in pruritus, when the somatic skin questions the efficiency of the psychological skin, and when the Skin Ego cannot be fully acquired, the psychoanalyst can symbolically propose to the patient a support replaying the attachment in these five main elements[16] and fulfil the function of an auxiliary Ego for a certain time[15,17] (cf. Part II, Subchapter 4, Psychological Approach). And here, with the analyst and his/her support, the path for each patient is unique, in touch with both his own body and his psychological life, leaning on both, in order to undertake work intended to provide him with greater welfare.

As an aid to all these therapies, from those that specifically intervene on the body to those that appeal to thinking, *psychotropic drugs* fulfil a very important function. Prescriptions for them are established according to the type of cutaneous symptom, its site and importance as well as the patient's psychological characteristics. While neuroleptics are used for psychosis, antidepressants and tranquillisers are more commonly used to chemically support a patient with dermatosis.[18] They can also be prescribed by the somatic doctor. Moreover, antidepressants have a specific action on pruritus[19] (cf. Part III, Subchapter 2, Antidepressants).

All the therapies shown, from therapeutic education to analysis-inspired psychotherapies to psychotropic drugs, represent a set of possibilities that can combine with each other depending on somatic signs, the patient's demand, and the possible support of the dermatologist.

## 50.4  On the Therapeutic Alliance: Between Professionals and Between the Doctor and Patient

If the patient comes to consult the dermatologist or the general practitioner, the fact is that what he exhibits may require a multiple treatment, involving a link between the latter and another professional, most often a specialist of the mind – a psychiatrist, psychologist or psychoanalyst.

And in this context of a specific consultation, the dermatologist–psychiatrist *joint consultation* can be a great help. At the Brest university hospital, France,[20] the patient is presented by his doctor with the understanding that he will consult a dermatologist in combination with a psychiatrist. The objective of this consultation is to allow both the cutaneous ailment and the psychological problems to be expressed, and to see their possible links in order to offer therapy for both. After a phase devoted to a clinical exam of the skin by the dermatologist, the transition is made smoothly to a conversation of a psychological nature initiated by the psychiatrist, although one where each of the two doctors has a place in the relationship with the patient. This entails a prescription on a single medium, uniting dermatological treatment and possibly psychiatric treatment. Over 1 year, while 50 patients have thereby benefited from this plan, 8 presented a pruritus sine materia (i.e., without visible lesion responsible for itch).

Depression and anxiety were frequently encountered. A new joint consultation was proposed to 23 patients out of these 50, and out of whom only 4 did not follow up. In 16 cases, a prescription for psychotropic drugs was written. Further, this consultation was taken as a filter for the most appropriate possible access to psychotherapy, as was proposed to 23 patients: analysis-inspired psychotherapy for 15, relaxation therapy for 4, hospitalization for 2, psychodrama therapy for 1, and cognitive therapy for 1. The complementary nature and simultaneity of medical expertise can allow the patient to see that he is being understood in his totality, without part of himself (the body or the mind) being sidelined. In addition, support on the cutaneous, clinical side represents a safeguard so that he does not experience this moment as mental interference. This fantasy can also lead to a refusal of a standard psychiatric consultation, while in this scenario the two doctors speak to the body and the patient authorizes or refuses to authorize sharing a little more of his psyche.

In addition, the joint consultation itself has a therapeutic effect through the link it offers between soma and psyche. While it has an impact – and in more ways than one – in the patient, it also has quite a bit of significance for the two practitioners. The psychiatrist is sensitized to the dermatological treatment and to the involvement of the body and the skin in her relationship with the patient. The dermatologist absorbs the psychological functioning of the patient in the disease and during the consultation. And because it is often difficult to lead the patient towards becoming aware of his psychological problems in order to offer him appropriate therapy, the support of a psychiatrist, psychologist or psychoanalyst colleague is invaluable for a dermatologist. Moreover, this support is also useful for the psychiatrist, psychologist, and psychoanalyst, since the dermatologist continues to give the patient attention on the state of his skin, which is therefore not neglected.[16] The patient is supported somatically and psychically. This is why communication and exchange between professionals is rewarding for more appropriate treatment.[15]

But isn't the first therapy initiated by the meeting between the dermatologist and the patient? *The doctor–patient relationship* is marked by cathexis on both the patient's and the doctor's part. Different elements can work towards facilitating communication.[21]

First of all, for the patient the duration of the consultation is, of course, a criterion for the dermatologist to take into account and take an interest in her subject;

however, it is the listening and availability of the doctor in the here and now that actually matters to him. Further, while the doctor takes 18 s on average before interrupting the patient, the latter could explain all of what led him there in 2 min. And the '*doorknob syndrome*' can be a symptom of this need for time or attention: while the consultation is coming to an end and farewells are approaching, the patient short-circuits this moment of transition to communicate important elements. If the dermatologist can welcome these remarks while maintaining the initial context and offering to touch on them more fully in the next consultation, the patient will be able to feel contained and understood. The approach is similar when the patient pours out a stream of uninterrupted words without limit, overflowing the context. In that case the doctor's attitude can aid in containing this wave – getting up and moving towards the door to signify the end of the exchange, while continuing to look at and listen to the patient.

This listening sought so much by the patient is also tested when the situation is exceptional, as in the case of delusional parasitosis. Dermatologists, even if they quickly identify the singularity of the problem, must first take into account the skin about which the patient (most often female) is complaining. He/she has certainly come to express psychological suffering, but with cutaneous support. And although speaking to a psychiatric colleague is appropriate, this is nonetheless difficult to propose and to have accepted. But in fact, it is very often the patient himself/herself who 'throws out a line' to the doctor by expressing mental suffering, even if it seems tenuous:[22] 'I can't take it anymore' or 'It's eating away at me from the inside….' Seizing on these remarks, then looking at them again from a distance during the following consultation, in soliciting the patient's explanation, initiates a path towards addressing the here and now, starting from the psychological suffering. In this context, having contacts in the psychiatric, psychoanalytic, or psychological sphere also allows the patient to take the step more confidently, feeling safety through the pre-existing link between dermatologists and their colleagues.

In a different, yet similarly delicate manner, caring for a patient suffering from a persistent pruritus confronts the doctor with the patient's dissatisfaction, his despondency, or his aggressiveness.[21] But in spite of all this, the patient is there in the dermatologist's office. Whether it may involve a difficulty in compliance that may be due to corticophobia, to weariness faced with the stress and the repetition of treatments, to social isolation, or to depressive elements (for example), the fact remains that the doctor can take this complaint as the point of departure for a conversation instead of a failure.[22] This situation may moreover solicit personal affect in the doctor, feeling himself/herself targeted personally by the patient, and for this reason provoking an annoyance or a certain distance with respect to the patient. But is it truly a matter of the doctor himself/herself, or something else?

In fact, the doctor–patient relationship is unequal since the patient, the one demanding care and relief, speaks to a doctor, the bearer of knowledge.[23] Further, each of them has an idealized representation of the other: 'the one who corresponds in every way to satisfying my conscious and my unconscious desires.' For the patient, the relationship seeks transference in the reactualization of past relationships, and particularly the parental bond. Similarly, for the dermatologist the countertransference in the relationship provokes her desires, fantasies, and representations – mechanisms that the analyzed and analyst both experience (cf. above). It is for this reason that being able to wonder about what this questions in oneself, while keeping in mind that, through oneself, it is an 'other' who is the recipient of the complaint, makes it possible in many cases to avoid the therapeutic rupture. Moreover, sensitising and training the dermatologist in the specific field of psychodermatology is in this sense an additional asset.[24]

To be capable of being amazed at what the patient is conveying, willing to follow him/her even if this runs counter to scientific and medical data and to support him tactfully and willingly can allow each one to take his/her proper place in order to build a genuine therapeutic alliance.[14]

# References

1. Misery L. Ne dites pas trop vite: "c'est psy" ou "c'est le stress". *Cutis et Psyché.* 2007;21:5–6.
2. Consoli SG. *Psychiatrie et Dermatologie. Encycl Méd Chir, Dermatologie, 98-874-A-10.* Paris: Elsevier; 2001.
3. Barbarot S, Gagnayre R, Bernier C, et al. and the members of the Therapeutic Education Group of the French Dermatology Society. Dermatite atopique: un référentiel d'éducation thérapeutique du malade. *Ann Dermatol Venereol.* 2007;134:121–127.
4. Staab D, Diepgen TL, Fartasch M, et al. Age related, structured educational programmes for the management of atopic dermatitis in children and adolescents: multicentre, randomised controlled trial. *BMJ.* 2006;332:933–938.
5. Van Os-Medendorp H, Eland-De Kok PC, Ros WJ, Bruijnzeel-Koomen CA, Grypdonck M. The nursing programme "Coping with itch": a promising intervention for patients with chronic pruritic skin diseases. *J Clin Nurs.* 2007;16(7):1238–1246.
6. Field T, Peck M, Hernandez-Reif M, Krugman S, Burman I, Ozment-Schenck L. Postburn itching, pain, and psychosocial symptoms are reduced with massage therapy. *J Burn Care Rehabil.* 2000;21(3):189–193.
7. Guelfi JD, Boyer P, Consoli SM, Olivier-Martin R. *Psychiatrie.* Paris: PUF; 1996.
8. Garat H. Dermatologie et hypnose médicale. *Cutis et psyché.* 2007;21:11–12.
9. Shenefelt PD. Hypnosis in dermatology. *Arch Dermatol.* 2000;136:393–399.
10. Rucklidge JJ, Saunders D. *The efficacy of hypnosis in the treatment of pruritus in people with HIV/AIDS: a time-series analysis. Int J Clin Exp Hypn.* 2002; 50(2):149–169.
11. Gieler U, Niemeier V, Brosig B, Kupfer J. Psychosomatic aspects of pruritus. *Dermatol Psychosom.* 2002;3:6–13.
12. Noren P. Habit reversal: a turning point in the treatment of atopic dermatitis. *Clin Exp Dermatol.* 1995;20(1):2–5.
13. Buchanan PI. Behavior modification: a nursing approach for young children with atopic eczema. *Dermatol Nurs.* 2001;13(1):15–25.
14. Consoli SG. Psychopathologie en dermatologie. *Nouv Dermatol.* 2000;19:582–585.
15. Consoli SG. Psychothérapie psychanalytique et dermatologie. *Nervure.* 2006;19(2):8–14.
16. Consoli SG. *Le moi-peau. Médecine/Sciences.* 2006;22: 197–200.
17. Consoli SG, Consoli SM. *Psychanalyse, dermatologie, prothèses – D'une peau à l'autre.* Paris: PUF; 2006.
18. Misery L. *La peau neuronale – Les nerfs à fleur de peau.* Paris: Ellipses; 2000.
19. Misery L. Symptomatic treatment of pruritus. *Ann Dermatol Venereol.* 2005 May;132(5):492–495.
20. Misery L, Chastaing M. Joint consultation by a psychiatrist and a dermatologist. *Dermatol Psychosom.* 2003;4: 160–164.
21. Poot F. La relation médecin-patient en dermatologie. *Cutis et Psyché.* 2005;18:12–17.
22. Consoli SG, Consoli SM. *Dermatologie... Et si c'était votre patient? Clés de communication médecin-patient-15 situations concrètes.* Paris: Editions scientifiques L et C; 2004.
23. Consoli SG. Le contre-transfert dans la relation dermatologue-malade. *Nouv Dermatol.* 2001;20(1):510–513.
24. Poot F, Sampogna F, Onnis L. Basic knowledge in psychodermatology. *J Eur Acad Dermatol Venereol.* 2007;21(2): 227–234.

# Chapter 51
# Ultraviolet Phototherapy of Pruritus

Joanna Wallengren

It has been known for more than 2000 years that several skin diseases improve upon exposure to the sun. However, it was not until the end of the 19th century before Niels R. Finsen started to use sunlight as well as electric light for the treatment of skin tuberculosis.[1] He was awarded the Nobel Prize in 1903 "in recognition of his contribution to the treatment of diseases, especially lupus vulgaris, with concentrated light radiation, whereby he has opened a new avenue for medical science." The carbon arc lamp initially used by Finsen was later shown to emit longwave ultraviolet radiation.[1] Another device, still successfully used in some circumscribed itchy skin diseases, was constructed by Gustav Bucky in 1929. This device produced ionizing radiation employing ultrasoft X-rays (0.07–0.4 nm), which Bucky called "grenz rays" since he believed that the biological effects of these rays resemble those of X-rays in some ways and ultraviolet rays in other ways.[2]

At the second International Congress of Light, held in Copenhagen in 1932, it was recommended that the ultraviolet (UV) spectrum should be divided into three defined spectral regions: UVA, UVB, and UVC.[3] The next milestone in the field of phototherapy was made by Ingram who introduced a combination treatment of tar and UV light (UVB) for psoriasis in 1953.[4] Twenty years later, psoralen in combination with UVA (PUVA) was recommended for severe psoriasis.[5] During the two decades that followed, broadband UVB (BB-UVB; 290–320 nm), UVA (UVA; 320–400 nm), UVA/UVB (UVAB; 290–400 nm) and psoralen UVA (PUVA) were the most common UV sources in modern phototherapy units. Gradually, new treatment modalities employing selected emission spectra such as narrowband UVB (NB-UVB; 311 nm) and long-wavelength ultraviolet A 1 (UVA1 340–400 nm) have found clinical applications. UVA1 phototherapy may be administered in high doses (HD-UVA1, 130 J/cm²), medium doses (MD-UVA1, 50 J/cm²), or low doses (LD-UVA1, 10 J/cm²). In addition, several types of targeted phototherapy devices are available; the most studied is an excimer laser, delivering 308 nm UVB to the affected skin areas.[6]

Phototherapy has been largely empirical. Thus, despite the long-term use its mechanisms of action are not quite clear. There is increasing evidence that the efficacy of phototherapy on itch results from structural changes in the skin including thickening of the epidermis and reduction of cutaneous nerve fibers as well as from induction of immune suppression and apoptosis of immunocompetent cells. The advantage of phototherapy is that the changes in the skin induced by UV exposures may last for months after cessation of treatment. They do not last for ever, however, and itch may recur. A possible approach is then maintenance therapy twice a week for a long time.

This chapter will focus on the effects of UV therapy on itchy skin conditions in inflamed skin, in noninflamed skin as well as in some systemic diseases associated with itch. The mechanisms of action of different UV wavelengths that may interact with transmission of itch will be discussed. Unfortunately, many reports on phototherapy for pruritic conditions are anecdotal or based on small and often uncontrolled studies.

## 51.1 Possible Mechanism of Action

Acute exposure to UV radiation (UVR) results in erythema, heat, edema, pain, and pruritus.[7] While UVB radiation-induced effects are mainly limited to the epidermis, UVA radiation affects both epidermal and dermal cell populations. Interestingly, the most acute effects of sun exposure are mainly due to wavelengths shorter than 320 nm (UVB). It would suggest that the mediators

L. Misery and S. Ständer (eds.), *Pruritus*,
DOI 10.1007/978-1-84882-322-8_51, © Springer-Verlag London Limited 2010

synthesized and released from epidermis upon UVB stimulation induce inflammation in the dermis. Several studies have pointed out a marked increase of the synthesis of several prostaglandins, mainly $PGE_2$, in both UVB- and UVA-treated skin.[7–10]

In addition, UVB induces expression of several cytokines on the surface of keratinocytes: the pro-inflammatory IL-6 and the anti-inflammatory IL-10 and TNF-$\alpha$.[11,12] The pro-inflammatory intercellular adhesion molecule ICAM-1 can either be stimulated or suppressed by UV radiation, depending on the time point after irradiation.[13] The immunosuppressive mediators released from keratinocytes upon UV irradiation contribute to the local as well as the systemic immunosuppression.[12] Another factor that contributes to immunosuppression is the reduction of the number of Langerhans cells in epidermis upon UVR, resulting in suppressed elicitation of eczema.[13]

Early studies of acute exposure to UVR have shown vascular changes in the dermis and mast cell degranulation which was preceded by $PGE_2$ that had been newly synthesized in epidermis.[7] Another study has shown that both histamine and bradykinin stimulate prostaglandin synthesis upon UV irradiation.[14] $PGE_2$ may be also synthesized by the leukocytes present in the skin as well as by the ones entering the skin in response to the inflammatory signals. Several mediators of inflammation also acting as neurotransmitters in sensory nerve fibers conducting itch, such as vaso-active intestinal peptide (VIP), substance P (SP) and calcitonin gene-related peptide (CGRP), have been shown to be released from nerve fibers following sunburn or phototherapy.[15–18] Neuropeptides have also immunoregulatory properties; while SP stimulates urticarial and eczematous reactions, VIP, and CGRP inhibit eczematous reactions.[14,19–21]

As histamine, bradykinin, cytokines, prostaglandins, and neuropeptides mentioned above (with the exception of CGRP) are pruritogenic, their release upon UV irradiation induces itch. The pruritogenic effect is partly mediated by mastcell degranulation.[22] It has been shown that both BB-UVB and NB-UVB induce apoptosis in a mast cell culture.[23]

This finding would explain why repeated treatment with UVB, UVA or PUVA inhibits responses induced by the histamine-liberator compound 48/80.[24] There may be, however, another explanation. Impairment of the sensory innervation may also contribute to a reduced histamine release as mast cells and sensory nerve fibers conducting the itch act as a functional unit.[25] Indeed, the number of intraepithelial nerve fibers (PGP 9.5-immunoreactive) was shown to be reduced after phototherapy in 13 patients treated with PUVA or NB-UVB.[26] In addition, the subepidermal nerve fibers became thicker.[26] Such swelling of nerve endings was shown previously in an electron microscopy study in two individuals after repeated UVA exposure; however, in this study intraepidermal nerve fibers proliferated.[27]

In addition, UVB exposure to one-half of the body induced a generalized reduction of pruritus in patients with uremia, suggesting an impact of phototherapy on circulating mediators.[28] The interactions of mediators synthesized and released following UVR are summarized in Fig. 51.1.

## 51.2 Itch in Inflamed Skin

In itchy skin disease with an ongoing inflammation, the inflammatory mediators will be continuously produced, fueling the firing of sensory nerve fibres. As inflammation fades, the associated itch will decrease. Therefore reduction of inflammation is often essential in combating itch. As UVA wavelengths penetrate into the dermis where inflammation takes place, UVA, PUVA as well as different doses of UVA1 would be the UV spectrum of choice. However, as the itch-conducting nerve fibers are localized in the subepidermal layer, and the majority of nerve endings penetrate into the epidermis where both cytokines and $PGE_2$ are released, different UVB modalities are also effective in the treatment of pruritus.

### 51.2.1 Atopic Dermatitis

Treatment of atopic dermatitis is a multifaceted approach that requires repair and maintenance of the barrier function, reduction of microbial skin flora, cessation of the itch–scratch cycle, and reduction of inflammation. Phototherapy can actually contribute to the treatment of all these symptoms.[29–31] The scope of this review is the effect of different modalities of UV therapy on pruritus, which is one of the three major criteria of atopic dermatitis.[32] Jekler and Larko performed several two-paired

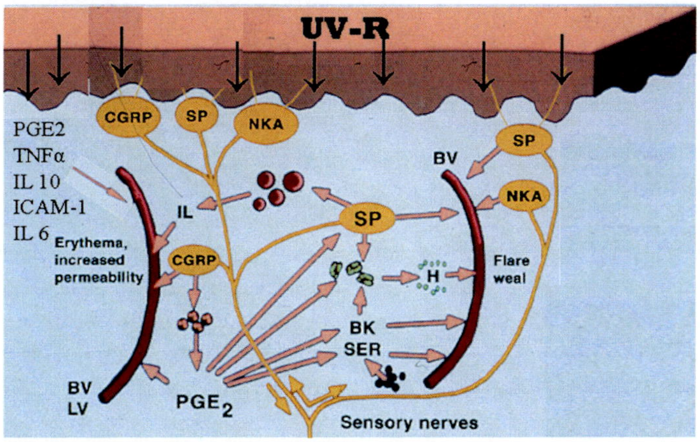

**Fig. 51.1**   The interactions of mediators synthesized and released following UVR are illustrated by the arrows

comparison studies: comparing different UV wavelengths on each half of the body in atopic patients. With respect to pruritus they found that BB-UVB is more effective than placebo, while UVAB is more effective than both BB-UVB and BB-UVA.[33–36] When Hjerppe et al. in a similar half-sided mode compared NB-UVB and UVAB in patients with atopic dermatitis, they found no difference in the effect on eczema but patients reported better effect of NB-UVB on pruritus.[37] In a half-side comparison study, the effect of 8-methoxypsoralen bath–PUVA was equal to that of NB-UVB in patients with severe chronic AD but the patients preferred NB-UVB because it was easier to perform.[37] The resolution of skin lesions in this study was always preceded by relief of pruritus, which generally occurred within the first 2 weeks of treatment.[38]

Today, MD-UVA1 is recommended for treatment of acute atopic eczema, while NB-UVB is recommended for treatment of chronic eczema (for a review see Ref. 39). MD-UVA1 has been shown to be as affective for AD as HD- UVA1 and more effective than LD-UVA1.[39] However, conventional UVA1 machines generate a great deal of heat, causing sweating during the treatment that lasts for more than half an hour. As sweating triggers pruritus in atopic patients, a "cold light" UVA1 equipped with a filtering and cooling system was used, which was shown to be better tolerated by the AD patients than conventional UVA1.[40]

In a placebo-controlled comparison between NB-UVB and BB-UVA for AD patients, 90% reported reduction of itch with NB-UVB and 63% with BB-UVA.[41] Also in a half-side comparison study of NB-UVB and MD-UVA1,

NB-UVB was shown to be more effective in combating pruritus.[42] In an uncontrolled study, 15 AD patients treated with excimer laser, delivering 308 nm UVB, twice weekly for 4 weeks reported 80% reduction of itch.[43] The conclusion of the studies taken together is that NB-UVB is the best choice for atopic pruritus.

## 51.2.2  Urticaria

Besides the disfiguring weals, burning and itching are the most disabling features of urticaria. Daily urticarial activity scores derived from weal numbers and itch can be used to monitor therapy for urticaria. However, this type of scoring has not been used in the studies on phototherapy for urticaria, and only a few of these studies monitor pruritus.

### 51.2.2.1  Chronic Urticaria

In a placebo-controlled study on 19 patients, UVA treatment was as good as PUVA showing improvement in about 60% of patients with chronic urticaria.[44] In another retrospective study on 88 patients, NB-UVB treatment produced clearance or improvement in 72% of cases.[45] Effects of BB-UVB were studied on 15 patients with different forms of chronic urticaria, 12 of who suffered from physical urticaria.[46] In this study 11 patients improved, none with idiopathic urticaria.[46] In another study using MD-UVA1, none of the four patients with chronic urticaria showed improvement. However, the number of treated cases was not high enough (a mean number of 8 ± 4 treatments).[47]

### 51.2.2.2 Urticaria Factitia

BB-UVB was employed in a study on 43 patients with symptomatic dermographism.[48] After 10–15 treatments (five times weekly for 2–3 weeks), 25 patients were freed from symptoms, while 14 improved.[48] In another study on 14 patients with severe dermographism treated with a 4-week course of PUVA, 5 reported clinically useful reduction of itch.[49]

### 51.2.2.3 Aquagenic Urticaria

One patient with aquagenic urticaria responded to BB-UVB and another to PUVA.[50,51]

### 51.2.2.4 Solar Urticaria

Solar urticaria can be induced by different UV waves ranging from UVB to visible light.[52]

Preventive therapy with different UV sources has been tried, but PUVA seems to be the most effective in inducing tolerance.[52]

### 51.2.2.5 Urticaria Pigmentosa (Mastocytosis)

Patients with urticaria pigmentosa may suffer from pruritus especially when the skin is rubbed or warm. Six of our patients with moderate itch were treated with NB-UVB, and five with severe itch were treated with oral PUVA. All patients improved with excellent results, particularly after PUVA, which also reduced the number of lesions in two patients (unpublished).

However, these skin lesions recurred some time after the discontinuation of PUVA treatment. In addition, PUVA induces pigmentation, which makes the primary lesions less visible.

Bath–PUVA was used in two studies on urticaria pigmentosa with good effect in five patients and no effect in four.[53,54] In the last study, oral PUVA was effective in 14 out of 20 patients with urticaria pigmentosa.[54] In another study on 19 patients, MD-UVA1 induced improvement in 45% of patients.[47] MD-UVA1 has been shown to be as effective as HD-UVA1 with respect to pruritus and quality of life in a study on 22 patients with urticaria pigmentosa.[55] As UVA1 rapidly induces tanning, it may also be of cosmetic value in these patients.

UV therapy in patients with urticaria pigmentosa and also in some other forms of urticaria triggers a massive mast cell degranulation which leads to vasodilation, itching, and sometimes headache or nausea. Therefore, the therapy should be performed with caution, possibly at least in the beginning, with the protection of nonsedative antihistamines.

### 51.2.3 Psoriasis

Although psoriasis has been the first skin disease to be treated with phototherapy, and patients with psoriasis are still frequent users of phototherapy units in countries with a temperate climate, the issue of associated pruritus has been poorly studied. In a questionnaire answered by 108 psoriatic patients, 84% revealed generalized pruritus.[56] Twenty patients were treated with BB-UVB and only seven reported relief of itch, two with a long-term effect.[56] Another study confirmed that pruritus in patients with psoriasis is generalized and not just confined to psoriasis plaques.[57] Some of the 20 patients studied, reported an improvement of itch following NB-UVB therapy.[57]

### 51.2.4 Cutaneous T-Cell Lymphoma

Cutaneous T-cell lymphoma is one of the major dermatologic conditions for which phototherapy continues to be a valuable treatment modality. Most studies published on the efficacy of different UV treatments determine histological and clinical response: clearing of the lesions to less than 50% being regarded as no response. Although pruritus is one of the most common initial manifestations of cutaneous lymphoma, it is seldom monitored in study outcomes. Mycosis fungoides is the most common form of cutaneous T-cell lymphoma, and its early patch or plaques stage is often treated with PUVA.[58] In a case report, the improvement of a patient with mycosis fungoides was slow, and pruritus disappeared successively after three months of treatment.[59] A patient with Sézary's syndrome with erythroderma and severe pruritus, which had been unreponsive to prednisone and cyclophosphamide, was cleared of the syndrome when PUVA was added to the treatment regimen.[58] However, PUVA may increase pruritus in patients with cutaneous T-cell lymphoma, and UVA exposures have to be increased more cautiously than with PUVA treatment for psoriasis.[58] In a study on eight patients with patch-stage mycosis fungoides treated with 19–42 NB-UVB exposures, all reported rapid and clinically significant improvement with abolition or reduction of pruritus.[60] MD- UVA1 "cold light" given five times weekly for 3 weeks was shown in a case report to improve erythema and itching of a patient with erythroderma with cutaneous T-cell lymphoma within a week.[61]

## 51.2.5 Prurigo

Prurigo is a condition of nodular cutaneous lesions that itch so fiercely that the condition is actually named itch-"pruire." While the rare acute form can be caused by insect stings, most of the subacute and chronic forms appear to be due to AD or of unknown origin.[62]

Subacute prurigo is often refractory to conventional treatment, and phototherapy is a treatment of choice. A comparison of oral PUVA, UVAB and BB-UVB in 11 patients with subacute prurigo has shown that 100% of the patients treated with PUVA showed at least some improvement compared with 66% of patients in the UVAB treatment group and 80% of patients in the BB-UVB treatment group.[63] However, in this study pruritus was not monitored, and only clearing of lesions was measured. In another study, 10 patients with subacute prurigo were treated with foil bath PUVA, requiring a median of 13 treatments to clear the pruritic lesions in all patients, the pruritus itself not being rated and no side effects being reported.[64] A randomized study on 33 patients with subacute prurigo was designed to investigate the efficacy of bath PUVA, MD-UVA1 and NB-UVB, respectively, using a PIP (papules, infiltration and pruritus) score for evaluation of the outcome.[65] Bath PUVA was performed four times weekly, and MD-UVA1 and NB-UVB five times weekly, the outcome being measured after 4 weeks of therapy. This study revealed significantly higher PIP score reduction in patients who were treated with bath PUVA and MD-UVA1 compared to NB-UVB.[65]

The genuine form of chronic prurigo is the prurigo nodularis of Hyde, who coined the term in 1909.[62]

In a Finnish study, 15 patients with prurigo nodularis were treated with bath PUVA daily for 1–4 weeks and then for 4 days every second month for 5 months.[66] The itching was reported to decrease markedly or to disappear completely within 4–6 days, while all lesions continued to heal and remained healed in 13 patients.[66] Hann et al. reported on a patient with generalized prurigo nodularis who was treated with 24 exposures of BB-UVB while most of the pruritic nodules as well as the itching sensation disappeared.[67] However, the remaining large itchy nodules were treated thereafter with 8-mehoxypsoralen topical PUVA three times weekly for 2 months with excellent results on lesions and pruritus.[67] In an English study, nodular prurigo in seven of eight patients improved with BB-UVB.[68] Only four of eight patients with chronic prurigo in our department improved on BB-UVB (unpublished observations). Maintenance therapy using NB-UVB once weekly in 10 patients with prurigo nodularis for about 6 months has been reported to notably improve the lesions and prevent relapse in 9 patients during an observation time of 1 year.[69]

Fourteen of 17 patients with prurigo nodularis treated with MD-UVA1 reported an improvement of pruritus, 41% reporting a marked improvement, 29% a moderate improvement, and 95% a slight improvement of pruritus.[47]

## 51.3 Itch in Noninflamed Skin

Itch in noninflamed skin may be either of neuropathic (secondary to morphological alterations of nerve fibers) or neurogenic (secondary to increased release of nerve transmitters or to circulating pruritogenic substances) origin, or due to both these mechanisms or none determined (pruritus of undetermined origin).

Proliferation of intraepidermal nerve fibers has been found in patients with pruritus of end-stage renal failure.[70,71] Neuropathic changes in cutaneous nociceptors may explain pruritus in patients on hemodialysis, although other factors such as increased numbers of cutaneous mast cells have been discussed.[23] Pruritus associated with HIV has been related to increased soluble mediators in plasma such as cytokines but may also appear as prurigo lesions in skin that does not seem inflamed.[62,72] As early as in 1899, Johnston wrote in the *Archives of Dermatology* that the number of hypertrophic nerve fibres in prurigo lesions is increased, which has been shown later to contain CGRP-positive nerve fibers.[73]

Experiments showing that UVB phototherapy to one-half of the body generates generalized improvement of uremic pruritus suggest circulating mediators as pathogenetic in pruritus in noninflamed skin.[28] Itch of cholestasis has been attributed to the increased intrahepatic synthesis of opioid peptides rather than to an accumulation of the bile salts in the tissues.[74] Itch induced by hot baths in patients with polycythemia vera has been proposed to be related to serotonin and to prostaglandins released from aggregating platlets.[75]

### 51.3.1 Chronic Renal Failure

Pruritus affects 12–20% of patients with chronic renal failure and 60–80% of patients undergoing peritoneal dialysis or hemodialysis.[76] The symptoms range from localized and mild to generalized and severe. Ultraviolet phototherapy is the treatment of choice in moderate to severe uremic pruritus and there are several controlled trials comparing UVB with UVA or placebo, while itch is assessed before and after the treatments.

In the first report by Gilchrest et al., 9 of 10 patients treated with BB-UVB two times weekly for 4 weeks improved as opposed to 2 of 8 in the UVA group.[77] However, in another controlled study by Simpson and Davison on 12 patients with the same protocol, both UVB and UVA appeared to have equal effect on uremic pruritus.[78] Seventeen chronic dialysis patients reporting severe pruritus, treated three times weekly, responded with resolution of pruritus after UVB, while UVA was without any significant effect.[79] This trial had, however, a limited duration of 2 weeks.[79]

In an uncontrolled study using BB-UVB in 14 patients with severe uremic pruritus, 8 had objective benefit and the itch intensity declined in all patients, mean itch scores being reduced from 7 to 5.[80]

In a recent study on 15 patients with uremic pruritus treated with NB-UVB three times weekly for 4 weeks, 9 reported 60% improvement of pruritus.[80]

The remission of pruritus after BB-UVB and NB-UVB seems to be equal ranging from 1 to 10 months after the phototherapy course.[28,80]

### 51.3.2 Cholestasis

Pruritus occurs in 25% of patients with cholestasis and in nearly 100% of patients with primary biliary cirrhosis where it is often the presenting symptom.[81] There are numerous approaches to control cholestatic pruritus including use of anticholestatic agents, opiate antagonists and antidepressants.[74] However, phototherapy is described mostly in case reports. Treatment with BB-UVB for 10 days induced remission of pruritus in five patients with primary biliary cirrhosis, and the symptoms relapsed 2 weeks after stopping the treatment and resolved again upon a new phototherapy course.[82] However, as the disease progresses, the effects of UVB treatment may cease as reported in two patients of Perlstein.[83] Another patient treated with UVA three to five times weekly reported a partial relief of pruritus.[84]

Johnston et al. described 14 cases of pruritus due to obstetric cholestasis in a 14-year survey and found the incidence to be approximately 1 in 1293 deliveries.[85] Although not reported, NB-UVB is suggested for the treatment of cholestatic pruritus. In addition, it can be safely used during pregnancy.[86]

### 51.3.3 Polycythemia Vera and Aquagenic Pruritus

Generalized pruritus occurs in 60% of patients with polycythemia vera and may appear either spontaneously or after a bath.[87] Patients with polycythemia vera may present with symptoms similar to those of aquagenic pruritus, and all patients with symptoms consistent with aquagenic pruritus should be investigated for the presence of polycythemia vera.

The first report on the success of photochemotherapy for pruritus secondary to polycythemia vera came from Oklahoma.[88] Two hours after the intake of 30 mg 8-methoxypsoralene, the patient exposed the skin to the midday sun, slowly increasing the time to a maximum of 25 min three times weekly during the summer. Two months after the discontinuation of the treatment, during autumn, pruritus returned.[88] In another study, oral PUVA at a phototherapy unit was given to 11 patients with pruritus due to polycythemia vera.[89] The patients received at least 15 treatments, given 2–3 times weekly, and then a maintenance therapy once every 1 or every 2 weeks. Upon this regimen, 8 of the 11 patients reported excellent results and 3 partial improvement of pruritus, respectively.[89] Menagé et al. described a patient with polycythemia vera whose itch was aggravated by BB-UVB phototherapy but who responded to eight treatments of PUVA and maintenance therapy every 2 weeks.[90] Baldo et al. described the good effect of treatment with NB-UVB in 10 patients with severe pruritus of polycythemia vera.[87] The patients were treated three times weekly and a complete remission of pruritus was achieved within 2–10 weeks of treatment in eight patients, the other two reporting only partial relief. Relapse of pruritus occurred within 8 months after stopping the treatment.[87]

Steinman et al. reported on 14 patients with aquagenic pruritus without polycythemia vera who were treated with BB-UVB.[91] Eight of these patients noted significant improvement but relapsed when the therapy was decreased in frequency or discontinued, requiring maintenance therapy with suberythemal doses two to three times weekly.[91] Oral PUVA therapy given to five patients with aquagenic pruritus twice weekly for up to 12 weeks resulted in complete remission of the disease.[90] However, relapse occurred within 2–24 weeks suggesting the need for a maintenance therapy. In another report, a patient with aquagenic pruritus responded to a course of oral PUVA given twice weekly for 6 weeks and remained on remission on bath-PUVA as maintenance therapy.[92]

## 51.4 HIV

Patients infected with human immunodeficiency virus (HIV) have a high prevalence of UVR responsive skin diseases including psoriasis, pruritus, eosinophilic filiculitis, and eczemas. Idiopathic generalized HIV pruritus is a diagnosis of exclusion.[93]

The first report on successful photochemotherapy for pruritus secondary to HIV used PUVA twice a week for 4 weeks followed by maintenance therapy once a week for 3 months.[94] Pruritus recurred 1 month after cessation of therapy. Another patient with HIV pruritus and prurigo was successfully treated with BB-UVB for 2 months.[95] When he discontinued therapy, pruritus returned promptly to resolve upon a new course of BB-UVB three times per week. Lim et al. treated 21 patients with intractable pruritus of HIV with BB-UVB three times weekly for 6–7 weeks, pruritus scores being reduced from 9 to 2.[96]

In view of the potential effects of UVR to increase HIV replication, viral plasma levels of HIV positive patients as well as their CD4 lymphocyte numbers before and after UVB or PUVA therapy were followed in several studies, which concluded that there were no adverse effects.[93,97]

## 51.5 Pruritus of Undetermined Origin and Pruritus of Senescence

Pruritus of undetermined origin is a diagnosis by exclusion when internal diseases have been ruled out. This group is probably larger than it appears, as many internal diseases known to be pruritogenic occur in patients with pruritus as a parallel phenomenon without being responsible for itching. Seckin et al. treated 25 patients with pruritus of undetermined origin with NB-UVB three times weekly for 6–7 weeks.[80] Seventeen patients completed the treatment, their pruritus grading score being decreased from 9 to 4 at the end of the treatment. Thirteen patients showed up for a follow-up six months later; eight were in remission and five reported relapse within 3 months.

Pruritus in the elderly is a common phenomenon.[98] Although there are no published trials, phototherapy is often suggested.[98,99] We have used NB-UVB successfully in several patients with pruritus of senescence. NB-UVB has been chosen because of the short exposure time in the booth and because it is almost as effective as PUVA but without the inconvenience of taking psoralene which may interact with other possible drugs.

## 51.6 General Aspects

At our department, a course of BB-UVB, NB-UVB or PUVA for pruritus is performed three times weekly for 6 weeks. Today NB-UVB is more frequently used than BB-UVB because it is less erythemogenic. Oral PUVA is offered in severe cases or when no sufficient effect has been obtained by the use of UVB. A less aggressive protocol, such as that suggested for cutaneous lymphoma rather than the one for psoriasis, is used because these patients have lower threshold of pruritus and erythema.[58,60]

Improvement of pruritus may be expected within the first 3 weeks and a complete resolution at the end of the course. As relapse is quite common after discontinuation, the patients are offered maintenance therapy twice and then once weekly for another 6 weeks. If the pruritus deteriorates, the number of sessions is increased to three times weekly. Sometimes the patients have to discontinue UV therapy after the first course of 6 weeks because of social reasons, but they may start again upon remittance. MD-UVA1 may be recommended to patients with pruritus secondary to exacerbation of atopic eczema.[61] Here the course is five times weekly for 3 weeks and has often to be followed up by NB-UVB in order to avoid relapse.

Although maintenance therapy is often necessary, generally patients with pruritus require much shorter durations of therapy than patients with chronic inflammatory skin diseases, where long-term effects of phototherapy have been studied.[100] Therefore, the chronic side effects of UV-based therapy are uncommon in patients with pruritus.

# References

1. Møller KI, Kongshoj B, Philipsen PA, Thomsen VO, Wulf HC. How Finsen's light cured lupus vulgaris. *Photodermatol Photoimmunol Photomed*. 2005;21(3):118–124.
2. Lindelöf B. Grenz ray therapy in dermatology. An experimental, clinical and epidemiological study. *Acta Derm Venereol Suppl (Stockh)*. 1987;132:1–67.
3. McGregor JM. The history of human photobiology. In: ED Hawk JLM. Arnold eds. *Photodermatology*. Oxford University Press; 1999.
4. Ingram JT. The approach to psoriasis. *Br Med J*. 1953;2(4836):591–594.
5. Parrish JA, Fitzpatrick TB, Tanenbaum L, Pathak MA. Photochemotherapy of psoriasis with oral methoxsalen and longwave ultraviolet light. *N Engl J Med*. 1974;291(23):1207–1211.
6. Rivard J, Lim HW. The use of 308-nm excimer laser for dermatoses: experience with 34 patients. *J Drugs Dermatol*. 2006;5(6):550–554.
7. Gilchrest BA, Soter NA, Stoff JS, Mihm MC Jr. The human sunburn reaction: histologic and biochemical studies. *J Am Acad Dermatol*. 1981;5(4):411–422.
8. Ruzicka T, Walter JF, Printz MP. Changes in arachidonic acid metabolism in UV-irradiated hairless mouse skin. *J Invest Dermatol*. 1983;81:300–303.
9. Black AK, Fincham N, Greaves MW, Hensby CN. Time course changes in levels of arachidonic acid and prostaglandins D2, E2, F2 alpha in human skin following UVB irradiation. *Br J Clin Pharmacol*. 1980;10:453–457.
10. Hawk JL, Black AK, Jaenicke KF, et al. Increased concentrations of arachidonic acid, prostaglandins E2, D2, and 6-oxo-F1α, and histamine in human skin following UVA irradiation. *J Invest Dermatol*. 1983;80:496–499.
11. Grandjean-Laquerriere A, Le Naour R, Gangloff SC, Guenounou M. Differential regulation of TNF-alpha, IL-6 and IL-10 in UVB-irradiated human keratinocytes via cyclic AMP/protein kinase A pathway. *Cytokine*. 2003;23(4–5):138–149.
12. Schwarz T. Mechanisms of UV-induced immunosuppression. *Keio J Med*. 2005;54(4):165–171.
13. Norris DA, Lyons MB, Middleton MH, Yohn JJ, Kashihara-Sawami M. Ultraviolet radiation can either suppress or induce expression of intercellular adhesion molecule 1 (ICAM-1) on the surface of cultured human keratinocytes. *J Invest Dermatol*. 1990;95(2):132–138.
14. Hruza LL, Pentland AP. Mechanisms of UV-induced inflammation. *J Invest Dermatol*. 1993;100(1):35S–41S.
15. Wallengren J, Ekman R, Möller H. Substance P and vasoactive intestinal peptide in bullous and inflammatory skin disease. *Acta Derm Venereol (Stockh)*. 1986;66:23–28.
16. Gillardon F, Moll I, Michel S, Benrath J, Weihe E, Zimmermann M. Calcitonin gene-related peptide and nitric oxide are involved in ultraviolet radiation-induced immunosuppression. *Eur J Pharmacol*. 1995;293(4):395–400.
17. Legat FJ, Griesbacher T, Schicho R, et al. Repeated subinflammatory ultraviolet B irradiation increases substance P and calcitonin gene-related peptide content and augments mustard oil-induced neurogenic inflammation in the skin of rats. *Neurosci Lett*. 2002;329:309–313.
18. Scholzen TE, Brzoska T, Kalden DH, et al. Effect of ultraviolet light on the release of neuropeptides and neuroendocrine hormones in the skin: mediators of photodermatitis and cutaneous inflammation. *J Investig Dermatol Symp Proc*. 1999;4(1):55–60.
19. Wallengren J. Substance P antagonist inhibits immediate and delayed type cutaneous hypersensitivity reactions.*Br J Dermatol*. 1991;124(4):324–328.
20. Bondesson L, Nordlind K, Mutt V. Lidén S. Vasoactive intestinal polypeptide inhibits the established allergic contact dermatitis in humans. *Ann N Y Acad Sci*. 1996;805:702–707.
21. Wallengren J. Dual effects of CGRP-antagonist on allergic contact dermatitis in human skin. *Contact Dermatitis*. 2000;43(3):137–143.
22. Wallengren J. Neuroanatomy and neurophysiology of itch. *Dermatol Ther*. 2005;18(4):292–303.
23. Szepietowski JC, Morita A. Tsuji T. Ultraviolet B induces mast cell apoptosis: a hypothetical mechanism of ultraviolet B treatment for uraemic pruritus. *Med Hypotheses*. 2002;58(2):167–170.
24. Fjellner B, Hagermark O. Influence of ultraviolet light on itch and flare reactions in human skin induced by histamine and the histamine liberator compound 48/80. *Acta Derm Venereol*. 1982;62:137–140.
25. Wallengren J. Vasoactive peptides in the skin. *J Investig Dermatol Symp Proc*. 1997;2(1):49–55.
26. Wallengren J, Sundler F. Phototherapy induces loss of epidermal and dermal nerve fibers. *Acta Derm Venereol (Stockh)*. 2004;84:111–115.

27. Kumakiri M, Hashimoto K, Willis I. Biological changes of human cutaneous nerves caused by ultraviolet irradiation: an ultrastructural study. *Br J Dermatol*. 1978;99(1):65–75.

28. Gilchrest BA, Rowe JW, Brown RS, Steinman TI, Arndt KA. Ultraviolet phototherapy of uremic pruritus. Long-term results and possible mechanism of action. *Ann Intern Med*. 1979;91(1):17–21.

29. Jekler J, Bergbrant IM, Faergemann J. Larkö O. The in vivo effect of UVB radiation on skin bacteria in patients with atopic dermatitis. *Acta Derm Venereol*. 1992;72(1):33–36.

30. Faergemann J, Larkö O. The effect of UV-light on human skin microorganisms. *Acta Derm Venereol*. 1987;67(1):69–72.

31. Samson Yashar S, Gielczyk R, Scherschun L, Lim HW. Narrow-band ultraviolet B treatment for vitiligo, pruritus, and inflammatory dermatoses. *Photodermatol Photoimmunol Photomed*. 2003;19(4):164–168.

32. Hanifin JM, Rajka G. Diagnostic features of atopic dermatitis. *Acta Derm Venereol*. 1980;92:44–47.

33. Jekler J, Larkö O. UVB phototherapy of atopic dermatitis. *Br J Dermatol*. 1988;119(6):697–705.

34. Jekler J, Larkö O. Combined UVA-UVB versus UVB phototherapy for atopic dermatitis: a paired-comparison study. *J Am Acad Dermatol*. 1990;22(1):49–53.

35. Jekler J, Larkö O. Phototherapy for atopic dermatitis with ultraviolet A (UVA), low-dose UVB and combined UVA and UVB: two paired-comparison studies. *Photodermatol Photoimmunol Photomed*. 1991;8(4):151–156.

36. Jekler J, Larkö O. UVA solarium versus UVB phototherapy of atopic dermatitis: a paired-comparison study. *Br J Dermatol*. 1991;125(6):569–572.

37. Hjerppe M, Hasan T, Saksala I, Reunala T. Narrow-band UVB treatment in atopic dermatitis. *Acta Derm Venereol*. 2001;81(6):439–440.

38. Der-Petrossian M, Seeber A, Hönigsmann H, Tanew A. Half-side comparison study on the efficacy of 8-methoxypsoralen bath-PUVA versus narrow-band ultraviolet B phototherapy in patients with severe chronic atopic dermatitis. *Br J Dermatol*. 2000;142(1):39–43.

39. Meduri NB, Vandergriff T, Rasmussen H, Jacobe H. Phototherapy in the management of atopic dermatitis: a systematic review. *Photodermatol Photoimmunol Photomed*. 2007;23(4):106–112.

40. von Kobyletzki G, Pieck C, Hoffmann K, Freitag M, Altmeyer P. Medium-dose UVA1 cold-light phototherapy in the treatment of severe atopic dermatitis. *J Am Acad Dermatol*. 1999;41(6):931–937.

41. Reynolds NJ, Franklin V, Gray JC, Diffey BL, Farr PM. Narrow-band ultraviolet B and broad-band ultraviolet A phototherapy in adult atopic eczema: a randomised controlled trial. *Lancet*. 2001;357(9273):2012–2016.

42. Legat FJ, Hofer A, Brabek E, Quehenberger F, Kerl H, Wolf P. Narrowband UV-B vs medium-dose UV-A1 phototherapy in chronic atopic dermatitis. *Arch Dermatol*. 2003;139(2):223–234.

43. Baltás E, Csoma Z, Bodai L, Ignácz F, Dobozy A, Kemény L. Treatment of atopic dermatitis with the xenon chloride excimer laser. *J Eur Acad Dermatol Venereol*. 2006;20(6):657–660.

44. Olafsson JH, Larkö O, Roupe G, Granerus G. Bengtsson U. Treatment of chronic urticaria with PUVA or UVA plus placebo: a double-blind study. *Arch Dermatol Res*. 1986;278(3):228–231.

45. Berroeta L, Clark C, Ibbotson SH, Ferguson J, Dawe RS. Narrow-band (TL-01) ultraviolet B phototherapy for chronic urticaria. *Clin Exp Dermatol*. 2004;29(1):97–98.

46. Hannuksela M, Kokkonen EL. Ultraviolet light therapy in chronic urticaria. *Acta Derm Venereol*. 1985;65(5):449–450.

47. Rombold S, Lobisch K, Katzer K, Grazziotin TC, Ring J, Eberlein B. Efficacy of UVA1 phototherapy in 230 patients with various skin diseases. *Photodermatol Photoimmunol Photomed*. 2008; 24(1):19–23.

48. Johnsson M, Falk ES. Volden G. UVB treatment of factitious urticaria. *Photodermatol*. 1987;4(6):302–304.

49. Logan RA, O'Brien TJ, Greaves MW. The effect of psoralen photochemotherapy (PUVA) on symptomatic dermographism. *Clin Exp Dermatol*. 1989;14(1):25–28.

50. Parker RK, Crowe MJ, Guin JD. Aquagenic urticaria. *Cutis*. 1992;50(4):283–284.

51. Juhlin L, Malmros-Enander I. Familial polymorphous light eruption with aquagenic urticaria: successful treatment with PUVA. *Photodermatol*. 1986;3(6):346–349.

52. Hönigsmann H. Mechanisms of phototherapy and photochemotherapy for photodermatoses. *Dermatol Ther*. 2003; 16(1):23–27.

53. Väätäinen N, Hannuksela M, Karvonen J. Trioxsalen baths plus UV-A in the treatment of lichen planus and urticaria pigmentosa. *Clin Exp Dermatol*. 1981;6(2):133–138.

54. Godt O, Proksch E, Streit V, Christophers E. Short- and long-term effectiveness of oral and bath PUVA therapy in urticaria pigmentosa and systemic mastocytosis. *Dermatology*. 1997;195(1):35–39.

55. Gobello T, Mazzanti C, Sordi D, et al. Medium versus high-dose ultraviolet A1 therapy for urticaria pigmentosa: a pilot study. *J Am Acad Dermatol*. 2003;49(4):679–684.

56. Yosipovitch G, Goon A, Wee J, Chan YH, Goh CL. The prevalence and clinical characteristics of pruritus among patients with extensive psoriasis. *Br J Dermatol*. 2000; 143(5):969–973.

57. Amatya B, Nordlind K. Focus groups in Swedish psoriatic patients with pruritus. *J Dermatol*. 2008;35(1):1–5.

58. Lowe NJ, Cripps DJ, Dufton PA, Vickers CF. Photochemotherapy for mycosis fungoides: a clinical and histological study. *Arch Dermatol*. 1979;115(1):50–53.

59. Pujol RM, Gallardo F, Llistosella E, et al. Invisible mycosis fungoides: a diagnostic challenge. *J Am Acad Dermatol*. 2000;42(2 pt 2):324–328.

60. Clark C, Dawe RS, Evans AT, Lowe G, Ferguson J. Narrowband TL-01 phototherapy for patch-stage mycosis fungoides. *Arch Dermatol*. 2000;136(6):748–752.

61. von Kobyletzki G, Dirschka T, Freitag M, Hoffman K, Altmeyer P. Ultraviolet-A1 phototherapy improves the status of the skin in cutaneous T-cell lymphoma. *Br J Dermatol*. 1999;140(4):768–769.

62. Wallengren J. Prurigo: diagnosis and management. *Am J Clin Dermatol*. 2004;5(2):85–95.

63. Clark AR, Jorizzo JL, Fleischer AB. Papular dermatitis (subacute prurigo, "itchy red bump" disease): pilot study of phototherapy. *J Am Acad Dermatol*. 1998;38(6 pt 1):929–933.

64. Streit V, Thiede R, Wiedow O, Christophers E. Foil bath PUVA in the treatment of prurigo simplex subacuta. *Acta Derm Venereol*. 1996;76(4):319–320.

65. Gambichler T, Hyun J, Sommer A, Stücker M, Altmeyer P, Kreuter A. A randomised controlled trial on photo(chemo) therapy of subacute prurigo. *Clin Exp Dermatol.* 2006; 31(3):348–353.

66. Väätäinen N, Hannuksela M, Karvonen J. Local photochemotherapy in nodular prurigo. *Acta Derm Venereol.* 1979;59(6):544–547.

67. Hann SK, Cho MY, Park YK. UV treatment of generalized prurigo nodularis. *Int J Dermatol.* 1990;29(6):436–437.

68. Divekar PM, Palmer RA, Keefe M. Phototherapy in nodular prurigo. *Clin Exp Dermatol.* 2003;28(1):99–100.

69. Tamagawa-Mineoka R, Katoh N, Ueda E, Kishimoto S. Narrow-band ultraviolet B phototherapy in patients with recalcitrant nodular prurigo. *J Dermatol.* 2007;34(10):691–695.

70. Fantini F, Baraldi A, Sevignani C, Spattini A, Pincelli C, Giannetti A. Cutaneous innervation in chronic renal failure patients. An immunohistochemical study. *Acta Derm Venereol.* 1992;72(2):102–105.

71. Johansson O, Hilliges M, Ståhle-Bäckdahl M. Intraepidermal neuron-specific enolase (NSE)-immunoreactive nerve fibres: evidence for sprouting in uremic patients on maintenance hemodialysis. *Neurosci Lett.* 1989;99(3):281–286.

72. Milazzo F, Piconi S, Trabattoni D, et al. Intractable pruritus in HIV infection: immunologic characterization. *Allergy.* 1999;54(3):266–272.

73. Vaalasti A, Suomalainen H, Rechardt L. Calcitonin gene-related peptide immunoreactivity in prurigo nodularis: a comparative study with neurodermatitis circumscripta. *Br J Dermatol.* 1989;120(5):619–623.

74. Bergasa NV. The pruritus of cholestasis. *J Hepatol.* 2005;43(6):1078–1088.

75. Fjellner B, Hägermark O. Pruritus in polycythemia vera: treatment with aspirin and possibility of platelet involvement. *Acta Derm Venereol.* 1979;59(6):05–12.

76. Stahle-Backdahl M. Uremic pruritus: clinical and experimental studies. *Acta Derm Venereol.* 1989;145(suppl): 1–38.

77. Gilchrest BA, Rowe JW, Brown RS, Steinman TI, Arndt KA. Relief of uremic pruritus with ultraviolet phototherapy. *N Engl J Med.* 1977;297(3):136–138.

78. Simpson NB, Davison AM. Ultraviolet phototherapy for uraemic pruritus. *Lancet.* 1981;1(8223):781.

79. Blachley JD, Blankenship DM, Menter A, Parker TF 3rd, Knochel JP. Uremic pruritus: skin divalent ion content and response to ultraviolet phototherapy. *Am J Kidney Dis.* 1985;5(5):237–241.

80. Seckin D, Demircay Z, Akin O. Generalized pruritus treated with narrowband UVB. *Int J Dermatol.* 2007; 46(4):367–370.

81. Martin J. Pruritus. *Int J Dermatol.* 1985;24(10):634–639.

82. Hanid MA, Levi AJ. Phototherapy for pruritus in primary biliary cirrhosis. *Lancet.* 1980;2(8193):530.

83. Perlstein SM. Phototherapy for primary biliary cirrhosis. *Arch Dermatol.* 1981;117(10):608.

84. Person JR. Ultraviolet A (UV-A) and cholestatic pruritus. *Arch Dermatol.* 1981;117(11):684.

85. Johnston WG, Baskett TF. Obstetric cholestasis. A 14 year review. *Am J Obstet Gynecol.* 1979;133(3):299–301.

86. Tauscher AE, Fleischer AB Jr, Phelps KC, Feldman SR. Psoriasis and pregnancy. *J Cutan Med Surg.* 2002;6(6): 561–570.

87. Baldo A, Sammarco E, Plaitano R, Martinelli V. Monfrecola. Narrowband (TL-01) ultraviolet B phototherapy for pruritus in polycythaemia vera. *Br J Dermatol.* 2002;147(5):979–981.

88. Swerlick RA. Photochemotherapy treatment of pruritus associated with polycythemia vera. *J Am Acad Dermatol.* 1985;13(4):675–677.

89. Jeanmougin M, Rain JD, Najean Y. Efficacy of photochemotherapy on severe pruritus in polycythemia vera. *Ann Hematol.* 1996;73(2):91–93.

90. Menagé HD, Norris PG, Hawk JL. Graves MW. The efficacy of psoralen photo-chemotherapy in the treatment of aquagenic pruritus. *Br J Dermatol.* 1993;129(2):163–165.

91. Steinman HK, Greaves MW. Aquagenic pruritus. *J Am Acad Dermatol.* 1985;13(1):91–96.

92. Smith RA, Ross JS, Staughton RC. Bath PUVA as a treatment for aquagenic pruritus. *Br J Dermatol.* 1994;131(4):584.

93. Gelfand JM, Rudikoff D. Evaluation and treatment of itching in HIV-infected patients. *Mt Sinai J Med.* 2001;68(4–5): 298–308.

94. Gorin I, Lessana-Leibowitch M, Fortier P, Leibowitch J, Escande JP. Successful treatment of the pruritus of human immunodeficiency virus infection and acquired immunodeficiency syndrome with psoralens plus ultraviolet A therapy. *J Am Acad Dermatol.* 1989;20(3):511–513.

95. Weiss DS, Taylor JR. Treatment of generalized pruritus in an HIV-positive patient with UVB phototherapy. *Clin Exp Dermatol.* 1990;15(4):316–317.

96. Lim HW, Vallurupalli S, Meola T, Soter NA. UVB phototherapy is an effective treatment for pruritus in patients infected with HIV. *J Am Acad Dermatol.* 1997;37(3 pt 1): 414–417.

97. Akaraphanth R, Lim HW. HIV, UV and immunosuppression. *Photodermatol Photoimmunol Photomed.* 1999;15(1): 28–31.

98. Ward JR, Bernhard JD. Willan's itch and other causes of pruritus in the elderly. *Int J Dermatol.* 2005;44(4):267–273.

99. Lonsdale-Eccles A. Carmichael AJ. Treatment of pruritus associated with systemic disorders in the elderly: a review of the role of new therapies. *Drugs Aging.* 2003;20(3): 197–208.

100. Lindelöf B, Sigurgeirsson B, Tegner E, et al. PUVA and cancer risk: the Swedish follow-up study. *Br J Dermatol.* 1999;141(1):108–112.

# Chapter 52
# Itch and Acupuncture

Laurent Misery and Laurence Potin-Richard

## 52.1 Definition

Acupuncture (from Latin "acus," "needle" and "pungere," "to prick") is a treatment from China which consists in pricking with needles in some specific points on the skin, along "meridians." Traditionally, it is based on energy fluxes but new pathophysiological data have led to a better understanding.

## 52.2 Pathophysiology

### 52.2.1 Traditional Concepts

Acupuncture is a very old technique and is only a part of traditional Chinese medicine. Hence, first explanations are based on philosophical rather than scientific concepts. Energy is supposed to circulate for 1 day in the human body, mainly along lines on the skin, which are called meridians. The human body (like the universe) is made of two opposite and complementary forces: Yin and Yang. There is a need to balance between Yin and Yang for good health. An excess of Yin or Yang may induce disease, and acupuncture could restore the equilibrium. But many other concepts are necessary to understand traditional Chinese medicine and acupuncture, like the four movements, the cycles, the five elements or the six levels of energy.

Each meridian is associated with one organ (or function). Twelve main meridians are defined: lung, large intestine, stomach, spleen-pancreas, heart, small intestine, bladder, kidney, heart master, triple warmer, gall bladder, and lever. Superficial meridians are cutaneous projection of these main meridians. That is why pricking on one skin point could treat visceral symptoms. These points are precisely defined and are depressible areas.

Hence, there is no meridian for the organ "skin." Skin is described as surface (Biao). Dermatology (Pi Fu Ke) is a part of external medicine (Wai Ke). Pruritus is linked to an excess of Yin. Some points are defined for treatment of skin diseases. The choice of acupuncture points is very complex. Point N°11GI (Gu Chi) is often used in patients with pruritus because it is known to chase out the Wind element. But there is no specific point against itch or against any disease or symptom. Several criteria are needed.

### 52.2.2 Current Concepts

Neurophysiological data bring new possibilities to understand the effects of acupuncture. Acupuncture points are small areas (<1 mm) which can be depressed by applying pressure with a finger. Sometimes, this pressure induces pain. The existence of an anatomical substratum is discussed. There could be a lower electrical resistivity[1] and there is often a plexus with amyelinic cholinergic fibers and myelinic fibers. A$\alpha$, A$\beta$, A$\delta$ and C fibers appear to end as cutaneous or muscular sensory receptors with a distribution that is closely associated with acupuncture points.[2] About 80% of points seem to be localized in the front of the split points between muscles or muscular fascia.[3]

A study on collagen lattice shows that the rotation of needles (as performed by acupunctors) induces mechanotransduction by fibroblasts probably followed by activation of nerve fibers.[4] Stimulation by needles in acupuncture points on rats has been shown to be followed by the local release of norepinephrin.[5]

L. Misery and S. Ständer (eds.), *Pruritus*,
DOI 10.1007/978-1-84882-322-8_52, © Springer-Verlag London Limited 2010

**Table 52.1** Differential effects according to frequency of stimulation (from Brown[8])

| Conducted at 50–200 Hz | Conducted at 2–4 Hz |
| --- | --- |
| Aβ fibers | Aδ fibers |
| Low-intensity stimulation | High-intensity stimulation |
| Effects: immediate | Effects: 20–30 min after stimulation |
| Duration: during stimulation | Duration: several hours or days after stimulation |
| Enhances dynorphin | Enhances met-enkephalin |
| Activation of κ receptors | Activation of μ receptors |

At the medullar level, acupuncture is supposed to activate gate control through effects on points of cutaneous projection of visceral sensitivity. Pain (or pruritus?) in an area is inhibited by pain in another area.

The stimulation of distant points seems to activate cerebral areas corresponding to areas that the acupunctor wants to treat: for example, acupuncture on feet in order to treat eye diseases is followed by activation of visual areas in the brain.[6] Acupuncture stimulates the release of opiods,[7] and its effects can be inhibited by opiod antagonists such as naloxone. Electroacupuncture at 50–200 Hz, induces release of dynorphin A, activates κ receptors and might inhibit pruritus, in contrast to 2–4 Hz (Table 52.1).

To assess the effects of acupuncture, there is a need to differentiate genuine acupuncture (with a specific movement of needle rotation) from a simple puncture, which could be defined as placebo. Indeed, cerebral activation is not the same with these two techniques[9] as assessed by functional magnetic resonance imaging (fMRI). The specific effects of acupuncture, by comparison with placebo, appear to be associated with the activation of insula.[10] Several studies versus placebo have shown effects against pain.

## 52.3 Effects on Pruritus

### 52.3.1 Pathophysiological Studies

The effects on pruritus, like on pain, are probably related to the inhibition of C fibers by gate control. The known effects of acupuncture on the mediators of inflammation (opiods, serotonin, prostaglandine E2,

substance P, calcitonin gene-related peptide (CGRP), vasoactive intestinal peptide (VIP), neuropeptide Y, tumor necrosis factor alpha (TNF-α), IgE, IL-1, IL-6, IL-8, IL-10, etc.)[11] suggest that acupuncture could be effective in many etiologies of pruritus. But the effects of acupuncture on neurogenic pruritus (brachio-radial pruritus, paresthetic nostalgia and parestethic meralgia)[12] indicate that there is also a neurogenic effect.

In a recent study,[13] 10 patients were treated by acupuncture for nondermatological reasons. Skin biopsies in areas where needles were introduced were performed before puncture and respectively 3 and 6 days after 10 following punctures. A prick test with histamine was used to induce pruritus in these areas and control areas. Skin innervation was dramatically reduced, as assessed by immunostainings against PGP9.5 and CGRP. Such a reduction may explain effects on pruritus. But no difference in responses to histamine was observed. Two hypotheses can be proposed: it could be due to the general effects of acupuncture on these patients; the effects of acupuncture may be prior to the histamine release.

Hence, the effects of acupuncture on pruritus may take place at two levels:

- Medullar and supramedullar level – gate control on C fibers;
- Cutaneous level – decrease of C-fiber density.

### 52.3.2 Clinical Studies

#### 52.3.2.1 Histamine-Induced Pruritus

Pruritus was induced by histamine on 10 healthy subjects.[14] Then placeboacupuncture, acupuncture or electroacupuncture at 2 or 80 Hz was performed. Four sessions were conducted spaced 1 week (4 weeks for electrostimulation). Pruritus was evaluated 5 and 20 min after puncture. There was a significant reduction of pruritus, according to the visual analog scale, after acupuncture and electroacupuncture at 2 and 80 Hz when puncture was realized on the same dermatome as histamine injection, but these results were not found when the puncture was performed on another dermatome.

Another study was performed on 32 healthy subjects.[15] Histamine was applied on forearms and then electroauriculoacupuncture was performed. Pruritus was measured 5 min after application, then auriculopuncture was performed and another measurement was made 5 min later. Another application of histamine was performed 4 weeks later but was not followed by auriculopuncture. There was a significant decrease of pruritus on the homolateral forearm. These results can be discussed because there was no placebopuncture.

A randomized controlled double-binded study was carried out.[16] Ten healthy volunteers without any previous experience of acupuncture were randomized into three groups: adapted acupuncture (11GI point), placeboacupuncture (puncture in another area on the same dermatome according to good practices of genuine acupuncture), and no acupuncture. Pruritus was evaluated for 20 s each. Significant results were obtained on the prevention of pruritus, and also wheal and flare, but only by picking at the 11GI point.

### 52.3.2.2  Uremic Pruritus

A study was performed on six patients.[17] No previous treatment was effective. After electroacupuncture, pruritus dramatically decreased and sleep improved. No result was obtained with superficial electric stimulation.

A randomized controlled double-blinded trial[18] including 40 patients with uremic pruritus was focalized on the point Quchi LI11/11GI. A first group of 20 patients was treated on this point twice a week, whereas a second group of 20 patients was treated in same conditions but at a point 2 cm away from it. In the first group, itch scores before treatment, after treatment and 3 months later were, respectively, $38.3 \pm 4.3$, $17.3 \pm 5.5$ and $16.5 \pm 4.9$. In the placebo group, they were, respectively, $38.3 \pm 4.3$, $37.5 \pm 3.2$ and $37.1 \pm 5$. Differences were significant ($p < 0.001$). There was no variation in the amounts of creatinine, magnesium, phosphate, calcium or parathyroid hormone in blood.

### 52.3.2.3  Senile Pruritus

Only one study has been carried out on patients suffering from senile pruritus.[19] Unfortunately, methodological imprecisions do not allow reaching any conclusions about its efficacy.

### 52.3.2.4  Neurogenic itch

A retrospective study about patients presenting with a segmentary pruritus without any dermatological cause and with normal biological data[12] was in favor of the disappearance of pruritus after acupuncture in paravertebral muscles corresponding to the involved dermatomes (Shu point). These results were obtained in 12/16 patients and four sessions were needed.

## 52.4  Conclusions

With pain and wound healing, pruritus is one of the three dermatological indications that appear to be validated by randomized studies.[20] But we can only accept a preventive effect on histamine-induced pruritus and a curative effect on uremic pruritus. Further studies are needed for other indications.

## References

1. Rabischong P, Niboyet JE, Terral C, Senelar R, Casez R. Bases expérimentales de l'analgésie acupuncturale. *Nouv Presse Med.* 1975; 4:2021–2026.
2. Li AH, Zhang JM, Xie YK. Human acupuncture points mapped in rats are associated with excitable muscle/skin–nerve complexes with enriched nerve endings. *Brain Res.* 2004;1012:154–159.
3. Langevin HM, Yandow JA. Relationship of acupuncture points and meridians to connective tissue planes. *Anat Rec.* 2002;269:257–265.
4. Kessler D, Dethlefsen S, Haase I, Plomann M, Hirche F, Krieg T. Fibroblasts in mechanically stressed collagen lattice assume a "synthetic" phenotype. *J Biol Chem.* 2001; 276:36575–36585.
5. Jia-Xu C, Basil OI, Sheng-Xing M. Nitric oxide modulation of norepinephrine production in acupuncture points. *Life Sci.* 2006;79:2157–2164.
6. Cho Z, Chung S, Jones J, et al. New findings of the correlation between acupoints and corresponding brain cortices using functional MRI. *Proc Natl Acad* Sci. 1998;95:2670–2673.
7. Kaptchuk TJ. Acupuncture: theory, efficacy, and practice. *Ann Intern Med.* 2002;136:374–383.
8. Brown JH. Stimulation-produced analgesia: acupuncture, TENS and alternative techniques. *Anaesth Intens Care Med.* 2005; 6:45–47.
9. Wu MT, Hsieh JC, Xion J, et al. Central nervous pathway for acupuncture stimulation: localization of processing with functional MRI of the brain-preliminary experience. *Radiology.* 1999;133:133–141.

10. Pariente J, White P, Richard S, Frackowiak J, Lewith G. Expectancy and belief modulate the neuronal substrates of pain treated by acupuncture. *Neuro Image*. 2005; 25:1161–1167.

11. Zijlstra FJ, Van den Berg-de Lange I, Huygen FJ, Klein J. Anti-inflammatory actions of acupuncture. *Mediators Inflamm*. 2003;12:59–69.

12. Stellon A. Neurogenic pruritus: an unrecognised problem? A retrospective case series of treatment by acupuncture. *Acupunct Med*. 2002;20:186–190.

13. Carlsson CP, Sundler F, Wallengren J. Cutaneous innervation before and after one treatment period of acupuncture. *Br J Dermatol*. 2006;155:970–976.

14. Lundeberg T, Bondesson L, Thomas M. Effect of acupuncture on experimentally induced itch. *Br J Dermatol*. 1987;117: 771–777.

15. Kesting MR, Thurmuller P, Holzle F, Wolff KD, Holland-Letz T, Stucker M. Electrical ear acupuncture reduces

16. histamine-induced itch (alloknesis). *Acta Derm Venereol*. 2006;86:399–403.

16. Pfab F, Hammes M, Bäcker M, et al. Preventive effect of acupuncture on histamine-induced itch: a blinded, randomized, placebo-controlled, crossover trial. *J Allergy Clin Immunol*. 2005;116:1386–1388.

17. Duo LJ. Electrical needle therapy of uremic pruritus. *Nephron*. 1987;47:179–183.

18. Chen-Yi C, Wen CY, Min-Tsung K, Chiu-Ching H. Acupuncture in haemodialysis patients at the Quchi (LI11) acupoint for refractory uraemic pruritus. *Nephrol Dial Transplant*. 2005;20:1912–1915.

19. Yang, Mingchang, Mao, Jinglie, Yu, Ju. Observation on therapeutic effect of acupuncture and moxibustion on senile cutaneous pruritus. *Chin Acupunct Moxib*. 2002;22.

20. Potin-Richard L, Peau et acupuncture. Medical Thesis, Brest, 2007.

# Section 5
# Future Perspectives

# Chapter 53
# Future Perspectives: Outlook

Sonja Ständer and Laurent Misery

The cutaneous and central neurobiology of pruritus is complex and underlies a regulation of variable and stress-vulnerable mechanisms. At present, not all mechanisms including neuromediators and receptors are known. Accordingly, the therapies and underlying mechanisms presented in this book represent only a part of the complex network of neuronal interactions. However, the current knowledge offers speculations about new and future possible therapies. For example, neuromediators inducing a peripheral or central sensitization of nerve fibers, such as neurotrophins, contribute to pruritus becoming chronic and may be a target for future therapies. Neurotrophins and their receptors play an important role in cutaneous nerve development and reconstruction after injury. They are released by non-neuronal inflammatory cells such as eosinophilic granulocytes. After binding to specific receptors on the peripheral nerve endings, they are transported along the axon on the cell bodies into the dorsal root ganglia where they regulate the expression of a variety of proteins involved in neuronal growth and sensitivity. Nerve growth factor (NGF) may lead to sensitization of peripheral neuroreceptors such as the histamine and capsaicin (TRPV1) receptor. It was demonstrated that NGF is overexpressed in prurigo nodularis and atopic dermatitis (AD). Moreover, it was speculated that NGF and its receptors contribute to the neurohyperplasia of the disease. Accordingly, substances targeting NGF could be a future option for treating prurigo nodularis or AD, preventing the pruritus from becoming chronic.

A decade ago, the proteinase activated receptor 2 (PAR-2) was described to be present on cutaneous sensory nerve fibers. It is activated by mast cell mediators such as tryptase. Activation leads to induction of pruritus and neurogenic inflammation comparable to effects induced upon histamine release from mast cells. In AD, PAR-2 was enhanced on primary afferent nerve fibers in lesional skin, suggesting that this receptor is involved in the pathophysiology of pruritus in AD. Accordingly, PAR-2-antagonists should be effective in the suppression of peripheral induced pruritus but these substances do not yet exist for therapeutic use.

Other recently discovered substances inducing peripheral pruritus may represent targets of new antipruritic drugs such as interleukin-31 (IL-31). Also, targeting of neuropeptides such as Substance P (SP) by neurokinin-1 (NK-1) antagonists was successful in pilot studies (Ständer and Luger, unpublished observation). Especially in severe forms of chronic pruritus, e.g., renal pruritus and aquagenic pruritus, new and effective therapies are essential because current therapy modalities are not sufficient in the long term. In summary, treatment of chronic pruritus is a challenge and demands knowledge of modern therapies acting directly at neuronal structures in the skin or in the central nervous system. Identifying the origin of pruritus as well as the early start of a specific therapy preventing the symptom from becoming chronic has high priority and is of greatest importance.

L. Misery and S. Ständer (eds.), *Pruritus*,
DOI 10.1007/978-1-84882-322-8_53, © Springer-Verlag London Limited 2010

# Index

## Atopic